Platelet Immunobiology

PLATELET IMMUNOBIOLOGY

MOLECULAR AND CLINICAL ASPECTS

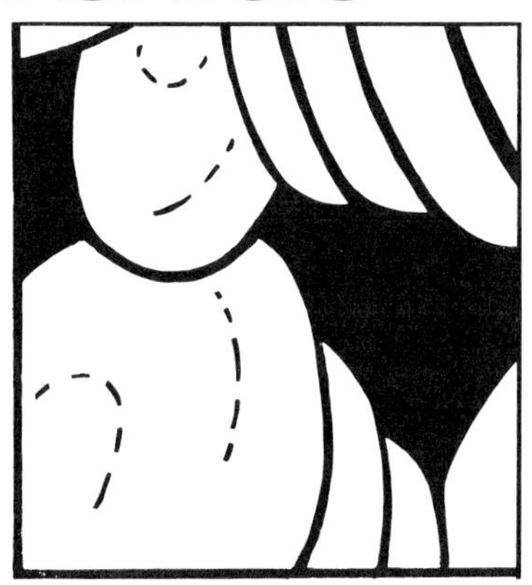

Edited by

THOMAS J. KUNICKI, Ph.D.
Senior Investigator, Platelet Research Section
The Blood Center of Southeastern Wisconsin
Milwaukee, Wisconsin

JAMES N. GEORGE, M.D.
Professor of Medicine
University of Texas Health Science Center
San Antonio, Texas

With 29 Contributors

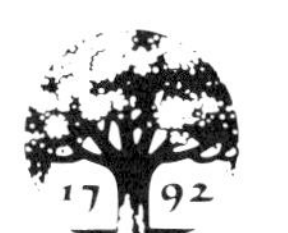

J. B. Lippincott Company

Philadelphia
Cambridge London
New York Singapore
St. Louis Sydney
San Francisco Tokyo

Acquisitions Editor: Lisa McAllister
Coordinating Editorial Assistant: Paula Callaghan
Project Editors: Patrick O'Kane, Dina Kamilatos
Manuscript Editor: Marguerite M. Hague
Indexer: Sandra King
Design/Production Coordinator: Caren Erlichman
Cover Design: Stephen Iwanczuk
Production Manager: Carol A. Florence
Compositor: Digitype
Printer/Binder: Halliday Lithograph

6 5 4 3 2 1

Library of Congress Cataloging-in-Publication Data
Platelet immunobiology : molecular and clinical aspects / [edited by] Thomas J. Kunicki, James N. George ; with 29 contributors.

p. cm.
Includes bibliographies and index.
ISBN 0-397-50872-7
1. Blood platelets—Immunology. I. Kunicki, Thomas J.
II. George, James N.
[DNLM: 1. Blood Platelets—immunology. 2. Glycoproteins—physiology. WH 300 P7173]
QP97.P54 1989
616.07'9—dc 19
DNLM/DLC
for Library of Congress 88-21630
CIP

The authors and publisher have exerted every effort to ensure that drug selection and dosage set forth in this text are in accord with current recommendations and practice at the time of publication. However, in view of ongoing research, changes in government regulations, and the constant flow of information relating to drug therapy and drug reactions, the reader is urged to check the package insert for each drug for any change in indications and dosage and for added warnings and precautions. This is particularly important when the recommended agent is a new or infrequently employed drug.

Contributors

CLARK L. ANDERSON, M.D.
Professor of Medicine
Department of Internal Medicine
The Ohio State University College of Medicine
Columbus, Ohio

ROBERT K. ANDREWS, Ph.D.
Postdoctoral Fellow
Department of Medicine
University of Sydney;
Research Fellow
Westmead Hospital
Sydney, New South Wales, Australia

RICHARD H. ASTER, M.D.
Clinical Professor of Medicine and Pathology
Medical College of Wisconsin;
President and Senior Investigator
Transfusion Medicine Section
The Blood Center of Southeastern Wisconsin
Milwaukee, Wisconsin

DIANA S. BEARDSLEY, M.D., Ph.D.
Assistant Professor of Pediatrics
Yale University School of Medicine;
Associate in Pediatrics
Yale–New Haven Hospital
New Haven, Connecticut

MICHAEL C. BERNDT, Ph.D.
Welcome Australian Senior Research Fellow
Department of Medicine
University of Sydney;
Senior Research Fellow
Westmead Hospital
Sydney, New South Wales, Australia

BENG H. CHONG, Ph.D.
Senior Lecturer in Medicine
University of New South Wales;
Consultant Hematologist
St. George Hospital
Sydney, New South Wales, Australia

BARRY S. COLLER, M.D.
Professor of Medicine and Pathology
Head
Division of Hematology, Department of Medicine;
Clinical Chief
Hematology Laboratory
University Hospital
State University of New York at Stony Brook
Stony Brook, New York

LAURENCE A. FITZGERALD, Ph.D.
Senior Scientist
COR Therapeutics, Inc.
Palo Alto, California

MARK H. GINSBERG, M.D.
Associate Member with tenure
Department of Immunology
Research Institute of Scripps Clinic
La Jolla, California

STEPHEN R. HANSON, Ph.D.
Assistant Member
Department of Basic and Clinical Research
Research Institute of Scripps Clinic
La Jolla, California

ELISABETH M. HODSON, M.D.
Royal Alexandra Hospital for Children;
The Prince of Wales Children's Hospital
Sydney, New South Wales, Australia

YOHKO KAWAI, M.D.
Clinical Associate
Department of Laboratory Medicine
Keio University
Tokyo, Japan

continued

VOLKER KIEFEL, M.D.
Senior Investigator
Institute for Clinical Immunology and Transfusion Medicine
Justus Liebig University
Giessen, Federal Republic of Germany

JOSEPH C. LOFTUS, Ph.D.
Senior Research Associate
Department of Immunology
Research Institute of Scripps Clinic
La Jolla, California

ROBERT R. MONTGOMERY, M.D.
Clinical Professor of Pediatrics and Pathology
Medical College of Wisconsin;
Vice-president and Director of Research
The Blood Center of Southeastern Wisconsin
Milwaukee, Wisconsin

CHRISTIAN MUELLER-ECKHARDT, M.D.
Professor and Director
Institute for Clinical Immunology and Transfusion Medicine
Justus Liebig University
Giessen, Federal Republic of Germany

PETER J. NEWMAN, Ph.D.
Investigator
Transfusion Medicine Section
The Blood Center of Southeastern Wisconsin
Milwaukee, Wisconsin

DIANE J. NUGENT, M.D.
Assistant Professor
Pediatric Hematology-Oncology;
Assistant Professor
Health Science Center
University of Wisconsin-Madison
Madison, Wisconsin

ALAN T. NURDEN
Directeur de Recherche
Centre National de la Recherche Scientifique
Section Pathologie Cellulaire de l'Hémostase
Hôpital Cardiologique
Bordeaux, France

DAVID R. PHILLIPS, Ph.D.
Vice-president and Director of Research
COR Therapeutics, Inc.
Palo Alto, California

DOMINIQUE PIDARD, Ph.D.
Chargé de Recherches
Centre National de la Recherche Scientifique
Hôpital Lariboisière
Paris, France

EDWARD F. PLOW, Ph.D.
Associate Member with tenure
Department of Immunology
Research Institute of Scripps Clinic
La Jolla, California

STEPHEN I. ROSENFELD, M.D.
Professor of Medicine
University of Rochester School of Medicine and Dentistry
Rochester, New York

ZAVERIO M. RUGGERI, M.D.
Associate Member (Associate Professor)
Department of Basic and Clinical Research
Research Institute of Scripps Clinic
La Jolla, California

BARBARA P. SCHICK, Ph.D.
Associate Professor
Cardeza Foundation for Hematologic Research
Jefferson Medical College
Thomas Jefferson University
Philadelphia, Pennsylvania

PAUL K. SCHICK, M.D.
Professor of Medicine
Cardeza Foundation for Hematologic Research
Jefferson Medical College
Thomas Jefferson University
Philadelphia, Pennsylvania

CHARLES A. SCHIFFER, M.D.
Professor of Medicine and Oncology
University of Maryland School of Medicine;
Chief
Division of Hematologic Malignancies
University of Maryland Cancer Center;
Chief
Division of Hematology, Department of Medicine
University of Maryland Hospital
Baltimore, Maryland

J. PAUL SCOTT, M.D.
Associate Clinical Professor
Medical College of Wisconsin;
Investigator
Hemostasis Research Section
The Blood Center of Southeastern Wisconsin
Milwaukee, Wisconsin

PETER J. SIMS, M.D., Ph.D.
Associate Member
Cardiovascular Biology Research
Oklahoma Medical Research Foundation;
Scientific Director
Oklahoma Blood Institute
Sylvan N. Goldman Blood Center
Oklahoma City, Oklahoma

Preface

Numerous scientists and clinicians have devoted their careers to the study of human blood platelet immunochemistry and immunohematology. The results of this effort have contributed immensely to our current understanding of the structure and function of platelet membrane constituents, particularly the plasma membrane glycoproteins. Given the breadth of information now accumulated, there is a need for a comprehensive review of *Platelet Immunobiology: Molecular and Clinical Aspects.* This book is a definitive text covering both the molecular and clinical aspects of platelet immunology. It also emphasizes the many ways in which the information gleaned from the study of the immunobiology of platelet glycoproteins has contributed to our understanding of their structure and function.

The human platelet plays a pivotal role in hemostasis, serving as the blood component that initially adheres to damaged areas of the vessel wall. Through its cohesive properties, the platelet forms a plug that prevents excessive loss of blood cells from the injured vessel. At the same time, the platelet serves as a nidus for coagulation and thereby promotes the formation of a durable fibrin clot. The platelet also figures in certain important pathological conditions, having been implicated in the pathogenesis of atherosclerotic plaques and thrombi. For these and many more reasons, it is evident that immunization against platelet glycoprotein antigens can result in acute and clinically relevant bleeding disorders characterized by clearance of antibody-coated platelets from the circulation or dysfunction of key platelet glycoprotein receptors. The production of antibodies specific for platelet membrane receptors, the pathology resulting from such antibody production, and the use of such antibodies to characterize platelet glycoprotein function are the subjects of this book.

We have enlisted the contributions of thirty-one major contributors to research in this field. They represent many leading academic and medical institutions in the United States, Europe, Japan, and Australia.

The chapters are organized in a sequence that develops the information on platelet membrane structure and function, antigenicity, applications of platelet-specific antibodies, immune receptors, and clinical relevance in an orderly, continuous manner. Each chapter is intended to be, first and foremost, a comprehensive review of the subject in question.

In the areas of human cell biology, immunology, and hematology, *Platelet Immunobiology* will appeal to both basic and clinical scientists. Indeed, both are represented among the contributors to the project. Moreover, the book will serve as a reference for researching and teaching the molecular basis of immune-mediated disease.

THOMAS J. KUNICKI, Ph.D.
JAMES N. GEORGE, M.D.

Acknowledgment

The production and editing of this book were successfully accomplished, in large part, because of the excellent assistance of Ms. Marcia Iverson of the Blood Center Research Department. The editors are grateful for her patience and her untiring effort on this project.

Contents

continued

Platelet Immunobiology

Part One Introduction

1

Platelet Immunology: Historical Perspective and Future Directions

RICHARD H. ASTER · THOMAS J. KUNICKI

THE DISCOVERY OF PLATELETS

Throughout the 19th century, the possible existence and function of circulating cells other than leukocytes and red cells attracted the attention of leading investigators, such as Addison, Gulliver, Osler, Hayem, Wharton Jones, and Beale[15] but, because of their small size, platelets tested the limits of early optical microscopes and were the last cellular element of the blood to be recognized. Unequivocal identification of platelets and clarification of their role in hemostasis is generally attributed to the Italian investigator, Giulio Bizzozero, who published a seminal paper on this subject in 1882.[4] James Homer Wright identified bone marrow megakaryocytes as the source of circulating platelets in 1906.[24]

PLATELET TRANSFUSIONS

The recognition that patients lacking blood platelets were at risk to bleed, often catastrophically, stimulated efforts to transfuse these blood elements. In 1910, Duke demonstrated elevation of the platelet count and shortening of the bleeding time after direct transfusion of fresh whole blood to a few patients with thrombocytopenia.[7] However, platelet transfusion therapy languished for many years, awaiting the development of plastic containers, which permitted manipulation of platelet-rich plasma, and the delineation of optimal methods for anticoagulation and storage.

As platelet transfusions became more widely used, it was recognized that patients sometimes became refractory after only a few treatments.[9,10] By testing recipient serum for immunologic reactivity against donor platelets, it was sometimes possible to find individual donors whose platelets produced good responses when transfused to such patients.[3] Pioneering studies by Yankee and his colleagues[25] showed that alloimmunization to class I HLA markers was a major cause of platelet transfusion refractoriness and that compatible donors could be found among relatives and unrelated persons by matching donor and recipient for these determinants.[13,25]

ALLOIMMUNE THROMBOCYTOPENIA

van Loghem and his colleagues were the first to identify an apparently platelet-specific alloantigen recognized by antibody from a previously transfused thrombocytopenic patient.[22] They called the determinant for which this antibody was specific Zw^a and showed that it was carried on platelets from about 98% of normal persons and was inherited. Shulman et al. independently discovered the same antigen,[20] called it $P1^{A1}$, provided partial immunochemical characterization, and showed that a new syndrome, posttransfusion purpura, was associated with sensitization to this marker. Shortly thereafter, it was found that neonatal alloimmune thrombocytopenia could result from maternal sensitization to $P1^{A1}$ and, possibly, HLA-A2 (then designated $P1GrLy^{B1}$).[21] Later studies of post-transfusion purpura and neonatal alloimmune thrombocytopenia led to recognition of a number of other inherited, platelet-specific, alloantigen systems (see Chap. 6, 9, 19, and 20).

DRUG-INDUCED THROMBOCYTOPENIA

For more than a century, it has been known that thrombocytopenia and hemorrhagic symptoms can be induced by drugs in certain sensitive individuals.[23] Rosenthal, in 1928, showed that the syndrome could be reproduced by administering the suspect drug after recovery.[16] Pioneering studies by Ackroyd demonstrated that serum from such patients contains a factor, later shown to be an immunoglobulin, capable of agglutinating and lysing normal platelets in the presence of drug.[1] Shulman first examined the molecular basis of drug–platelet–antibody interaction in this disorder.[17–19] Although literally hundreds of drugs have now been implicated as causes of drug-induced thrombocytopenia,[2] the pathogenesis of this remarkable condition is not yet fully understood and offers important challenges for investigators.

AUTOIMMUNE THROMBOCYTOPENIA

Thrombocytopenic purpura, triggered by prior viral infection in children or occurring "spontaneously" in adults, is generally thought to have an autoimmune basis. For many years, arguments raged over whether reduced platelet levels in this condition resulted from defective platelet production[5,8] or from excessive platelet destruction.[6,11,14] Even today, the relative importance of these two mechanisms in reducing platelet levels is not fully established. Autoimmune thrombocytopenia is a common condition—it may be that platelets are attacked by autologous immune mechanisms more often than any other tissue. Despite recent advances, much remains to be learned about the defect in immune regulation that presumably underlies the disease, the character of the cellular and humoral processes that act on platelets in this condition, the target molecules against which the autologous immune response is directed, mechanisms by which platelets are destroyed, and optimal therapeutic approaches for this sometimes life-threatening condition.

OTHER ASPECTS OF PLATELET IMMUNOLOGY

Platelets present numerous other exciting challenges for investigators. At a basic level, immunologic probes and methods have provided exquisite new tools with which to study platelet structure and function. At a clinical level, studies of the importance of the immune complexes in mediating platelet destruction in "idiopathic" thrombocytopenia and in alloimmunized patients are needed. Manipulation of the immune system for treatment of immune-mediated platelet disorders is becoming feasible and may lead the way to effective management of conditions affecting other blood cells and tissues.

FUTURE DIRECTIONS

Contributors to this book have addressed structural elements of the platelet plasma membrane; antigens of the platelet surface, with emphasis on those known to have clinical significance; applications of modern immunochemical and molecular biologic techniques to the study of platelet surface determinants; platelet-associated immunoglobulins and complement components; and immunologic disorders affecting platelets. The text has been organized such that readers are allowed an opportunity to review a spectrum of information relating to platelet immunology, from basic studies of structure/function to clinical application.

This text summarizes the state of platelet immunology in late 1987. Newly developed immunologic and biochemical tools are likely to lead to a further explosion of knowledge in the near future. It is reasonable to predict, for example, that the next decade will see complete molecular characterization of the protein and carbohydrate alloantigens of platelets and their corresponding gene sequences. Improved immunochemical techniques should provide important new tools with which to detect and characterize platelet-reactive allo-, auto-, and drug-dependent antibodies. The newly acquired information will almost certainly lead to improved understanding of the pathogenesis of immunologically mediated platelet disorders. New platelet alloantigen systems are likely to be identified. The target molecules for platelet autoantibodies and the possible role of cellular immunologic processes in the pathogenesis of autoimmune thrombocytopenia will undoubtedly be understood more fully. It is reasonable to hope that these developments will translate into improved methods of diagnosing, treating, and preventing immunologic conditions of platelets and will be applicable to disorders affecting tissues other than platelets. Long-term platelet transfusion support, unaccompanied by alloimmunization and other complications, may also become a reality. We hope readers will find the current volume useful as a "snapshot" of the current state of platelet immunology and as a summary of the future challenges and opportunities available to investigators.

REFERENCES

1. Ackroyd JF: The pathogenesis of thrombocytopenic purpura due to hypersensitivity to Sedormid. Clin Sci 7:249, 1949
2. Aster RH: Thrombocytopenia due to enhanced platelet destruction. In Williams WJ et al (eds): Hematology, New York, McGraw-Hill, 1983
3. Aster RH, Cooper HC, Singer D: Simplified complement fixation test for detection of platelet antibodies in human serum. J Lab Clin Med 63:161, 1964
4. Bizzozero G: Ueber einer neuen Formbestandtheil-Blutes und Desser Role bei der Thrombose und der Blutgerinnung. Arch Pathol Anat Physiol 90:261, 1881
5. Dameshek W, Miller EB: The megakaryocytes in idiopathic thrombocytopenic purpura: A form of hypersplenism. Blood 1:27, 1946
6. Doan CA, Bouroncle BA, Wiseman BK: Idiopathic and secondary thrombocytopenic purpura: Clinical study and evaluation of 381 cases over a period of 28 years. Ann Intern Med 53:861, 1960
7. Duke WW: The relation of blood platelets to hemorrhagic disease: Description of a method for determining the bleeding time and coagulation time and report of three cases of hemorrhagic disease relieved by transfusion. J Am Med Assoc 55:1185, 1910
8. Frank E: die essentielle thrombopinie. Berl Klin Wochenschr 52:454, 1915
9. Freireich EJ, Kliman A, Gaydos L: Response to repeated platelet transfusion from the same donor. Ann Intern Med 59:277, 1983
10. Grumet FC, Yankee RA: Long-term platelet support of patients with aplastic anemia. Effect of splenectomy and steroid therapy. Ann Intern Med 73:1, 1970
11. Harrington WJ, Minnich V, Hollingsworth JW, Moore CV: Demonstration of a thrombocytopenic factor in the blood of patients with thrombocytopenic purpura. J Lab Clin Med 38:1, 1951
12. Hirsch EO, Gardner FH: The transfusion of human blood platelets with a note on the transfusion of granulocytes. J Lab Clin Med 39:556, 1952
13. Lohrmann HP, Bull MI, Decter JA, Yankee RA, Graw RG: Platelet transfusion from HL-A compatible unrelated donors to alloimmunized patients. Ann Intern Med 80:9, 1974
14. Minot GR: Studies on a case of idiopathic purpura hemorrhagica. Am J Med Sci 152:48, 1916
15. Robb-Smith AHT: Why the platelets were discovered. Br J Haematol 13:618, 1967
16. Rosenthal N: The blood picture in purpura. J Lab Clin Med 13:303, 1928
17. Shulman NR: Immunoreactions involving platelets. I. A steric and kinetic model for formation of a complex from a human antibody, quinine as a haptene, and platelets, and for fixation of complement by the complex. J Exp Med 107:665, 1958
18. Shulman NR: Immunoreactions involving platelets. III. Quantitative aspects of platelet agglutination, inhibition of clot retraction, and other reactions caused by the antibody of quinidine purpura. J Exp Med 107:697, 1958
19. Shulman NR: Immunoreactions involving platelet. IV. Studies on the pathogenesis of thrombocytopenia in drug purpura using test doses of quinidine in sensitized individuals. Their implications in idiopathic thrombocytopenic purpura. J Exp Med 107:711, 1958
20. Shulman NR, Aster RH, Leitner A, Hiller MD: Post-transfusion purpura due to a complement-fixing antibody against a genetically controlled platelet antigen: A proposed mechanism for thrombocytopenia and its relevance in "autoimmunity." J Clin Invest 40:1597, 1961
21. Shulman NR, Aster RH, Pearson HA, Hiller MC: Reactions of maternal isoantibodies responsible for neonatal purpura. Differentiation of a second antigen system. J Clin Invest 41:1059, 1962
22. van Loghem JJ, Dorfmeyer H, van der Hart M, Schreuder F: Serological and genetical studies on a platelet antigen (Zw). Vox Sang 4:161, 1959
23. Vipan WH: Quinine as a cause of purpura. Lancet 2:37, 1865
24. Wright JH: Die Enstehung der Blutplattchen. Arch Pathol Anat Physiol 186:55, 1906
25. Yankee RA, Grumet FC, Rogentine GN: Platelet transfusion therapy. The selection of compatible platelet donors for refractory patients by lymphocyte HLA typing. N Engl J Med 281:1208, 1969

Part Two Structural Profile of the Platelet Plasma Membrane

2

Structure and Function of Platelet Membrane Glycoproteins

LAURENCE A. FITZGERALD • DAVID R. PHILLIPS

An understanding of platelet membrane glycoprotein structure and function is of central importance to an appreciation of the role of platelets in primary hemostasis. Platelet membrane glycoproteins (GP) mediate two principal events in primary hemostasis, adhesion and aggregation, by acting as receptors for adhesive glycoproteins. Adhesion occurs primarily through the von Willebrand factor (VWF)-dependent binding of unstimulated platelets to the subendothelium of damaged vessels. The GPIb–IX complex is the receptor for VWF on unstimulated platelets. Aggregation, or platelet cohesion, involves the binding of fibrinogen to agonist-stimulated cells. The GPIIb–IIIa complex is the platelet receptor for fibrinogen, and this complex on stimulated platelets can also act as a receptor for fibronectin and VWF. The GPIb–IX and GPIIb–IIIa complexes are the most studied platelet membrane components. The focus of this chapter will be on recent studies of these two receptor complexes. Platelet membrane glycoproteins have been discussed in several recent reviews[22,36,44,46,88,89] and a book.[47] The reader is referred to these sources for background information and detailed discussions of techniques.

Table 2-1 lists the characterized platelet membrane glycoproteins and gives some of their biochemical and functional properties. Over 30 different surface proteins have been described by two-dimensional electrophoresis of surface-labeled cells.[9,22] Many of these glycoproteins are noncovalently associated in the form of 1 : 1 heterodimeric complexes.[32,35,69,74] A number of glycoproteins, such as GPIb, GPIc, and GPIIb, consist of two polypeptide chains. An understanding of the functional roles of the GPIb–IX and GPIIb–IIIa complexes has come from studies of the congenital abnormalities Glanzmann's thrombasthenia and Bernard-Soulier syndrome[44,45] and from the use of certain murine monoclonal antibodies. These types of studies are described in detail in Chapters 5 and 12. In the following sections, we will review (1) some of the general methods used to study platelet membrane glycoproteins, (2) the GPIIb–IIIa complex and the mechanism of platelet aggregation, (3) the GPIb–IX complex and the mechanism of platelet adhesion, and (4) other platelet membrane glycoproteins that are less well characterized.

METHODS USED TO STUDY PLATELET MEMBRANE GLYCOPROTEINS

As new methods have been developed, they have been applied to the study of platelet membrane glycoproteins. In comparison with nucleated cells, it is easier in several respects to isolate membrane glycoproteins in platelets. Platelets are readily obtained as viable, purified cell suspensions, and the membrane glycopro-

Table 2-1
Platelet Membrane Glycoproteins: Biochemical Properties and Receptor Function

Glycoprotein	M_r nonreduced (kDa)	M_r reduced (kDa)	Characteristics	Analogous Proteins	Functions
Ia	150	165	Complexed with GPIIa*	VLA-2 α subunit	Collagen receptor
Ib	160	128–141 22	Heavily sialylated, 25,000 per platelet complexed with GPIX		VWF receptor on unstimulated platelets; thrombin receptor
Ic	148	145 25	Complexed with GPIIa	VLA-5†, α subunit	Fibronectin receptor
IIa	130	150	Complexed with GPIa, Ic	FnR, VLA, β subunit	
IIb	145	130 23	Ca^{2+}-dependent heterodimer complexed with GPIIIa, 50,000 per platelet		Fibrinogen, fibronectin, VWF receptor on stimulated platelets (IIb and IIIa)
IIIa	95	105	Cysteine-rich complexed with GPIIb	VnR, β subunit	
IV	85	85	Highly glycosylated protease-resistant		Thrombospondin receptor
V	82		Thrombin substrate		
IX	17		Complexed with GPIb		
GMP-140 or PADGEM	138	148	α-Granule membrane protein on surface of stimulated platelets		

*Abbreviations used: GP, glycoprotein; VLA, very late activation antigen; FnR, fibronectin receptor; GMP, granule membrane protein; PADGEM, platelet activation-dependent granule external membrane; VWf, von Willebrand factor; VnR, vitronectin receptor.

†See editor's note, p. 30.

teins represent approximately 5% of total platelet protein. In general, platelet surface proteins remain stable after detergent lysis. An exception is GPIb, which is cleaved by the calcium-dependent protease. This protease can be inhibited by leupeptin; other proteases in platelet lysates can be inhibited by benzamidine and phenylmethylsulfonyl fluoride. A preliminary centrifugation at 100,000 × *g* for 1 to 3 hr will remove the cytoskeletal components,[39] which in unstimulated platelets are primarily of actin filaments. The initial fractionation of platelet lysates can then be readily performed by lectin affinity columns, gel filtration, or ion-exchange resins to isolate a glycoprotein-enriched fraction.[36]

Several approaches have been used to identify and study platelet membrane glycoproteins. First, cell-surface labeling and electrophoretic separation have been used to characterize these components.[97] In general, lactoperoxidase-catalyzed iodination is most effective in labeling GPIIb–IIIa, whereas the periodate/sodium [^{3}H]borohydride method detects GPIb and GPV most readily. Figure 2-1 shows some of the major platelet membrane glycoproteins, which were fractionated by sodium dodecyl sulfate–polyacrylamide gel electrophoresis (SDS–PAGE) from detergent lysates of surface-labeled cells. The roman numeral classification was originated by Phillips and coworkers[43,97] and modified to its present form as described by Clemetson.[22] Two-dimensional nonreduced–reduced gels are useful for detecting surface glycoproteins consisting of either disulfide-linked subunits (e.g., GPIb, GPIIb, GPIc) or those glycoproteins having intrachain disulfides (e.g., GPIIa, GPIIIa).[22] Crossed-immunoelectrophoresis can be used to detect glycoprotein complexes[74] (e.g., GPIIb-IIIa), and this technique is reviewed in Chapter 11. Electrophoretic transfer of proteins from polyacrylamide gels to nitrocellulose, termed *Western blotting*, is often useful for analyzing the specificity of polyclonal antibodies.[33,36] Western blotting has recently been used to determine the specificity of human platelet alloantibodies, as described in Chapter 6. Glycoprotein Ib and IIb–IIIa can be selectively detected on Western blots of total platelet lysates by use of the lectins wheat germ agglutinin and concanavalin A, respectively.[36]

Second, several platelet membrane glycoproteins have been purified to study their structural and functional properties. The GPIIb-IIIa complex can be readily purified from either whole platelet lysates or from isolated platelet membranes by standard biochemical techniques.[34,69,85] The purified GPIIb–IIIa complex has been reconstituted into phospholipid vesicles to investigate its ligand-binding properties[7,92–94,106] and to examine its physical structure by rotary-shadow electron microscopy.[92] Glycoprotein Ib has been purified from membranes by monoclonal antibody affinity chromatography.[9] Functional

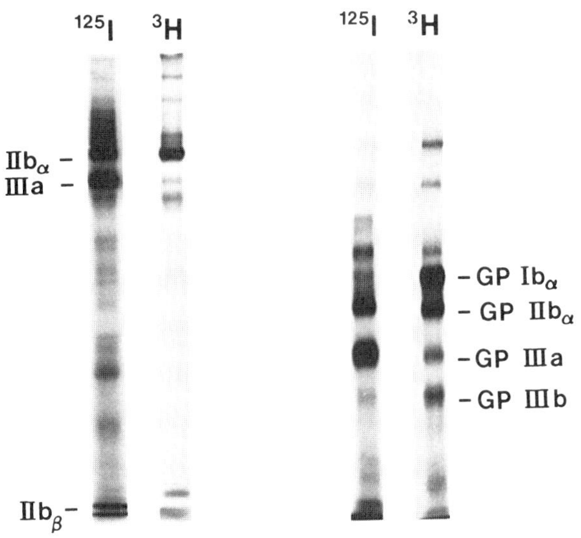

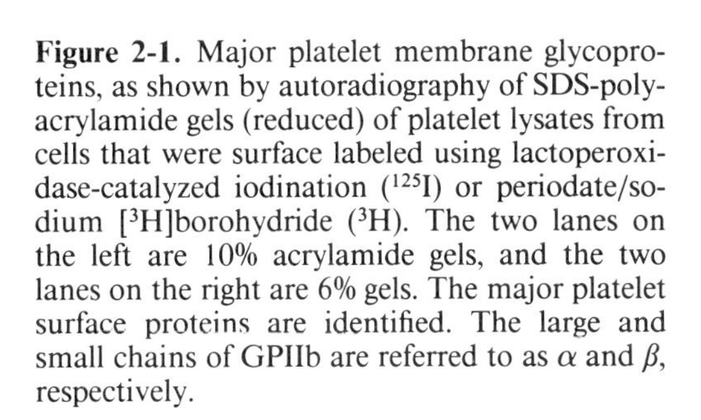

Figure 2-1. Major platelet membrane glycoproteins, as shown by autoradiography of SDS-polyacrylamide gels (reduced) of platelet lysates from cells that were surface labeled using lactoperoxidase-catalyzed iodination (^{125}I) or periodate/sodium [^{3}H]borohydride (^{3}H). The two lanes on the left are 10% acrylamide gels, and the two lanes on the right are 6% gels. The major platelet surface proteins are identified. The large and small chains of GPIIb are referred to as α and β, respectively.

proteolytic products of GPIb have been identified,[57] and the purified GPIb has also been examined by electron microscopy.[39] The amino-terminal sequences of several glycoproteins have been reported.[21,52,57]

A third, widely employed method used to study platelet membrane glycoproteins is the use of murine monoclonal antibodies. These antibodies can be used, for example, to study glycoprotein function on intact platelets,[36] to study conformational changes in GPIIb-IIIa,[25,51,117] to purify glycoproteins,[5,10,36] and to identify inherited deficiencies of membrane glycoproteins.[46,88] In most respects, these antibodies have replaced earlier techniques for purification of platelet membrane glycoproteins.

Finally, platelet membrane glycoproteins can be studied by the methods of molecular biology, beginning with the isolation of specific complementary DNA (cDNA) clones. We have used these methods extensively. Because platelets contain little, if any, messenger RNA (mRNA), it was necessary to obtain these clones from cDNA libraries derived from cultured cell lines that synthesize platelet membrane glycoproteins. Human umbilical vein endothelial (HUVE) cells were used as a source for cloning a GPIIIa cDNA,[38] and human erythroleukemia (HEL) cells for isolating GPIb and IIb cDNAs.[81,105] For these studies, total mRNA was isolated from the respective cell lines and double-stranded cDNA generated, with reverse transcriptase and DNA polymerase.[65] The cDNA libraries are often prepared in the versatile expression vector λgt11.[65] Specific cDNAs can be obtained either through the design of oligonucleotide probes based on peptide sequences[76] or by the expression of fusion proteins that contain epitopes that are detected by using specific antibodies.[65] The techniques of isolating specific cDNA clones by expression screening are reviewed in Chapter 15. For GPIIIa, cDNAs were obtained by screening a HUVE cell cDNA library with a 42-mer oligonucleotide probe. This probe was designed from an internal cyanogen bromide-derived peptide sequence that was obtained from purified platelet GPIIIa by using a codon utilization table.[38,76] For GPIb and GPIIb, and HEL cell λgt11 libraries were "expressed" as the bacterial β-galactosidase fusion gene proteins, and specific epitopes were detected on individual clones by use of polyclonal antibodies.[81,105] These platelet glycoprotein-specific cDNAs were sequenced to obtain an open-reading frame, which represents the entire protein sequence. The cDNA-deduced protein sequences were used to predict membrane spanning regions, likely cytoplasmic and extracellular domains, potential glycosylation and phosphorylation sites, putative Ca^{2+}-binding domains, repeating segments, and certain aspects of secondary structure. In addition, the deduced sequences can be used to compare the receptors on platelets with those of other cells that also mediate adhesion.

THE GLYCOPROTEIN IIb-IIIa COMPLEX AND THE MECHANISM OF PLATELET AGGREGATION

General Properties

Because of its abundance and its importance to platelet functioning, and because its deficiency causes bleeding disorders in humans, the GPIIb-IIIa complex has been the most extensively studied platelet receptor. Glycoproteins IIb and IIIa are the most abundant surface glycoproteins, at about 50,000 copies of each per platelet, and represent 1% to 2% of the total platelet protein.[36,44,46,89] A substantial amount of GPIIb-IIIa, perhaps as much as 50% of the total platelet content, appears to be present in the surface-connected canalicular system,[48] which under certain conditions is not accessible to extracellular protein ligands or probes (e.g., antibodies).[131] However, the role that this "intracellular" form of GPIIb-IIIa plays in the larger cell-surface pool is not clearly understood. The general properties of GPIIb and IIIa are given in Table 2-1. These glycoproteins have several other important characteristics: (1) the GPIIb-IIIa complex is present as a Ca^{2+}-dependent heterodimer, noncovalently associated on the platelet surface;[35,74,98] (2) GPIIb appears to bind Ca^{2+};[36,40] and (3) by rotary-shadow electron microscopy, the GPIIb-IIIa complex has two sites of membrane attachment.[19,92] The GPIIb-IIIa complex appears to interact with the platelet cytoskeleton in stimulated and aggregated platelets.[36]

The receptor functions of the GPIIb-IIIa complex have been established in three ways: by studies using thrombasthenic platelets, which lack these glycoproteins;[46,88] by inhibition of ligand binding with monoclonal antibodies;[36,46] and by reconstitution of the purified GPIIb-IIIa complex into phospholipid vesicles.[7,93,94] These experiments and others have established that the GPIIb-IIIa complex is the receptor on activated platelets for fibrinogen,[92,104,106] fibronectin,[41,53,94,104] and VWF.[31,96,104,110,129] Three major developments for GPIIb-IIIa have emerged in the last 2 years. First, the mechanism of ligand binding appears to operate primarily by an Arg-Gly-Asp (RGD)-dependent process;[43,53,59,103,106] this mechanism is similar to that found in certain adhesion receptors of nucleated cells,[106] such as the fibronectin receptor (FnR).[107] Second, GPIIb-IIIa-like membrane proteins have been identified on endothelial[33,78,86,102,127] and other nucleated cells.[12,21,102,118,122,123] Third, some of the other adhesion receptors of nucleated cells, such as the FnR[107] and the vitronectin receptor (VnR),[108] have been isolated, and their protein sequence has been determined from their α and β subunit cDNAs. The VnR and FnR are similar to GPIIb-IIIa biochemically and structurally.[106] Thus, the GPIIb-IIIa complex appears to be a member of a family of adhesion receptors.[21,102,106] In this context, *adhesion* refers to the interaction of cells with components of the extracellular matrix, not to the platelet-VWF binding that initiates primary hemostasis.

Receptor Function

The adhesive ligands (e.g., fibrinogen, fibronectin, and VWF) are large, multisubunit proteins. Thus, it was unexpected that the receptor recognition sequences for these ligands could be localized to small peptides. For fibronectin, the cell adhesion-binding domain was initially identified in a small peptic fragment of 11.5 kDa.[111] Synthetic peptides corresponding to regions of this fragment eventually identified the cell-binding domain as an Arg-Gly-Asp-Ser (RGDS) sequence.[100] Synthetic peptides containing this sequence could support fibroblast adhesion, and these peptides would block cell adhesion to fibronectin-coated surfaces.[100] The RGD sequence was subsequently found on other adhesive proteins, such as the α chain of fibrinogen,[111] VWF,[112] thrombospondin,[77] laminin,[111] and vitronectin.[121] Collagen contains several RGD sequences. This sequence is widely distributed in proteins and is found even in those with no known adhesive function.[111]

The binding of ligands involved in platelet aggregation also operates via an RGD-type mechanism. Peptides that contain the RGD sequence in solution block platelet aggregation[43] and inhibit the binding of fibrinogen, fibronectin, or VWF to the GPIIb-IIIa complex on stimulated platelets.[43,53,59,103] In addition to the RGD sequence, a second sequence has been shown to be involved in the binding of fibrinogen to GPIIb-IIIa. This sequence of 12 amino acids is located at the carboxyl-terminus of the γ chain of fibrinogen and is referred to as the *dodecapeptide*.[72] The dodecapeptide sequence is not found in other adhesive proteins. Similarly to the RGDS sequence, the dodecapeptide in solution can inhibit platelet aggregation and fibrinogen binding.

Considerable evidence suggests that the adhesive proteins either share a binding site on the GPIIb-IIIa complex or that the binding of one adhesive protein affects GPIIb-IIIa such that other binding sites are lost. First, the binding of fibrinogen, fibronectin, and VWF is mutually exclusive.[104] Second, the RGDS peptides and dodecapeptides appear to recognize sites that are in close proximity or are conformationally associated. For example, the dodecapeptide will inhibit the binding of both fibronectin and VWF to stimulated platelets,[75] even though these ligands do not contain the dodecapeptide sequence. Third, it was found that peptides that contained either immobilized RGD or immobilized dodecapeptides could be selectively used to retain GPIIb-IIIa from platelet lysates.[75] Interestingly, GPIIb-IIIa bound to an RGDS column can be eluted with dodecapeptide, and vice versa.[75] In addition, the dodecapeptide and RGD peptides compete for binding sites on intact platelets.[75] Fourth, ^{125}I-labeled dodecapeptide and RGD peptides can be covalently cross-linked to either whole platelets or to the purified GPIIb-IIIa complex.[115] It was reported that the derivitized RGDS peptides cross-link to both GPIIb and GPIIIa, whereas the derivitized dodecapeptide appeared to label GPIIb selectively. However, the dodecapeptide inhibits the binding of RGD to GPIIIa. These data indicate that the binding of the peptides, and by inference the ligands themselves, to GPIIb-IIIa is a complex interaction that may be characterized by multiple binding sites.[115] The binding of VWF to stimulated platelets, although RGD-dependent, may take place at a site different from that of fibrinogen. A monoclonal antibody, LJ-P5, will selectively inhibit VWF binding to ADP-stimulated platelets (see Chap. 12). It would be of great interest to identify specific ligand-binding regions on the GPIIb–IIIa complex because the primary structure of these proteins has now been obtained from their cDNAs (see later discussion).

The GPIIb–IIIa complex located on unstimulated platelets has no ligand-binding activity: adhesive proteins bind to this complex only after platelet stimulation. The mechanism by which platelet stimulation regulates the receptor function of GPIIb–IIIa is of great importance. Two general hypotheses attempt to explain this phenomenon. First, a conformational change in the GPIIb–IIIa complex may occur upon platelet stimulation, before ligand binding. Alternatively, platelet stimulation could involve the removal of inhibitory membrane proteins, exposing a cryptic binding site.[25] One method to study the expression of receptor function of the GPIIb–IIIa complex is to use certain monoclonal antibodies. The PAC-1 antibody selectively binds to stimulated platelets.[116] Whereas another antibody, 7E3, has an enhanced rate of binding after stimulation.[25] These studies show that there is an increased expression of a GPIIb–IIIa epitope after platelet stimulation. A third antibody, PMI-1, binds to intact platelets only in the presence of EDTA under conditions in which adhesive proteins will not bind.[51] The use of the antibodies indicates that the GPIIb–IIIa complex can exist in a number of conformational states, for example, after platelet stimulation or Ca^{2+} chelation.

Another method to study conformational changes involves the use of the purified GPIIb–IIIa complex itself. The binding of the RGDS peptide will alter the sedimentation and gel filtration properties of GPIIb–IIIa and expose thrombin-sensitive sites on GPIIb.[95] Electron microscopic studies, using a colloidal gold immunolabeling technique, have shown that unstimulated platelets have a uniform distribution of cell-surface GPIIb–IIIa. Following fibrinogen or RGDS peptide binding to stimulated platelets, the GPIIb–IIIa distribution becomes clustered.[67] This is a particularly critical observation for the peptide because RGDS is not multivalent, unlike fibrinogen. Thus, the clustering of GPIIb–IIIa complexes must occur by a ligand-independent mechanism, either by direct interaction of the conformationally altered complexes themselves or through involvement of components of the cytoskeleton.

Interesting work on stimulus–response coupling has been reported using platelets that have been permeabilized with detergents or electric discharge. Such techniques are now being applied to the study of GPIIb–IIIa receptor function, specifically to investigate how the acquisition of receptor activity is coupled to the general mechanisms of platelet stimulation. Studies with saponin-permeabilized platelets, as monitored by the binding of PAC-1, would suggest that there are two independent pathways for the induction of GPIIb–IIIa receptor function.[117] One pathway, induced by thrombin, is dependent on polyphosphoinositide (PIP_2) hydrolysis, which results in the release of Ca^{2+} from the dense tubular system.[116] The Ca^{2+} is thought to transform the GPIIb–IIIa complex into a receptor-active form, apparently by activating the arachidonate metabolism pathway. Another pathway must be independent of Ca^{2+} because PAC-1 binding is induced by epinephrine, an agonist that does not release intracellular Ca^{2+}. A G protein inhibitor blocks the stimulus-dependent binding of PAC-1. Thus, the G proteins may also be involved in coupling platelet agonists to the adhesive protein–receptor interaction required for platelet aggregation.[116]

The Adhesion Receptor Family

A major advance in our understanding of the role of GPIIb–IIIa was the discovery of immunologically or structurally related receptors on nucleated cells. Membrane proteins apparently identical with GPIIb and GPIIIa have been described on HEL cells[123] and K562 cells.[122] In HEL cells, the two glycoproteins were found to be synthesized from separate mRNAs.[12,118] The two chains of GPIIb result from posttranslational processing of a single polypeptide chain from a single message.[12,105] Glycoproteins IIb and IIIa appear to become assembled into a heterodimer before their expression on the cell surface.[109] Although human monocytes have been reported to express GPIIb-IIIa,[6,17,55] recent studies have failed to demonstrate that these cells synthesize these glycoproteins, and isolation of monocytes free from platelet contamination appears to eliminate GPIIb-IIIa.[23,68,80] Thus, the appearance of these glycoproteins on monocytes, noted in the previous reports, was probably due to platelet contamination. Furthermore, in a recent study of GPIIb-IIIa on leukocytes, synthesis of these proteins was not established.[18]

A number of groups have described GPIIb-IIIa-like membrane components on HUVE cells.[33,78,86,102,127] The HUVE cell and platelet components are similar in relative molecular mass (M_r) on SDS-polyacrylamide gels, and are synthesized by HUVE cells in culture. The HUVE cell GPIIb-IIIa-like components are present as a heterodimer complex, but this complex cannot be dissociated by Ca^{2+} chelation.[33,78] The HUVE cell GPIIb-like component binds Ca^{2+} but has a slightly different isoelectric point on two-dimensional gels compared with platelet GPIIb.[21] The HUVE cell complex can be purified by the monoclonal antibody 7E3,[20] which was originally developed against platelet GPIIb-IIIa.[25] Antibody 7E3 inhibits the attachment of HUVE cells in suspension to fibrinogen- and VWF-coated surfaces but not to fibronectin-coated surfaces.[20] Other work has also shown that fibrinogen can mediate endothelial cell adhesion,[28] and fibrinogen binding to HUVE cells has been demonstrated.[29,30] Thus, the HUVE cell GPIIb-IIIa-like complex is both similar to and different from the platelet glycoproteins. Recently, it has become evident that the HUVE cell GPIIb-IIIa-like complex is probably identical with another membrane receptor, the VnR,[107] which is discussed in the following paragraph. First, amino-terminal sequence analysis has shown that GPIIb-IIIa and the VnR have an apparently identical small β subunit, GPIIIa.[52] Second, polyclonal antibodies specific for platelet GPIIb do not bind the HUVE cell GPIIb-IIIa-like complex, whereas polyclonal antibodies specific for platelet GPIIIa bind the complexes of both cells.[52] Finally, although we have been able to obtain cDNA clones for GPIIIa from a HUVE cell cDNA library,[38] we could not obtain clones for GPIIb. Rather, clones for the VnR α subunit (VnR_α) have been obtained.[37]

As shown in Table 2-2, a number of other cell-surface receptors are structurally similar to platelet GPIIb-IIIa.[66,106] These adhesion receptors all consist of noncovalently associated α and β subunits, which are thought to be in the form of α/β heterodimers. The mammalian FnR and VnR complexes are most similar to the platelet GPIIb-IIIa complex and have α and β subunits with M_rs of 140,000/140,000[13,14,107] and 125,000/115,000,[108] respectively, on reduced gels. The FnR is often referred to as the 140-kDa complex.[14,107] The VnR and GPIIb-IIIa complexes can be purified by affinity chromatography using RGD-containing peptides.[107] The FnR does not bind to RGD peptides, but can be purified by affinity columns of the cell-binding domain of fibronectin.[107] Polyclonal and monoclonal antibodies to the FnR complex will inhibit cell attachment to fibronectin-coated substrates.[14] The purified FnR and VnR have been reconstituted into phospholipid vesicles to study ligand specificity.[108] The FnR is specific for fibronectin, and will not bind to fibrinogen, VWF, or thrombospondin.[106] The VnR was first believed to bind only vitronectin,[106] but is now thought to be capable of interacting with fibrinogen and VWF also.[20] Vitronectin is a 70-kDa plasma protein, previously termed the "serum-spreading factor." Vitronectin has been cloned and sequenced and has an RGD sequence in its primary structure.[121]

A related receptor complex that binds laminin in addition to fibronectin has been identified on chicken embryo fibroblasts by using the monoclonal antibodies CSAT and JG22.[2,15,16,63] These antibodies immunoprecipitate three cell-surface glycoproteins of M_rs 155,000, 135,000, and 120,000 on nonreduced SDS-polyacrylamide gels. This receptor complex is often referred to as the CSAT antigen.[15] It seems likely that the CSAT antigen is in the form of two separate α/β heterodimers, with the 120-kDa component, often referred to as band 3, as the common β subunit.[16] Band 3 is the avian homologue of the β subunit of the mammalian FnR.[66,124] It is not known which of the α subunits, the 155-kDa or 135-kDa one, of the chicken fibronectin/laminin receptor is analogous to the mammalian FnR 140-kDa α subunit. The CSAT complex is a low-affinity receptor for laminin,[63] fibronectin,[2,63] and the cytoskeletal protein talin.[64] Thus, the term *integrin* was proposed for this receptor complex, referring to its ability to integrate

Table 2-2
Adhesion Receptor Family

Name	α Subunits* (kDa)	β Subunits† (kDa)	Distribution
GPIIb-IIIa	GPIIb (125 + 25)	GPIIIa (115)	Platelets, HEL cells
Vitronectin receptor (VnR)	VnR_α (125 + 25)		Widely distributed (e.g., endothelial cells)
Fibronectin receptor (FnR), 140-kDa complex	FnR_α (140 + 25)	FnR_β (140)	Widely distributed (e.g., fibroblasts)
Very late activation Antigens (VLA)	VLA-1 (200) VLA-2 (165) VLA-3 (135 + 25) VLA-4 (150) VLA-5 (135 + 25)‡		T lymphocytes and other cells (e.g., VLA-2 and VLA-3 on platelets)
CSAT antigen	Band 1 (155) Band 2 (135)	Band 3 (120)	Chicken embryo fibroblasts
Leukocyte adhesion receptors	Mac-1 (170) p150 (150) LFA-1 (180)	β (95)	Leukocytes

*Bands 1 and 2 and leukocyte adhesion receptors are non-reduced; all others are reduced. Some α subunits are composed of large and small chains.
†β subunit is nonreduced, all others are reduced.
‡VLA-5 is equivalent to FnR_β (see text).

the extracellular and cytoplasmic compartments.[126] More recently, the term integrin has been expanded to include all α/β adhesion receptors, including platelet GPIIb–IIIa.[66]

Another group of adhesion receptors, termed the *very late activation* (VLA) antigens, were described on stimulated T lymphocytes: VLA-1 and VLA-2.[61] However, more recent studies show that there are five VLA antigens and that they are widely distributed.[60] All five have a common β subunit of 120 and 140 kDa on nonreduced and reduced gels, respectively. Three of the VLA antigens (VLA-1, 2, and 4) have single-chain α subunits, and two (VLA-3 and 5) have two-chain α subunits.[60] Recently, it was reported that the VLA and FnR β subunits are identical.[124] One of the VLA antigens (VLA-5) is identical with the mammalian 140-kDa FnR,[37,125] and another VLA antigen (VLA-3) probably corresponds to the chicken fibronectin/laminin receptor bands 2 and 3.[124] As shown in Table 2-1, platelet GPIa and Ic correspond to the α subunits of VLA-2 and VLA-5*, respectively. Platelet GPIIa corresponds to the VLA/FnR β subunit.

A final group of α/β subunit adhesion receptors, the Mac-1, LFA-1, and p150/95 antigens, are found in leukocytes. These receptors also share a 95-kDa β subunit, but they have structurally and immunologically distinct α subunits.[3,113] The Mac-1 and p150/95 complexes mediate the binding of the C3bi protein from complement to monocytes, which is necessary for phagocytosis and granulocyte adherence.[3,84] The C3bi primary structure contains an RGD sequence,[27] and RGD-containing peptides from C3bi mediate the binding of cultured monocytes to peptide-coated erythrocytes.[132,133] Interestingly, Mac-1 and p150/95 are present in an intracellular, vesicular compartment as well as on the cell surface.[3] Inflammatory agents, such as C5a and *f*-Met-Leu-Phe, stimulate a five- to ten-fold increase in cell-surface Mac-1 and 150/95.[3] The LFA-1

*See editor's note, p. 30.

complex is widely distributed in leukocytes and is involved in T-lymphocyte killer and adhesive function.[3] Leukocyte adhesion deficiency (LAD), an inherited defect of these receptors, is characterized by a deficiency or alteration in the β subunit of LFA-1.[3,26,82] This disorder is characterized by life-threatening infections resulting from impaired leukocyte adhesion at sites of inflammation.

Evidence for an adhesion receptor family initially developed when the amino-terminal sequences were determined for several of the α subunits, including GPIIb, Mac-1, LFA-1, the VLA antigens, and VnR_α. These peptide sequences could be aligned to give about a 40% homology.[21,52,99,120,125] Particularly striking is the conservation in amino-terminal positions 2 to 4, which almost invariably have an Asn-Leu-Asp sequence. Recently, the complete cDNA-deduced protein sequences for three of the adhesion receptor α subunits and three of the β subunits have become known. Ten α subunits and three β subunits have been identified in humans; Table 2-2 also includes the CSAT antigen from chicken cells.[37,66] The adhesion receptor family is divided into three subfamilies, each of which is defined by a single β subunit.[66] Each of the β subunits is complexed with two to five different α subunits. No α subunit is complexed with more than one β subunit. For example, GPIIIa is the β subunit for both the VnR and the platelet GPIIb-IIIa complex.[52] Four of the α subunits (GPIIb, VnR_α, FnR_α, and VLA-3_α) consist of two chains, a 125-kDa to 140-kDa large chain and a 25-kDa small chain, which are linked by an interchain disulfide.[4,37,105,120] The remaining six α subunits—VLA-1, VLA-2, and VLA-4 and all of the leukocyte adhesion receptors—are single-chain polypeptides that are somewhat larger (150-kDa-200-kDa) than the nonreduced two-chain α subunits.[60]

Structure of the Glycoprotein IIb-IIIa Complex and Its Relationship to Other Adhesion Receptors

All three β-subunits in the adhesion receptor family have been sequenced from their cDNAs: GPIIIa,[38] the human leukocyte β subunit,[71] and the chicken CSAT antigen β subunit (band 3).[126] Their overall predicted protein structures are strikingly similar, as shown in Figure 2-2 and Table 2-3. The mature proteins range in size from 747 to 779 amino acids, and each has a putative single hydrophobic transmembrane segment near the carboxyl terminus. Thus, it would appear that all of the β subunits consist of a short, 40- to 46-amino acid cytoplasmic domain and a large (>680-amino acid) extracellular domain. The extracellular domain contains 56 cysteines, 31 of which are clustered into four tandemly repeated segments of about 40 amino acids each. The chicken fibronectin/laminin receptor β subunit (band 3) has 12 potential *N*-linked glycosylation sites in the extracellular domain, whereas GPIIIa and the leukocyte β subunit have only six. This difference largely accounts for the larger size (by 15 to 20 kDa) of band 3 on SDS-polyacrylamide gels.

The protein sequences of the α subunits can

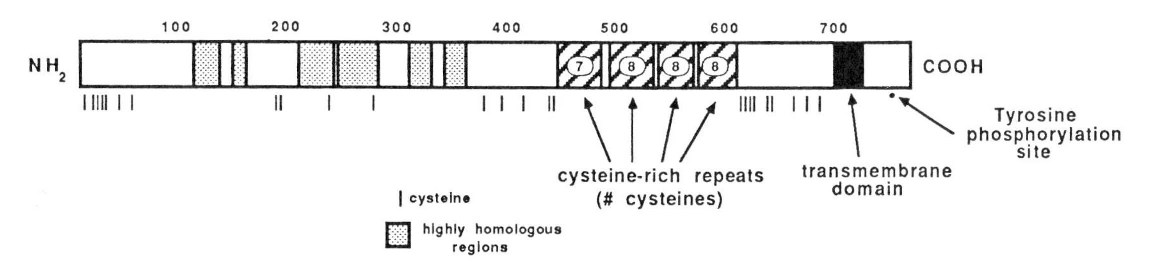

Figure 2-2. Model of the overall cDNA-derived structure of the three β subunits of the adhesion receptor family. The amino acid numbers, the positions of cysteine residues, and the major domains are indicated.

Table 2-3
Properties of Adhesion Receptor Subunits

α Subunits	GPIIb	VnR	FnR
Number of amino acids, total	1008	1018	1008
Large chain	871	860	858
Small chain	137	158	150
Number of cysteines, total	17	18	20
Large chain	14	15	16
Small chain	3	3	4
Potential *N*-linked glycosylation sites (Asn-Xaa-Ser/Thr)	5	13	14
Large chain	4	10	14
Small chain	1	3	0
Putative Ca^{2+}-binding repeats	4	4	4
Length of cytoplasmic domain (No. of amino acids)	20	32	28

β Subunits	GPIIIa	Band 3	Leukocyte β
Number of amino acids (mature protein)	762	779*	747*
Potential *N*-linked glycosylation sites in extracellular domain	6	12	6
Number of cysteincs	56	56	56
Length of cytoplasmic domain (No. of amino acids)	41–46	41–46	40–45
Number of cysteine repeats	4	4	4

*Amino terminus uncertain, but predicted from likely cleavage site for signal peptide.

be easily aligned by placing the cysteines in register. Glycoprotein IIIa and the leukocyte β subunit are more homologous with band 3 than they are with each other (Table 2-4). The majority of identical positions are shared by all three proteins. The homologies indicate that the three proteins evolved by a process of separate gene duplications from the precursor to band 3. The region of greatest homology extends from amino acid position 110 to 350 (*see* Fig. 2-2), where over 45% of the positions are identical in all three proteins. Within this region there are six segments of 14 to 38 amino acids that are 56% to 76% conserved (Fig. 2-3). These regions are predicted to be of critical importance in common functions and structures for these receptor complexes, such as ligand binding or formation of a noncovalent association with an α subunit. One method of assigning functions to a given peptide sequence is to prepare antibodies against synthetic peptides from the β subunit sequences and to determine the effects of such antibodies on, for example, ligand binding or subunit reassociation.

The four cysteine-rich repeats for each β subunit can be aligned and a consensus sequence can be derived.[38,71,126] The repeats have a core structure of *Cys*-Xaa-*Cys*-Xaa-Xaa-*Cys*-Xaa-*Cys*. A number of other cell membrane receptors are characterized by the presence of cysteine-rich repeated segments, including those for the low-density lipoprotein, epidermal growth factor, and insulin.[56] The cysteine repeats in the low-density lipoprotein receptor are believed to occur in the site of ligand binding. The β subunit protein sequences have no homology to these other receptors in their cysteine repeats.[38,71,126] The cysteine repeats in the β subunits are a region of relatively low overall homology apart from the cysteines themselves. The cytoplasmic domain of band 3 and GPIIIa has a tyrosine residue in a sequence that is homologous to other receptors known to become phosphorylated, such as the insulin and epidermal growth fac-

Table 2-4
Protein Sequence Identities in the Adhesion Receptor Subunits

α Subunits	Large Chain No.	Large Chain %	Small Chain No.	Small Chain %	Overall No.	Overall %*
Common	261	28.9	27	17.0	288	27.1
GPIIb vs FnR	359	39.8	43	27.1	402	37.9
GPIIb vs VnR	340	37.7	43	27.0	383	36.1
FnR vs VnR	424	47.0	49	30.8	473	44.5
β Subunits					**No.**	**%†**
Common					248	31.4
GPIIIa vs Band 3					358	45.3
GPIIIa vs Leuk. β					304	38.5
Band 3 vs Leuk. β					359	45.4

*Based on total positions in alignment: 1062.
†Positions in alignment: 790.

tor receptors.[38,126] The chicken fibronectin/laminin receptor has been shown to become phosphorylated in virally transformed cells.[62]

Only three of the ten α subunits of the adhesion receptor family have been completely sequenced from their cDNAs: GPIIb from HEL cells,[104] the FnR_α from fibroblasts and HUVE cells,[4,37] and the VnR_α from placenta and HUVE cells.[37,120] The overall structural features of these three proteins are shown in Figure 2-4 and Table 2-3. The large- and small-chain nucleotide sequences were obtained from a single cDNA, which indicates that both chains are synthesized from a single mRNA.[4,105,120] The small chain is 3′ (carboxyl-terminal) relative to the large chain. Each protein has a single hydrophobic stretch of amino acids near the carboxyl terminus of the small chain; this sequence represents a transmembrane domain. The large chains have no comparable putative transmembrane domain. Our interpretation of this data is that the large chains are entirely extracellular and linked to the small chains by one or more interchain disulfides.[37] Thus, GPIIb and the other β subunits have very short cytoplasmic regions of 20 to 32 amino acids. The large chains contain four repeated segments of about 30 amino acids, which are separated from each other by about 30 residues (*see* Fig. 2-4).[37,105] Within each repeat is a sequence of 12 amino acids having aspartyl and other residues in a spacing that is characteristic of Ca^{2+}-binding regions of proteins such as calmodulin, troponin C, and parvalbumin.[42,73] These Ca^{2+}-binding proteins have the so-called EF hand structure,[73] with Ca^{2+}-binding coordinates as shown in Figure 2-5. In the EF hand structure, the Ca^{2+}-binding coordinates are located in a β turn, which is flanked by segments with an α-helical secondary structure.[42] Interestingly, these putative α-helical segments are missing in the α subunits of the adhesion receptors.[37] Extracellular Ca^{2+} in the micromolar concentration range is necessary for maintaining the GPIIb–IIIa complex,[35,40,98] and millimolar concentrations of Ca^{2+} are required for ligand binding. The role of Ca^{2+} in the other adhesion receptor complexes is not as well defined. However, many cell adhesion functions are known to be Ca^{2+}-dependent.

Glycoprotein IIb and the VnR and FnR α subunits are homologous (*see* Table 2-4),[37] and their cDNA-deduced protein sequences can be aligned most easily by placing the cysteines in register. The FnR_α has 20 cysteines, 16 in the large chain and four in the small chain (*see* Table 2-3). If the cysteines are numbered consecutively, then the VnR_α is missing cysteine 15 and 20 and GPIIb is missing cysteines 11, 15, and 20 (*see* Fig. 2-4). The putative Ca^{2+}-binding regions from amino acid residues 225 to 460 have no cysteines. We believe that the two chains of GPIIb are linked by a single disulfide bond. When ^{125}I-labeled platelet lysates are incubated with increasing concentra-

```
                                         Percent Overall
 GP              Sequence                   Homology                       Position

            ** * ********** ***
GP IIIa    EDYPVDIYYLMDLSYSMKDDL                                           108-128
           |||| | |||||||||||||
Band 3     EDYPIDLYYLMDLSYSMKDDL             76.2%
             ||||||||||||||| |||
Leuk. β    KGYPIDLYYLMDLSYSMLDDL

           ***** ** * * *
GP IIIa    RIGFGAFVDKPVSP                                                  150-163
           ||||| || | | |
Band 3     RIGFGSFVEKTVMP                    71.4%
           |||||||| ||| |
Leuk. β    RIGFGSFVDKTVLP
                   |
           * **   * * * **** ** **
GP IIIa    VKKQSVSRNRDAPEGGFDAIMQ                                          207-228
           | ||   | | | |||||||||
Band 3     VGKQHISGNLDSPEGGFDAIMQ            63.6%
           |||| |||||| |||| || ||
Leuk. β    VGKQLISGNLDAPEGGLDAMMQ
                      |
           *****    **** **    * * *   *   *  **** **
GP IIIa    IGWRNDASHLLVFTTDAKTHIALDRGLAGIVQPNDGQCH                         236-274
           |||||    |||| |||  | | |    | ||| |||| ||
Band 3     IGWRN-VTRLLVFSTDAGFHFAGDGKLGGIVLPNDGKCH             56.4%
           ||||| ||||||| || |||||||||||  |  |||| ||
Leuk. β    IGWRN-VTRLLVFATDDGFHFAGDGKLGAILTPNDGRCH

           **   **  *****
GP IIIa    KLSQKNINLIFAVT                                                  298-311
           |||  ||  |||||
Band 3     KLSENNIQTIFAVT                    64.3%
           || ||||| |||||
Leuk. β    KLAENNIQPIFAVT

           **   ** **  ****  **  **
GP IIIa    IPGTTVGVLSMDSSNVLQLIVDAY                                        325-348
           ||   || ||  |||| ||| |||
Band 3     IPKSAVGTLSSNSSNVIQLIIDAY          58.3%
           ||||||| ||  ||||  ||  ||
Leuk. β    IPKSAVGELSEDSSNVVHLIKNAY
                     |
```

Figure 2-3. Amino acid sequences of six strongly conserved segments in the three β subunits. Positions of identity (|) between individual subunits and among all three subunits (*) are indicated. The identity symbols (|) at the bottom of each segment indicate identities between GPIIIa and the leukocyte β subunit.

tions of β-mercaptoethanol, the large and small chains of GPIIb separate, followed by a single M_r shift in electrophoretic mobility for the small chain.[38] Thus, of the three cysteines in the small chain, two must be in an intrachain disulfide linkage, leaving only one to form an interchain disulfide bond. We predict that the other two-chain α subunits also are joined by a single disulfide. When the three protein sequences are aligned (*see* Table 2-4), 288 positions (27%) are identical in all three α subunits. The FnR_α has more homology to GPIIb and the VnR_α than does GPIIb to the VnR_α. The putative Ca^{2+}-binding repeats of the large chains are the most homologous regions of the protein sequence, with over 60% of the positions having identical residues in all three proteins.[38] Outside the Ca^{2+}-binding region, iden-

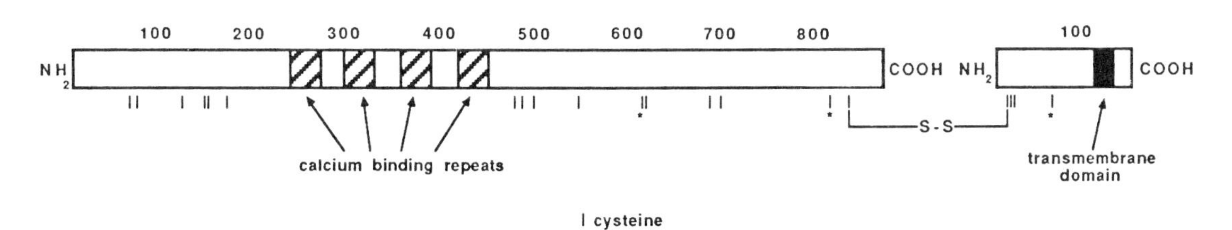

Figure 2-4. Model of the overall cDNA-derived structure of three two-chain α subunits (GPIIb, VnRα, and FnRα). The positions of cysteine residues are indicated (|), and those cysteines missing in GPIIb and the VnRα are marked (*). The positions of the cysteines involved in the interchain disulfide linkage (S–S) have not been determined.

tical residues are generally clustered into segments of four to eight residues.[38]

It seems likely that the α subunits of the adhesion receptor family also evolved by a process of independent gene duplications from a common precursor. We speculate that GPIIb and the VnR_α evolved separately from the precursor of the FnR_α.[37] Despite the fact that GPIIb and the VnR_α have similar ligand-binding properties and relative molecular masses and that both are complexed with the same β subunit (GPIIIa), they are less homologous with each other than with the FnR_α. It is our opinion that the α and β subunits in the FnR/VLA subfamily of the adhesion receptors[66] were the source of gene duplications for all of the other α and β subunits. The protein sequencing of additional α subunits will clarify this issue.

Another interesting group of receptors are found in *Drosophilia* and are termed *position-specific antigens.*[130] These proteins are involved in cell positioning and movement in embryonic development of this fly. The proteins appear to have a common β subunit and several distinct α subunits that have about the

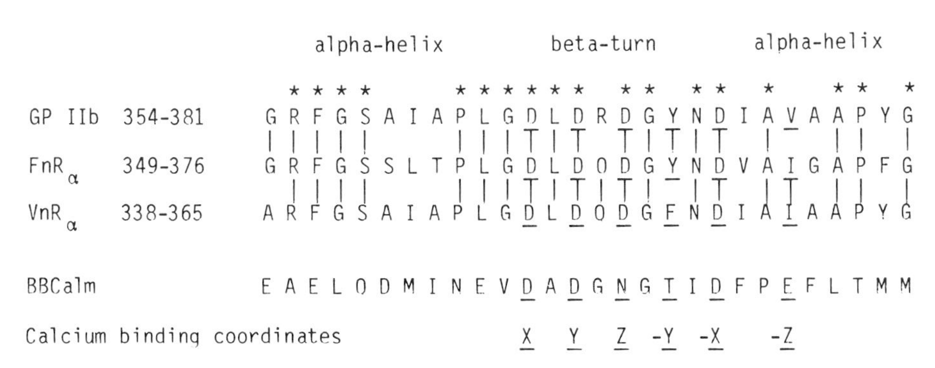

Figure 2-5. Comparison of amino acid sequence of the Ca^{2+}-binding repeats of the three α subunits of the adhesion receptor family *versus* a representative "EF hand" structure, bovine brain calmodulin (BBCalm).[41] The six Ca^{2+}-binding coordinates (*X, Y, Z, -Y, -X, -Z*) are in a β-turn secondary structure as shown. Note the presence of Gly (*G*) and Pro (*P*) residues in the segments flanking the β turn in the adhesion receptors; these segments are not predicted to form α helices. Positions of identity are denoted as before.

same molecular masses as the adhesion receptor subunits described previously. The amino-terminal sequence of one of the α subunits of the position-specific antigens can be aligned with the amino-terminal sequences of some of the adhesion receptor α subunits.[125] It seems likely that these fly antigens are another subfamily of α/β adhesion heterodimers.[79]

Given the cDNA-deduced protein sequences, we can now speculate about the organization of the GPIIb–IIIa complex in the platelet membrane. Over 95% of the protein is extracellular, with GPIIb and GPIIIa each having only a single transmembrane domain. On the basis of rotary-shadow electron micrographs of the purified GPIIb–IIIa complexes reconstituted into phospholipid vesicles,[92] it appears that there is a large globular domain distal to the membrane and that it is the region where the α and β subunits are complexed. This region could also be the site of ligand binding. This globular region is extended from the membrane by two regions of filamentous structure in each subunit. Previously, both of the filamentous "arms" were described as GPIIIa.[19,92] In light of the cDNA-deduced protein sequences described earlier, however, it seems more likely that the filamentous arms represent portions of GPIIb and GPIIIa.

THE GLYCOPROTEIN Ib–IX COMPLEX AND THE MECHANISM OF PLATELET ADHESION

The GPIb–IX complex is the second major glycoprotein complex on platelets; about 25,000 copies of this complex are found per platelet.[36,44,46] Glycoprotein Ib (M_r, 145,000) is composed of disulfide-linked large (M_r, 125,000) and small (M_r, 23,000) chains. The GPIb–IX complex has been purified by monoclonal antibody affinity chromatography,[9] and GPIb and GPIX appear to be in a 1 : 1 heterodimer complex.[32] Glycoprotein Ib is heavily glycosylated, with up to 60% of its mass consisting of *O*-linked and *N*-linked carbohydrate.[36] A large, water-soluble fragment of GPIb, termed glycocalicin, is released by the Ca^{2+}-dependent protease (calpain) present in the platelet cytoplasm. Amino-terminal sequence analysis has shown that glycocalicin represents the amino-terminal part of the large chain.[57] Rotary-shadowed electron microscopy has shown that the purified GPIb–IX complex consists of a globular, membrane-associated domain and an elongated, extracellular domain.[39]

A major function of the GPIb–IX complex is to link the plasma membrane with a submembranous "membrane skeleton," which is composed of short actin filaments and actin-binding protein (ABP).[39,91] Over 50% of the cell-surface-labeled GPIb of unstimulated platelets can be immunoprecipitated by polyclonal antibodies to ABP in nonionic detergent lysates.[39] In contrast, platelets stimulated by ionophore A23187 or dibucaine, which activate calpain, have no cytoskeleton-associated GPIb.[39] The release of GPIb from the membrane skeleton is accompanied by the hydrolysis of ABP.[39] Thus, the cytoplasmic portion of GPIb apparently associates with a protease-labile portion of ABP. This association is important in the maintenance of the platelets discoid shape and in the expression of VWF-binding sites.[39] Interestingly, Bernard-Soulier platelets, which lack GPIb–IX, are very large, polymorphic cells[46] whose size and shape may be due to a lack of membrane–cytoskeleton association. The small chain of GPIb, often referred to as $GPIb_\beta$, has been shown to become phosphorylated in intact platelets.[134] Recently, HEL cells were shown to have a GPIb-like protein, since a protein of M_r 60,000 could be detected on metabolically labeled and surface-labeled HEL cells, using platelet GPIb-specific polyclonal and monoclonal antibodies.[70] However, HEL proteins corresponding to the $GPIb_\beta$ and GPIX were not detected.

The protein sequence of the large chain of GPIb was recently determined from a cDNA clone obtained from an HEL cDNA expression library.[81] The mature protein consists of 610 amino acids, with a single transmembrane segment toward the carboxyl terminus and an intracellular domain of about 100 amino acids. In the extracellular domain of GPIb are five repeating segments of nine amino acids each that are rich in serine and threonine and appear to be likely sites for *O*-linked carbohydrate attachment. Glycoprotein Ib also has seven tandem 24-amino acid repeats, each of which is homologous to a plasma leucine-rich α_2-glycoprotein. The significance of this observation is uncertain. The small subunit of GPIb is apparently translated from a separate mRNA. No homology has been found between GPIb and the α/β subunit adhesion receptors described previously. It remains possible that other GPIb-like proteins are present on nucleated cells, although recently it has been shown that in HUVE cells the VnR binds VWF.[20]

The GPIb-IX complex is involved in VWF binding, a process necessary for platelet adhesion. Bernard-Soulier platelets, which lack the GPIb-IX complex, are defective in adhesion and do not bind VWF.[46] Certain monoclonal antibodies to GPIb also block adhesion and VWF binding to normal platelets.[129] In vitro, the antibiotic ristocetin acts as a cofactor to mediate the GPIb-VWF interaction, possibly by inducing a change in GPIb or VWF.[46] In vivo, this conformational change in VWF is presumably mediated by the attachment of VWF to components of the subendothelial matrix.[24] The amino-terminal region of GPIb is the site of VWF binding,[57] and the mechanism of this binding is different from the RGD-dependent VWF binding to GPIIb-IIIa.[95,129] The GPIb-binding region of VWF has been localized to the amino-terminal region of the protein, which does not contain an RGD sequence.[54,112] The GPIb-VWF interaction is responsible for platelet adhesion under high shear conditions.[129] Glycoprotein Ib also contains the moderate- and high-affinity platelet binding sites for thrombin[58] that may be involved in platelet stimulation.

OTHER PLATELET MEMBRANE GLYCOPROTEINS

Recent studies have shown that platelets have surface glycoproteins that correspond to certain of the FnR and VLA antigen heterodimers on nucleated cells (*see* Table 2-1). The VLA-2 antigen has been detected on platelets,[60,125] and it appears likely that the subunits of this receptor correspond to platelet GPIa (α subunit) and GPIIa (β subunit).[44] The α subunit of VLA-2 has an M_r of 165,000 and 150,000 on reduced and nonreduced SDS-polyacrylamide gels, respectively,[60] which correspond to those of GPIa.[22] It has been reported that GPIa was absent from platelets in a patient who has a defect in collagen binding,[87] and GPIa has been identified as the receptor mediating the divalent cation-dependent binding of collagen to platelets.[114] Recently, it was reported that a 160-kDa protein was immunoprecipitated from labeled platelets by using a polyclonal antibody specific for the β subunit of the FnR.[49] This antibody also specifically detects GPIIa by Western blotting of total platelet lysates. Thus, GPIa and GPIIa appear to be complexed with each other. Platelets also contain VLA-5*,[44,101] which probably corresponds to a GPIc-IIa complex.[44] Glycoprotein Ic has a two-chain structure whose disulfide-linked subunits are similar in size to those of GPIIb.[22] The platelet GPIc-IIa complex apparently does not correspond to the 140-kDa FnR complex on nucleated cells (e.g., HUVE cells). Instead, GPIc is possibly homologous to band 2 of the chicken fibronectin/laminin receptor complex. Thus, at least five platelet glycoproteins—GPIa, GPIc, GPIIa, GPIIb, and GPIIIa—are members of the α/β adhesion receptor family, and these glycoproteins form at least three separate heterodimer complexes (*see* Table 2-1). The report of platelet GPIIa on HUVE cells[128] can now be explained because both platelets and HUVE cells have the FnR/VLA β subunit.[20]

Three other platelet membrane glycoproteins deserve mention. All of these components are single-chain polypeptides that are not complexed to other platelet glycoproteins and have been characterized with monoclonal antibodies. An α-granule membrane protein, called GMP-140[119] or PADGEM,[8] is present on the plasma membrane only after α-granule secretion. About 8000 to 12,000 copies of this glycoprotein are found on stimulated platelets. Quantitation of this component is a useful indicator of platelet stimulation.[48] Glycoprotein IV, also called GPIIIb, is a highly glycosylated, protease-resistant component of M_r 85,000.[36,47] A monoclonal antibody reported to bind to platelet GPIV, called OKM5, inhibits thrombospondin binding to stimulated platelets.[5] Although thrombospondin contains an RGD sequence,[77] its binding to platelets apparently occurs through a GPIIb-IIIa-independent mechanism.[1] Glycoprotein IV is also present on HUVE cells.[5]

The platelet receptor GPV is shrouded in controversy.[36,44] This 82-kDa component is the

*See editor's note, p. 30.

only major platelet membrane glycoprotein that is a thrombin substrate. A water-soluble fragment of GPV, GPV_{fl} (M_r, 69,000) is released from the platelet by thrombin.[36] Thus, GPV was initially interpreted to be a thrombin receptor involved in platelet stimulation. However, GPV_{fl} release does not necessarily correlate with platelet stimulation, which has led investigators to suggest that GPV is not the thrombin receptor involved in platelet stimulation.[11,83] Glycoprotein V is also deficient in patients with Bernard-Soulier syndrome, which suggests that it is associated with the GPIb-IX complex.[10,46] However, an association of GPV with the GPIb-IX complex has not been directly proved. It is not known if proteins corresponding to GPV are present in nucleated cells.

SUMMARY AND PROSPECTIVE

Our understanding of the structure and function of platelet membrane glycoproteins, particularly the GPIIb-IIIa complex and GPIb, has increased considerably in the last 2 years. The structure and amino acid sequence of GPIIb and GPIIIa are homologous to those of other members of a family of adhesion receptors having an α/β heterodimeric structure.[37,38,66,105] It is currently believed that these receptors bind their ligands primarily through an RGD-dependent mechanism.[111] However, a second sequence on fibrinogen, the decapeptide sequence at the carboxyl terminus of the γ-chain, is also important in receptor interaction on platelets.[71,75,115] In addition, unlike the adhesion receptors in nucleated cells, the GPIIb-IIIa receptor activity is not expressed constitutively, but only as a consequence of platelet stimulation.

Three other platelet glycoproteins, Ia, Ic, and IIa, also appear to be members of the adhesion receptor family. In vivo, only GPIIb appears to be restricted to platelets. The two other platelet adhesion receptor complexes, GPIa-IIa and GPIc-IIa, could be involved in functions such as platelet spreading on collagen and fibronectin, respectively. Although antibodics that block these receptor functions on other cells have been shown to cross-react with selected platelet glycoproteins, direct evidence that these glycoproteins possess such receptor functions on platelets is still lacking.

A number of experimental approaches are likely to provide useful information about the function of GPIIb-IIIa and other platelet membrane glycoproteins. Detailed analysis of the congenital defects in patients with Glanzmann's thrombasthenia and Bernard-Soulier syndrome is likely to identify functionally important sites in these receptors. Glanzmann's thrombasthenia now appears to be a more complex disorder than previously described. Platelets from a number of patients with this disease have significant amounts of GPIIb-IIIa, but this residual complex is often defective either in forming the native heterodimer or in ligand binding[89] (*see* Chap. 5). Because GPIIIa is also present as the β subunit of the VnR,[53] we suspect that most of the GPIIb-IIIa defects in thrombasthenia will ultimately be traced to GPIIb. In support of this speculation, normal amounts of the endothelial cell GPIIb-IIIa-like proteins (VnR) have been reported from thrombasthenic patients.[50] As mentioned earlier, a second approach to study platelet membrane glycoproteins further would entail the generation of antibodies specific for peptide sequences of GPIIb-IIIa and GPIb to localize functional domains. Finally, we would like to understand how members of the adhesion receptor family are selectively expressed in given cell types. Many cell types, including platelets, HUVE cells, and osteosarcoma cells, express two β subunits.[20,106] One means of examining this selective expression will be to analyze the 5′ regulatory elements (i.e., promoters and enhancers) associated with the genes of the adhesion receptor subunits. The results of these studies could also elucidate how the cell can coordinately express different α and β subunits that ultimately associate into the cell-surface heterodimer.

Although the other platelet membrane glycoproteins discussed in this review are presently less well understood, we can predict that many will also have counterparts on other cells. Thus, in the last few years we have witnessed the integration of our knowledge about platelet ligand-receptor processes with our understanding of more generalized cell receptor phenomena that are relevant to the biology of cell-cell and cell-substrate interactions.

This work was supported by National Institutes of Health grants HL28947 and HL32254 (to D. R. P.).

REFERENCES

1. Aiken ML, Ginsberg MH, Plow EF: Identification of a new class of inducible receptors on platelets. Thrombospondin interacts with platelets via a GP IIb–IIIa-independent mechanism. J Clin Invest 78:1713, 1986

2. Akiyama SK, Yamada SS, Yamada KM: Characterization of a 140-kD avian cell surface antigen as a fibronectin-binding molecule. J Cell Biol 102:442, 1986

3. Anderson DC, Springer TA: Leukocyte adhesion deficiency: An inherited defect in the Mac-1, LFA-1, and p150,95 glycoproteins. Annu Rev Med 38:175, 1987

4. Argraves WS, Pytela R, Suzuki S, Millán JL, Pierschbacher MD, Ruoslahti E: cDNA sequences from the α subunit of the fibronectin receptor predict a transmembrane domain and a short cytoplasmic peptide. J Biol Chem 261:12922, 1986

5. Asch AS, Barnwell J, Silverstein RL, Nachman RL: Isolation of the thrombospondin membrane receptor. J Clin Invest 79:1054, 1987

6. Bai Y, Durbin H, Hogg N: Monoclonal antibodies specific for platelet glycoproteins react with human monocytes. Blood 64:139, 1984

7. Baldassare JJ, Kahn RA, Knipp MA, Newman P: Reconstitution of platelet proteins into phospholipid vesicles. Functional proteoliposomes. J Clin Invest 75:35, 1985

8. Berman CL, Yeo EL, Wencel-Drake JD, Furie BC, Ginsberg MH, Furie B: A platelet alpha granule membrane protein that is associated with the plasma membrane after activation. Characterization and subcellular localization of platelet activation-dependent granule-external membrane protein. J Clin Invest 78:130, 1986

9. Berndt MC, Gregory C, Kabral A, Zola H, Fournier D, Castaldi PA: Purification and preliminary characterization of the glycoprotein Ib complex in the human platelet membrane. Eur J Biochem 151:637, 1985

10. Berndt MC, Phillips DR: Platelet membrane proteins: Composition and receptor function. In Gordon JL (ed): *Platelets in Biology and Pathology*, pp 43–75. Amsterdam, Elsevier/North-Holland Biomedical Press, 1981

11. Bienz D, Schnippering W, Clemetson KJ: Glycoprotein V is not the thrombin activation receptor on human blood platelets. Blood 68:720, 1986

12. Bray PF, Rosa J-P, Lingappa VR, Kahn YW, McEver RP, Shuman MA: Biogenesis of the platelet receptor for fibrinogen: Evidence for separate precursors for glycoproteins IIb and IIIa. Proc Natl Acad Sci USA 83:1480, 1986

13. Brown PJ, Juliano RL: Selective inhibition of fibronectin-mediated cell adhesion by monoclonal antibodies to a cell-surface glycoprotein. Science 228:1448, 1985

14. Brown PJ, Juliano RL: Expression and function of a putative cell surface receptor for fibronectin in hamster and human cell lines. J Cell Biol 103:1595, 1986

15. Buck CA, Knudsen KA, Damsky CH, Decker CL, Greggs RR, Duggan KE, Bozyczko D, Horwitz AF: Integral membrane protein complexes in cell-matrix adhesion. In Edelman GM, Thiery J-P (eds): *The Cell in Contact. Adhesions and Junctions as Morphogenetic Determinants*, pp 345–364. New York, John Wiley & Sons, 1985

16. Buck CA, Shea E, Duggan K, Horwitz AF: Integrin (the CSAT antigen): Functionality requires oligometric integrity. J Cell Biol 103:2421, 1986

17. Burckhardt JJ, Anderson WHK, Kearny JF, Cooper MD: Human blood monocytes and platelets share a cell surface component. Blood 60:767, 1982

18. Burns GF, Cosgrove L, Triglia T, Bealle JA, López AF, Werkmeister JA, Begley CG, Haddad AP, d'Apice AJF, Vadas MA, Cawley JC: The IIb–IIIa glycoprotein complex that mediates platelet aggregation is directly implicated in leukocyte adhesion. Cell 45:269, 1986

19. Carrell NA, Fitzgerald LA, Steiner B, Erikson HP, Phillips DR: Structure of human platelet membrane glycoproteins IIb and IIIa as determined by electron microscopy. J Biol Chem 260:1743, 1985

20. Charo IF, Bekeart LS, Phillips DR: Platelet glycoprotein IIb–IIIa-like proteins mediate endothelial cell attachment to adhesive proteins and the extracellular matrix. J Biol Chem 262:9935, 1987

21. Charo IF, Fitzgerald LA, Steiner B, Rall SC Jr, Bekeart LS, Phillips DR: Platelet glycoproteins IIb and IIIa: Evidence for a family of immunologically and structurally related glycoproteins in mammalian cells. Proc Natl Acad Sci USA 83:8351, 1986

22. Clemetson KJ: Glycoproteins of the platelet plasma membrane. In George JN, Nurden AT, Phillips DR (eds): *Platelet Membrane Glycoproteins*, pp 51–85. New York, Plenum Press, 1985

23. Clemetson KJ, McGregor JL, McEver RP, Jacques YV, Bainton DF, Domzig W, Baggiolini M: Absence of platelet membrane glycoproteins IIb/IIIa from monocytes. J Exp Med 161:972, 1985

24. Coller BS: Platelet–von Willebrand factor interactions. In George JN, Nurden AT, Phillips DR (eds): *Platelet Membrane Glycoproteins*, pp 215–257. New York, Plenum Press, 1985

25. Coller BS: Activation affects access to the

platelet receptor for adhesive proteins. J Cell Biol 103:451, 1986

26. Dana N, Clayton LK, Tennen DG, Pierce MW, Lachmann PJ, Law SA, Arnaout MA: Leukocytes from four patients with complete or partial Leu-CAM deficiency contain the common β-subunit precursor and β-subunit messenger RNA. J Clin Invest 79:1010, 1987

27. de Bruijn MHL, Fey GH: Human complement component C3: cDNA coding sequence and derived primary structure. Proc Natl Acad Sci USA 82:708, 1985

28. Dejana E. Colella S, Languino LR, Balconi G, Corbascio GC, Marchisio PC: Fibrinogen induces adhesion, spreading, and microfilament organization of human endothelial cells in vitro. J Cell Biol 104:1403, 1987

29. Dejana E, Languino LR, Polentarutti N, Balconi G, Ryckewaert JJ, Larrieu MJ, Donati MB, Montovani A, Marguerie G: Interaction between fibrinogen and cultured endothelial cells. Induction of migration and specific binding. J Clin Invest 75:11, 1985

30. Delvos U, Preissner KT, Müller-Berghaus G: Binding of fibrinogen to cultured bovine endothelial cells. Thromb Haemostasis 53:26, 1985

31. De Marco L, Girolami A, Zimmerman TS, Ruggeri ZM: von Willebrand factor interaction with the glycoprotein IIb–IIIa complex. Its role in platelet function as demonstrated in patients with congenital afibrinogenemia. J Clin Invest 77:1272, 1986

32. Du X, Beutler L, Ruan C, Castaldi PA, Berndt MC: Glycoprotein Ib and glycoprotein IX are fully complexed in the intact platelet membrane. Blood 69:1524, 1987

33. Fitzgerald LA, Charo IF, Phillips DR: Human and bovine endothelial cells synthesize membrane proteins similar to human platelet glycoproteins IIb and IIIa. J Biol Chem 260:10893, 1985

34. Fitzgerald LA, Leung B, Phillips DR: A method of purifying the platelet membrane GPIIb–IIIa complex. Anal Biochem 151:169, 1985

35. Fitzgerald LA, Phillips DR: Calcium regulation of the platelet membrane glycoprotein IIb–IIIa complex. J Biol Chem 260:11366, 1985

36. Fitzgerald LA, Phillips DR: Platelet membrane glycoproteins. In Colman RW, Hirsh J, Marder VJ, Salzman EW (eds): *Hemostasis and Thrombosis: Basic Principles and Clinical Practice*, 2nd ed, pp 572–593. Philadelphia, JB Lippincott, 1987

37. Fitzgerald LA, Poncz M, Steiner B, Rall SC Jr, Bennett JS, Phillips DR: Comparison of cDNA-derived protein sequences of the human fibronectin and vitronectin receptor α-subunits and platelet GPIIb. Bochemistry 26:8158, 1988

38. Fitzgerald LA, Steiner B, Rall SC Jr, Lo S-S, Phillips DR: Protein sequence of endothelial glycoprotein IIIa dervied from a cDNA clone. Identity with platelet glycoprotein IIIa and similarity to "integrin." J Biol Chem 262:3936, 1987

39. Fox JEB, Boyles JK: Characterization of the platelet membrane skeleton. In *Proceedings of the UCLA Conference on Signal Transduction in Cytoplasmic Organization and Cell Motility*. New York, Alan R. Liss, (in press)

40. Fujimura K, Phillips DR: Calcium cation regulation of glycoprotein IIb–IIIa complex formation in platelet plasma membranes. J Biol Chem 258:10247, 1983

41. Gardner JM, Hynes RO: Interaction of fibronectin with its receptor on platelets. Cell 42:439, 1985

42. Gariépy J, Hodges RS: Primary sequence analysis and folding behavior of EF hands in relation to the mechanism of action of troponin C and calmodulin. FEBS Lett 160:1, 1983

43. Gartner TK, Bennett JS: The tetrapeptide analogue of the cell attachment site of fibronectin inhibits platelet aggregation and fibrinogen binding to activated platelets. J Biol Chem 260:11891, 1985

44. George JN: The role of membrane glycoproteins in platelet function. Transfusion Med Rev 1:34, 1987

45. George JN, Nurden AT: Inherited disorders of the platelet membrane: Glanzmann's thrombasthenia and Bernard-Soulier syndrome. In Colman RW, Hirsh J, Marder VJ, Salzman EW (eds): *Hemostasis and Thrombosis. Basic Principles and Clinical Practice*, 2nd ed, pp 726–740. Philadelphia, JB Lippincott, 1987

46. George JN, Nurden AT, Phillips DR: Molecular defects in interactions of platelets with the vessel wall. N Engl J Med 311:1084, 1984

47. George JN, Nurden AT, Phillips DR: *Platelet Membrane Glycoproteins*. New York, Plenum Press, 1985

48. George JN, Pickett EB, Saucerman S, McEver RP, Kunicki TJ, Kieffer N, Newman PJ: Platelet surface glycoproteins. Studies on resting and activated platelets and platelet membrane microparticles, and observations in patients during adult respiratory distress syndrome and cardiac surgery. J Clin Invest 78:340, 1986

49. Giancotti FG, Languino LR, Zanetti A, Peri G, Tarone G, Dejana E: Platelets express a membrane protein complex immunologically related to the fibroblast fibronectin receptor and distinct from GPIIb/IIIa. Blood 69:1535, 1987

50. Giltay JC, Leeksma OC, Breederveld C, van Mourik JA: Normal synthesis and expression of en-

dothelial IIb/IIIa in Glanzmann's thrombasthenia. Blood 69:809, 1987

51. Ginsberg MH, Lightsey A, Kunicki TJ, Kaufmann A, Marguerie G, Plow EF: Divalent cation regulation of the surface orientation of platelet membrane glycoprotein IIb. Correlation with fibrinogen binding function and definition of a novel variant of Glanzmann's thrombasthenia. J Clin Invest 78:1103, 1986

52. Ginsberg MH, Loftus J, Ryckwaert J-J, Pierschbacher M, Pytela R, Ruoslahti E, Plow EF: Immunochemical and amino-terminal sequence comparison of two cytoadhesins indicates they contain similar or identical β subunits and distinct α subunits. J Biol Chem 262:5437, 1987

53. Ginsberg M, Pierschbacher MD, Ruoslahti E, Marguerie G, Plow EF: Inhibition of fibronectin binding to platelets by proteolytic fragments and synthetic peptides which support fibroblast adhesion. J Biol Chem 260:3931, 1985

54. Girma J-P, Kalafatis M, Piétu G, Lavergne J-M, Chopek MW, Edgington TS, Meyer D: Mapping of distinct von Willebrand factor domains interacting with platelet GPIb and GPIIb/IIIa and with collagen using monoclonal antibodies. Blood 67:1356, 1986

55. Gogstad G, Hetland O, Solum NO, Prydz H: Monocytes and platelets share the glycoproteins IIb and IIIa that are absent from both cells in Glanzmann's thrombasthenia type I. Biochem J 214:331, 1983

56. Goldstein JL, Brown MS, Anderson RGW, Russell DW, Schneider WJ: Receptor-mediated endocytosis: Concepts emerging from the LDL receptor system. Annu Rev Cell Biol 1:1, 1985

57. Handa M, Titani K, Holland LZ, Roberts JR, Ruggeri ZM: The von Willebrand factor-binding domain of platelet membrane glycoprotein Ib. Characterization by monoclonal antibodies and partial amino acid sequence analysis of proteolytic fragments. J Biol Chem 261:12579, 1986

58. Harmon JT, Jamieson GA: The glycocalacin portion of platelet glycoprotein Ib expresses both high and moderate affinity receptor sites for thrombin. A soluble radio-receptor assay for the interaction of thrombin with platelets. J Biol Chem 261:13224, 1986

59. Haverstick DM, Cowan JF, Yamada KM, Santoro SA: Inhibition of platelet adhesion to fibronectin, fibrinogen, and von Willebrand factor substrates by a synthetic tetrapeptide derived from the cell-binding domain of fibronectin. Blood 66:946, 1985

60. Hemler ME, Huang C, Schwarz L: The VLA protein family. Characterization of five distinct cell surface heterodimers each with a common 130,000 molecular weight β subunit. J Biol Chem 262:3300, 1987

61. Hemler ME, Jacobson JG, Strominger JL: Biochemical characterization of VLA-1 and VLA-2. Cell surface heterodimers on activated T cells. J Biol Chem 260:15246, 1985

62. Hirst R, Horwitz A, Buck C, Rohrschneider L: Phosphorylation of the fibronectin receptor complex in cells transformed by oncogenes that encode tyrosine kinases. Proc Natl Acad Sci USA 83:6470, 1986

63. Horwitz A, Duggan K, Greggs R, Decker C, Buck C: The cell substrate attachment (CSAT) antigen has properties of a receptor for laminin and fibronectin. J Cell Biol 101:2134, 1985

64. Horwitz A, Duggan K, Buck C, Beckerle MC, Burridge K: Interaction of plasma membrane fibronectin receptor with talin–a transmembrane linkage. Nature 320:531, 1986

65. Huynh TV, Young RA, Davis RW: Constructing and screening cDNA libraries in λgt10 and λgt11. In Glover DM (ed): *DNA Cloning. Volume 1. A Practical Approach*, pp 49–78. Washington, IRL Press, 1985

66. Hynes RO: Integrins: A family of cell surface receptors. Cell 48:549, 1987

67. Isenberg WM, McEver RP, Phillips DR, Shuman MA, Bainton DF: The platelet fibrinogen receptor: An immunogold-surface replica study of agonist-induced ligand binding and receptor clustering. J Cell Biol 104:1655, 1987

68. Jennings LK, Ashmun RA, Phillips DR, Fitzgerald LA, Dockter MA: Binding of human platelets to circulating blood monocyte occurs after venipuncture and is inhibited by prostacyclin. Thromb Haemostasis 54:232a, 1985

69. Jennings LK, Phillips DR: Purification of glycoproteins IIb and III from human platelet membranes and characterization of a calcium-dependent glycoprotein IIb–III complex. J Biol Chem 257:10458, 1982

70. Kieffer N, Debili N, Wicki A, Titeux M, Henri A, Mishal Z, Breton-Gorius J, Vainchenker W, Clemetson KJ: Expression of platelet glycoprotein Ib_{α} in HEL cells. J Biol Chem 261:15854, 1986

71. Kishimoto TK, O'Connor K, Lee A, Roberts TM, Springer TA: Cloning of the β subunit of the leukocyte adhesion proteins: Homology to an extracellular matrix receptor defines a novel supergene family. Cell 48:681, 1987

72. Kloczewiak M, Timmons S, Lukas TJ, Hawiger J: Platelet receptor recognition site on human fibrinogen. Synthesis and structure-function relationship of peptides corresponding to the carboxyterminal segment of the γ chain. Biochemistry 23:1767, 1984

73. Kretsinger RH, Nockolds CE: Carp muscle calcium-binding protein. II. Structure determination and general description. J Biol Chem 248:3313, 1973

74. Kunicki TJ, Pidard D, Rosa J-P, Nurden AT: The formation of Ca^{2+}-dependent complexes of platelet membrane glycoproteins IIb and IIIa in solution as determined by crossed immunoelectrophoresis. Blood 58:268, 1981

75. Lam SC-T, Plow EF, Smith MA, Andrieux A, Ryckwaert J-J, Marguerie G, Ginsberg MH: Evidence that arginyl-glycyl-aspartate peptides and fibrinogen γ chain peptides share a common binding site on platelets. J Biol Chem 262:947, 1987

76. Lathe R: Synthetic oligonucleotide probes deduced from amino acid sequence data. Theoretical and practical considerations. J Mol Biol 183:1, 1985

77. Lawler J, Hynes RO: The structure of human thrombospondin, an adhesive glycoprotein with multiple calcium-binding sites and homologies with several different proteins. J Cell Biol 103:1635, 1986

78. Leeksma OC, Zandbergen-Spaargaren J, Giltay JC, van Mourik JA: Cultured human endothelial cells synthesize a plasma membrane protein complex immunologically related to the platelet glycoprotein IIb/IIIa complex. Blood 67:1176, 1986

79. Leptin M: The fibronectin receptor family. Nature 321:728, 1986

80. Levene RB, Rabellino EM: Platelet glycoproteins IIb and IIIa associated with blood monocytes are derived from platelets. Blood 67:207, 1986

81. Lopez JA, Chung DW, Fujikawa K, Hagen FS, Papayannopoulou T, Roth GJ: Cloning of the α chain of human platelet glycoprotein Ib: A transmembrane protein with homology to leucine-rich α_2-glycoprotein. Proc Natl Acad Sci USA 84:5615, 1987

82. Marlin SD, Morton CC, Anderson DC, Springer TA: LFA-1 immunodeficiency disease. Definition of the genetic defect and chromosomal mapping of α and β subunits of the lymphocyte function-associated antigen 1 (LFA-1) by complementation in hybrid cells. J Exp Med 164:855, 1986

83. McGowan EB, Ding A-H, Detwiler TC: Corrrelation of thrombin-induced glycoprotein V hydrolysis and platelet activation. J Biol Chem 258:11243, 1983

84. Micklem KJ, Sim RB: Isolation of complement-fragment-iC3b-binding proteins by affinity chromatography. The identification of p150,95 as an iC3b-binding protein. Biochem J 231:233, 1985

85. Newman PJ, Kahn RA: Purification of human platelet membrane glycoproteins IIb and IIIa using high performance liquid chromatography gel filtration. Anal Biochem 132:215, 1983

86. Newman PJ, Kawai Y, Montgomery RR, Kunicki TJ: Synthesis by cultured human umbilical vein endothelial cells of two proteins structurally and immunologically related to platelet membrane glycoproteins IIb and IIIa. J Cell Biol 103:81, 1986

87. Nieuwenhuis HK, Sakariassen KS, Houdijk WPM, Nievelstein PFEM, Sixma JJ: Deficiency of platelet membrane glycoprotein Ia associated with a decreased platelet adhesion to subendothelium: A defect in platelet spreading. Blood 68:692, 1986

88. Nurden AT: Abnormalities of platelet glycoproteins in inherited disorders of platelet function. In Gordon JL (ed): *Platelets in Biology and Pathology*, Vol. 3. Amsterdam, Elsevier/North-Holland Medical Press, 1988 (in press)

89. Nurden AT, George JN, Phillips, DR: Platelet membrane glycoproteins: Their structure, function, and modification in disease. In Phillips DR, Shuman MA (eds): *Biochemistry of Platelets*, pp 159–224. Orlando, Academic Press, 1986

90. Nurden AT, Rosa J-P, Fournier D, Legrand C, Didry D, Parquet A, Pidard D: A variant of Glanzmann's thrombasthenia with abnormal glycoprotein IIb–IIIa complexes in the platelet membrane. J Clin Invest 79:962, 1987

91. Okita JR, Pidard D, Newman PJ, Montgomery RR, Kunicki TJ: On the association of glycoprotein Ib and actin-binding protein in human platelets. J Cell Biol 100:317, 1985

92. Parise LV, Phillips DR: Platelet membrane glycoprotein IIb–IIIa complex incorporated into phospholipid vesicles. Preparation and morphology. J Biol Chem 260:1750, 1985

93. Parise LV, Phillips DR: Reconstitution of the purified platelet fibrinogen receptor. Fibrinogen binding properties of the glycoprotein IIb–IIIa complex. J Biol Chem 260:10698, 1985

94. Parise LV, Phillips DR: Fibronectin-binding properties of the purified platelet glycoprotein IIb–IIIa complex. J Biol Chem 261:14011, 1986

95. Parise LV, Helgerson SL, Steiner B, Nannizzi L, Phillips DR: Synthetic peptides from fibrinogen and fibronectin change the conformation of purified platelet glycoprotein IIb–IIIa. J Biol Chem 262:12597, 1987

96. Parker RI, Gralnick HR: Identification of platelet glycoprotein IIb/IIIa as the major binding site for released platelet–von Willebrand factor. Blood 68:732, 1986

97. Phillips DR: Surface labeling of platelet membrane glycoproteins. *Methods Enzymol.* (in press)

98. Pidard D, Didry D, Kunicki TJ, Nurden AT: Temperature-dependent effects of EDTA on the

membrane glycoprotein IIb-IIIa complex and platelet aggregability. Blood 67:604, 1986

99. Pierce MW, Remold-O'Donnell E, Todd RF III, Arnaout MA: *N*-terminal sequence of human leukocyte glycoprotein Mo1: Conservation across species and homology to platelet IIb/IIIa. Biochim Biophys Acta 874:368, 1986

100. Pierschbacher MD, Ruoslahti E: Cell attachment activity of fibronectin can be duplicated by small synthetic fragments of the molecule. Nature 309:30, 1984

101. Pischel KD, Bluestein HG, Woods VL Jr: Lymphocytes bear molecules (VLA) that are antigenically and structurally similar to platelet GPIa, GPIcα, and GPIIa. Blood 63:311a, 1985

102. Plow EF, Loftus JC, Levin EG, Fair DS, Dixon D, Forsyth J, Ginsberg MH: Immunologic relationship between platelet membrane glycoprotein GPIIb/IIIa and cell surface molecules expressed by a variety of cells. Proc Natl Acad Sci USA 83:6002, 1986

103. Plow EF, Pierschbacher MD, Ruoslahti E, Marguerie G, Ginsberg MH: The effect of Arg-Gly-Asp-containing peptides on fibrinogen and von Willebrand factor binding to platelets. Proc Natl Acad Sci USA 82:8057, 1985

104. Plow EF, Srouji AH, Meyer D, Marguerie G, Ginsberg, MH: Evidence that three adhesive proteins interact with a common recognition site on activated platelets. J Biol Chem 259:5388, 1984

105. Poncz M, Eisman R, Heidenreich R, Silver SM, Vilaire G, Surrey S, Schwartz E, Bennett JS: Structure of the platelet membrane glycoprotein IIb. Homology to the α subunits of the vitronectin and fibronectin membrane receptors. J Biol Chem 262:8476, 1987

106. Pytela R, Pierschbacher MD, Ginsberg MH, Plow EF, Ruoslahti E: Platelet membrane glycoprotein IIb/IIIa: Member of a family of Arg-Gly-Asp-specific adhesion receptors. Science 231:1559, 1986

107. Pytela R, Pierschbacher MD, Ruoslahti E: Identification and isolation of a 140 kD cell surface glycoprotein with properties expected of a fibronectin receptor. Cell 40:191, 1985

108. Pytela R, Pierschbacher MD, Ruoslahti E: A 125/115-kDa cell surface receptor specific for vitronectin interacts with the arginine-glycine-aspartic acid adhesion sequence derived from fibronectin. Proc Natl Acad Sci USA 82:5766, 1985

109. Rosa J-P, Cevallos M, McEver RP: Fibrinogen receptor assembly in human erythroleukemia (HEL) cells. Blood 68:325a, 1986

110. Ruggeri ZM, Bader R, De Marco L: Glanzmann thrombasthenia: Deficient binding of von Willebrand factor to thrombin-stimulated platelets. Proc Natl Acad Sci USA 79:6038, 1982

111. Ruoslahti E, Pierschbacher MD: Arg-Gly-Asp: A versatile cell recognition signal. Cell 44:517, 1986

112. Sadler JE, Shelton-Inloes BB, Sorace JM, Harlan JM, Titani K, Davie EW: Cloning and characterization of two cDNAs coding for human von Willebrand factor. Proc Natl Acad Sci USA 82:6394, 1985

113. Sanchez-Madrid F, Nagy JA, Robbins E, Simon P, Springer TA: A human leukocyte differentiation antigen family with distinct α-subunits and a common β-subunit: The lymphocyte function-association antigen (LFA-1), the C3bi complement receptor (OKM1/Mac-1), and the p150,95 molecule. J Exp Med 158:1785, 1983

114. Santoro SA: Identification of a 160,000 dalton platelet membrane protein that mediates the initial divalent cation-dependent adhesion of platelets to collagen. Cell 46:913, 1986

115. Santoro SA, Lawing WJ Jr: Competition for related but nonidentical binding sites on the glycoprotein IIb-IIIa complex by peptides derived from platelet adhesive proteins. Cell 48:867, 1987

116. Shattil SJ, Brass LF: Induction of the fibrinogen receptor on human platelets by intracellular mediators. J Biol Chem 262:992, 1987

117. Shattil SJ, Hoxie JA, Cunningham M, Brass LF: Changes in the platelet membrane glycoprotein IIb•IIIa complex during platelet activation. J Biol Chem 260:11107, 1985

118. Silver SM, McDonough MM, Vilaire G, Bennett JS: The in vitro synthesis of polypeptides for the platelet membrane glycoproteins IIb and IIIa. Blood 69:1031, 1987

119. Stenberg PE, McEver RP, Shuman MA, Jacques YV, Bainton DF: A platelet alpha-granule membrane protein (GMP-140) is expressed on the plasma membrane after activation. J Cell Biol 101:880, 1985

120. Suzuki S, Argraves WS, Pytela R, Arai H, Krusius T, Pierschbacher MD, Ruoslahti E: cDNA and amino acid sequences of the cell adhesion protein receptor recognizing vitronectin reveal a transmembrane domain and homologies with other adhesion protein receptors. Proc Natl Acad Sci USA 83:8614, 1986

121. Suzuki S, Oldberg A, Hayman EG, Pierschbacher MD, Ruoslahti E: Complete amino acid sequence of human vitronectin deduced from cDNA. Similarity of cell attachment sites in vitronectin and fibronectin. EMBO J 4:2519, 1985

122. Tabilio A, Pelicci PG, Vinci G, Mannoni P, Civin CI, Vainchenker W, Testa U, Lipinski M, Rochant H, Breton-Gorius J: Myeloid and mega-

karyocytic proteins of K-562 cell lines. Cancer Res 43:4569, 1983

123. Tabilio A, Rosa J-P, Testa U, Kieffer N, Nurden AT, Del Canizo MC, Breton-Gorius J, Vainchenker W: Expression of platelet membrane glycoproteins and α-granule proteins by a human erythroleukemia cell line (HEL). EMBO J 3:453, 1984

124. Takada Y, Huang C, Hemler ME: Fibronectin receptor structures in the VLA family of heterodimers. Nature 326:607, 1987

125. Takada Y, Strominger JL, Hemler ME: The very late antigen family of heterodimers is part of a superfamily of molecules involved in adhesion and embryogenesis. Proc Natl Acad Sci USA 84:3239, 1987

126. Tamkun JW, DeSimone DW, Fonda D, Patel RS, Buck C, Horwitz AF, Hynes RO: Structure of integrin, a glycoprotein involved in the transmembrane linkage between fibronectin and actin. Cell 46:271, 1986

127. Thiagarajan P, Shapiro SS, Levine E, DeMarco L, Yalcin A: A monoclonal antibody to human platelet glycoprotein IIIa detects a related protein in cultured human endothelial cells. J Clin Invest 75:896, 1985

128. van Mourik JA, Leeksma OC, Reinders JH, de Groot PG, Zandbergen-Spaargaren J: Vascular endothelial cells synthesize a plasma membrane protein indistinguishable from the platelet membrane glycoprotein IIa. J Biol Chem 260:11300, 1985

129. Weiss HJ, Turitto VT, Baumgartner HR: Platelet adhesion and thrombus formation on subendothelium in platelets deficient in glycoproteins IIb-IIIa, Ib, and storage granules. Blood 67:322, 1986

130. Wilcox M, Leptin M: Tissue-specific modulation of a set of related cell surface antigen in *Drosophila.* Nature 316:351, 1985

131. Woods VL Jr, Wolff LE, Keller DM: Resting platelets contain a substantial centrally located pool of glycoprotein IIb-IIIa complex which may be accessible to some but not other extracellular proteins. J Biol Chem 261:15242, 1986

132. Wright SD, Meyer BC: Fibronectin receptor of human macrophages recognizes the sequence Arg-Gly-Asp-Ser. J Exp Med 162:762, 1985

133. Wright SD, Reddy PA, Jong MTC, Erickson BW: C3bi receptor (complement receptor type 3) recognizes a region of complement protein C3 containing the sequence Arg-Gly-Asp. Proc Natl Acad Sci USA 84:1965, 1987

134. Wyler B, Bienz D, Clemetson KJ, Luscher EF: Glycoprotein Ib_{β} is the only phosphorylated major membrane glycoprotein in human platelets. Biochem J 234:373, 1986

135. Kunicki TJ, Nugent DJ, Staats SJ, Orchekowski RP, Wayner EA, Carter WG: The human fibroblast class II extracellular matrix receptor mediates platelet adhesion to collagen and is identical to the platelet glycoprotein Ia-IIa complex. J Biol Chem 263:4516, 1988

136. Hemler ME, Crouse C, Takada Y, Sonnenberg A: Multiple very late antigen (VLA) heterodimers on platelets: Evidence for distinct VLA-2, VLA-5 (fibronectin receptor) and VLA-6 structures. J Biol Chem 263:7660, 1988

137. Wayner EA, Carter WG, Piotrowicz RS, Kunicki TJ: The function of multiple extracellular matrix receptors in mediating cell adhesion to extracellular matrix: Preparation of monoclonal antibodies to the fibronectin receptor that specifically inhibit cell adhesion to fibronectin and react with platelet glycoproteins Ic-IIa. J Cell Biol 107:1881, 1988

EDITOR'S NOTE: Initial studies[101] led to the tentative identification of the platelet fibronectin receptor as VLA-3. However, more recent studies have determined that there are at least three VLA heterodimers that function as adhesion receptors on platelets. GPIa-IIa functions as a receptor for types I and III collagen[135] and is identical to VLA-2. Two forms of GPIc-IIa may exist on platelets, each having an apparently identical beta subunit (GPIIa) and one of two very similar but antigenically distinguishable alpha subunits (GPIc and a "GPIc-like" glycoprotein)[136]. One of these GPIc-IIa complexes functions as an activation-independent receptor for fibronectin and is identical to VLA-5[137]; the other is antigenically related to VLA-6[136]. In light of this new data, the activation-independent fibronectin receptor discussed in this manuscript is referred to as VLA-5.

3

Platelet Glycolipids

PAUL K. SCHICK

Platelets, like most mammalian cells, contain small amounts of glycolipids. Glycolipids are a heterogenous group of molecules that differ from other lipids in that they contain carbohydrates. They may be neutral or negatively charged molecules and may contain sialic acid or sulfate groups. These lipids are membrane components that are usually oriented on the cell surface. Glycolipids have also been reported to be present within intracellular organelles and may, thus, be involved in cellular secretion.

Glycolipids are believed to be involved in receptor-mediated activities, such as cell adhesion, immune responses, and cellular maturation and differentiation. Many of these cellular activities are important for platelet function and, therefore platelet glycolipids would be expected to be vital for platelet physiologic activities.

Although glycolipids have been demonstrated in platelets, the physiologic role of the platelet glycolipids has not been extensively investigated. However, there is evidence that these lipids are involved in serotonin binding and the platelet response to thrombin. Sulfatides, sulfated glycolipids, have been recently detected in platelets. Available information on the composition, structure, and physiologic importance of glycolipids in platelets will be reviewed in this chapter. In addition, a perspective on glycolipid biochemistry, recent developments in methodology, and the role of glycolipids in cellular maturation will be considered.

GLYCOLIPID BIOCHEMISTRY

Most glycolipids are composed of three basic components: sphingosine, a fatty acid, and one or more monosaccharides. The basic structure of glycolipids is illustrated in Figure 3-1, which depicts a simple glycolipid, glycosyl ceramide or galactosyl cerebroside. The lipid is composed of galactose, sphingosine, and a fatty acid. The sphingosine base, an aminoalcohol, is acylated at its amine group. The sphingosine and fatty acid component of the molecule is known as a ceramide, which is an integral component of all glycolipids.[23,31,76] Free ceramides, however, have been detected in several mammalian cells.[6,34,49,59,66] One or more monosaccharides may be linked to the ceramide backbone to form a large variety of glycolipid species.

Sphingosines are long-chain hydroxylated secondary amines that are synthesized from serine and palmitate. There are several species of sphingosine, which differ in chain length, number of double bonds, or the branching of the alkyl chain. 4-Sphingenine (sphingosine), sphinganine (dihydrosphingosine), and 4-hydroxysphinganine (phytosphingosine) are the three 18-carbon chain sphingosines that are most commonly found in cells and tissues.

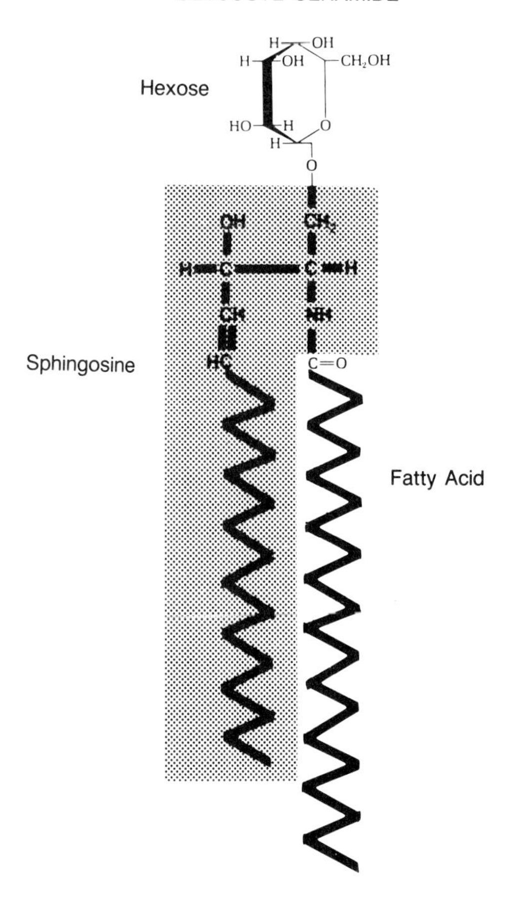

Figure 3-1. A simple glycolipid.

Sphingosine is the most abundant base in mammalian cells, whereas phytosphingosine is found primarily in plants. Free sphingosine is present in only trace amounts and is thought to be toxic to cells.[76]

Fatty acids in glycolipids usually have long carbon chains and are likely to be C_{16}, C_{18}, C_{22}, or C_{24} fatty acids. Fatty acids in glycolipids are usually either saturated or monounsaturated, but they are unlikely to be polyunsaturated fatty acids. α-Hydroxyfatty acids also have been detected in ceramides and glycolipids in several tissues and are considerably more polar than nonhydroxy-fatty acids, which are more commonly found in glycolipids.[76]

There are a limited number of monosaccharide species that may be present in glycolipids. The most commonly found monosaccharides in glycolipids are galactose, glucose, *N*-acetyl-D-galactosamine, *N*-acetyl-D-glucosamine, fucose, and *N*-acetylneuraminic or *N*-glycolylneuraminic acid.[76]

Glycolipids can be classified into neutral and acidic lipids by virtue of their monosaccharide composition. There are over 120 known glycolipids, which vary in the number, type, and sequence of monosaccharides. Most glycolipids can be subclassified as neutral glycolipids. Representative neutral glycolipids are depicted in Figure 3-2. A neutral glycolipid, which contains nine monosaccharides and thus is more complex than galactosyl ceramide shown in Figure 3-1, is illustrated. This glycolipid is A_1 blood group alloantigen and resembles other ABO, Lewis, and H alloantigen, which also contain multiple and branched monosaccharide moieties.[23] Evidence that these glycolipid blood group alloantigens are present in platelets is reviewed in Chapter 6.

There are two types of acidic glycolipids: gangliosides and sulfatides. They are considered acidic because the former contains one or

A Neutral Glycolipid (A1 Blood Group Alloantigen)

```
NAcGal—Gal—NAcGal—Gal—NAcGlu—Gal—Glu—Ceramide
        |          |
      Fucose     Fucose
```

Gangliosides

```
     NANA—Gal—Glu—Ceramide              GM3 (Hematoside)

NANA—NANA—Gal—Glu—Ceramide              GD3

Gal—NAcGal—Gal—Glu—Cermaide             GM1
            |
           NANA
```

Bovine Brain Sulfatide

Sulfate-Gal-Ceramide

NAcGal: N-Acetylgalactosamine
NAcGlu: N-Acetylglucosamine
NANA: Sialic Acid
Gal: Galactose
Glu: Glucose

Figure 3-2. Examples of neutral glycolipids and gangliosides and bovine sulfatide. Blood group A_1 alloantigen is illustrated and is an example of a neutral glycolipid with multiple and branched monosaccharides. Acidic glycolipids, gangliosides, are distinguished from neutral glycolipids by the presence of sialic acid. Three gangliosides are depicted: two are monosialo-gangliosides and one a disialoganglioside. Sulfatides are also acidic glycolipids because the sulfation of monosaccharides results in a negatively charged lipid. Bovine sulfatide is illustrated.

more sialic acid moieties and the latter are sulfated. Gangliosides and sulfatides are considered to be critical for cellular physiology and maturation. Examples of gangliosides are illustrated in Figure 3-2. Monosialic acid gangliosides, such as hematoside G_{M3}, are distinguished from other gangliosides that contain several sialic acid residues. Hematoside G_{M3} is the major ganglioside present in platelets and can bind serotonin.[42] A disialoganglioside, G_{D3}, is reported to also bind serotonin.[63] G_{M1}, which contains an internally located sialic acid, can bind cholera toxin and is considered to be important for cellular maturation. However, G_{D3} and G_{M1} have not been detected in platelets. Bovine brain sulfatide is also depicted in Figure 3-2. Preliminary evidence suggests that sulfatides are present in human platelets and differ from bovine brain sulfatide.[55]

Glycolipid molecules contain both hydrophobic and hydrophilic regions and thus are amphipathic. The fatty acid and sphingosine moieties shown in Figure 3-1 are hydrophobic and thus are implanted in the lipid core of cellular membranes, whereas the carbohydrate portion are hydrophilic and exposed on the membrane surface. There is considerable variability in the species of sphingosine, fatty acid, and carbohydrate species in glycolipids, and this variability would be expected to markedly influence the orientation of glycolipids within cellular membranes and, thereby, to regulate cellular activities.

METHODOLOGY

There have been several important technological advances that have facilitated the isolation and identification of glycolipids, despite that these lipids are relatively minor components of cells and tissues. Myelin contains more glycolipid than other mammalian tissue but, even here, glycolipids represent only about 20% of the total myelin lipid. On the other hand, glycolipids represent less than 5% of the lipid content of platelets and of most other mammalian cells.[23,42,66,71,77]

The introduction of methods for the isolation and analyses of small quantities of glycolipids has provided an opportunity to investigate the structure and function of these important membrane lipid components.

Glycolipids can be extracted by either the Folch or Fligh-Dyer methods. In these procedures, lipids are extracted from tissues with chloroform and methanol, and after aqueous partitioning, most lipids are present in the organic phase.[54,56,71] However, glycolipids with multiple monosaccharides and certain gangliosides will partition in the aqueous phase because these glycolipids are more amphipathic than other lipids. For example, certain granulocyte glycolipids[19] and about 40% of hematoside,[71] the major ganglioside found in platelets, are known to partition in the aqueous phase of the Bligh-Dyer extraction. However, the major platelet neutral glycolipids are present in the lower organic phase. Therefore, both the upper and lower phases of a Folch or Bligh-Dyer extract should be analyzed to assess the total glycolipid content of tissues and cells.[19,71] Alternately, lipids may be extracted by procedures that avoid partitioning.[35]

It is important to separate glyclolipids from phospholipids and neutral lipids by methods such as silicic acid chromatography.[56,71] Ceramides, neutral glycolipids, and acidic glycolipids are effectively purified by this procedure. Gangliosides and sulfatides can be separated from neutral glycolipids by DEAE silica gel chromatography.[35]

Glycolipids can be quantitatively analyzed by high-performance thin-layer chromatography (HPTLC).[36] The separation of platelet glycolipids by HPTLC is depicted in Figure 3-3. High-performance liquid chromatography (HPLC) of derivitized glycolipids can be used to analyze glycolipids in small samples of tissues, and methods for the analyses of benzoylated glycolipids have been reported.[30,68] The fatty acid and carbohydrate composition of glycolipids is best analyzed by gas-liquid chromatography.[37] The structure of glycolipids can be evaluated by selective enzymatic hydrolysis, chemical and immunological assays, as well as by mass-spectrometry.[2,10,19,20,25,50,74]

PLATELET CERAMIDES AND GLYCOLIPIDS

Several studies have defined the neutral glycolipid, ganglioside, and ceramide composition of human platelets and have shown that glycolipids represent about 3.2% of total platelet lipids.[42,66,71] The amount of free ceramides in platelets is greater than in most other mammalian cells.[6,34,49,59,66] Radiolabeled acetate and palmitate are readily incorporated into platelet

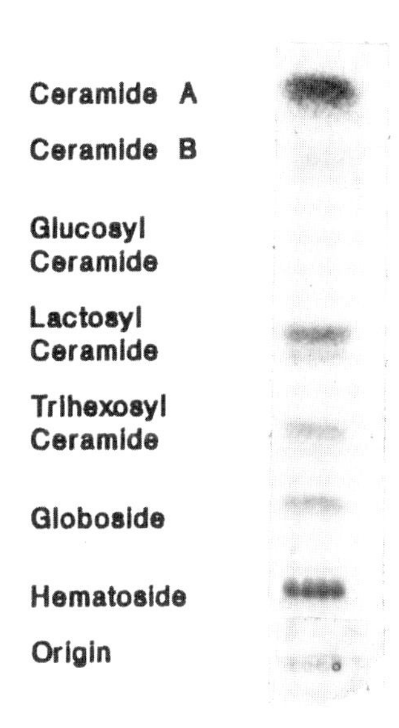

Figure 3-3. Human platelet glycolipids. Glycolipids were isolated from human platelets. Lipids were extracted by the Folch method and glycolipids were purified by a silicic acid column and alkaline methanolysis. Glycolipids were separated by TLC and visualized by charring.

ceramides.[14] Human ceramides have been well characterized, and the predominant fatty acid is generally lignoceric acid (24:0), whereas the most common base is sphingosine.[24,52] α-Hydroxy fatty acids were not detected in these studies. Three ceramides have been detected in porcine platelets, and each was found to have a specific fatty acid and sphingosine composition.[27] Two ceramides have been identified in human platelets, and they differ in their content of sphingosine species.[71]

Four major neutral glycolipids are present in human platelets.[61,66,71] The structure of platelet glycolipids is illustrated in Figure 3-4. Lactosylceramide represents about 64% of the total neutral glycolipids. Trihexosylceramide, globoside, and glucosylceramide account for the balance of neutral glycolipids in human platelets. The principal fatty acids in human platelet glycolipids are arachiditic acid (20:0), behenic acid (22:0), and lignoceric acid (24:0).

Gangliosides account for about 0.5% of total platelet lipids but contain 6% of total platelet sialic acid. Three gangliosides, acidic glycolipids, and traces of two additional gangliosides have been identified in human platelets.[42] Ganglioside I has been identified as hematoside (G_{M3}) and represents 92% of total platelet gangliosides. Hematoside is a simple ganglioside, composed of glucose, galactose, and sialic acid, as depicted in Figure 3-2. Ganglioside II represents about 5% of platelet gangliosides and appears to be a lacto-*N*-neotetraose, composed of glucose, galactose, sialic acid, and hexosamines in a molor ratio of 1:2:1:1.

The ceramide and glycolipid composition of platelets differs from that in other blood cells and plasma. The most abundant neutral glycolipid in plasma is glycosylceramide,[13,52] whereas globoside is the primary glycolipid in erythrocytes and leukocytes.[13,44] As mentioned earlier, the predominant glycolipid in human platelets is lactosylceramide. The content of gangliosides in human platelets is greater than in other blood cells.[13,41,66,71] The specific content of glycolipids in platelets and other blood cells most likely reflects the specialized functions of these cells.

Figure 3-4. Major glycolipids and gangliosides present in human platelets. The structure and amount of the major glycolipids present in human platelets are depicted. Ceramide, which consists of sphingosine and a fatty acid, is an integral component to all glycolipids.

Species	Structure	nmol/10^9 Platelets
Ceramides	Cer	3.48
Glucosylceramide	Cer—Glu	0.02
Lactosylceramide	Cer—Glu—Gal	1.39
Trihexosylceramide	Cer—Glu—Gal—Gal	0.56
Globoside	Cer—Glu—Gal—Gal—NAcGal	0.42
Hematoside (GM3)	Cer—Glu—Gal—NANA	0.63

Glu: Glucose
Gal: Galactose
NANA: Sialic acid
NAcGal: N-Acetyl-galactosamine

GLYCOLIPID SYNTHESIS AND CATABOLISM IN HUMAN PLATELETS

Sphingosine is synthesized in the endoplasmic reticulum and then acylated to form ceramides. Glycosylation of ceramides and glycolipids is mediated by specific enzymes termed glycosyltransferases, and ceramides as well as neutral glycolipids. Gangliosides can be degraded by several enzymes such as ceramidase, galactosidases, β-*N*-acetylhexosamidinidases, and neuraminidase.[39]

Human platelets can synthesize ceramides as assessed by the incorporation of radiolabeled acetate and palmitate.[14] In experiments in which platelets were incubated with radiolabeled glucose in vitro, it was demonstrated that platelets can glycosylate ceramides for the production of glycosylceramide.[28]

Several hydrolytic enzymes have been detected in platelets, including *N*-acetylhexosaminidase A and B, and α- and β-galactosidase.[3,61] Platelet hexosaminidase has been shown to be decreased in platelets from patients with Sandoff's disease and platelet α-galactosidase is decreased in Fabry's disease.[61] Patients with Sandoff's disease are likely to have dementia, seizures, and ocular changes. Fabry's disease is characterized by skin rashes, renal deficiency, and hypertension. The estimation of platelet enzyme levels in the homozygote may serve as a means for the early diagnosis of these disorders.[61] The effects of these enzyme deficiencies on platelet function have not been studied.

Sphingosine can inhibit protein kinase C in platelets and may be involved in platelet biologic activities.[26] Sphingosine may be generated either by synthesis or by catabolism of glycolipids and, thus, glycolipid metabolism may represent a mechanism for the regulation of cellular activities.

LOCALIZATION OF GLYCOLIPIDS IN PLATELET: RECEPTOR-MEDIATED ACTIVITIES

Formerly, it was thought that glycolipids were present primarily in membranes on the surface of mammalian cells. There is evidence, however, that these lipids may also be present in membranes of intracellular structures. In general, the hydrophilic carbohydrate components of glycolipids are probably exposed on the external surface of plasma membranes or the cytoplasmic surface of intracellular membranes. Thus, glycolipids would be available for receptor-mediated and immunologic activities.

The exposure of glycolipids on the platelet surface has been investigated with an external-labeling technique, the oxidation of externally exposed glycolipid carbohydrates by galactose oxidase, followed by reduction and labeling with tritiated sodium borohydride.[71] This study suggested that hematoside, globoside, and trihexosylceramide are available on the platelet surface, whereas lactosylceramide is not exposed. These data are shown in Figure 3-5.

The stimulation of human platelets with thrombin causes marked changes in the exposure of platelet glycolipids on the platelet surface, as assessed by the external-labeling technique described earlier.[71] There is a reduction in the exposure of trihexosylceramide and globoside but more than a 100% increase in the availability of hematoside on the platelet surface after thrombin treatment as shown in Figure 3-5. These observations indicate that thrombin causes an unmasking of gangliosides and a masking of selected neutral glycolipids or, possibly, extensive reorganization of the platelet plasma membrane. It is also possible that hematoside located in intracellular structures may emerge on the platelet surface in activated platelets. Platelet hematoside is a negatively charged molecule owing to its content of sialic acid, and its exposure on the surface of thrombin-activated platelets most likely is important for platelet activation. There is evidence that there is an increase in the absolute amount of hematoside and a decrease in lactosylceramide in thrombin-treated platelets.[9,66] Our study confirmed that there is an increase in hematoside, but we could not demonstrate a significant reduction in lactosylceramide in thrombin-treated platelets.[71] In view of the potential involvement of gangliosides in the binding of agonists and macromolecules, the exposure of hematoside (G_{M3}) on the surface of activated platelets probably facilitates the modulation and regulation of platelet responses.[71]

The effects of thrombin on the availability of glycolipids on the platelet surface are considerably greater than they are on aminophospholipids. Thrombin induced only a 12% increase in exposure of phosphatidylethanolamine on the platelet surface.[54] We have not studied the effects of thrombin–collagen combination on

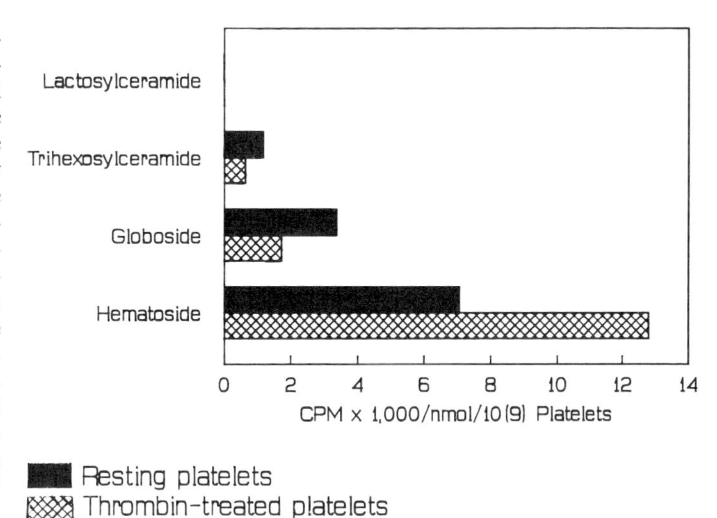

Figure 3-5. The exposure of gangliosides and neutral glycolipids on the surface of resting and thrombin-activated human platelets. Glycolipids on the surface of resting platelets and of those treated with thrombin were assessed by an external-labeling method, galactose oxidase followed by reduction and labeling with tritiated borohydride. Platelets were incubated with 1.25 U thrombin per milliliter of incubation medium at 37°C for 30 mins. Platelet lipids were extracted, and the glycolipids were isolated and separated by thin-layer chromatography. Bands were scraped and labeling measured by scintillation spectrometry. The results are expressed as specific activity (CPM $\times 10^{-3}$ nmol/10^9 platelets).

the exposure of glycolipids, but both agents together increase the availability of phosphatidylserine, also a negatively charged lipid.[4] One can speculate about whether or not hematoside, which similarly to phosphatidylserine is an acidic lipid, is important for platelet coagulant activities.

Several studies have indicated that gangliosides can bind serotonin.[42,63] It has been shown that serotonin can bind to human platelet gangliosides, and this binding was irreversible and specific because serotonin bound to hematoside (G_{M3}) and to a minor platelet ganglioside but not to other glycolipids and phospholipids.[42] Recent studies have confirmed that specific gangliosides, e.g., G_{M3} and G_{D3}, can bind serotonin.[63] There has been concern about the significance of these observations because only small amounts of serotonin bound to gangliosides in these experiments, and low-affinity binding was demonstrated. However, serotonin-binding proteins have been isolated from several tissues and, when both the serotonin-binding protein and gangliosides were present in binding studies, there was a fivefold increase in the binding of serotonin to this protein.[64] A serotonin-binding protein has recently been isolated from platelets,[46,64] but gangliosides did not increase the binding of serotonin to the serotonin-binding protein.[64] The extent and relevance of the binding of serotonin to platelet gangliosides are not yet defined.

The G_{M1} ganglioside is thought to mediate cholera toxin binding to G_{M1} and result in the stimulation of adenylate cyclase.[18] Cholera toxin has been shown to bind to platelets, but it did not have any effect on platelet cyclic nucleotides.[30]

The concept that gangliosides serve as receptors has been questioned because the binding of various bioactive substances to gangliosides has been of low affinity and specificity in most cells and tissues. However, there is increasing evidence that gangliosides serve as cofactors, modulators, or auxilliary receptors for stimulus–response coupling.[7,12] For example, gangliosides are thought to act as modulators or auxilliary receptors for thyrotropin, interferon, and chorionic gonadotropin.[21,38,70]

Gangliosides may affect membrane receptors or cell–cell interactions by regulating tyrosine kinase activity.[8] Exogenous gangliosides can inhibit protein kinase C phosphoration of rat myelin basic protein. The effect is specific to certain intact gangliosides because asialogangliosides and sialic acid did not affect the phosphorylation of myelin basic protein.[32] In other tissues, gangliosides can stimulate phosphorylation of proteins, as noted in certain rat brain membranes.[21] It is interesting that both gangliosides[8,21,32] and sphingosine,[26] as previously described in this paper, can modify protein kinase C activity.

One can speculate about the mechanisms involved in the ability of glycolipids to modulate phosphorylation of proteins and receptor-mediated activities. Glycolipids, particularly gangliosides and sulfatides, because of their negative charge, would be expected to exert a marked influence on membrane conformation and the membrane environment of receptors and enzymes, and, thereby, regulate membrane activities.

IMMUNOLOGY

Glycolipids, particularly gangliosides, are immunogenic,[2,10,24,43,69] and antiplatelet glycolipid antibodies undoubtedly would modify platelet function. Antiglycolipid antibodies have been shown to cause neurologic impairment.[2,10] A recent study suggested that antiglycolipid and antisulfatide antibodies are present in the plasma of some patients with chronic idiopathic thrombocytopenic purpura and, possibly, are instrumental in the genesis of thrombocytopenia and platelet dysfunction.[69]

COMPONENTS OF PLATELET CYTOSKELETONS

It has been shown that glycolipids and phospholipids are associated with isolated human platelet cytoskeletons.[56] Only two of the major platelet glycolipids are present in cytoskeletons prepared by Triton X-100 precipitation, representing about 7% of total platelet trihexosylceramide and 2% of total hematoside. The amounts of glycolipids in platelet cytoskeletons are significant, considering that 5% of total platelet protein is present in these structures. Thus, there is a specific composition of glycolipids in cytoskeletons. This selective inclusion of lipid species in cytoskeletons is not limited to glycolipids because two of the five major phospholipids, phosphatidylcholine and sphingomyelin, as well as cholesterol also were detected in platelet cytoskeletons.[56] The presence of lipids in cytoskeletons did not represent lipids trapped in the course of the preparation of these structures because radiolabeled cholesterol added just before the addition of the detergent was not incorporated into the cytoskeletal preparations.[56]

Phospholipids have been detected in platelet cytoskeletons in two other studies.[67,77] In one study, about 12% of total platelet protein and 2% of total lipid phosphorus were detected in cytoskeletons prepared from unclumped platelets, whereas 16% of total protein and 20% of total platelet lipid phosphorus were present in cytoskeletons prepared from aggregated and clumped platelets. The increase of both proteins and lipids in cytoskeletons from clumped platelets was most likely due to the inaccessibility of membrane to Triton extraction in clumped platelets.[76] This artifact was avoided in our study of the lipid species in cytoskeletons because cytoskeletons were prepared from unclumped platelets and only 5% of total platelet protein was present in the cytoskeletal preparations.[56]

Glycolipids have been shown to be associated with cytoskeletons and microtubules in other cells. With the use of immunohistologic techniques, cholera toxin was shown to bind to BALB/c-3T3 cells.[62] This study also demonstrated significant binding of cholera toxin to isolated 3T3 cytoskeletons. These experiments suggest that ganglioside G_{M1} is present in 3T3 cytoskeletons because cholera toxin is thought to recognize G_{M1}. In another study, antiactinin affinity-purified antibody and cholera toxin were used to show that capping of G_{M1} in mouse lymphocytes was associated with the reorganization of lymphocyte cytoskeletal structures.[32] Glycolipids have also been shown to be integral components of cholchicine-sensitive microtubules in a number of cells and tissues in two other studies.[45,61]

There are several implications of the presence of glycolipids in cytoskeletons in platelets and in other cells. The plasma membrane is a likely source of lipids that become associated with the cytoskeleton. Because the plasma membrane serves as an anchor for cytoskeletal elements, a portion of the plasma membrane with its specific content of lipids may be intimately associated with the cytoskeleton. Ankyrin, a protein of the erythrocyte plasma membrane, is known to serve as an anchor for erythrocyte cytoskeletons.[40] An alternate possibility is that lipids are integral components of cytoskeletons and provide structural support to cytoskeletons or mediate physiologic activities.[45,67]

SULFATIDES

Sulfatides are negatively charged molecules as they contain a sulfate group. Small amounts of these acid glycolipids have been detected in several tissues. These lipids have been implicated in several physiologic activities such as cellular maturation[60] and ATPase activity.[75] There is recent evidence that sulfatides are important for the initiation of coagulation. Sulfatides also bind to adhesive proteins such as thrombospondin and von Willebrand factor (VWF).[47,48]

Sulfatides have been shown to provide a negatively charged surface for the autoactivation and cleavage of factor XII[16,65] and for the activation of prekallikrein.[58] These acidic lipids are a diverse group of sulfated glycolipids that vary in their ability to activate prekallikrein or factor XII.[58] As opposed to kaolin, celite, and glass, sulfatides are the only potential biologic surface yet identified that would be available for the initiation of contact and intrinsic blood coagulation systems.

Platelets are a potential source of sulfatides. However, early studies did not detect sulfatides in human platelets.[42,66] On the other hand, several sulfatides had been detected in porcine platelets.[27] Because most cells contain only trace amounts of sulfatides, one would expect that it would be extremely difficult to demonstrate these compounds in platelets unless large numbers of platelets were analyzed and the sulfatides were separated from other acidic glycolipids.

Methods, such as the binding of adhesive proteins to sulfatides, can be used to provide indirect evidence for the presence of these molecules in cells. Along these lines, recent studies have used the binding of radioiodinated VWF and thrombospondin to demonstrate that sulfatides are present in platelets.[47,48] These studies showed that the binding of these adhesive proteins to sulfatides was specific because the proteins did not bind to neutral glycolipids, gangliosides, or to phospholipids, and the binding of thrombospondin or VWF could be inhibited by the respective unlabeled adhesive protein. These studies are the first to demonstrate that platelets contain sulfatides and that sulfatides may be components of the platelet surface receptor for thrombospondin and VWF.

We have used the same experimental approach to demonstrate that sulfatides are also present in endothelial cells.[55] Acidic glycolipids purified from human umbilical vein endothelial cells were separated by thin-layer chromatography and overlayed with ^{125}I-labeled thrombospondin, and the binding was then detected by autoradiography. The preliminary studies suggest that thrombospondin binds to one lipid band, which presumably is endothelial sulfatide.

Currently, it is thought that glycoprotein IIb–IIIa complexes are the receptor for thrombospondin, and glycoprotein Ib can function as a receptor for VWF. The binding of adhesive proteins to sulfatides has been detected only in the aforementioned experimental systems, and it would be premature to suggest that this binding occurs in vivo. Nevertheless, it is possible that sulfatides are intimately associated with glycoproteins within platelet membranes and serve as modulators of the binding of adhesive proteins to platelet glycoprotein complexes.

The demonstration that platelets and endothelial cells contain sulfatides is important because these cells are involved in hemostasis and, when activated, may provide sulfatides for the initiation of coagulation or for the binding of adhesive proteins.

ROLE OF CERAMIDES AND GLYCOLIPIDS IN CELLULAR MATURATION

Several observations indicate that glycolipids are involved in cellular maturation and differentiation. There is a distinct difference in the composition of neutral glycolipids and gangliosides that are present in immature versus mature tissues and cells.[5,20,41] The composition of glycolipids, i.e., fatty acids, carbohydrate, and sphingosine species, can vary according to cellular maturity. For example, small amounts of α-hydroxy fatty acids and sialic acid differ during the course of intestinal cellular maturation.[5] The species of fatty acids, carbohydrates, and sphingosine bases most likely are critical for maturation. Additional evidence for a role of glycolipids in maturation is that there are significant changes in the glycolipid composition of transformed and malignant cells.[22,24,33,72] Generally, it has been noted that simple glycolipids predominate in transformed or malignant cells. These changes have been attributed to the modification of glycosyltransferase activity that results in the decreased formation of complex glycolipids. It is interesting that the therapeutic administration of antiglycolipid antibodies has induced remissions of murine lymphoma and other experimental neoplasias.[73]

Glycolipids appear to influence the activity of growth factors. Several studies have indicated that the addition of exogenous gangliosides can stimulate the growth of neurites in vitro.[17,57] It has been reported that glycolipids are involved in the maturation of erythroblasts. This study showed that ceramides and glycolipids with lingnoceric acid (24:0) stimulated erythrocyte maturation, whereas those with benehic acid (22:0) were less effective.[11] A recent study indicates that G_{M1} and G_{M3} can inhibit cell proliferation by modulating platelet-derived growth factor receptor phosphorylation through effect upon tyrosine phosphorylation.[8] This inhibitory effect is specific to G_{M1} and G_{M3} because other gangliosides did not have the same action. In this study gangliosides inhibited receptor activity, possibly by a structural interaction with the receptor within the platelet membrane. There are other examples of the ability of gangliosides to enhance the activity of receptors.[23] Gangliosides are intimately associated with other membrane components and receptors, and this glycolipid environment most likely can modulate receptor sensitivity. It would appear that gangliosides limit excessive growth and differentiation under normal circumstances. There is a decrease in gangliosides in neoplastic cells and conceivably a loss of the control of cell growth that is modulated by these lipids.[8,23]

Several studies have indicated that glycolipids are important for hemopoiesis. It has been reported that radiolabeled glucosamine is incorporated into a glycolipid in bone marrow and that erythropoeitin stimulates glycolipid synthesis.[15] Glycolipids present in bone marrow cells in relation to maturity have been investigated with anticholera toxin IgG–F(ab')$_2$.[1] The study indicated that G_{M1}, detected by anticholera toxin, progressively increases with the maturity of granulocyte precursors and is present in the greatest amounts of G_{M1} that decrease during the maturation of erythrocytes.

There is little information about the role of glycolipids in megakaryocyte maturation and platelet synthesis. The observation that wheat germ agglutinin reacts with more mature megakaryocytes indicates that sialic acid becomes exposed on the surface of more mature megakaryocytes.[53] Because 6% of total platelet sialic acid is present in hematoside, hematoside as well as glycoproteins may become exposed on the surface of mature megakaryocytes.

CONCLUSION

Small amounts of glycolipids are present in human platelets. The major glycolipids in platelets have been characterized and found to be relatively simple molecules in that they do not contain a large number of branched oligosaccharides. Hematoside, which is present in platelets, is a monoganglioside, but the disialogangliosides have not been detected in platelets. Platelets have been found to contain more free ceramides than most other cells. There is little information about the physiologic roles of platelet glycolipids and ceramides. However, serotonin can preferentially bind to hematoside. Also, thrombin can induce an exposure of hematoside on the platelet surface that may be important for receptor-mediated activities or platelet activation. Specific glycolipids are present in platelet cytoskeletons, which may be important for the structure and function of these structures. Small amounts of sulfatides have recently been detected in human platelets, and these negatively charged molecules may be involved in the initiation of coagulation and the binding of thrombospondin and VWF. Glycolipids, particularly gangliosides, are immunogenic and it would be important to investigate the possibility that antiplatelet glycolipid antibodies are responsible for certain cases of immunogenic thrombocytopenia. Glycolipids have been shown to be critical for cellular maturation and differentiation. The role of glycolipids in megakaryocytes and platelet maturation and in platelet activation is a virtually unexplored area but a potentially vital aspect of platelet biology.

This work was supported by National Institutes of Health grant HL25455, BRSG support from Temple University, and from the American Health Association, Pennsylvania Affiliate.

REFERENCES

1. Ackerman GA, Wolken KW, Gelder FG: Differentiation expression of surface monosialoganglioside G_{M1} in various hemic cell lines of normal human bone marrow. J Histochem Cytochem 28:1334, 1980

2. Ariga T, Kohriyama T, Freddo L et al: Characterization of sulfated glucoronic acid containing glycolipids reacting with IgM M-proteins in patients with neuropathy. J Biol Chem 15:848, 1987

3. Beutler E, Kuhl W: The diagnosis of adult type Gaucher's disease and its carrier state by demonstration of deficiency of beta-glucosidase activity in pe-

ripheral blood leukocytes. J Lab Clin Med 76:747, 1970

4. Bevers EM, Comformius JP, van Rijn JL et al: Generation of prothrombin-converting activity and the exposure of phosphatidylserine on the outer surface of platelets. Eur J Biochem 122:429, 1982

5. Bouhours D, Bouhours J-F: Developmental changes of hematoside of rat small intestine: Postnatal hydroxylation of fatty acids and sialic acid. J Biol Chem 258:299, 1983

6. Bouhours J-F, Bouhours D: Identification of free ceramide in human erythrocyte membrane. J Lipid Res 25:613, 1984

7. Bremer EG, Hakomori S-I: Gangliosides are receptor modulators. Adv Exp Med Biol 174:381, 1984

8. Bremer EG, Hakomori S-I, Bowen-Pope DF et al: Ganglioside-mediated modulation of cell growth factor binding and receptor phosphorylation. J Biol Chem 259:6818, 1984

9. Chatterjee S, Sweeley CC: The effect of thrombin induced aggregation on human platelet sphingolipids. Biochem Biophys Res Commun 53:1310, 1973

10. Chow KH, Ilyas AA, Evans JE et al: Structure of a glycolipid reacting with monoclonal IgM in neuropathy and with HNK-1. Biochem Biophys Res Commun 128:383, 1985

11. Clayton RB, Cooper JM, Curstedt T et al: Stimulation of erythroblast maturation in vitro by sphingolipids. J Lipid Res 15:557, 1974

12. Dawson G, Berry-Kravis E: Gangliosides as modulators of the coupling of neurotransmitters to adenylate cyclase. Adv Exp Med Biol 174:341, 1984

13. Dawson G, Sweeley, CC: In vivo studies on glycosphingolipid metabolism in porcine blood. J Biol Chem 245:410, 1970

14. Deykin D, Desser RK: The incorporation of acetate and palmitate into lipids by human platelets. J Clin Invest 47:1590, 1968

15. Dukes PP: Erythropoietin-stimulated incorporation of 1-^{14}G-glucosamine into glycolipids in bone marrow cells in culture. Biochem Biophys Res Commun 31:345, 1968

16. Espana F, Ratnoff OD: Activation of Hagemen factor (factor XII) by sulfatides and other agents in the absence of plasma proteases. J Lab Clin Med 102:31, 1983

17. Ferrari G, Fabris M, Gorio A: Gangliosides enhance neurite outgrowth in PC12 cells. Brain Res 284:215, 1983

18. Fishman PH: Role of membrane gangliosides in the binding and action of bacterial toxins. J Membr Biol 69:85, 1982

19. Fukuda MN, Dell A, Oates JE et al: Structures of glycosphingolipids isolated from human granulocytes. J Biol Chem 260:1067, 1985

20. Fukuda MN, Levery SB: Glycolipids in fetal, newborn, and adult erythrocytes: Glycolipid pattern and structural study of H3-glycolipid from newborn erythrocytes. Biochemistry 22:5034, 1983

21. Gardas A, Aldler G, Lewartowska A et al: Influence of anti-ganglioside antibodies on thyrotropin binding and adenylate cyclase activity in thyroid plasma membranes. Acta Endocrinol 104:333, 1983

21b. Goldenring JR, Otis LC, Yu RK, DeLorenzo RJ: Calcium/ganglioside-dependent protein kinase activity in rat brain membrane. J Neurochem 44:1129, 1985

22. Hakomori S-I: Glycolipids in cellular interaction, differentiation and oncogenesis. Ann Rev Biochem 50:733, 1981

23. Hakomori S-I: Glycosphingolipids. Sci Am 254:44, 1986

24. Hakomori S-I, Young WW Jr, Patt LM et al: Cell biological and immunological significance of ganglioside changes associated with transformation. Adv Exp Med Biol 125:247, 1980

25. Handa S, Kushi Y: Application of field desorption and secondary ion mass spectrometry for glycolipid analysis. Adv Exp Med Biol 174:65, 1984

26. Hannum YA, Loomis CR, Merrill AH, Bell RM: Sphingosine inhibition of protein kinase C activity in vitro and in human platelets. J Biol Chem 261:12604, 1986

27. Heckers H, Stoffel W: Sphingolipids in blood platelets of the pig. Hoppe Seylers Z Physiol Chem 353:407, 1972

28. Hughes HN, Liberti JP: In vitro synthesis of glycosylceramide in rabbit platelets. Biochem Biophys Res Commun 63:555, 1975

29. Hughes RJ, Insel PA: Human platelets are defective in processing of cholera toxin. Biochem J 212:669, 1983

30. Jungalwala FB, Hayes L, McCluer RH: Determination of less than a nanomol of cerebrosides by high performance liquid chromatography with gradient elution analysis. J Lipid Res 18:285, 1977

31. Kanfer JN, Hakomori S (eds): Handbook of Lipid Research, Vol 3, Sphingolipid Biochemistry. New York, Plenum Press, 1983

32. Kellie S, Patel B, Pierce EJ, Critchley DR: Capping of cholera toxin ganglioside G_{M1} complexes on mouse lymphocytes is accompanied by co-capping of alpha-actinin. J Cell Biol 97:447, 1983

32b. Kim, JYH, Goldenring JR, DeLorenzo RJ, Yu RK: Gangliosides inhibit phospholipid-sensitive Ca^{2+} dependent kinase phosphorylation of rat myelin basic proteins. J Neurosci Res 15:159, 1986

33. Klock JC: Chemical characterization of neutral glycosphingolipids in human myeloid leukemia. J Lipid Res 22:1079, 1981

34. Krivit W, Hammarstrom S: Indentification

of free ceramide in human erythrocyte membrane. J Lipid Res 13:525, 1972

35. Kundu SK: DEAE-silica gel and DEAE-controlled porous glass as ion exchangers for the isolation of glycolipids. Methods Enzymol 72:74, 1981

36. Kundu SK: Thin-layer chromatography of neutral glycosphingolipids and gangliosides. Methods Enzymol 72:185, 1981

37. Laine RA, Esselman WJ, Sweeley CC: Gas-liquid chromatography of carbohydrates. Methods Enzymol 28:159, 1972

38. Lee G, Aloj SM, Brady RO, Kohn LD: The structure and function of glycoprotein hormone receptors: Ganglioside interactions with human chorionic gonadotropin. Biochem Biophys Res Commun 73:370, 1976

39. Li Y-T, Li S-C: Biosynthesis and catabolism of glycosphingolipids. Adv Carbohydr Chem Biochem 40:235, 1982

40. Lux SE: Spectrin–actin membrane skeleton of normal and abnormal red blood cells. Semin Hematol 16:21, 1979

41. Mannson JE, Vanier MT, Svennerholm L: Changes in the fatty acid and sphingosine composition of the major gangliosides of human brain with age. J Neurochem 30:273, 1978

42. Marcus AJ, Ullman HL, Safier LB: Studies on human platelet gangliosides. J Clin Invest 51:2602, 1972

43. Marcus DM, Schwarting GA: Immunological properties of glycolipids and phospholipids. Adv Immunol 23:203, 1976

44. Miras CJ, Mantzos JD, Levis GM: The isolation and partial characterization of glycolipids of normal human leukocytes. Biochem J 98:782, 1966

45. Nagai Y, Sakakibara K: Cytoskeleton-associated glycolipid (CAG) and its cell biological implication. Adv Exp Med Biol 152:425, 1982

46. Pignatti PF, Cavalli-Sforza LL: Serotonin binding proteins from human blood platelets: An experimental model system for studies on properties of synaptic vesicles. Neurobiology 5:65, 1975

47. Roberts DD, Haverstick DM, Dixit VM: The platelet glycoprotein thrombospondin binds specifically to sulfated glycolipids. J Biol Chem 260:9405, 1985

48. Roberts DD, Williams SB, Gralnick HR, Ginsberg V: von Willebrand factor binds specifically to sulfated glycolipids. J Biol Chem 261:3306, 1986

49. Royer M, Foote JL: The identification or ceramides and glycerol esters in unsaponifiable lipid of human aorta. Chem Phys Lipids 7:266, 1971

50. Saito M, Kasai N, Yu RK: In situ immunological determination of basic carbohydrate structures of gangliosides on thin-layer platelets. Anal Biochem 148:54, 1985

51. Sakakibara K, Momoi T, Uchida T, Nagai Y: Evidence for association of glycosphingolipid with a colchicine-sensitive microtubule-like cytoskeleton structure of cultured cells. Nature 293:76, 1981

52. Samuelson K: Identification and quantitative determination of ceramides in human plasma. J Clin Lab Invest 27:371, 1971

53. Schick PK, Filmyer W: Sialic acid on the surface of mature megakaryocytes: Detected by wheat germ agglutinin. Blood 65:1120, 1985

54. Schick PK, Kurica KB, Chacko GK: Location of phosphatidylethanolamine and phosphatidylserine in the human platelet plasma membrane. J Clin Invest 57:1221, 1976

55. Schick PK, Shapiro S. Tuszynski G, Slawek J: Sulfatides and glycolipids in platelets and endothelial cells. Thromb Haemostasis 58:842a, 1987

56. Schick PK, Tuszynski GP, Vander Voort PW: Human platelet cytoskeletons: Specific content of glycolipids and phospholipids. Blood 61:163, 1983

57. Schwartz M, Spirman N: Sprouting from chicken embryo dorsal root ganglia induced by nerve growth factor is specifically inhibited by affinity purified antiganglioside antibodies. Proc Natl Acad Sci USA 70:6080, 1983

58. Shimada T, Sugo T, Kato H et al: Activation of factor XII and prekallikrein with polysaccharide sulfates and sulfatides: Comparison with kaolin-mediated activation. J Biochem (Tokyo) 97:429, 1985

59. Shimojo TA, Kataura A, Yamaguchi H, Ohno K: Studies on pig erythrocyte lipids. Fractionation of erythrocyte lipid by the simple combination of silicic acid and cellulose column chromatography. Sapporo Med J 28:85, 1965

60. Singh H, Pfeiffer SE: Myelin-associated galactolipids in primary cultures from dissociated fetal rat brain: Biosynthesis, accumulation, and cell surface expression. J Neurochem 45(5):1371, 1985

61. Snyder PD Jr, Desnick RJ, Krivit W: Glycosphingolipids and gycosyl hydrolases of human blood platelets. Biochem Biophys Res Commun 46:1857, 1972

62. Streuli CH, Patel B, Critchely DR: The cholera toxin receptor ganglioside G_{M1} remains associated with Triton-X-100 cytoskeletons of BALB/c-3T3 cells. Exp Cell Res 136:247, 1981

63. Tamir H, Brunner W et al: Enhancement of gangliosides of the binding of serotonin to serotonin binding protein. J Neurochem 34:1719, 1980

64. Tamir H, Gershon MK. Storage of serotonin and serotonin binding protein in synaptic vesicles. J Neurochem 33:35, 1979

65. Tans G, Rosing J, Griffen JH: Sulfatide-dependent autoactivation of human blood coagulation factor XII (Hagemen factor). J Biol Chem 258:8215, 1983

66. Tao RV, Sweeley CC, Jamieson GA: Sphingolipid composition of human platelets. J Lipid Res 14:16, 1973

67. Tuszynski GP, Mauco GP, Koshy A et al: The platelet cytoskeleton contains elements of prothrombinase complex. J Biol Chem 259:6947, 1984

68. Ullman MD, McCluer RH: Quantitative analysis of brain gangliosides by high performance liquid chromatography of their perbenzoyl derivatives. J Lipid Res 26:501, 1985

69. van Vliet HHDM, Kappers-Klunne MC, van der Hel JWB, Abels J: Antibodies against glycosphingolipids in sera of patients with idiopathic thrombocytopenic purpura. Br J Haematol 67:103, 1987

70. Vengris VE, Fernie BF, Pitha PM: The interaction between gangliosides and interferon. Adv Exp Med Biol 125:479, 1980

71. Wang CT, Schick PK: The effect of thrombin on the organization of human platelet glycosphingolipids: The sphingosine composition of platelet glycolipids and ceramides. J Biol chem 256:752:1981

72. Yogeeswaren G: Cell surface glycolipids and glycoproteins in malignant transformation. Adv Cancer Res 38:289, 1983

73. Young WW Jr, Hakomori, S-I: Therapy of mouse lymphoma with monoclonal antibodies to glycolipid: Selection of low antigenic variants in vivo. Science 211:487, 1981

74. Yu RK: Gangliosides: Structure and analysis. Adv Exp Med Biol 174:39, 1984

75. Zambrano F, Rojas M: Sulfatide content in a membrane fraction isolated from rabbit gastic mucosal: Its possible role in the enzyme involved in H^+ pumping. Arch Biochem Biophys 253:87, 1987

76. Zubay G: Biochemistry, 1st ed. p 527. Reading, Mass, Addison-Wesley, 1983

77. Zucker MB, Masiello NC: The Triton-X-100 residue ("cytoskeleton") of aggregated platelets contain increased lipid phosphorus as well as ^{125}I-labeled glycoproteins. Blood 61:676, 1983

4

Platelet Proteoglycans and Sulfated Proteins

BARBARA P. SCHICK

The sulfated macromolecules of platelets consist of the proteoglycans and the sulfated proteins. The existence of platelet proteoglycans, called mucopolysaccharides (MPS) in the early literature, has been known since the work of Odell and collaborators.[2,56–60] The platelet proteoglycans consist of chondroitin sulfate–containing molecules, as will be discussed in detail. Most of the proteoglycans appear to be localized in the α granules, and the functional importance of these molecules is suggested by their release when cells are stimulated with thrombin or ADP.[4,89] The platelet surface has been shown by electron microscopy to contain a dense glycocalix that is highly negatively charged, and although this is primarily due to the presence of sialic acid, surface proteoglycan probably is also involved.

Our recent studies, using in vivo labeling of the molecules of megakaryocytes and platelets by injecting guinea pigs with [^{35}S]sulfate, have demonstrated for the first time the existence of another class of sulfated macromolecules, the sulfated proteins, in platelets. We do not have any information about the subcellular localization of these molecules, but it is reasonable to suggest that they could comprise a substantial portion of the negative charge of the platelet surface in either resting or activated platelets. Their contribution to the antigenicity of the platelet surface is yet to be determined.

This chapter will focus on the characterization and metabolism of the sulfated proteoglycans and the sulfated proteins of platelets and megakaryocytes. Although there have not yet been any reports concerning the immunogenicity of these molecules in platelets, this chapter may provide a stimulus for future investigations on whether or not these molecules have a role in platelet-related immunologic disorders.

STRUCTURE AND FUNCTION OF PROTEOGLYCANS AND SULFATED PROTEINS

Proteoglycans

Structure

Proteoglycans, referred to in the early literature as mucopolysaccharides (MPS), are rather large protein- and carbohydrate-containing molecules whose structures differ considerably from glycoproteins. The general structure of a chondroitin sulfate proteoglycan is shown in Figure 4-1. The proteoglycans contain a core protein, which typically accounts for 10% to 20% of the weight of the molecule, to which varying numbers of glycosaminoglycan (GAG) chains are attached to serine residues via the trisaccharide linkage region Xyl-Gal-Gal. The glycosaminoglycan chains consist of numerous repeating disaccharide units, each containing a uronic acid and an *N*-acetylhexosamine. Each *N*-acetylhexosamine, and in some cases the

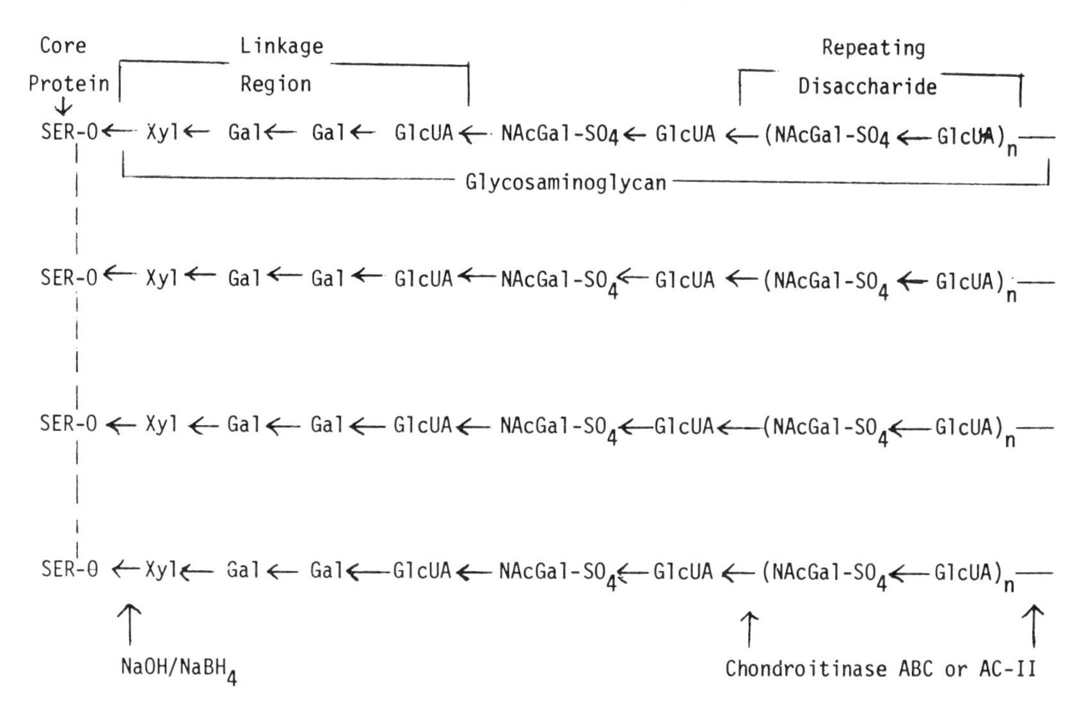

Figure 4-1. General structure of a chondroitin sulfate proteoglycan. The proteoglycan is made up of a core protein to which glycosaminoglycan chains are attached at serine residues. Chondroitin-4-sulfate and chondroitin-6-sulfate contain the sulfate residues at the C-4 and C-6 positions, respectively, of the *N*-acetylgalactosamine. The glycosaminoglycans can be released from the core protein by treatment with 0.05 N NaOH/1 M $NaBH_4$ or with 0.5 N NaOH. The chondroitinase enzymes cleave the glycosaminoglycan chains to the component disaccharides by an elimination reaction that results in formation of a 4,5-unsaturated bond in the glucuronic acid residue.

uronic acid moiety as well, contains a sulfate residue, and the uronic acid has a carboxyl group. There are typically in the range of 25 to 100 repeating disaccharide units on each chain, and the presence of a carboxyl group and at least one sulfate group on each disaccharide unit impart an extraordinarily high negative charge density to the molecule. The most common cellular proteoglycans are the chondroitin sulfates (dissaccharides of glucuronic or iduronic acid and 4- or 6-sulfated *N*-acetylgalactosamine) and heparan sulfates (sulfated glucuronic or iduronic acid and sulfated *N*-acetylglucosamine.)[93]

Figure 4-1 also indicates the positions at which the proteoglycan molecules can be cleaved into their constituent parts for characterization. The glycosaminoglycan chains can be cleaved from the core protein at the serine-xylose linkage point by treatment with 0.1 M NaOH or 0.05 M NaOH/1 M $NaBH_4$, and then can be characterized by gel filtration[91] or gel electrophoresis[55] for size, or by ion-exchange chromatography or cellulose acetate electrophoresis for charge density. In addition, the core protein can be cleaved by some proteases, producing fragments similar in size to those of the free GAG chains. The GAG chains can be broken down into their constituent disaccharides by the chondroitinase enzymes, and the position of the sulfate group can be identified by specific removal of the 4- or 6-sulfate by chondro-4- or chondro-6-sulfatase. The intact proteoglycan can also be digested with chondroitinase ABC or AC-II, but a hexasaccharide containing the tetrasaccharide Xyl-Gal-Gal-GlcUA and the terminal disaccharide with a 4,5-unsaturated bond on the uronic acid are left as stubs on the core protein. Chondroitinase digestion of the intact proteoglycan has proved to be the best way to obtain intact core protein for size estimation. For detailed discussion of proteoglycan analysis the reader is referred to the review of Hascall and Kimura.[26]

Chondroitin sulfate proteoglycans vary greatly in relative molecular mass (M_r) from about 70,000 to several million. It should be noted that the molecules that are associated with cell granules or membranes are usually on the order of perhaps a few hundred thousand daltons at most, and are considerably smaller than the proteoglycan monomers from cartilage or from extracellular matrix. These large proteoglycans form very large aggregates with the nonsulfated GAG hyaluronic acid. Their general structure has been well reviewed in a number of texts, including Alberts[1] and further discussion is beyond the scope of this chapter.

Subcellular Localization and Functions

Proteoglycans are found in granules of cells and in plasma membranes, and are also secreted by a number of cells to contribute to the formation of extracellular matrix or basement membranes. Proteoglycans are associated with catecholamines and ATP in the chromaffin granules of the adrenal medulla;[49] with acetylcholine and ATP in granules of the electric organ of marine rays;[12] in prolactin storage granules;[96] and with proteolytic enzymes in pancreatic zymogen granules[67] and lysosomes of the cells of the immune system.[82,85] In platelets proteoglycans are thought to reside in the α granules with the nonproteolytic secretory proteins.[4,5,48,50] Proteoglycans are released from secretory granules of all these cells in response to an appropriate stimulus. The function of the proteoglycans in secretory granules is thought to be to package the protein or amine constituents of the granules.[49] The role of the released proteoglycans in the target tissues or in tissues in which they are released is not known.

Cell surface proteoglycans are thought to be involved in such functions as permeability and cell–cell adhesion. Vascular wall proteoglycans are thought to be responsible for repulsion of platelets,[93] possibly owing to interactions with platelet surface proteolgycans. Behnke has shown recently that the attachment of platelets to collagen is mediated by initial attachment of the cells to proteoglycans present on the collagen fibrils and probably involves carbohydrate–carbohydrate recognition between the cells and the fibrils.[6] Cell surface proteoglycans may be important for regulating the adhesion to and movement of cells through a substratum, for example, in the bone marrow,[17] and may play a role in hematopoiesis.[19,94] Cell surface proteoglycan appears to interact with cellular cytoskeletons in at least two cell types.[11,65]

The amount and types of proteoglycans synthesized by cells at different stages of development can vary,[18,21,40,41] and these molccules can play a critical role in determining tissue structure.[9] An immune function for proteoglycan on the cell surface is suggested by the finding that a small proteoglycan is associated with the class II molecules of the HLA system in human lymphoblastoid B-cell lines, in human tonsil cells and normal peripheral mononuclear cells,[73] and in mouse spleen cells.[72] The core protein of this proteoglycan is the same as the invariant chain of the Ia antigen in mouse spleen cells.[72,73]

Sulfated Proteins

In the last few years, sulfated proteins have been identified in several cell types. The sulfation of the protein can occur either on a tyrosine residue[8,30,32–34,38,42,45,46,83] or on the terminal sugars of the carbohydrate side chains, most commonly *N*-acetylgalactosamine.[7,10,22,23,30,51] Thus far, the immunogenicity of sulfated proteins has only been explored in brain tissue, where it has been found that the HNK antibody that recognizes a uronic acid-containing glycolipid also recognizes a sulfated glycoprotein[78] and also a chondroitin sulfate proteoglycan.[50] Sulfation of tyrosine residues as well as sulfation of *N*-linked and *O*-linked oligosaccharides has been found on secretory proteins.[30,83] Tyrosine sulfation has been found on molecules relevant to coagulation and the complement system, including fibrinogen,[8] α-2-antiplasmin,[45] heparin cofactor II,[34] fibronectin,[46] the fourth component of complement,[33] and also on type III procollagen.[38] Tyrosine sulfation[42] and sulfation of carbohydrate[22] have both been accomplished in vitro.

IMMUNOCHEMISTRY OF PROTEOGLYCANS

Antibodies have been raised against several types of proteoglycans. The antigenicity of the molecule appears to reside in the core protein rather than in the glycosaminoglycan chain. There can be cross-reactivity between cell types; for example, an antibody against basement membrane heparan sulfate[27] was found to react with colon carcinoma heparan sulfate.[36] A novel approach to the generation of antiproteoglycan antibodies was to use chondroitinase-digested proteoglycan, which leaves the trisaccharide linkage region and a small portion of the chondroitin sulfate attached to the core protein as "stubs." The stubs appear to be a part of the antigen against which the antibody is directed. This antibody has been used to detect chondroitin-6-sulfate in several chondroitinase-digested tissues.[13] To our knowledge, there have been no reports in the literature of naturally occurring antiproteoglycan antibodies in humans, but anti-GAG antibodies were found in arthritic rabbits[63] and in other situations.[88] Interestingly, these antibodies in the arthritic rabbits appear to be directed against the unsaturated uronic acid residues of partially degraded hyaluronic acid and chondroitin sulfate, and to the latter, especially, when the carbohydrate chain was still attached to the core protein. It was suggested that this humoral immunity might develop after the GAGs are degraded by eliminases or hydrolases produced by bacteria or other cells. It is possible that bacterial infection might result in production of antigenic sites on proteoglycans; for instance, the bacteria present in periodontal pockets can produce a hyaluronidase that degrades both hyaluronic acid and chondroitin sulfate.[87] In addition, murine T-lymphocytes secrete a proteoglycan-degrading enzyme in vitro,[39] and it is conceivable that enzymes secreted in inflammatory states could produce proteoglycan degradation products that would be antigenic. Such an autoimmune response might affect platelets.

PLATELET PROTEOGLYCANS: REVIEW OF THE LITERATURE

Characterization

The earliest characterizations of platelet proteoglycans, or mucopolysaccharides (MPS), were reported by Odell and coworkers in the late 1950s.[2,57,60] Cytochemical evidence was obtained for the presence of MPS in platelets,[24] and the accumulation of [^{35}S]sulfate in megakaryocytes and isolated platelets was demonstrated by autoradiography.[60] The sulfated mucopolysaccharide was isolated by Odell and Anderson[2,57] from 0.5 N NaOH digests of platelets, which had been labeled in vivo by injection of rats with [^{35}S]sulfate, and was identified as chondroitin sulfate by paper electrophorcsis. Almost all of the ^{35}S-labeled material was solubilized by the NaOH treatment, but about half was lost during dialysis and was not identified. A nonsulfated mucopolysaccharide material was also seen on the electrophoretograms.[57] Riddell and Bier[68] found that a chondroitin sulfate mucopolysaccharide was released by thrombin from ^{35}S-labeled pig platelets, representing about half of the radioactivity that had been incorporated into the cells, and that some residual chondroitin sulfate remained with the platelets. Olsson and Gardell[62] isolated chondroitin-4-sulfate and small amounts of hyaluronic acid from human platelets that had been digested with papain. Chondroitin-4-sulfate had been identified in [^{35}S]sulfate-labeled rabbit platelets by Ward et al,[90] and chondroitin-6-sulfate has been found in guinea pig platelets in our laboratory.[75,76]

Odell and McDonald[59] found that the incorporation of radioactivity into protein-containing molecules of platelets increased gradually over a 24-hr period following injection of rats with [^{35}S]sulfate, and because the platelets themselves appeared to be unable to incorporate [^{35}S]sulfate into large molecules, it was inferred that the radiolabeled material was incorporated first into the megakaryocytes and later found in the circulating platelets. In rats,[25] rabbits,[64] and guinea pigs,[76] platelet labeling with [^{35}S]sulfate is maximal 3 days after injection of the radioisotope. The time course of incorporation of [^{35}S]sulfate into platelets in vivo has been taken as a measure of the rate of platelet production, and can be altered by inducing thrombocytopenia or thrombocytosis.[25,58]

The studies just described were performed using NaOH or papain digests of platelets and, thus, were able to characterize only the glycosaminoglycan portion of the proteoglycans, because the NaOH treatment cleaves the GAG chains from the core protein and the protease cleaves the core protein (*see* Fig. 4-1). The first study on intact platelet proteoglycan molecules was that of Barber et al.[4] The intact proteoglycan was isolated from the releasate of thrombin-treated platelets and characterized by sedimentation equilibrium as a molecule of M_r 56,000, with four chondroitin-4-sulfate chains of M_r 12,000. The core protein would thus represent about 14% of the weight of the molecule. The proteoglycan was thought to be the carrier for platelet factor 4, and to be released as a complex containing 8 mol of platelet factor 4 and 2 mol of proteoglycan. The distribution of chondroitin sulfate (determined as hexuronic acid) among subcellular fractions paralleled that of platelet factor 4, with about 55% in the granule-rich fractions, 43% in the soluble fraction, and only 2% in the membrane fraction. The latter finding is in agreement with a previous report of low recovery of chondroitin sulfate from platelet membranes.[2] In agreement with the aforementioned studies, small amounts of hyaluronic acid were also found in the human platelets by Barber et al.[4]

A second isolation and characterization of human platelet proteoglycans was reported by Huang et al.[35] A proteoglycan was isolated from the supernatant of frozen-thawed, outdated, human platelet-rich plasma using a polylysine-Sepharose CL-4B column followed by affinity chromatogaphy on a platelet factor 4-ω-aminobutyl agarose column. In close agreement with the findings of Barber et al.,[4] the proteoglycan was found to have a M_r of 53,000 as determined by sedimentation equilibrium. The sedimentation equilibrium profile showed a single symmetrical peak. The identity of the glycosaminoglycan moiety as chondroitin-4-sulfate was confirmed by chondro-4-sulfatase and chondro-6-sulfatase digestion. This study was also the first attempt to analyze the amino acid composition of the core protein. Five amino acids, aspartic acid, glutamic acid, leucine, glycine, and serine, accounted for 55% of the amino acids of the core protein.

A third study of human platelet proteoglycans by Okayama et al.[61] used a different isolation methodology and obtained results that were different from those obtained in the two studies just cited. The methods of Okayama et al. were based on those in general use in recent years for proteoglycan analysis.[26] Platelets were extracted with 4 M guanidine HCl in the presence of protease inhibitors, the extract was dialyzed against 7 M urea, and the proteoglycan was purified by DEAE-Sephacel ion-exchange chromatography, cesium chloride density gradient centrifugation, gel filtration, and rechromatography on DEAE-Sephacel. The relative proportions of uronic acid, hexosamine, sulfate, and protein were similar to those found by Barber et al.,[4] but the M_r was estimated by equilibrium sedimentation to be 136,000. The glycosaminoglycans were again found to be chondroitin-4-sulfate, but their chain length was estimated to be >22,000 by reference to heparin standards using Bio-Gel A-0.5-m column chromatography. The appearance of a single compact spot on cellulose acetate electrophoresis when the glycosaminoglycans from the major CsCl fraction were analyzed was interpreted to mean that the chondroitin sulfate chains were homogeneous in chain length and charge density. However, the glycosaminoglycans from the "retarded" portion of the peak from the gel filtration column migrated somewhat differently on cellulose acetate electrophoresis. The size of glycosaminoglycans of the platelet proteoglycan suggested to these authors that the platelet was the source of the C1q inhibitor proteoglycan described by Silvestri et al.[80] This interpretation is in contrast to the suggestion by Huang et al.[35] that the platelet proteoglycan was much smaller than the C1q inhibitor. The predominant five amino acids of the core protein were found to be the same as those determined by Huang et al.,[27] but with some differences in the proportions, and to comprise 64% of the total amino acids, with minor differences in the remaining amino acid composition found in the two studies. The reason for the differences between the study of Okayama et al. and the other two studies cited is not clear. Possibilities are the source of the material (extracted whole platelets versus releasates or lysates of outdated platelets), and the methods used to calibrate the M_r. Unfortunately, the diversity in proteoglycan structure in number, length, and spacing of GAG chains results in great variability in the size of the highly hydrated molecules and, thus, standardized calibration of proteoglycan M_r is difficult to achieve. The data from our laboratory are closest to the data of Okayama et al.[61]

Subcellular Localization of Proteoglycans in Platelets

The question of the subcellular localization of platelet proteoglycans has been addressed by morphologic studies. Three studies have compared platelets and megakaryocytes. Behnke compared the staining of the surface membranes of megakaryocytes and platelets using ruthenium red, which does not permeate intact plasma membranes, and found that the demarcation membrane system of the megakaryocyte and the platelet surface membranes were labeled.[5] Although ruthenium red staining is commonly considered to indicate the presence of proteoglycans, this dye can also label other anionic substances and, thus, cannot be considered a specific label for proteoglycans. Spicer and coworkers[81] examined human and rabbit platelets stained with dialyzed iron and antimonate. In the cells from both humans and rabbits, the dialyzed iron stained the "nucleoids" of the α granules of platelets and megakaryocytes, the outer surface of the plasma membranes of platelets and megakaryocytes, and the luminal surface of the platelet demarcation membrane system of the megakaryocytes. The dialyzed iron stain suggested the presence of MPS on the platelet plasma membrane and in the α granules. Antimonate, which reacts with cations, stained the dense bodies, presumably the site of amines and other cations. In another study, pyroantimonate stained the nucleoid of the α granule and was thought to have recognized a thrombin-sensitive pool of calcium associated with mucopolysaccharide.[74] MacPherson[48] determined the location of ^{35}S labeling in megakaryocytes and platelets by autoradiography. Rat marrow was labeled by in vitro incubation for 10 min, and radioactivity was found in the Golgi, where sulfation is presumed to take place, and to a lesser degree in granules and the demarcation membranes. When rats were injected with [^{35}S]sulfate, after 3 or 12 hr the sulfate was found to only a small extent in the Golgi and predominantly in granules and the demarcation membranes. When platelets were analyzed 3 days after sulfate injection, i.e., at the point of maximal labeling, grains were seen primarily over the granules but also to a significant degree above the plasma membrane. Thus, the morphologic studies would suggest that most of the platelet proteoglycans are located in the α granules, but some proteoglycan is present on the platelet surface membranes.

The only study, thus far, that has attempted to isolate subcellular fractions from platelets to determine the chondroitin sulfate distribution is that of Barber et al.,[4] and the finding of small amounts of proteoglycan in the plasma membrane (2% of total platelet glycosaminoglycan) appears to underestimate what might have been expected from the morphologic studies. The reason for this is not clear. It could be due to loss of loosely bound material from the platelet plasma membrane during the separation procedure, to a substantial labeling of nonproteoglycan anionic molecules by the staining reagents, or to labeling on nonproteoglycan sulfated molecules on the surface with [^{35}S]sulfate. There are no data available to ascertain whether or not any of these situations indeed exist.

Packham and coworkers have tried to distinguish between granule and surface membrane proteoglycans by studying proteoglycan release in response to ADP, which they have found to activate rabbit platelets without release of known α granule proteins, and in response to thrombin, which is known to release the α-granule constituents.[89,90] They found that platelets isolated from rabbits 3 days after injection of the animals with [^{35}S]sulfate released about 15% of the ^{35}S radioactivity in response to ADP, and suggested that this represented release of the membrane proteoglycans.[90] About 70% of the remainder was released by thrombin and was taken to represent α-granule release. Both the material released by ADP and the material released by thrombin eluted in the void volume of a Sephadex G-200 column, and both releasates were completely digested with chondroitinase to produce the disaccharide characteristic of chondroitin-4-sulfate. Because the proteoglycan molecules from both releasates eluted in the void volume of the Sephadex G-200 column, no information could be obtained concerning possible differences in molecular size between the putative membrane and granule proteoglycans or their glycosaminoglycans.[90] No conclusive evidence was presented in these studies that the proteoglycan released by ADP was, in fact, derived from the membrane.

In summary, platelets from all species thus far examined contain chondroitin sulfate proteoglycans, and the platelet proteoglycans are synthesized during megakaryocyte development in the bone marrow. The proteoglycans appear to be found primarily in the α granules but to a significant extent in the surface membranes, and proteoglycans are released from α granules and possibly from the plasma membrane by agents that induce platelet aggregation. Although three studies have each characterized what the authors considered to be relatively homogeneous proteoglycans, there is some disagreement on the molecular mass of the intact proteoglycan molecule and of the glycosaminoglycan chains.

GUINEA PIG PLATELET PROTEOGLYCAN AND SULFOPROTEIN METABOLISM

Two of the studies cited earlier[4,35] suggested that platelets contain a single homogeneous proteoglycan, whereas the third[61] presented data that suggested some diversity in platelet proteoglycans. In contrast, data from our laboratory[76] suggest that the proteoglycan content of platelets and megakaryocytes is much more diverse than has been suggested previously. Our decision to undertake studies of platelet proteoglycans was based on the observations that megakaryocytes of all stages of development appeared to contain and to synthesize proteoglycans,[48] that a number of cells exhibit changes in proteoglycan content and synthesis during maturation,[15,18,21,40,41] and that platelets appear to contain both granule and membrane proteoglycans, suggesting that at least two species might be present. It is important to note that the methodology used in the previous studies precluded characterization of all the proteoglycans in the platelets. For example, about 15% of the hexuronic acid-containing material in the study of Huang et al.[35] was lost on the initial ion-exchange column procedure and, therefore, the nature of that material is not known. More importantly, material left behind in the platelet membrane was also lost, so that a major portion, if not all, of the membrane-bound material was not characterized. It is probable that membrane-bound proteoglycans would be more likely to remain associated with the membrane under these conditions than under the conditions of cell lysis used by Barber et al.[4] The same is true of the studies of Ward et al.[89,90] which characterized only material that was released from the platelets. In addition, the complex isolation procedure used by Barber et al.[4] involved precipitation steps that could have resulted in the loss of some proteoglycan material. Also, in the study of Okayama et al.,[61] again 15% of the uronic acid of 4 M Gdn HCl-solubilized platelets was bound to the DEAE-Sephacel column and was eluted under hydrolytic conditions by treatment of the column with 0.5 N NaOH. Thus this material could be studied only as free GAG chains and not in the context of its intact proteoglycan. Our studies have characterized this proteoglycan fraction, and we have found it to be different in several ways from the major proteoglycan fraction. In addition, we have established that the major proteoglycan fraction contains considerable structural, as well as metabolic, diversity.

Our work has characterized platelet and megakaryocyte proteoglycan structure using proteoglycans radiolabeled in vivo by injection of guinea pigs with [^{35}S] sulfate. This approach has two advantages. First, it enables us to work with reasonably small numbers of animals compared with doing studies requiring large amounts of proteoglycan mass for characterization, and second, it has enabled us to monitor the time course of synthesis of the various portions of the proteoglycan population, as well as their behavior during platelet activation. We have established the validity of this approach by determining that the nonradioactive uronic acid-containing molecules from both guinea pig and human platelets coelute from Sepharose CL-6B columns and comigrate on sodium dodecyl sulfate-polyacrylamide gel electrophoesis (SDS-PAGE) with the radiolabeled material obtained from guinea pig platelets at the time of maximal labeling, i.e., 3 days after injection. In addition, the radiolabeling approach has led us to the discovery of substantial amounts of what appear to be sulfated proteins in guinea pig platelets and megakaryocytes.[75,76]

Changes in Proteoglycan Synthesis During Megakaryocyte Maturation

The rationale for our in vivo experiments[76] is shown in Figure 4-2. The assumptions were that the [^{35}S]sulfate injection would serve as a pulse label, because free [^{35}S]sulfate would be available at high specific activity in plasma for only a short time, and would be taken up by megakaryocytes at all stages of development. Then, if different molecules were synthesized by cells at different stages of maturation (i.e., molecules A-D in Fig. 4-2), we should be able to see their appearance sequentially with time in the platelets and their concurrent loss from the megakaryocytes. In addition, we would be able to see molecules synthesized by very young megakaryocytes (molecule D), which are not isolatable by the methods we use for megakaryocyte isolation,[43,56] as these cells become larger ("isolatable"), and eventually in the platelets as these megakaryocytes yielded their platelets to the circulation.

The [^{35}S]sulfate whole-cell labeling of megakaryocytes and platelets was determined over a

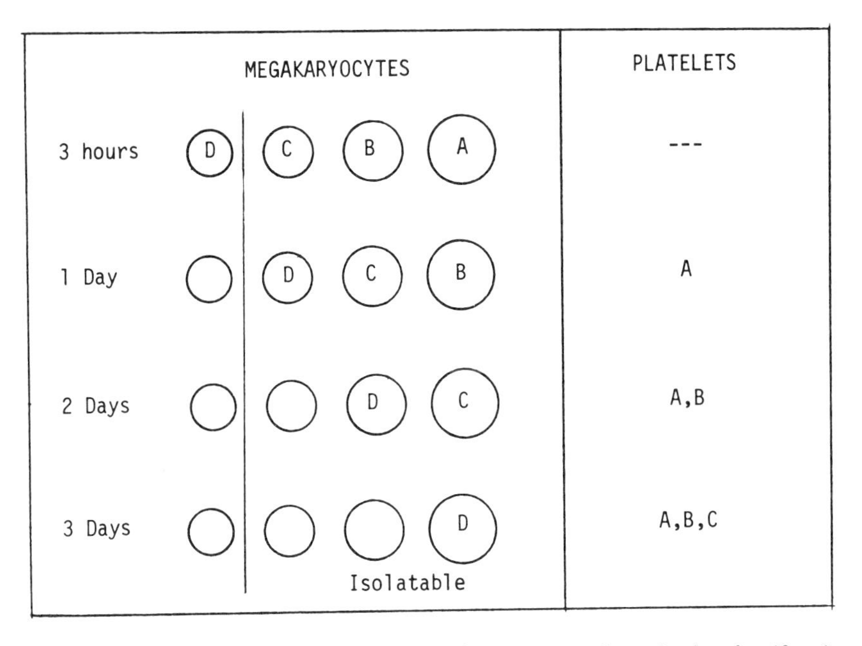

Figure 4-2. Rationale for studying the time course of synthesis of sulfated macromolecules by megakaryocytes in vivo. The times indicated represent time elapsed after a single ip injection of $Na_2{}^{35}SO_4$. The increasing size of the circles represents maturation of megakaryocytes, and the letters represent the different molecules presumably synthesized at the different stages of maturation. As the cells mature, the molecules that are synthesized at the time of injection appear in increasingly mature megakaryocytes and then in platelets. The smallest megakaryocytes cannot be isolated by the methodology used in these experiments;[43] thus, a molecule (e.g., *D*) synthesized by very immature megakaryocytes can be identified in "isolatable" megakaryocytes only at 1–3 days after the injection, and in the platelets only at 3–4 days after injection.

5-day period by passing extracts made by solubilizing whole cells in 4 M Gdn HCl/4% Zwittergent 3–12 through Sepharose CL-6B columns. The data are shown in Figures 4-3 and 4-4 and are presented in terms of K_{av}, where K_{av} 0.0 is the void volume (V_o) and K_{av} 1.0 is the total volume (V_t) of the column. At 3 hr there was virtually no labeling of platelet proteins or proteoglycans, although a broad range of sulfated macromolecules was already present in megakaryocytes. The megakaryocyte extract showed a very broad peak with K_{av} 0 to 0.2. At 24 hr after injection, a peak with K_{av} to 0.18 to 0.20 was seen in the platelet extracts, and the higher K_{av} portion of the peak had disappeared from the megakaryocyte extract. At 48 hr the K_{av} of the platelet peak was about 0.14, and the peak was much broader and larger than at 24 hr. Over the next 2 days there was a gradual shift to lower K_{av} in platelets, and the appearance of specific portions of the platelet-labeling curve could be correlated with the disappearance of the same material from the megakaryocytes. In addition to this major peak, there were peaks from K_{av} 0.3 to 0.6 that increased with time in the isolatable megakaryocytes and later in the platelets. We presume that these molecules were synthesized by very young megakaryocytes that were too small to be isolated by our procedure[33,43] at 3 hr after the injection, but that had matured sufficiently 24 hr to 72 hr later to be isolated.

The initial step in proteoglycan purification is separation of these molecules from proteins by ion-exchange chromatography on DEAE-Sephacel columns. We found that the cells could be completely solubilized in the buffer used to equilibrate the DEAE-Sephacel columns, namely, 8 M urea/50 mM TRIS/0.1 M NaCl/0.2% Triton X-100 and, thus, the whole-cell extract could then be fractionated by ion-exchange chromatography. This procedure en-

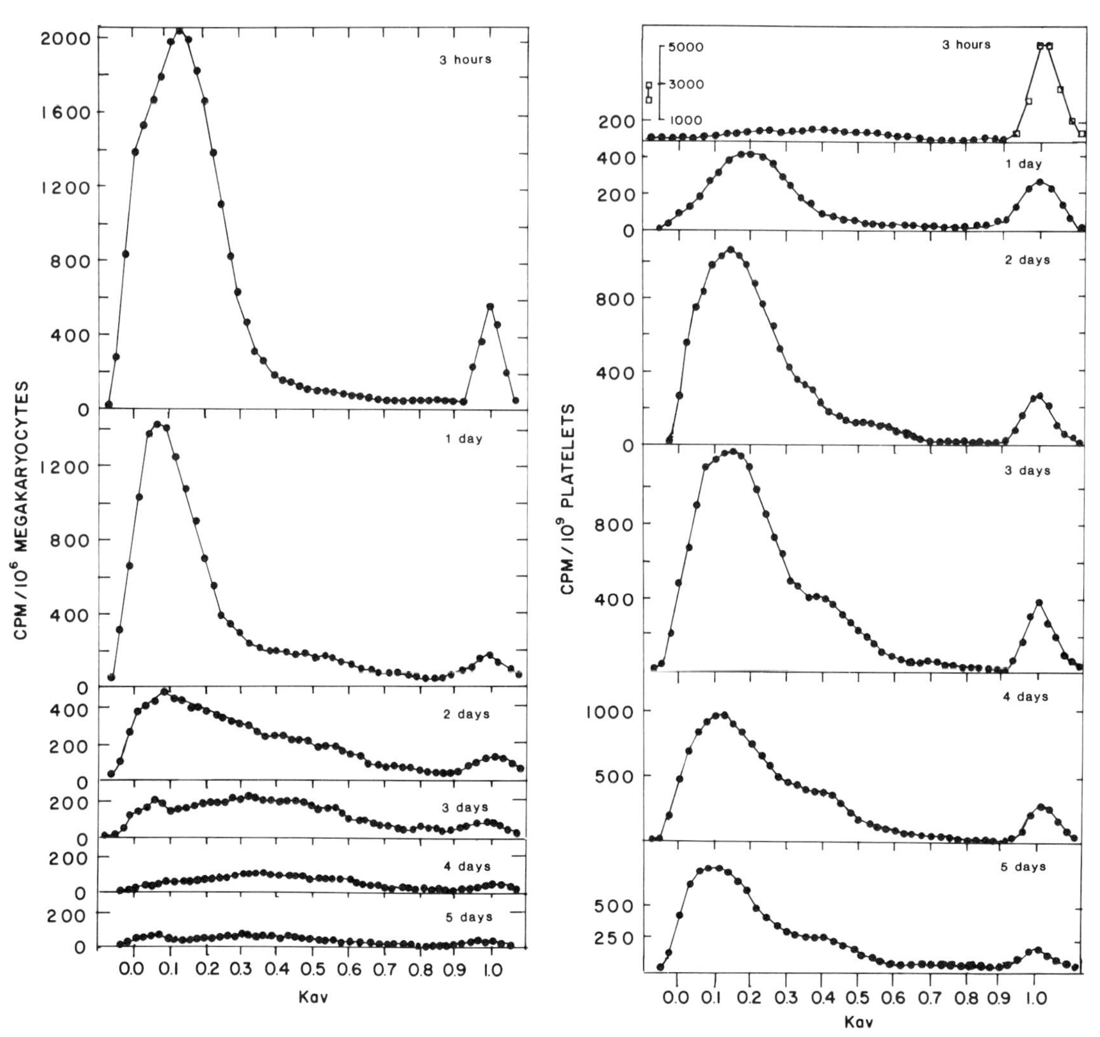

Figure 4-3 (*Left*). Time course of labeling of sulfated molecules in megakaryocytes: Sepharose CL-6B elution profiles of whole-cell extracts. Megakaryocytes were solubilized in 2% Zwittergent 3-12/4 M guanidine HCl.[26] This whole-cell extract was applied to a Sepharose CL-6B column that had been equilibrated with 4 M Gdn HCl/0.2% Triton X-100/50 mM NaAc, and elution was performed with this same buffer. K_{av} 0 = void volume, K_{av} 1 = total volume of the column. Note that the maximal cell labeling occurs at 3 hr after injection. Each time point represents a single animal.

Figure 4-4 (*Right*). Time course of labeling of sulfated molecules in platelets: Sepharose CL-6B elution profiles of whole-cell extracts. Platelets were solubilized and chromatographed as in Figure 4-3. Note maximal labeling at 3 days after injection.

abled us to bypass the transfer of proteoglycans from the 4 M guanidine HCl into the urea buffer, which in our hands (as also in the study of Okayama et al.[61]) caused extensive precipitation. About 25% to 35% of the radioactivity eluted at 0.1 M NaCl, 3% to 4% at 0.23 M NaCl, 60% to 65% with 4 M Gdn HCl, and the remainder with 4 M Gdn HCl and 2% CHAPS or 2% Triton X-100 (Fig. 4-5). The Sepharose CL-6B elution patterns of each of these four fractions is shown in Figure 4-6. About two-thirds of the radioactivity in the first fraction was found in molecules that appeared to be sulfated proteins (*see* later discussion), and the remainder was associated with dialyzable low-molecular-weight molecules. The 0.23 M NaCl eluate also contained sulfated proteins. The 4 M Gdn HCl fraction contained about 85% of the proteoglycans and the 4 M Gdn/CHAPS the remainder. The proteoglycans in the 4 M

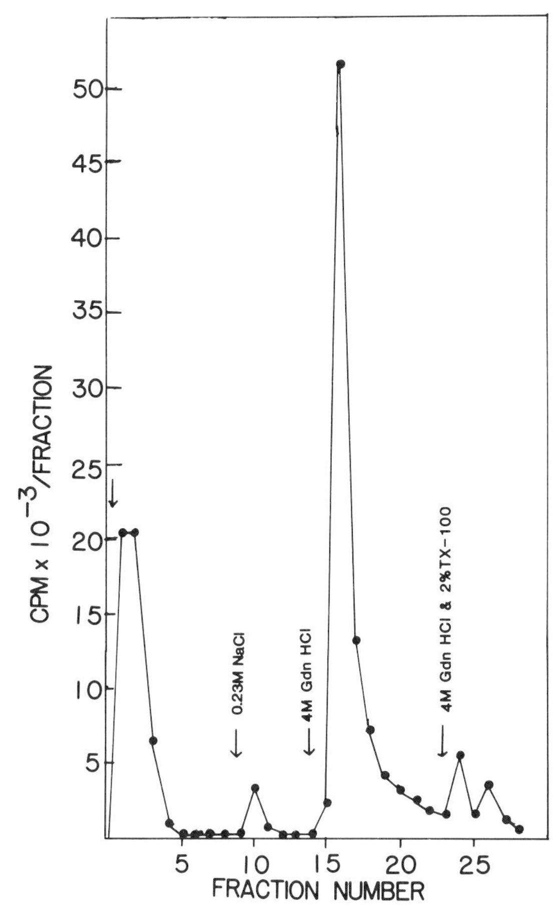

Figure 4-5. DEAE-Sephacel chromatography of platelets 3 days after [^{35}S]sulfate injection. Platelets were solubilized in 8 M urea/50 mM TRIS/0.2% Triton X-100/0. 1 M NaCl and applied to a DEAE-Sephacel column equilibrated in the same buffer. Elution was as indicated in the text.

Gdn HCl fraction eluted from Sepharose CL-6B at K_{av} 0.18 to 0.20 at 24 hr after injection, and shifted to 0.10 to 0.12 over the next 3 days, thus reflecting the changes in the major peak in Figures 4-3 and 4-4. In contrast, the detergent-eluted proteoglycan at 3 days had a K_{av} of 0.07, and was virtually absent at 24 hr. The different proteoglycans could be nearly resolved on SDS-PAGE (Figure 4-7). Two bands of core protein were seen on SDS-PAGE of chondroitinase digests (Figure 4-8) at 3 days after ^{35}S injection, but only the lower band was present at 24 hr, suggesting the presence of two different proteoglycans in this fraction. The size of the proteoglycans in the 4 M Gdn HCl fraction was found to be directly related to GAG chain length by analysis of different portions of the proteoglycan CL-6B eluate (Fig. 4-9). In addition, the GAGs labeled at 24 hr were considerably smaller than those labeled at 3 days (Fig. 4-10). Despite the much larger size of the detergent-solubilized proteoglycan, its GAGs were the same average chain length as the 4 M Gdn HCl eluate, and thus did not correspond to the proteoglycan size and GAG chain length correlation found in the 4 M Gdn HCl eluate (*see* bottom panel, Fig. 4-4). A number of controls showed that this larger molecule was not an aggregate of the smaller proteoglycans. Calibration based on data obtained for intact proteoglycan[29] and free chondroitin sulfate[91] suggested that the mean M_r of proteoglycans in the 4 M Gdn eluate was about 200,000, and that of the GAGs about 50,000.

To determine the relevance of our findings to human platelets, we isolated human platelet proteoglycans by the same protocol used for the guinea pig molecules. The human platelet proteoglycans from the 4 M Gdn HCl fraction from DEAE-Sephacel cochromatographed with the tracer amount of ^{35}S-labeled proteoglycans from the guinea pig platelets (Fig. 4-11). In addition, the 4 M Gdn HCl/2% CHAPS eluate from the human platelets contained a large proteoglycan that was seen by alcian blue staining to comigrate on SDS-PAGE with the radiolabeled material from the guinea pig cells.

Thus, these experiments show that platelets have at least three chondroitin sulfate proteoglycans that differ in their mean molecular masses and in behavior on ion exchange chromatography, and that these differences evolve as a function of megakaryocyte maturation.

Fate of Proteoglycans During Platelet Activation

When platelets that have been radiolabeled in vivo are treated with thrombin, about 60% of the total cellular radioactivity is released from the cells. Most of this activity is associated with proteoglycans corresponding to those eluting from the DEAE-Sephacel column with 4 M Gdn HCl, and the remainder with very low molecular mass material (i.e., the V_t of the Sepharose CL-6B column). The large proteoglycan that requires detergent for elution from the ion exchange column (K_{av} 0.04–0.07) appears to be retained by the cells (Fig. 4-12). The

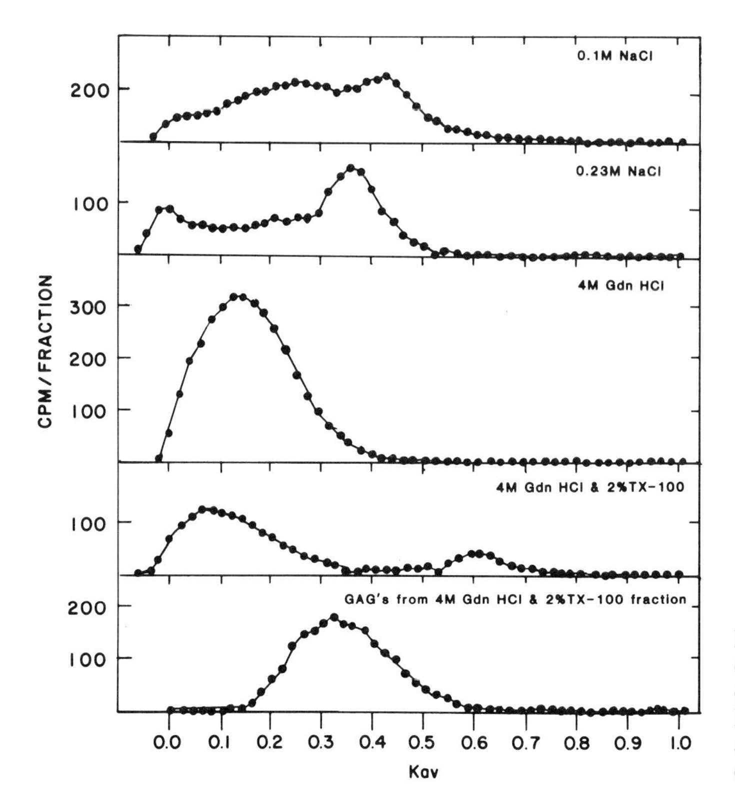

Figure 4-6. Sepharose CL-6B profiles of fractions from the DEAE-Sephacel column. The four fractions obtained in Figure 4-5 were dialyzed, lyophilized, and analyzed by gel filtration under the conditions described in Figure 4-3.

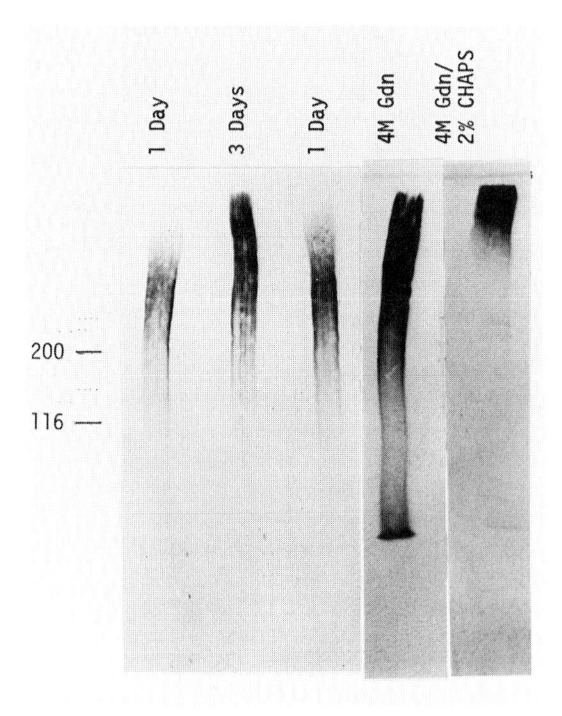

Figure 4-7. Fluorography of SDS-PAGE of proteoglycans from the 4 M Gdn HCl eluate and the 4 M Gdn HCl/2% CHAPS eluate from the DEAE-Sephacel column. Proteoglycans in the 4 M Gdn HCl fraction, which were labeled at 1 and 3 days after [^{35}S] sulfate injection, are shown in the *left panel*; proteoglycans in the 4 M Gdn HCl and 4 M Gdn HCl/2% CHAPS, which were labeled at 3 days, are shown in the *right panel*. No radiolabel was seen in the 4 M Gdn HCl/2% CHAPS fraction at 1 day. Alcian blue stain of the 4 M Gdn HCl fraction encompasses the areas of the gel labeled at 1 and 3 days (not shown).

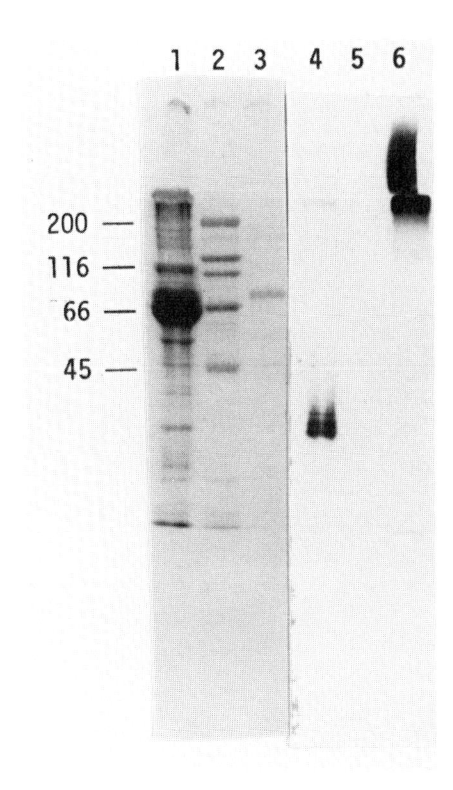

Figure 4-8. Demonstration of core proteins by SDS-PAGE and fluorography. Proteoglycans in the 4 M Gdn HCl fraction from DEAE-Sephacel analysis of platelets obtained 3 days after [^{35}S]sulfate injection were digested with chondroitinase ABC in the presence of protease inhibitors. *Lanes 1–3*: Coomassie Blue stain; *lanes 4–6*: fluorography. Lanes 1 and 4 are the chondroitinase digest (bands in lane 1 represent enzyme preparation and carrier albumin), lanes 2 and 5 are protein standards, and lanes 3 and 6 are the undigested material. At 1 day after injection the lowest band predominates in lane 4 (not shown).

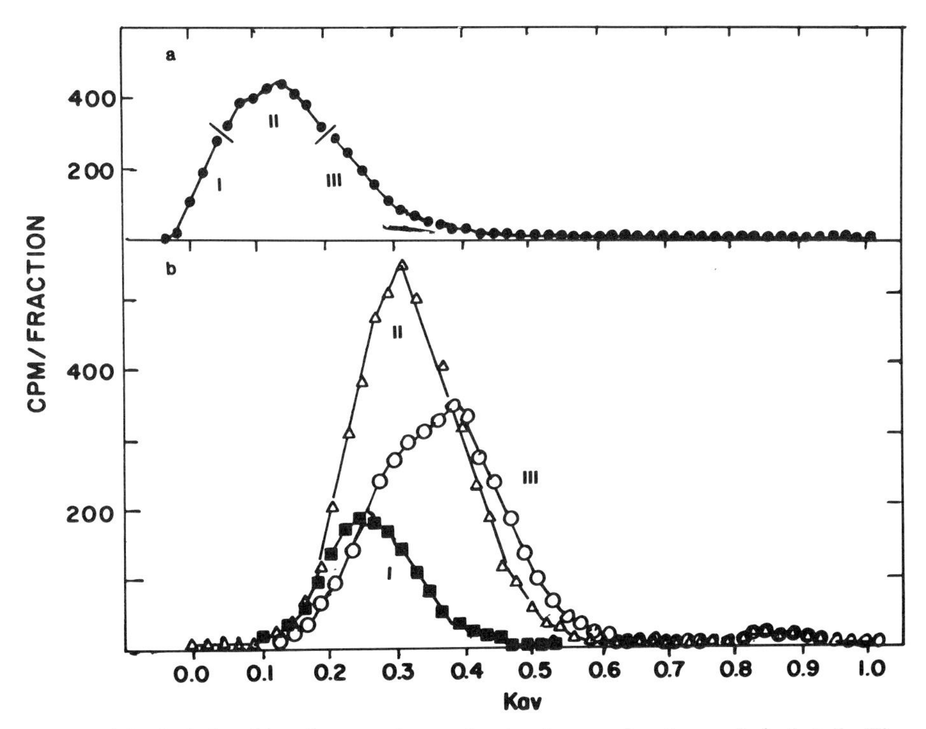

Figure 4-9. Relationship of proteoglycan size to glycosaminoglycan chain length. The Sepharose CL-6B eluate was subfractionated as shown in the *upper panel*, and each subfraction was digested separately with mild alkaline borohydride. The digests were chromatographed on the same column (*lower panel*).

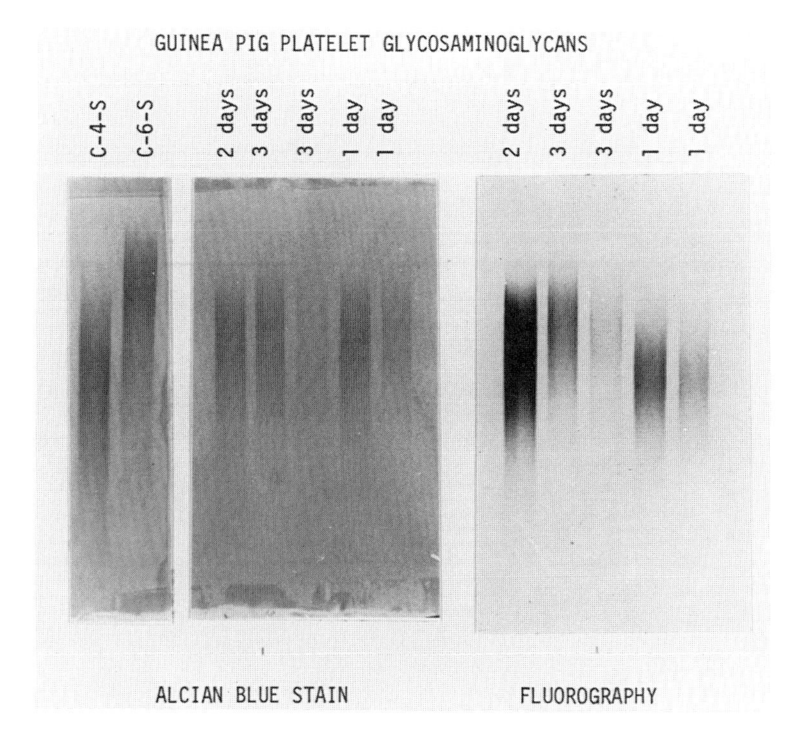

Figure 4-10. Comparison of glycosaminoglycans labeled in platelets at different times after [^{35}S]sulfate injection. Proteoglycans from the 4 M Gdn HCl fraction from the DEAE-Sephacel column were digested with mild alkaline borohydride, the digests were dialyzed and lyophilized, and the glycosaminoglycans were subjected to electrophoresis using the system of Min and Cowman.[55] Chondroitin-6-sulfate (nominal M_r range 40,000–80,000) and chondroitin-4-sulfate standards (*left panel*) were obtained from Miles Laboratories. *Center panel* shows alcian bluc stain and *right panel* shows fluorography of each sample.

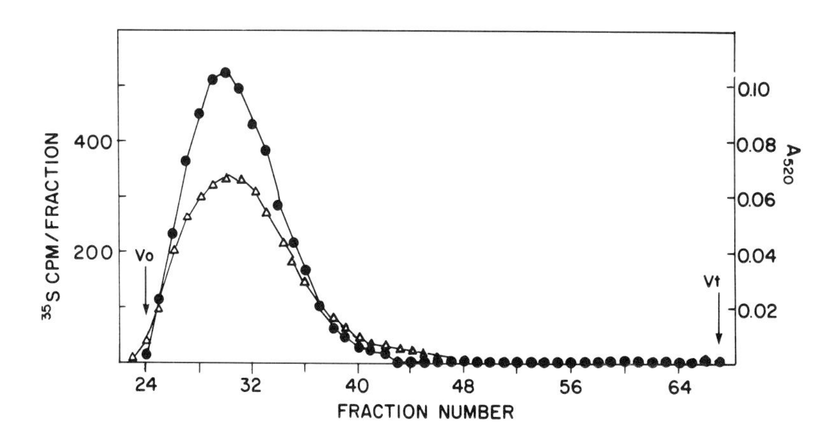

Figure 4-11. Cochromatography of [^{35}S]sulfate-labeled guinea pig platelet proteoglycans and unlabeled human platelet proteoglycans on Sepharose CL-6B. Proteoglycans from guinea pig platelets obtained 3 days after [^{35}S]sulfate injection and proteoglycans from human platelets were isolated by DEAE-Sephacel chromatography as described in Figure 4-5. Guinea pig platelet proteoglycans were mixed with proteoglycans from 10 times the number of human platelets, and radioactivity and uronic acid were determined for each column fraction. The elution was performed with 0.2 M NaCl/0.05 M NaAc. ● Human platelets, uronic acid; △ guinea pig platelets, ^{35}S CPM.

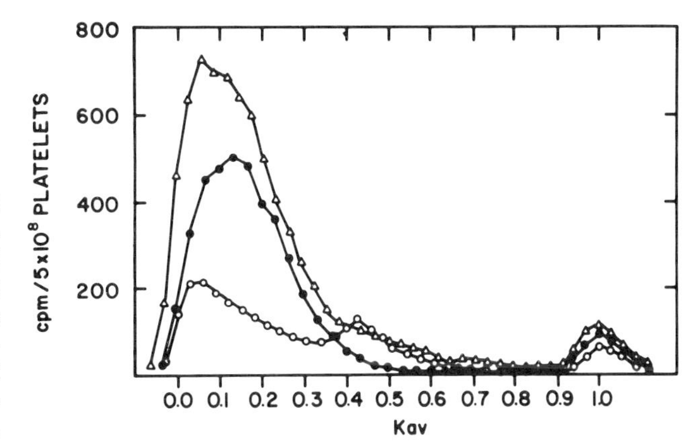

Figure 4-12. Comparison of ^{35}S-labeled molecules released and retained by thrombin-treated platelets. Platelets, obtained 4 days after ^{35}S injection, were treated with 2 U/ml thrombin, and the releaseates and cells were analyzed by Sepharose CL-6B chromatography as described in Figure 4-3. △ Intact platelets; ● released material; ○ residual material left in cells after thrombin treatment.

hydrophobic properties of this molecule would suggest that it is derived from membranes. When the platelets are stimulated with ADP, about 15% of the radioactivity is released and is associated with the same size range of proteoglycans and small molecules that are released by thrombin. Thus, it is not clear whether there is α-granule release of proteoglycans in the absence of release of other markers, whether a portion of these small proteoglycans is associated with the membrane, or whether these molecules originate from an as yet unidentified subcellular location. Investigation of the specific localization of this proteoglycan is in progress in this laboratory. It is of interest to note also that the molecules that we have characterized as sulfated proteins are not released from the platelets to a significant extent by either ADP or thrombin.

Sulfated Proteins in Guinea Pig Platelets and Megakaryocytes

About 20% of the total cellular radioactivity eluted at low salt from DEAE-Sephacel and appeared on Sepharose CL-6B as several broad peaks either near the V_o or from K_{av} 0.3 to 0.6 (*see* Fig. 4-5). These molecules are not proteoglycans because digestion with $NaBH_4$/NaOH, papain, or pronase produce small ^{35}S-labeled fragments that elute at K_{av} >0.80 on CL-6B and are mostly in the included volume of Bio-Gel P-2 columns. There are several distinct bands that can be seen on fluorograms of SDS polyacrylamide gels, and different bands appear at different times after [^{35}S]sulfate injection. The complete characterization of these molecules will appear elsewhere.* To our knowledge, this is the first report of sulfated proteins in platelets. The presence of small sulfated oligosaccharides on platelet glycoproteins would explain the finding of Anderson and Odell[3] that 50% of the radioactivity in NaOH-digested rat platelets was dialyzable. These sulfated proteins remain almost entirely with the platelets after thrombin and ADP treatment. We are attempting to determine whether they are part of the surface membrane or whether they are located in the granules.

COMPARISON OF PLATELET PROTEOGLYCANS WITH PROTEOGLYCANS FROM CELLS OF THE IMMUNE SYSTEM

Because proteoglycans have been shown to be involved in immune reactions of white cells, it would be of interest to compare proteoglycans of platelets with those of white cells. For more comprehensive information, the reader is referred to the recent review of Stevens.[82]

A number of recent studies have shown that different types of mast cells and different types of cells of the hematopoietic system contain different types of proteoglycans. These proteoglycans differ in molecular mass, the dissaccharide units making up the glycosaminoglycan chains, the length of the glycosaminochains, and the size and nature of the core protein. For example, rat serosal mast cell proteoglycans have an M_r of 750,000 with heparin glycosaminoglycan chains of 80,000, and a peptide core of about 20,000.[52,69] Rat mucosal mast cells have disulfated chondroitin sul-

*Schick B: Unpublished data.

fate B proteoglycans of M_r 150,000, with the M_r of the GAG chains and core proteins as yet undetermined.[83] The rat basophilic leukemia cell line RBL-1 contains a proteoglycan of 150,000 M_r with GAG chains of disulfated chondroitin sulfate B or heparan sulfate chains of M_r 12,000.[53,79] The mouse bone marrow-derived mast cell has a proteoglycan of M_r 200,000 with chondroitin sulfate E (chondroitin 4,6-disulfate) chains of M_r 25,000 and a peptide core of about 10,000.[84] The human natural killer (NK) cell has a proteoglycan of M_r 200,000 with chondroitin-4-sulfate chains of about 50,000.[47] These proteoglycans are thought to be located in the metachromatic secretory granules. The evidence for this includes x-ray dispersion studies that demonstrated that the secretory granules of rat serosal heparin mast cells were the only areas of the cell that contained substantial amounts of sulfur-containing molecules,[28] and the finding of parallel exocytosis of histamine and ^{35}S-labeled heparin proteoglycans from these cells upon immunological stimulation. Similarly, the chondroitin sulfate E proteoglycans of rat mucosal ChS-mast cells have been shown to reside in the metachromatic granules by transmission electron microscopy and autoradiography of ^{35}S-labeled molecules,[20] x-ray dispersion analysis,[86] and exocytosis of the proteoglycans in soluble form when cells were activated.[66]

The mast cell granules that contain the proteoglycans are very different from the platelet α granules. The mast cell proteoglycans just described reside in lysosomes that contain numerous proteases, and they are secreted along with the proteases when the cells are activated. It is thus interesting to note that the core proteins of all these proteoglycans appear to be extremely resistant to proteases: for example, the mouse ChS-mast cell proteoglycans cannot be degraded by collagenase, clostripain, trypsin, chymotrypsin, elastase, chymopapain, V8 protease, proteinase K, or pronase.[79] In contrast, we[76] and others have found the platelet proteoglycans to be susceptible to papain and pronase. The immune cell peptide cores that have been analyzed have been shown to be rich in serine and glycine (rat serosal HP-mast cell),[52] serine, glycine, and alanine (RBL-1),[79] and serine, glycine, and glutamic acid (mouse bone-marrow derived ChS-mast cell).

The principal components of the secretory granules of HP-mast cells, ChS-mast cells, and basophils are the serine proteases, vasoactive amines, and proteoglycans.[82] The proteoglycans most likely are bound to the positively charged serine proteases and vasoactive amines. The purpose for this organization is not known, but it may be related to protection of the cell from nonspecific proteolysis and for directing the proteases to their targets after exocytosis. The role of proteoglycans in organizing the contents of the secretory granules is suggested by electron microscopic studies demonstrating highly ordered crystalline arrays in human eosinophils[54] and human lung heparin mast cells.[14] Three laboratories have provided evidence for the organization of the contents of the α granules of platelets: Cramer et al. have demonstrated specific organization of proteins within the α granules,[16] Spicer et al. have shown that proteoglycanlike material forms a "nucleoid" in the α granule,[81] and Sato et al.[74] have found that calcium is associated with this "nucleoid." It has also been proposed that secretory granule proteoglycans regulate the osmotic pressure of the granules. It has been shown that an influx of water into the granules of human lung HP-mast cells precedes fusion of the granule membranes with the plasma membrane and exocytosis of the granule contents.[14]

Levitt and Ho[44] have shown that human and mouse peripheral blood mononuclear cells and their major subpopulations (B cells, T cells, and monocytes) and mouse spleen cells synthesize and secrete proteoglycans, and that these processes were enhanced by treatment with conconavalin A or phorbol-12-myristate-3-acetate. The chondroitin sulfate proteoglycan secreted by these cells had a M_r of about 130,000 with GAG chains of 25,000. In addition, these cells were found to synthesize large amounts of heparan sulfate. In an intriguing study of mouse spleen cells, Sant et al.[72] showed that the cells synthesize a small chondroitin sulfate proteoglycan, M_r 45 kDa to 75 kDa, that has a core protein identical with the invariant chain of the Ia antigen of the mouse MHC class II system, and that this proteoglycan was found in a complex with glycoprotein in the plasma membrane.

The function of the proteoglycans once they are released from any of these cells is not understood. Some studies have suggested that mast cell proteoglycans can regulate the alternative complement pathway[92,95] and the Hageman factor-dependent contact activation system.[31] The role of platelet proteoglycans in these processes remains to be determined, but the obvious importance of platelet procoagulant activity and the role of platelets in certain stages of complement activation (*see* Chap. 18), lead one to speculate that much of this functional activity may be mediated in part by proteoglycans.

CONCLUSION

In conclusion, the platelet granule proteoglycans appear to be quite different from the proteoglycans of the white blood cells or the cells of the immune system, in terms of size, glycosaminoglycan content, glycosaminoglycan chain length, protease susceptibility, and the types of granules in which they are located. The platelet plasma membrane may also contain proteoglycans, and the proteoglycan that we have tentatively suggested to be the membrane proteoglycan is also different from the molecules that have been described for the other cells. The role of these molecules in platelet immunology and their fate after platelet secretion are unknown as yet, but this represents an intriguing area of study that begs attention.

The platelet sulfated proteins also represent a new aspect of platelet protein chemistry, and their identity, subcellular localization, and function are currently under study in our laboratory.

REFERENCES

1. Alberts A (ed): Molecular Biology of the Cell, pp 705-707. New York, Garland Press, 1983

2. Anderson B, Odell TT Jr: Chemical studies of mucopolysaccharides of rat blood platelets. Proc Soc Exp Biol Med 99:765, 1958

3. Barber AJ, Jamieson GA: Isolation of glycopeptides from low and high density platelet plasma membranes. Biochemistry 10:4711, 1970

4. Barber AJ, Kaser-Glanzmann R, Jakabova M, Luscher EF: Characterization of a chondroitin-4-sulfate proteoglycan carrier for heparin neutralizing activity (platelet factor 4) released from human blood platelets. Biochim Biophys Acta 286:312, 1972

5. Behnke O: An electron microscope study of the megakaryocyte of the rat bone marrow. 1. The development of the demarcation membrane system and the platelet surface coat. J Ultrastruc Res 24:412, 1968

6. Behnke O: Platelet adhesion to native collagens involves proteoglycans and may be a two-step process. Thromb Haemostasis 58:786, 1987

7. Bernfield M: Dependence of salivary epithelial morphology and branching morphogenesis upon acid mucopolysaccharide-protein (proteoglycan) at the epithelial surface. J Cell Biol 52:674, 1972

8. Bertrand F, Veissiere D, Picard J: Sulphated glycoproteins and proteoglycans from rat liver plasma membranes: Partial characterization of a sulphated glycopeptide and glycosaminoglycans. Eur J Biochem 18:17, 1983

9. Bettelheim FR: Tyrosine-*O*-sulfate in a peptide from fibrinogen. J Am Chem Soc 76:2838, 1954

10. Bhat NR, Brunngraber EG: Synthesis and release of sulfated glycoproteins by cultured glial cells. Biochem Biophys Res Commun 126:778, 1985

11. Carey DJ, Todd MS: A cytoskeleton-associated plasma membrane heparan sulfate proteoglycan in Schwann cells. J Biol Chem 261:7518, 1986

12. Carlson SS, Kelly RB: A highly antigenic proteoglycan-like component of cholinergic synaptic vesicles. J Biol Chem 258:11082, 1983

13. Caterson B, Christner J, Baker JR, Couchman JR: Production and characterization of monoclonal antibodies directed against connective tissues proteoglycans. Fed Proc 44:386, 1985

14. Caulfield JP, Lewis RA, Hein A, Austen KF: Secretion in dissociated pulmonary mast cells. Evidence for solubilization of granule contents before discharge. J Cell Biol 85:299, 1980

15. Cohn RH, Banerjee SD, Bernfield MR: Basal lamina of embryonic salivary epithelia. Nature of glycosaminoglycans and organization of extracellular materials. J Cell Biol 73:464, 1977

16. Cramer EM, Martin JF, Vainchenker W, Breton-Gorius J: Production and localization of alpha-granule proteins in maturing megakaryocytes: An overview on ultrastructural aspects of megakaryocyte maturation. Thromb Haemostasis 58:43, 1987

17. Del Rosso M, Cappelletti R, Dini G, Fibbi G, Vannucchi S, Chiarugi V, Guazzelli C: Involvement of glycosaminoglycans in detachment of early myeloid precursors from bone marrow stromal cells. Biochim Biophys Acta 676:129, 1981

18. Dietrich K, Armelin H, Nogueira YL, Nader HB, Michelacci S: Turnover, change of composition with rate of cell growth, and effect of phenylxyloside on synthesis and structure of cell surface sulfated glycosaminoglycans of normal and transformed cells. Biochim Biophys Acta 717:387, 1982

19. Gallagher JT, Spooncer E, Dexter TM: Role of the cellular matrix in haemopoiesis. I. Synthesis of glycosaminoglycans by mouse bone marrow cell cultures. J Cell Sci 63:155, 1983

20. Galli SJ, Dvorak AM, Marcum JA, Ishizaka T, Nabel G, Der Simonian H, Pyne K, Goldin JM, Rosenberg RD, Cantor H, and Dvorak HF: Mast cell clones: A model for the analysis of cellular maturation. J Cell Biol 95:435, 1982

21. Glant TT, Mikecz K, Roughley PR, Buzaz EM, Poole AR: Age-related changes in protein-related epitopes of human articular cartilage proteoglycans. Biochem J 236:71, 1986

22. Green ED, Baenziger JU, Boime I: Cell-free sulfation of human and bovine pituitary hormones. Comparison of the sulfated oligosaccharides of lutropin, follitropin, and thyrotropin. J Biol Chem 260:15631, 1985

23. Green ED, van Halbeek H, Boime I, Baenziger JU: Structural elucidation of the disulfated oligosaccharide from bovine lutropin. J Biol Chem 260:15623, 1985

24. Gude WD, Upton AK, Odell TT Jr: Blood platelets of humans and rat: A cytochemical study. Lab Invest 5:348, 1956

25. Harker LA: Regulation of thrombopoiesis. Am J Physiol 218:1386, 1970

26. Hascall VC, Kimura J: Proteoglycans: Isolation and characterization. Methods Enzymol 82:769, 1982

27. Hassell JR, Robey PG, Barach HJ, Wiliczek J, Rennard SI, Martin GR: Isolation and characterization of a heparan sulfate-containing proteoglycan from basement membrane. Proc Acad Matl Sci USA 77:4494, 1980

28. Hein A, Caulfield JP: Sulfur and calcium in rat peritoneal mast cell granules. J Biol Chem 95:397, 1982

29. Heinegard D, Hascall VC: Characterization of chondroitin sulfate isolated from trypsin-chymotrypsin digests of cartilage proteoglycans. Arch Biochem Biophys 165:427, 1974

30. Herzog V: Secretion of sulfated thyroglobulin. Eur J Cell Biol 39:399, 1985

31. Hojima Y, Cochrane CG, Wiggins RC, Austen KF, Stevens RL: In vitro activation of the contact (Hageman factor) system of plasma by heparin and chondroitin sulfate E. Blood 63:1453, 1984

32. Horton G, Folz R, Gordon JI, Strauss AW: Characterization of sites of tyrosine sulfation in proteins and criteria for predicting their occurrence. Biochem Biophys Res Commun 141:326, 1986

33. Hortin G, Sims H, Strauss AW: Identification of the site of sulfation of the fourth component of human complement. J Biol Chem 261:1786, 1986

34. Hortin G, Tollefson DM, Strauss AW: Identification of two sites of sulfation of human heparin cofactor II. J Biol Chem 261:15827, 1986

35. Huang SS, Huang JS, Deuel TF: Proteoglycan carrier of human platelet factor 4: Isolation and characterization. J Biol Chem 257:11546, 1982

36. Iozzo RV: Biosynthesis of heparan sulfate proteoglycan by human colon carcinoma cells and its localization at the cell surface. J Cell Biol 99:403, 1984

37. Jenkins RB, Hall T, Dorfman N: Chondroitin-6-sulfate oligosaccharides as immunological determinants of chick proteoglycans. J Biol Chem 256:8279, 1981

38. Jukkola A, Risteli J, Niemela O, Risteli L: Incorporation of sulphate into type III procollagen by cultured human fibroblasts. Identification of tyrosine-*O*-sulfate. Eur J Biochem 154:219, 1986

39. Kammer GM, Sapolsky AI, Malemud CJ: Secretion of an articular cartilage proteoglycan-degrading enzyme activity by murine T-lymphocytes in vitro. J Clin Invest 76:395, 1985

40. Kölset SO, Kjellen L: Effect of in vitro differentiation on proteoglycan structure in cultured human monocytes. Glycoconj J 4:73, 1986

41. Kölset SO, Kjellen L, Seljelid R, Lindahl U: Changes in glycosaminoglycan biosynthesis during differentiation in vitro of human monocytes. Biochem J 210:661, 1986

42. Lee REWH, Huttner WB: Tyrosine-*O*-sulfated proteins of PC-12 pheochromocytoma cells and their sulfation by a tyrosylprotein sulfotransferase. J Biol Chem 258:11326, 1983

43. Levine RF, Fedorko ME: Isolation of intact megakaryocytes from guinea pig femoral marrow. J Cell Biol 69:159, 1976

44. Levitt D, Ho P-L: Induction of chondroitin sulfate proteoglycan synthesis and secretion in lymphocytes and monocytes. J Cell Biol 97:351, 1983

45. Lijnen HR, van Hoef B, Wiman B, Collen D: Modification of a tyrosine residue in the carboxyterminal portion of human α-2 antiplasmin. Thromb Res 39:625, 1985

46. Liu M-C, Yu S, Sy J, Redman CM, Lipman F: Tyrosine sulfation of proteins from the human hepatoma cell line Hep G-2. Proc Natl Acad Sci USA 82:7160, 1985

47. MacDermott RP, Schmidt RE, Caulfield JP, Hein A, Bartley GT, Ritz J, Schlossman SF, Austen KF, Stevens RL: Proteoglycans in cell-mediated toxicity. Identification, localization and exocytosis of a chondroitin sulfate proteoglycan from human cloned natural killer cells during target cell lysis. J Exp Med 162:1771, 1985

48. MacPherson GG: Synthesis and location of sulphated mucopolysaccharide in megakaryocytes and platelets of the rat. An analysis by electron-microscope autoradiography. J Cell Sci 10:705, 1972

49. Margolis RU, Margolis RK: Isolation of chondroitin sulfate and glycopeptides from chromaffin granules of adrenal medulla. Biochem Pharmacol 22:2195, 1973

50. Margolis RK, Ripellino JA, Goossen B, Steinbrich R, Margolis RU: Occurrence of the HNK-1 epitope (3-sulfoglucuronic acid) in PC-12 pheochromocytoma cells, chromaffin granule membranes, and chondroitin sulfate proteoglycans. Biochem Biophys Res Commun 145:1142, 1987

51. Merkle RK, Heifetz A: Enzymatic sulfation of *N*-glycosidically linked oligosaccharides by endothelial cell membranes. Arch Biochem Biophys 234:460, 1984

52. Metcalfe DD, Smith JA, Austen KF, Silbert JE: Polydispersity of rat mast cell heparin. Implications for proteoglycan assembly. J Biol Chem 255:11753, 1980

53. Metcalfe DD, Wasserman SI, Austen KF: Isolation and characterization of sulfated mucopolysaccharides from rat leukemic (RBL-1) basophils. Biochem J 185:367, 1980

54. Miller F, DeHarven E, Palade GE: The structure of eosinophil leukocyte granules in rodents and in man. J Cell Biol 31:349, 1966

55. Min H, Cowman MK: Combined alcian blue and silver staining of glycosaminoglycans in polyacrylamide gels: Application to electrophoretic analysis of molecular weight distribution. Anal Biochem 155:275, 1986

56. Nachman RL, Levine RF, Jaffe E: Synthesis of factor VIII antigen by cultured guinea pig megakaryocytes. J Clin Invest 60:914, 1977

57. Odell TT Jr, Anderson B: Isolation of a sulfated mucopolysaccharide from blood platelets of rats. Proc Soc Exp Biol Med 94:151, 1957

58. Odell TT Jr, Jackson CW, Reiter RS: Depression of the megakaryocyte-platelet system in rats by transfusion of platelets. Acta Haematol 38:34, 1967

59. Odell TT Jr, McDonald TP: Two mechanisms of sulfate ^{35}S-uptake by blood platelets of rats. Am J Physiol 206:580, 1964

60. Odell TT Jr, Tausche FG, Gude WD: Uptake of radioactive sulfate by elements of the blood and bone marrow rats. Am J Physiol 180:491, 1955

61. Okayama M, Oguri K, Fujiwara Y, Nakanishi H, Yonekura H, Kondo T, Ui N: Purification and characterization of human platelet proteoglycan. Biochem J 233:73, 1986

62. Olsson I, Gardell S: Isolation and characterization of glycosaminoglycans from human leukocytes and platelets. Biochim Biophys Acta 141:348, 1967

63. Poole AR, Reiner A, Roughley P, Champion B: Rabbit antibodies to degraded and intact glycosaminoglycans which are naturally occurring and present in arthritic rabbits. J Biol Chem 260:6020, 1985

64. Rand ML, Greenberg JP, Packham MA, Mustard JF: Density subpopulations of rabbit platelets: Size, protein and sialic acid content, and specific radioactivity changes following labeling with ^{35}S-sulfate in vivo. Blood 57:741, 1981

65. Rapraeger A, Jalkanen M, Bernfield M: Cell surface proteoglycan associates with the cytoskeleton at the basolateral surface of mouse mammary epithelial cells. J Cell Biol 103:2683, 1986

66. Razin E, Mencia-Huerta J-M, Stevens RL, Lewis RA, Liu F-T, Corey EJ, Austen KF: IgE-mediated release of leukotriene C4, chondroitin sulfate E proteoglycan, β-hexosaminidase, and histamine from cultured bone marrow-derived mast cells. J Exp Med 157:189, 1983

67. Reggio HA, Palade GE: Sulfated compounds in the zymogen granules of the guinea pig pancreas. J Cell Biol 77:288, 1978

68. Riddell PE, Bier AM: Electrophoresis of ^{35}S-labeled material released from clumping platelets. Nature 205:711, 1965

69. Robinson HC, Horner AA, Höök M, Ogren S, Lindahl U: A proteoglycan form of heparin and its degradation to single-chain molecules. J Biol Chem 253:6687, 1978

70. Rosa P, Hille A, Lee RWH, Zanini A, de Camilli P, Huttner W: Secretogranins I and II. Two tyrosine-sulfated secretory proteins common to a variety of cells secreting peptides by the regulated pathway. J Cell Biol 101:1999, 1985

71. Rosenberg LC, Choi HU, Tang L-H, Johnson TL, Pal S, Webber C, Reiner A, Poole AR: Isolation of dermatan sulfate proteoglycans from mature bovine articular cartilages. J Biol Chem 260:6304, 1985

72. Sant AJ, Cullen SE, Giacoletto KS, Schwartz BD: Invariant chain is the core protein of the Ia-associated chondroitin sulfate proteoglycan. J Exp Med 162:1916, 1985

73. Sant AJ, Cullen SE, Schwartz BD: Identification of a sulfate-bearing molecule associated with HLA class II antigens. Proc Natl Acad Sci USA 81:1534, 1984

74. Sato T, Herman L, Changler JA, Stracher A, Detwiler TC: Localization of a thrombin-sensitive calcium pool in platelets. J Histochem Cytochem 23:103, 1975

75. Schick BP, Walsh CJ, Breslin DL: Megakaryocyte and platelet proteoglycans. In Levine RF, Williams N, Levin J, Evatt B (eds): Megakaryocyte Development and Function, pp 287-292. New York, Alan R. Liss, 1986

76. Schick BP, Walsh CJ, Jenkins-West T: Sulfated proteoglycans and sulfated proteins in guinea pig megakaryocytes and platelets in vivo: Relevance to megakaryocyte maturation and platelet activation. J Biol Chem 263:1052, 1988

77. Schmidt RE, MacDermott RP, Bartley G, Bertovich M, Amato DA, Austen KF, Schlossman SF, Stevens RL, Ritz J: Specific release of proteoglycans from human natural killer cells during target lysis. Nature 318:289, 1985

78. Schwarting GA, Jungalwala FB, Chou DKH, Boyer AM, Yamamoto M: Sulfated glucuronic acid-containing glycoconjugates are temporally and spatially related antigens in the developing mammalian nervous system. Dev Biol 120:65, 1987

79. Seldin DC, Austen KF, Stevens RL: Purification and characterization of protease-resistant secretory granule proteoglycans containing chondroitin sulfate di-β and heparin-like glycosaminglycans from rat basophilic leukemia cells. J Biol Chem 260:1131, 1985

80. Silvestri L, Baker JR, Roden L, Stroud RM: The C1q inhibitor in serum is a chondroitin-4-sulfate proteoglycan. J Biol Chem 256:7383, 1981

81. Spicer SS, Greene WB, Hardin JH: Ultrastructural localization of acid mucosubstance and antimonate-precipitable cation in human and rabbit platelets and megakaryocytes. J Histochem Cytochem 17:781, 1969

82. Stevens RL: Intracellular proteoglycans in cells of the immune system. In Wight, TN (ed): Biology of the Extracellular matrix. New York, Academic Press, 1986

83. Stevens RL, Katz HR, Seldin DC, Austen KF: Bochemical characteristics distinguish subclasses of mammalian mast cells. In Befus AD, Bienenstock J, Denburg J (eds): New York, Raven Press (in press)

84. Stevens RL, Otsu K, Austen KF: Purification and analysis of the core protein of the protease-resistant intracellular chondroitin sulfate E proteoglycan from the interleukin 3-dependent mouse cell. J Biol Chem (in press) 1987

85. Stevens RL, Otsu K, Weis JH, Tantravahi RV, Austen KF, Henkart PA, Galli MC, Reynolds CW: Co-sedimentation of chondroitin sulfate A glycosaminoglycans and proteoglycans with the cytolytic secretory granules of rat large granular lymphocyte (LGL) tumor cells, and identification of an mRNA in normal and transformed LGL that encodes proteoglycans. J Immunol 139:863, 1987

86. Stevens RL, Razin E, Austen KF, Hein A, Caulfield JP, Seno N, Schmid K, Akiyama F: Synthesis of chondroitin sulfate E glycosaminoglycan onto p-nitrophenyl-β-D-xyloside and its localization to the secretory granules of rat serosal mast cells and mouse bone marrow-derived mast cells. J Biol Chem 258:5977, 1983

87. Tam Y-C, Chan ECS: Hyaluronidase-producing peptostreptococci associated with peridontal disease. J Dental Res 62:1009, 1983

88. Underhill CB: Naturally occurring antibodies which bind hyaluronate. Biochem Biophys Res Commun 108:1488, 1982

89. Ward JV, Packham MA: Characterization of the sulfated glycosaminoglycan on the surface and in the storage granules of rabbit platelets. Biochim Biophys Acta 583:196, 1979

90. Ward JV, Radojewski-Hutt M, Packham MA, Haslam RJ, Mustard JF: Loss of sulfated proteoglycan from the surface of rabbit platelets during adenosine-5′-diphosphate-induced aggregation. Lab Invest 35:337, 1976

91. Wasteson A: A method for the determination of the molecular weights and molecular weight distribution of chondroitin sulfate. J Chromatogr 59:87, 1971

92. Weiler J-M, Yurt RW, Fearon DT, Austen KF: Modulation of the formation of the amplification convertase of complement, C3b, Bb, by native and commercial heparin. J Exp Med 147:409, 1978

93. Wight TN: Vessel proteoglycan and thrombogenesis. Prog Haemostasis Thromb 5:1, 1982

94. Wight TN, Kinsella MG, Keating A, Singer JW: Proteoglycans in human long-term bone marrow cultures: Biochemical and ultrastructural analyses. Blood 67:1333, 1986

95. Wilson JG, Fearon DT, Stevens RL, Seno N, Austen KF: Inhibition of the function of activated properdin by squid chondroitin sulfate E glycosaminoglycan and murine bone marrow-derived mast cell chondroitin sulfate E proteoglycan. J Immunol 132:3058, 1984

96. Zanini A, Giannattasio G, Nussdorfer G, Margolis RK, Margolis RU, Meldolesi J: Molecular organization of prolactin granules. II. Characterization of glycosaminoglycans and glycoproteins of the bovine prolactin matrix. J Cell Biol 86:260, 1980

5

Congenital Abnormalities of Platelet Membrane Glycoproteins

ALAN T. NURDEN

Historically, it was the discovery of the molecular defects in platelets of patients with inherited bleeding syndromes that led to the identification of membrane glycoproteins as mediators of platelet adhesion and platelet aggregation. In this chapter, I will review the glycoprotein defects in inherited platelet syndromes. Emphasis will be placed on recent advances and several interesting patients with variant-type defects will be described. An attempt will be made to present the results in the context of interpreting the significance of membrane glycoproteins and their active sites in normal platelet function.

GLANZMANN'S THROMBASTHENIA

Glanzmann's thrombasthenia was first recognized in 1918 by Glanzmann who noted the failure of platelets to clump on a blood smear or retract a clot.[52] Classically, Glanzmann's thrombasthenia has an autosomal-recessive mode of inheritance and its occurrence is most common within ethnic groups in which consanguinity may occur. Patients generally have a normal platelet count and platelet structure. An extensive literature search was reported in the review of George and Nurden[44] who found clinical descriptions of 105 patients representing 90 families in English-language references published between 1964 and 1984. Although thrombasthenia is certainly rare, its frequency in some countries may be underestimated. For example, the diagnosis has been made in over 50 patients in the author's laboratory over the past 10 years. Bleeding is usually noted from birth and primarily occurs from small blood vessels in mucocutaneous tissues. The bleeding time is prolonged as a result of the platelet functional defect. As will be discussed, this results from the failure of thrombasthenic platelets to aggregate when stimulated. It is for this reason that Glanzmann's thrombasthenia is viewed with such interest in cell biology as a model for studies on the mechanisms of cell–cell interaction. Further background information on the clinical basis of the disease can be obtained from the reviews of Bellucci et al.,[9] George et al.,[45] and George and Nurden.[44]

Platelet Function

A key feature of Glanzmann's thrombasthenia is the absent or decreased platelet aggregation when ADP or other physiologic agonists are added to stirred, citrated platelet-rich plasma.[25] Nonetheless, thrombasthenic platelets respond to stimulation by forming pseudopodia. They are also able to secrete. Thus, primary receptors for stimuli are present in the membrane and function normally (reviewed in Nurden[100]).

Platelet Aggregation Defect

Platelet aggregation occurs through the formation of linking bonds that bind adjacent platelets together. As I shall outline, thrombasthenic platelets have a decreased ability to form these bonds. In a platelet aggregometer, the formation of large macroaggregates is primarily responsible for the optical density change that accompanies aggregation. It is this process that is defective in Glanzmann's thrombasthenia. Small clusters of platelets were noted in early studies when platelets of some patients were stirred with ADP or collagen.[25] More recently, Burgess-Wilson et al.[22] confirmed this phenomenon by electronically counting the single platelets that remained after the addition of physiologic agonists to whole blood. However, optical density tracings in a platelet aggregometer barely changed from their background level. The lack of formation of macroaggregates is a specific defect. Thus, thrombasthenic platelets are agglutinated by ristocetin, although the process has been noted to be reversible and may occur in cycles.

Platelet Interaction with Subendothelium

The lack of macroscopic platelet aggregation in vitro suggested that bleeding resulted from a defective thrombus formation in response to vessel injury. This was confirmed in studies in which blood from thrombasthenic patients was circulated over everted, de-endothelialized rabbit vessel segments (early studies are reviewed in George et al.[45] and Nurden[100]). Platelets were observed on the exposed surface as a monolayer, but thrombi were absent. Thus, the initial attachment of platelets to subendothelium was seen to occur. This further confirms the normal functioning of the GPIb receptor for von Willebrand factor (VWF) (*see* Chap. 2) and, additionally, indicates the presence of receptors for other vessel wall constituents in the thrombasthenic platelet membrane. Nonetheless, Sakariassen et al.,[130] who studied four patients, have recently shown that whereas platelet adherence in citrated blood was within the normal range at shear rates below 1000 s^{-1}, there was some decrease in adhesion at higher shear rates. Furthermore, platelet spreading, an event that follows the initial platelet attachment, was impaired at the high shear rates. These authors also noted that the absence of thrombus formation allowed an increased number of single platelets to be in contact with the vessel wall. In parallel studies, Weiss et al.,[148] who used anticoagulated and nonanticoagulated blood, also noted that the percentage of single platelets in the contact phase was increased and highlighted an abnormality of platelet spreading.

Clot Retraction

Clot retraction is often abnormal in Glanzmann's thrombasthenia. In fact, it was the functional heterogeneity in clot retraction that led Caen[23] to distinguish between two subgroups of patients. Type I thrombasthenia is characterized by a lack of platelet aggregation and a profound defect in clot retraction. In the less common type II subgroup, a lack of platelet aggregation is accompanied by a moderately defective or even normal clot retraction. Although platelets of type I patients may become trapped in a polymerizing fibrin clot, they do not form clumps or serve as foci for radiating fibrin strands.[125] The result is an inability of the platelets to organize contractile force and bring about retraction.

Discovery of the Glycoprotein IIb–IIIa Lesion

The discovery of membrane glycoprotein (GP) deficiencies in platelets in this disorder is an interesting story. My first approach to understanding the role of membrane glycoproteins in platelet function was to perform comparative studies on mammalian platelets. The logic was that if membrane glycoproteins were crucial to the role of platelets in hemostasis then glycoproteins of comparable size and abundance would be common to the platelets of all mammalian species. A fairly wide survey proved this to be so but did not give information concerning the role of the individual glycoproteins.[99,106] In 1972 I became aware of the existence of Glanzmann's thrombasthenia, and it was immediately apparent to me that the glycoproteins of thrombasthenic platelets should be studied. However, working in London, I was unable to find such a patient. A chance meeting with Dr. Simon Karpatkin (Dept. of Medicine, New York University Medical School) led to the suggestion that I contact Professor Jacques Caen at the Hôpital Saint-Louis, Paris. Professor Caen agreed to make his patients available, and this is how the initial studies on membrane glycoproteins of thrombasthenic platelets came to be performed in Paris. These early studies pointed to deficiencies in membrane GPII and III[103,104] which are now recognized as GPIIb and GPIIIa. Subsequently, it was recognized that GPIIb and GPIIIa were present in the normal platelet membrane as the heterodimeric GPIIb-IIIa complex (*see* Chap. 2). Our, and other early studies on the glycoprotein defects of thrombasthenic platelets, have been reviewed in detail by Nurden and Caen[105] and by Nurden.[100]

The Type I Subgroup

In this subgroup, GPIIb–IIIa complexes are either absent or are present in barely detectable amounts. A typical finding is illustrated in Figure 5-1. Such patients represent about 70% of those studied in Paris. As a result of this severe deficiency, the patients' platelets fail to bind monoclonal antibodies to GPIIb–IIIa complexes (Table 5-1), a property that permits a rapid screening for the disorder.[92] McGregor et al.[89] suggested that thrombasthenic platelets also contained glycoprotein deficiencies unrelated to their low content of GPIIb–IIIa complexes. For example, a high molecular mass (M_r) glycoprotein of 200 kDa was described as being absent. However, this band had now been shown to represent the GPIIIa dimer occasionally present in detergent-solubilized platelet extracts prepared for electrophoresis.[26] Overwhelming evidence suggests that the primary defect of thrombasthenic platelets concerns GPIIb–IIIa complexes.

Inheritance of the Defect

The inheritance of GPIIb–IIIa in type I thrombasthenia was studied among 20 kindred of two large gypsy families from the Strasbourg region of France.[80] Platelets from obligate heterozygotes were analyzed by crossed-immunoelectrophoresis and were shown to contain approximately 50% levels of GPIIb–IIIa. This finding was subsequently confirmed for a Norwegian family.[139] In this way, a direct link be-

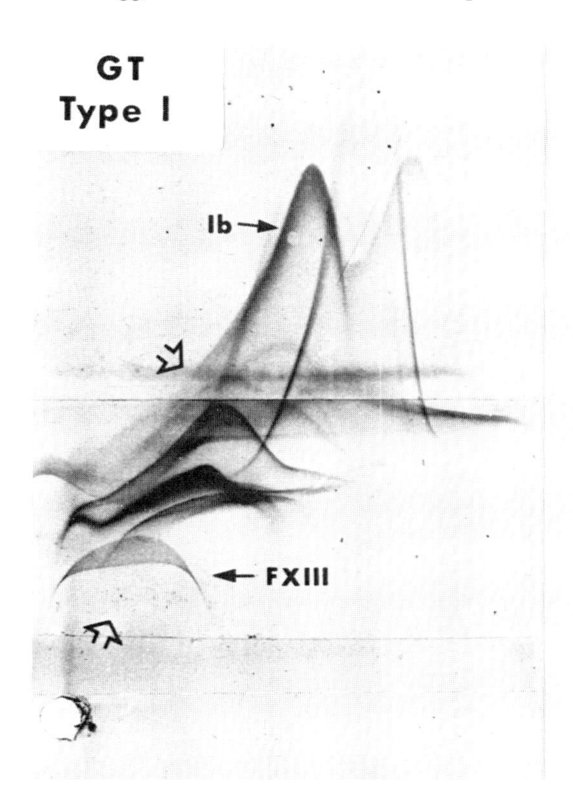

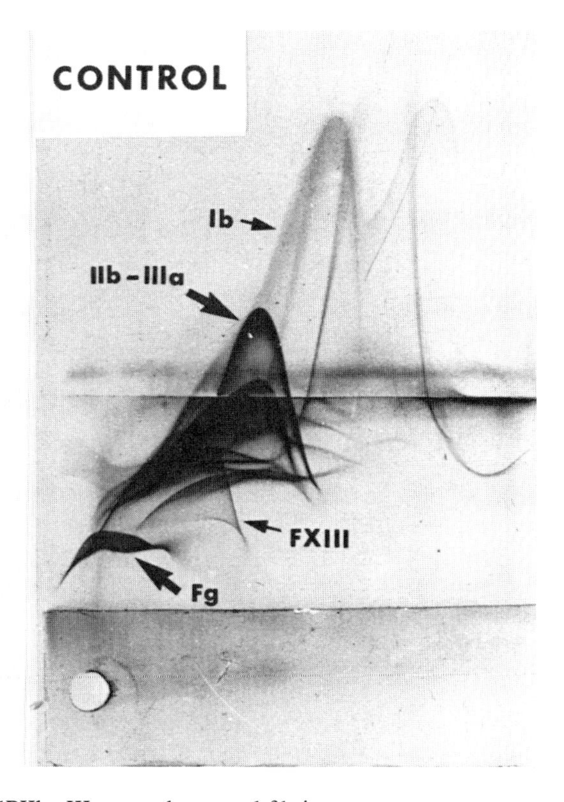

Figure 5-1. Demonstration of a severe deficiency of GPIIb–IIIa complexes and fibrinogen in the platelets of a patient with type I Glanzmann's thrombasthenia (GT) by crossed-immunoelectrophoresis. Samples of Triton X-100-soluble protein (100 μg) were electrophoresed in the second-dimension agarose gel against a rabbit antihuman platelet antibody preparation. Precipitates were located by Coomassie Blue R250 staining. Full details of the methods used were given by Hagen et al.[57] and by Kunicki et al.[80,81] Open arrows highlight the missing precipitates.

Table 5-1
Binding of the Monoclonal Antibody AP-2 to Platelets of Thrombasthenia Patients. *

Donors	Number of Binding Sites (per platelet)	Effect of EDTA†
Normal population ($n = 27$)	37,100 ± 8,600 (range 22,400–58,600)	Unchanged
Type I		
C.B.	<2%	ND‡
M.T.	<2%	ND
Type II		
J.H.	7,300	ND
M.P.	5,200	ND
Variant		
Lille I (C.M.)	38,900	2,540
Paris I (R.P.)	17,200	Unchanged

*Selected studied performed with the monoclonal antibody AP-2 using the binding assay of Pidard et al.[118]
†Incubation of platelets with 5 mM EDTA was for 30 min at room temperature.
‡ND, not determined.

tween the glycoprotein abnormalities and the inheritance of the thrombasthenic trait was established.

Binding studies with monoclonal antibodies have also been used to detect heterozygotes in Glanzmann's thrombasthenia. By using ^{125}I-labeled Tab, McEver et al.[86] showed that platelets from four patients bound less than 5% of the normal amount of antibody and those from obligate heterozygotes intermediate amounts. More recently, Coller et al.[35] have used the antibody IOE5 to test the platelets of a large number of thrombasthenics and their kindred from 19 families in Israel. The obligate carriers were found to bind 63% of the mean value for the controls. However, a feature of both of the preceding studies was the detection of an occasional normal donor whose number of antibody-binding sites fell within the range of the obligate carriers. This is something that we, too, have observed (*see* Table 5-1). It may reflect a normal variability. Alternatively, these donors may represent unsuspected heterozygotes for the disease. The frequency of carriers for thrombasthenia in a normal population has yet to be calculated. Such a finding could also be the result of a secondary defect (presence of a naturally occurring masking antibody, for example).

Nature of the Defect

As described in Chapter 2, GPIIb and GPIIIa are the products of separate genes. A key element is whether or not platelets of type I patients lack all traces of GPIIb and GPIIIa. We used polyclonal rabbit antibodies to GPIIb and GPIIIa in an immunoblot procedure able to detect trace amounts of these glycoproteins. Of the 12 type I patients so far examined, all but two have platelets with amounts of GPIIIa detectable by this procedure. The initial results were presented by Nurden et al.[108] A semiquantitative analysis of autoradiographs revealed GPIIIa levels of up to 15% of the normal amount. In contrast, GPIIb levels were lower (<3%) and the glycoprotein was often not detected. Such results imply that in the type I subgroup platelets may contain GPIIIa noncomplexed with GPIIb. They also suggest that the genetic defect may often principally concern GPIIb. It should be emphasized that of the aforementioned patients, ten were from unrelated families. Coller et al.[34] subsequently used a similar procedure to study GPIIIa in platelets of a large number of patients from Israel. No traces of GPIIIa were detected for 14 of 15 Iraqi-Jewish patients, whereas residual amounts of GPIIIa were detected in platelets of each of four Arabs. The results of this study nicely confirm the existence of biochemical heterogeneity among the type I subgroup. The fact that so many Iraqi-Jewish patients possessed platelets lacking GPIIIa should not be overinterpreted for, after generations of intramarriage, these patients could share the same genetic defect.

Platelet Immunology

The presence of residual GPIIIa in the platelets of type I patients has implications for the immunology of the platelets. As discussed in Chapter 6, GPIIb-IIIa complexes carry a number of platelet-specific alloantigens. In particular, GPIIb carries the Bak^a (Lek^a) antigen, whereas P1^{A1} is to be found on GPIIIa. Kunicki and Aster[77] first reported that thrombasthenic platelets had a defective expression of the P1^{A1} antigen. Of five patients studied, three were severely deficient and two were markedly deficient in the antigen. The degree to which P1^{A1} was decreased correlated with the amount of residual GPIIIa in the patients' platelets. Subsequently, van Leeuwen et al.[146], and then Boizard and Wautier[18], reported decreased levels of both Bak^a and P1^{A1} alloantigens in platelets in thrombasthenia. An immunofluorescent procedure, used by van Leeuwen et al.[146] showed that 11/11 patients were negative with anti-Bak^a serum and 8/11 patients negative with anti-P1^{A1} serum. The three remaining patients were weakly positive for the P1^{A1} antigen. Interestingly, these authors reported an abnormally high incidence of Bak^a negativity among family members of the patients. This suggested a close association between the gene for GPIIb synthesis and that responsible for Bak^a expression. In the past, we have examined two patients who were referred to us as P1^{A1}-positive type I Glanzmann's thrombasthenia. Immunoblotting with anti-P1^{A1} antibody confirmed that residual GPIIIa was responsible for this diagnosis (illustrated in Nurden[100]). A positive immunofluorescent test with anti-P1^{A1} antibody implies that at least some of the GPIIIa is exposed at the platelet surface.

The Type II Subgroup

In the type II subgroup, GPIIb-IIIa complexes are not lacking, but they are present in subnormal amounts. This was first shown for two French patients by Hagen et al.[57] and Kunicki et al.,[79] who measured GPIIb-IIIa complexes in Triton X-100 extracts with crossed-immunoelectrophoresis. Platelets of these patients were adjudged to contain 13% and 15% of the normal levels of the complex. Rocket immunoelectrophoresis, as first used by Kristopeit and Kunicki,[76] allows a precise measurement of the residual GPIIb-IIIa. This procedure is illustrated in Figure 5-2. A separate examina-

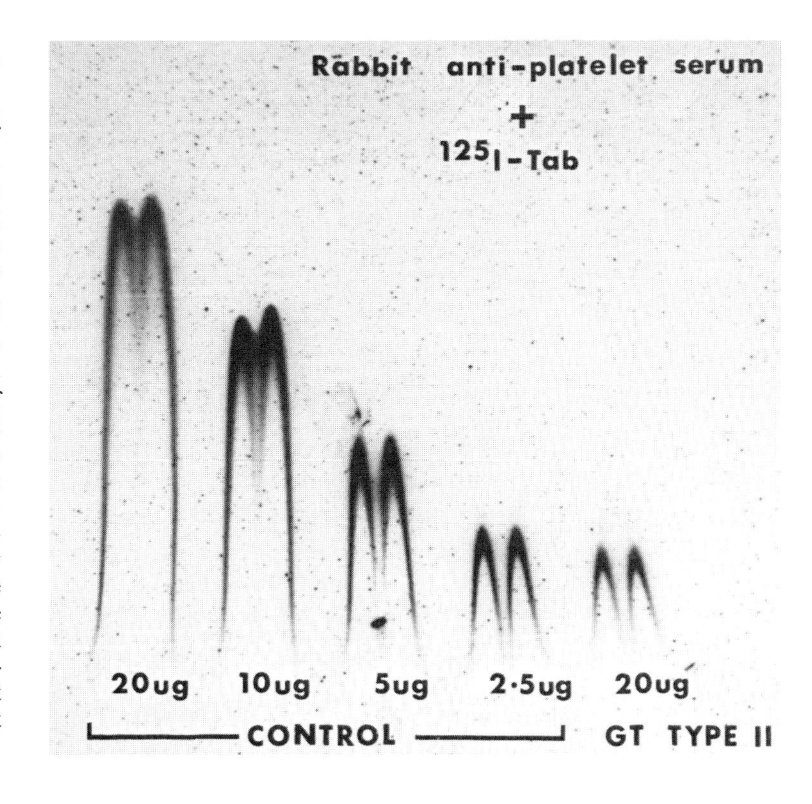

Figure 5-2. Quantitative analysis of GPIIb-IIIa complexes by electroimmunoassay. Duplicate samples (5 μl) of Triton X-100-soluble extracts of washed platelets were electrophoresed into an agarose gel containing precipitating amounts of a rabbit antihuman platelet antibody preparation to which had been added ^{125}I-labeled Tab (10^6 cpm), a monoclonal antibody to GPIIb.[86] Antigen wells contained a series of dilutions of control platelet protein and the Triton X-100-soluble extract of platelets isolated from a patient with type II Glanzmann's thrombasthenia. Procedures were as described by Kristopeit and Kunicki.[76] The autoradiograph shows the GPIIb-IIIa peaks identified by ^{125}I-Tab. This patient possessed platelets with about 10% of the normal platelet content of GPIIb-IIIa.

tion of platelets of two type II patients by immunoblotting showed GPIIb and GPIIIa to be present in the same proportion as that found in normal platelets and to have a usual migration pattern.[108]

Significant labeling when platelets of type II patients were incubated with ^{125}I during lactoperoxidase-catalyzed iodination shows that GPIIb-IIIa complexes are present in the surface membrane.[79] In our studies, the relative proportion of radioactivity incorporated into GPIIb and GPIIIa was similar to that observed with control platelets. However, others have reported a much increased labeling of GPIIb compared with GPIIIa in platelets of type II thrombasthenic patients.[98] The significance of a possible heterogeneity in the organization of GPIIb-IIIa complexes in the platelets of different type II patients is unknown. Binding studies with monoclonal antibodies enable quantitation of the GPIIb-IIIa complexes in the plasma membrane of platelets of type II patients. Results for two patients are given in Table 5-1. Flow cytometry is particularly suitable for the diagnosis of thrombasthenia and has been used to study the distribution of residual complexes in the type-II subgroup.[69,70] A low level of fluorescence was observed on all platelets, showing that the abnormality was not due to a gene deletion in a selected population of megakaryocytes. Figure 5-3 illustrates the result obtained for a typical type II patient.

The presence of small amounts of $P1^{A1}$ on the platelets of type II patients was first noted by Kunicki et al.[80] Later, Nurden[100] used an immunoblot assay to directly demonstrate Bak^a (Lek^a) antigen and $P1^{A1}$ antigen on the residual GPIIb and GPIIIa of platelets of a type II patient. These results confirm that the residual GPIIb and GPIIIa have been normally processed.

The inheritance of type II thrombasthenia was first studied by Hermann et al.[62] Among the patients examined were three whose platelets contained small amounts of GPIIb-IIIa complexes (~5%) in whom a residual capacity to undergo a limited clot retraction was apparent. The parents of each of these patients possessed platelets with intermediate levels of GPIIb-IIIa. Subsequently, Jennings et al.[69] found similar results when using flow cytometry to analyze the binding of GPIIb-IIIa-specific antibodies to platelets of members of three families with the thrombasthenia trait. Of particular interest, here, was a patient whose platelets contained 33% GPIIb-IIIa and whose father possessed platelets with 61% of the normal levels of these glycoproteins. The other parent was not examined. Recently, in collaboration with Dr. B. Schlegelberger (University of Kiel), we were able to examine the parents of a type II patient whose platelets contained 12% of the GPIIb-IIIa content of the corresponding control. Figure 5-4 illustrates that intermediate levels of GPIIb-IIIa complexes were present in the platelets of both parents and nicely illustrates how crossed-immunoelectrophoresis, in combination with a monospecific radiolabeled monoclonal antibody, can be used in quantitative studies.

Defective Binding of Adhesive Proteins

A crucial observation was made independently by Bennett and Vilaire[10] and Mustard et al.[94] who demonstrated that ADP-stimulated thrombasthenic platelets failed to bind fibrinogen. For details of how it was subsequently shown that GPIIb-IIIa complexes constitute the receptor for fibrinogen on activated platelets, the reader is referred to the reviews of Plow et al.,[122] Peerschke,[113] and Hawiger.[60] Fibrinogen has different sequences that are able to interact with GPIIb-IIIa complexes. As detailed in the preceding reviews, these consist of a dodecapeptide (γ 400-411) from the COOH-terminus of the γ chain and the Arg-Gly-Asp-Ser (RGDS) sequence that occurs at two intervals in the α chain. In type I thrombasthenia, the severe decrease of GPIIb-IIIa complexes means that neither of these interactions can occur. Typical fibrinogen-binding studies to stimulated platelets of two thrombasthenia patients are illustrated in Figure 5-5.

Fibronectin and VWF also bind to GPIIb-IIIa complexes on activated normal platelets, although their binding characteristics are not identical. For example, fibronectin binds to thrombin-stimulated platelets but not to those activated by ADP. In contrast, VWF binds to both ADP- and thrombin-stimulated platelets. RGD-containing sequences in both proteins appear to mediate this interaction.[60,122] Again, the absence of GPIIb-IIIa complexes means that thrombasthenic platelets do not bind VWF or fibronectin when stimulated by the appropriate agonist.[49,128]

Thus, in Glanzmann's thrombasthenia, the primary functional platelet defect arises

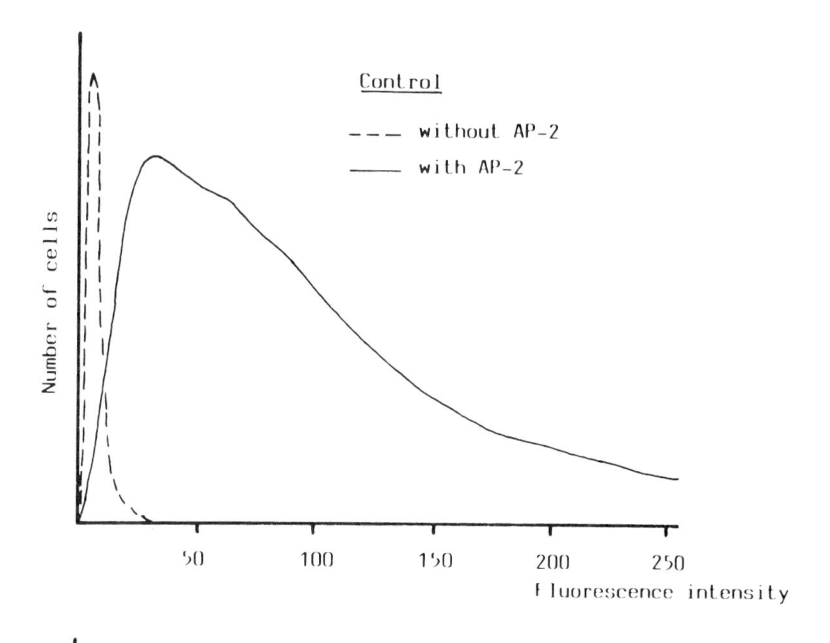

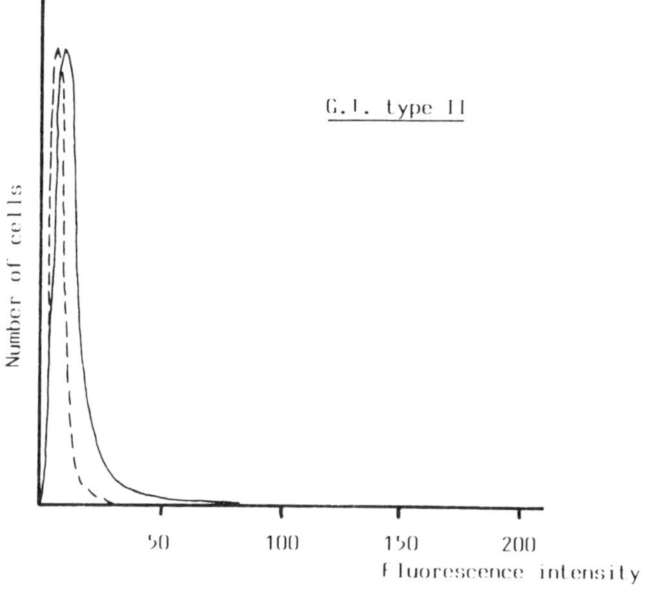

Figure 5-3. Fluorescence intensity profile of washed platelets incubated with the monoclonal antibody AP-2 followed by FITC-conjugated goat antimouse IgG. *Upper panel*, normal donor; *lower panel*, a patient with type II Glanzmann's thrombasthenia (G.T.), whose platelets were assessed at 12% of the normal platelet content of GPIIb-IIIa complexes. Quantitative measurements were made on a linear scale using an ODAM ATC 3000 flow cytometer linked to an ODAM Aspect 3000 computer.

through the failure of a family of adhesive proteins (fibrinogen, fibronectin, VWF and, perhaps, vitronectin) to interact with GPIIb-IIIa complexes on the activated platelet surface. As fibrinogen is the principal cofactor for platelet aggregation in plasma, the defective binding of fibrinogen to GPIIb-IIIa complexes is the principal cause of the aggregation defect. Here, it should be emphasized that the GPIIb-IIIa complex is an *inducible* receptor. Activation of platelets by a physiologic agonist is required for exposure of the binding epitope(s) for adhesive proteins. Other, noninducible, platelet receptors for VWF and fibronectin are present and function normally on thrombasthenic platelets. Thus, as detailed in the earlier section on the platelet aggregation defect, the GPIb-mediated attachment of platelets to bound VWF in the vessel wall proceeds normally. Furthermore, recent evidence suggests a normal functioning of the GPIc-IIa receptor for fibronectin on thrombasthenic platelets.[47,120] This

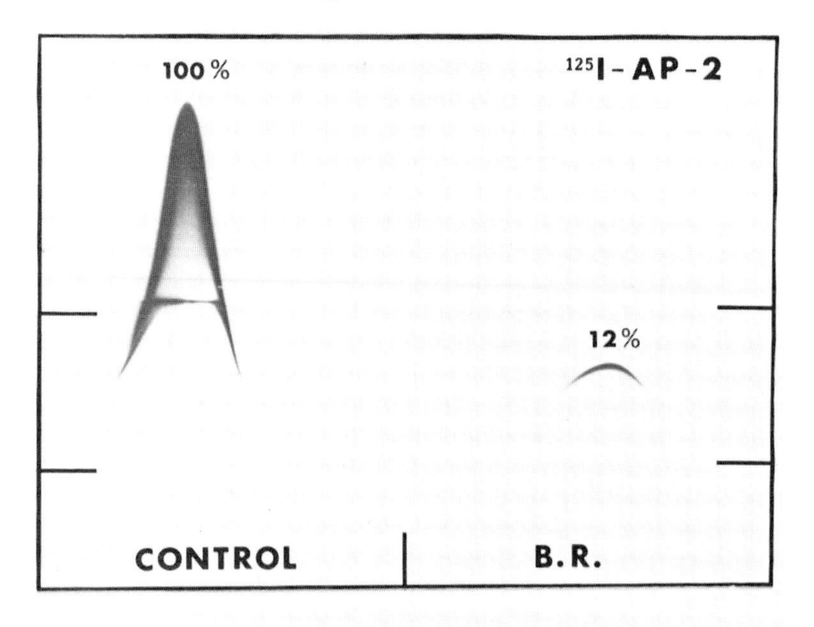

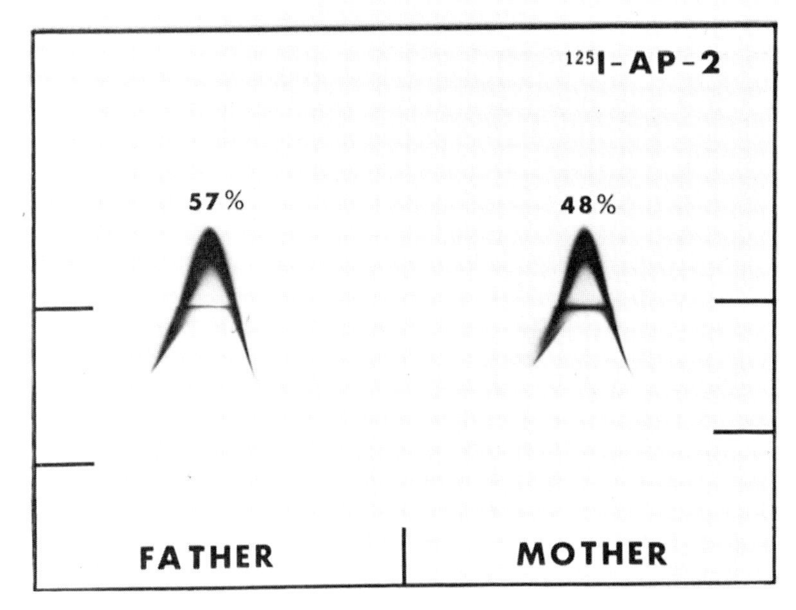

Figure 5-4. Inheritance of the membrane GPIIb-IIIa deficiency of platelets in type II Glanzmann's thrombasthenia. Triton X-100 extracts of platelets from the patient (B.R.) and from her mother and father were analyzed by crossed-immunoelectrophoresis as outlined in the legend to Figure 5-1. Here, trace amounts of ^{125}I-labeled AP-2 (10^6 cpm), a murine monoclonal antibody to GPIIb-IIIa complexes, were incorporated into the intermediate gel present in the second dimension. Additional methodology involved in using AP-2 in this way is detailed by Pidard et al.[118] Immunoprecipitates containing ^{125}I-AP-2 and, therefore, GPIIb-IIIa complexes, were revealed by autoradiography and are illustrated. Note that intermediate levels of GPIIb-IIIa were present in the platelets of both parents.

receptor attaches platelets to surface-bound fibronectin by a RGDS-dependent mechanism and, as for GPIb and VWF, platelet stimulation is not required. The normal functioning of the GPIc-IIa receptor can, therefore, account at least in part, for the attachment of thrombasthenic platelets to the vessel wall at low shear rates.[130,148]

In hemostasis, binding of VWF to GPIb is sufficient to induce platelet activation and fibrinogen receptor expression on GPIIb-IIIa complexes.[36,55] Thus, the active site(s) on GPIIb-IIIa complexes are exposed after platelet attachment to the vessel wall. The absence of GPIIb-IIIa complexes from thrombasthenic platelets therefore means that thrombus formation cannot be so initiated in this disorder. The defective platelet spreading in thrombasthenia also suggests that GPIIb-IIIa complexes participate in other stages of the platelet-vessel wall interaction.

Partial Binding to Platelets of Type II Patients

Lee et al.[82] compared the binding of fibrinogen to platelets from four patients with type I

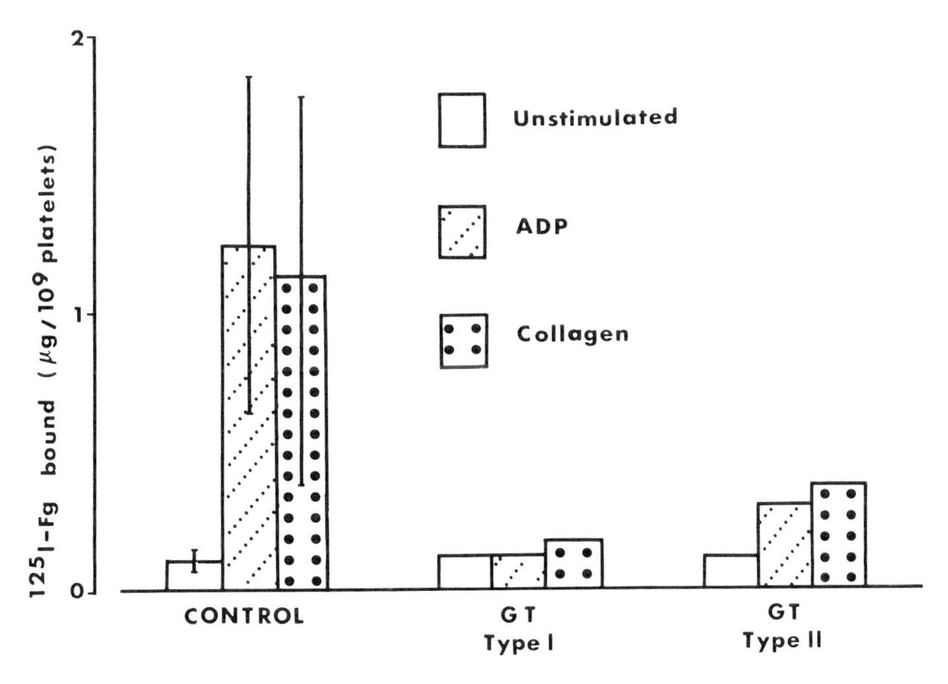

Figure 5-5. The binding of fibrinogen to stimulated platelets of patients with type I and type II Glanzmann's thrombasthenia (G.T.) Washed platelets (4×10^8/ml) were incubated with 0.1 μM ^{125}I-labeled fibrinogen at room temperature and with mild agitation in the presence of buffer (unstimulated), 10 μM ADP or 50 μg/ml type I collagen from calf skin. Fibrinogen binding was assessed after 30 min by centrifuging triplicate samples through a layer of inert oil and measuring the ^{125}I-radioactivity in the pellets. Further details are given in Legrand and Nurden[83] (adapted from Legrand and Nurden,[83] with permission).

thrombasthenia and two individuals of the type II subgroup. Platelets of the type II patients bound significant amounts of fibrinogen, although platelet aggregation did not occur. A patient with the type II subgroup was later reexamined by Legrand and Nurden.[83] The results are illustrated in Figure 5-5. With both ADP and collagen, the amount of fibrinogen that was bound was approximately 15% to 20% of the normal and paralleled the platelet content of GPIIb–IIIa complexes. This implies that the residual GPIIb–IIIa complexes in the platelets of these patients are functionally active. Their density is, however, insufficient to support platelet aggregation.

Chymotrypsin-Induced Binding of Fibrinogen

Controversy was raised when Kornecki et al.[75] reported that thrombasthenic platelets treated by chymotrypsin expressed a limited number of high-affinity binding sites for fibrinogen. These authors implied the presence of fibrinogen receptors other than those carried by GPIIb–IIIa complexes. The interest of these studies is related to the fact that when normal platelets are treated with the enzyme, the fibrinogen-binding sites become exposed and platelet aggregation occurs independently of ADP (reviewed by Peerschke).[113] Subsequent studies have now clarified the situation. Reexamination of the platelets of each patient showed residual GPIIb–IIIa complexes in those platelets aggregated by chymotrypsin.[98] Their concentration ranged from 3% to 12% of the normal value. Significantly, chymotrypsin-induced aggregation of these platelets was inhibited by monoclonal antibodies to GPIIb–IIIa complexes. A patient whose platelets were completely lacking GPIIb and GPIIIa failed to respond to chymotrypsin. Thus, this aggregation is mediated through the binding of fibrinogen to residual GPIIb–IIIa. As the platelets were not aggregated by ADP, an additional effect of chymotrypsin other than the expression of fibrinogen binding sites may be required.

Secretion and α Granule Fibrinogen Deficiency

It has been known for some time that thrombasthenic platelets may be deficient in fibrinogen. In fact, Caen[23] used platelet fibrinogen content as one of his distinguishing characteristics in defining the type I and type II subgroups. Thus, platelets of the type I patients are severely deficient in fibrinogen, whereas those of type II patients contain readily detectable amounts. This was estimated as 30% and 50% of normal levels for two French patients.[100] Of over 50 thrombasthenic patients studied in the author's laboratory, the proportion of type I to type II patients is about 7:3. Examination of the platelets of each type I patient by sodium dodecyl sulfate-polyacrylamide gel electrophoresis (SDS-PAGE) or crossed-immunoelectrophoresis always showed a severely decreased fibrinogen content, thus confirming Caen's report. Typical results for three type I and one type II patient were illustrated in Figure 12 of Nurden.[100] It was a surprise, therefore, when Karpatkin et al.[72] published a purported type I patient whose platelets contained 11.7 μg fibrinogen per milligram protein compared with 12.5 μg/mg for the control. Although this result may indicate patient heterogeneity, our results suggest that this patient is the exception to the general rule.

Secreted Fibrinogen

Immunocytochemical studies have shown that when normal platelets are stimulated with agonists, such as thrombin or collagen, platelet secretion is followed by the expression of part of the secreted fibrinogen (and other adhesive proteins) in patches on the platelet surface.[65,138] This is illustrated in Figure 5-6, by which a severely decreased surface expression of fibrinogen on the thrombin-stimulated platelets of a type I thrombasthenia patient is confirmed. Clearly, this deficiency may participate in the lack of platelet aggregation and thrombus formation observed in thrombasthenia. An interesting question is whether or not the residual fibrinogen in the platelets of type II patients is normally organized in the α granules. This appears to be so for, in preliminary studies, the platelets of two type II French patients readily secreted their residual fibrinogen when stimulated with collagen or thrombin, and part of this fibrinogen was expressed on the platelet surface.*

*Nurden AT and Legrand C: Unpublished results

Biosynthesis of Platelet Fibrinogen

The striking parallel between the absence of fibrinogen in the α granules of type I thrombasthenic platelets and their severe decrease in GPIIb-IIIa complexes suggests a role for the latter in the packaging of fibrinogen in α granules of normal platelets. One mechanism whereby this may occur is by endocytosis of plasma fibrinogen bound to GPIIb-IIIa complexes in the surface membrane of platelets or megakaryocytes. A second mechanism is through the direct synthesis of fibrinogen by megakaryocytes.[145] Although uptake by endocytosis cannot yet be excluded, structural studies favor the suggestion that platelet fibrinogen is megakaryocytic in origin.[93] Gogstad et al.[53] reported that GPIIb-IIIa complexes are a normal constituent of α-granule membranes of platelets. Their absence from these membranes, or from other intracellular membranes such as the Golgi apparatus, could result in a defective packaging of newly synthesized fibrinogen in type I thrombasthenia. Although most synthesis of platelet proteins occurs in megakaryocytes, platelets contain mRNA and are capable of a vestigial synthesis. This led Belloc et al.[7] to investigate whether or not the platelets of a patient with type I thrombasthenia possessed the capacity to synthesize fibrinogen. The patient possesses an estimated 1.05 μg fibrinogen per 10^8 platelets as compared with a normal range of 10-14 μg/10^8 platelets. In vitro metabolic-labeling experiments showed that platelets of this patient were able to synthesize fibrinogen. However, when the fate of the radioactive fibrinogen was examined, it was found to be degraded to the same extent as neosynthesized cytoplasmic proteins, whereas in control platelets less degradation had occurred. This points to a storage abnormality for fibrinogen in type I thrombasthenia. Nonetheless, it should be emphasized that the fibrinogen synthesis was not quantitated, and it is not known whether this is a major pathway in normal platelets or megakaryocytes.

Other Adhesive Proteins

Interestingly, VWF and fibronectin are normally present in the α granules of thrombasthenic platelets (discussed in Nurden[101]). This suggests that these two proteins are targeted toward α granules by mechanisms that are independent of GPIIb-IIIa complexes. Nonetheless, Ginsberg et al.[49] showed that thrombin-

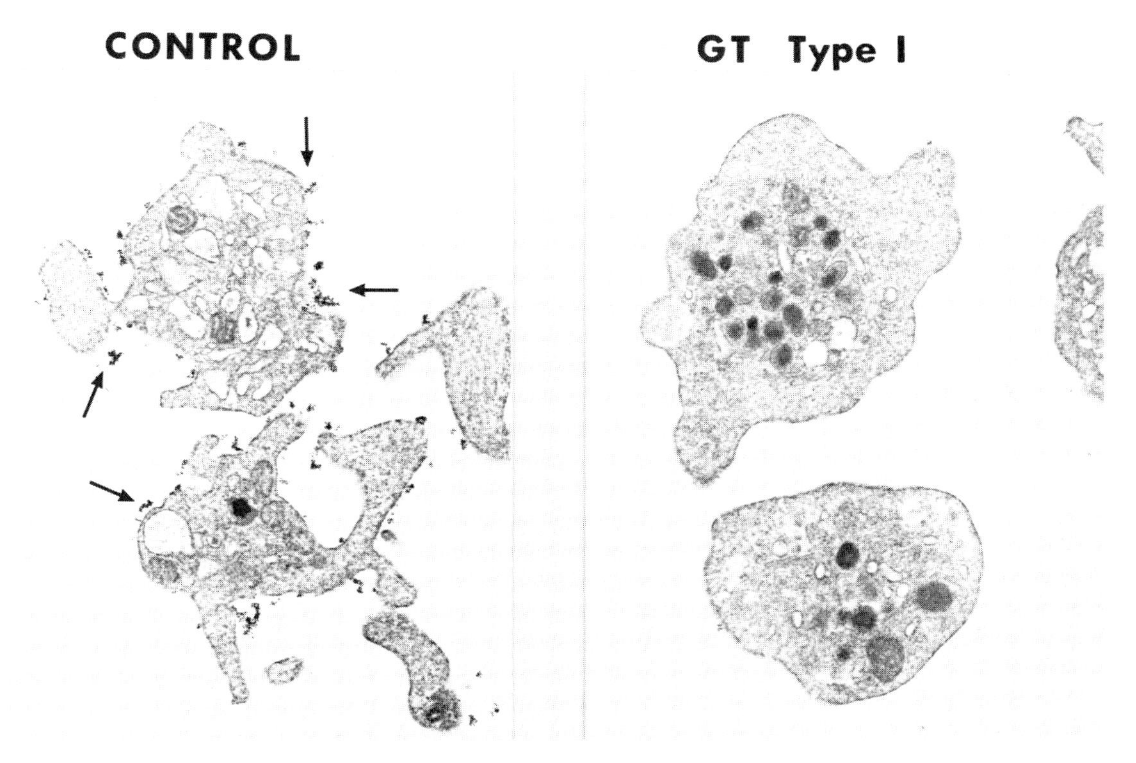

Figure 5-6. Localization of secreted fibrinogen on the surface of thrombin-stimulated normal platelets and its absence from the platelets of a patient with type I Glanzmann's thrombasthenia. Washed platelets suspended at 3×10^8/ml in a Tyrode buffer, *p*H 7.4, containing 2 mM $CaCl_2$, and 1 mM $MgCl_2$, were incubated with 0.05 U/ml thrombin for 3 min at 37°C. After glutaraldehyde fixation, the platelets were incubated with affinity-purified IgG of a rabbit antifibrinogen serum, and bound antibody was visualized using the IgG of a goat antirabbit IgG antibody coupled to 5 nm gold particles. Abundant large particle clusters located on the surface of normal platelets were rarely seen on the platelets isolated from the type I thrombasthenia patient (original magnification × 30,000; Hourdillé et al.,[65] with permission).

stimulated thrombasthenic platelets failed to express secreted fibronectin on their surface, suggesting that GPIIb–IIIa complexes normally mediate this expression.

Thrombospondin

Thrombospondin (TSP), an abundant protein of α granules, is expressed on the normal platelet surface after platelet activation by agonists such as thrombin and collagen.[6,65] Here, TSP is thought to play a role in platelet aggregation, perhaps by stabilizing the fibrinogen–GPIIb–IIIa interaction.[84] Controversy exists concerning the interaction between TSP and thrombasthenic platelets. Examination of Triton X-100 lysates of platelets of type I or type II patients by crossed-immunoelectrophoresis reveals a normal TSP content (shown in George et al.[45]) and the protein is normally secreted (Fig. 5-7). By use of a direct-binding assay and purified ^{125}I-labeled TSP, Aiken et al.[1] demonstrated normal binding to the platelets of two thrombasthenic patients. As with normal platelets, two types of binding sites were located. A low number of noninducible receptors were expressed on the unstimulated platelets of both patients (1400 and 3300, respectively). After stimulation by thrombin this number rose to 12,400 and 32,200 sites. Thus, the majority of the receptors were inducible. This result implies the presence of a receptor(s) on thrombasthenic platelets other than GPIIb–IIIa complexes.

As well as studying the binding of ^{125}I-TSP, Aiken et al.[1] studied the surface expression of secreted TSP by measuring the binding of the monoclonal antibody TSP-1 to thrombin-stimulated thrombasthenic platelets. A normal TSP

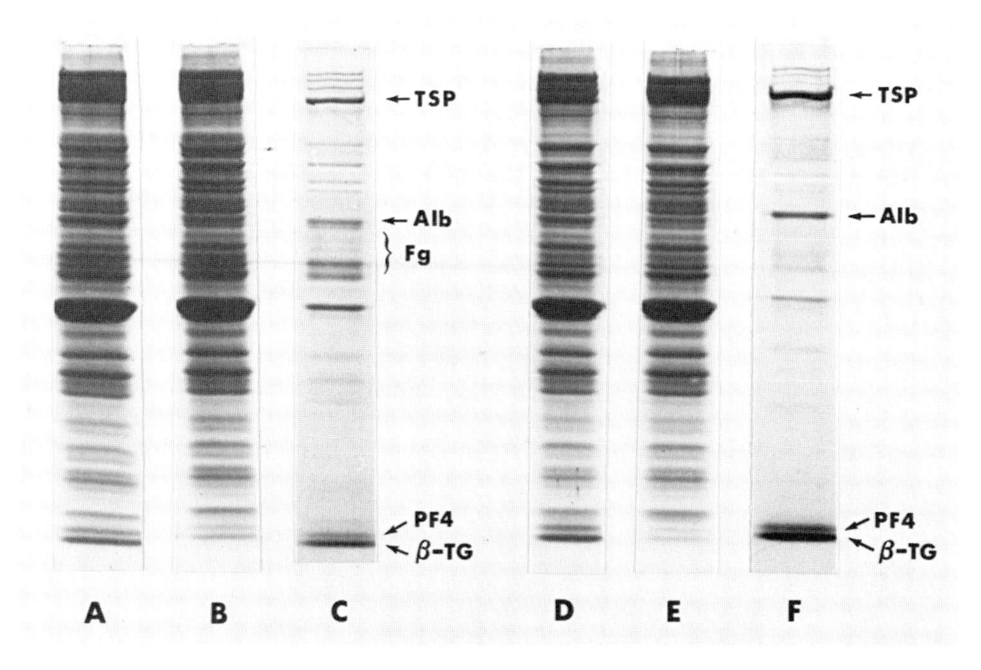

Figure 5-7. Release of α-granule proteins from washed platelets by thrombin. Platelet suspensions (10^9/ml) in Tyrode buffer containing 5 mM EDTA, pH 7.4, were incubated with thrombin (0.1 U/ml) for 5 min at 37°C. Hirudin (1 U/ml) was then added and the platelets sedimented by centrifugation. Samples of untreated or thrombin-treated platelets (100 μg protein) and of the supernatant fractions (80 μl) were incubated with SDS and 2-mercaptoethanol and electrophoresed on 7–20% gradient acrylamide slab gels as described by Hourdillé et al.[63] Proteins were visualized by Coomassie Blue R250 staining. Compared are the results obtained for normal platelets (*A–C*) and those obtained using platelets isolated from a patient with type I Glanzmann's thrombasthenia (*D–F*). Samples are: untreated platelets (*A,D*), treated platelets (*B,E*), and supernatants (*C,F*). TSP, thrombospondin; F, fibrinogen; Alb, albumin; PF4, platelet factor 4; and β-TG, β-thromboglobulin.

expression was observed. This result differed from that reported by Hourdillé et al.,[65] who used immunocytochemical procedures to compare the expression of TSP on the surface of thrombin-stimulated normal and thrombasthenic platelets. Here, TSP was visualized by electron microscopy when bound polyclonal anti-TSP antibody was located by an anti-IgG antibody adsorbed onto gold particles. Whereas TSP was located in patches on thrombin-stimulated normal platelets, thrombasthenic platelets exhibited significantly less labeling. The number of gold particle clusters was lower and their size reduced. The pattern resembled that observed on normal platelets that had been stimulated in the presence of EDTA. The presence of divalent cation-dependent and cation-independent binding sites for TSP on platelets was a feature of the studies of Aiken et al.[1,2] Although the situation requires further clarification, it appears from these studies that the binding of secreted TSP to activated platelets is largely divalent cation-dependent, provided that the concentration of TSP exceeds that required to saturate the noninducible sites that bind the protein with higher affinity. Immunocytochemical studies suggest that secreted TSP and fibrinogen colocalize on the stimulated platelet surface. Thus, a possible explanation for the results obtained by Hourdillé et al.[65] is that in the absence of GPIIb–IIIa complexes and bound fibrinogen, surface expressed TSP on thrombasthenic platelets may be more widely distributed and, therefore, less easy to visualize by immunocytochemical procedures.

One important conclusion from the preceding studies is that surface expressed TSP alone is unable to support platelet aggregation.

Patient Heterogeneity

Up to now, I have described those patients who fit into the classic pattern of thrombasthenia. Although the original classification of the type I and type II patients has been useful, it is an artificial distinction, for there is no clear division between the two subgroups. Quite simply, our studies suggest that patients range from those who lack GPIIb and GPIIIa to those whose platelets contain 20% or more of the complex. An important question is: Why are the aggregation and clot retraction mechanisms affected differently? I will speculate that this may be a function of the extent of the GPIIb-IIIa deficiency. Although the mechanism of clot retraction is unknown, it clearly involves the interaction of polymerizing fibrin with membrane receptors. Accumulating evidence suggests that GPIIb-IIIa complexes mediate the interaction of fibrin with platelets.[58] Fibrin is a much larger molecule than native fibrinogen; thus, it can cross-link dispersed residual GPIIb-IIIa complexes, which may still be able to provide an anchoring support through which platelets can effect contractile force (*see* under section on clot retraction). But, at the same concentration of receptors, fibrinogen molecules may not bind at a sufficient density to promote stable platelet-platelet linking forces.

The minimum concentration of GPIIb-IIIa complexes that can support platelet aggregation is unknown. Heterozygotes with intermediate levels of GPIIb-IIIa aggregate normally, yet platelets with 10% to 15% of the normal concentration fail to aggregate. A clue may be provided by a patient recently studied by Hardisty et al.[59] Platelets of this patient contain 25% to 50% of the normal levels of GPIIb-IIIa as determined by crossed-immunoelectrophoresis, and 12% to 20% of the normal-binding sites for monoclonal antibodies to the GPIIb-IIIa complex. In comparison with normal platelets,[151] an increased proportion of his GPIIb-IIIa complexes may be intracellular. Studies with ^{125}I-fibrinogen showed the surface-orientated complexes to be functional after platelet stimulation. Clot retraction was normal but the platelet aggregation response was slow and incomplete. This patient appears to have a platelet content of GPIIb-IIIa at the borderline of that required for platelet aggregation. Interestingly, a population of his platelets were larger than normal. When his parents were examined, his father was shown to have enlarged platelets, with a normal GPIIb-IIIa content. In contrast, his mother possessed normal-sized platelets and was an apparent heterozygote for Glanzmann's thrombasthenia. This patient may, therefore, be a double heterozygote and carry two different genetic defects.* He nicely illustrates the variability that may be encountered in this disease.

Newly Described Variants of the Disease

I have mainly considered those patients whose platelet function defects are due to a lack or decreased concentration of GPIIb-IIIa complexes. Another category of patient possesses platelets in which a functional platelet defect accompanies structural defects of the GPIIb-IIIa complexes.

The Guam Family

The first such report was by Lightsey et al.[85] who studied three members of a family from Guam. Both GPIIb and GPIIIa were normally radiolabeled with ^{125}I during lactoperoxidase-catalyzed iodination and exhibited a normal *p*I during isoelectric focusing. However, a thrombasthenia-like trait was present and the platelets failed to bind fibrinogen or fibronectin when stimulated.[49] Interestingly, both platelet aggregation and clot retraction were modified. More recent studies have confirmed the presence of a near-normal platelet content of GPIIb-IIIa complexes but a virtual absence of platelet fibrinogen.[50] Although the exact nature of the abnormality is unknown, an altered reactivity of the patients' platelets with the monoclonal antibody PMI-1, which binds to the GPIIb α chain, suggests a structural or organizational defect of GPIIb-IIIa complexes.

Variant Lille I

This patient (C.M.) belongs to a family with no previous history of a bleeding disorder. Platelet aggregation and clot retraction were defective since birth, despite the presence of a normal platelet content of GPIIb and GPIIIa.[111] This latter finding is illustrated in Figure 5-8 for

*Nurden AT and Hardisty RM: Unpublished results.

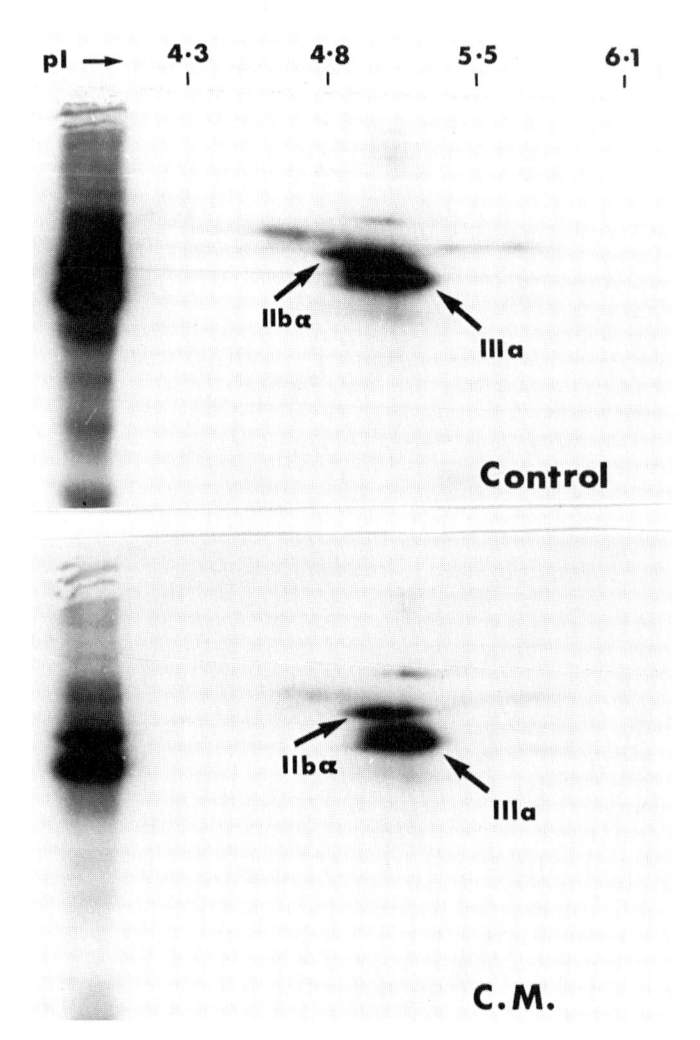

Figure 5-8. Two-dimensional electrophoresis of the ^{125}I-labeled surface proteins of normal platelets and those isolated from the Glanzmann's thrombasthenia variant Lille I (C.M.) The SDS-soluble extracts (200 μg protein) of radiolabeled platelets were made 9 M with urea and Triton X-100 was added to give a 4:1 ratio with the SDS. After first-dimension separation by isoelectric focusing, the gels were incubated with 2% SDS and 5% 2-mercaptoethanol during 1 hr at room temperature. Second-dimension separation of the reduced proteins was by SDS-PAGE using 7–12% gradient acrylamide slab gels. Typical autoradiographs obtained from dried Coomassie Blue R-250-stained slab gels are illustrated. Only those areas of the autoradiographs that show the major membrane glycoproteins are shown (Nurden et al.,[111] with permission).

platelets surface-labeled with ^{125}I by the lactoperoxidase-catalyzed procedure. However, although GPIIb–IIIa complexes were normally detected in platelets isolated in Ca^{2+}-containing buffers, the dissociated glycoproteins predominated when platelets were isolated in the presence of EDTA. This was unusual, for the dissociation of GPIIb–IIIa complexes of normal platelets by EDTA occurs at 37°C but not at room temperature.[119] An instability of the GPIIb–IIIa complexes toward divalent cation chelation was then confirmed in monoclonal antibody-binding studies (illustrated in Table 5-1). As with the Guam family, platelets from the variant totally failed to bind fibrinogen when stimulated, and secretable α-granule fibrinogen was severely decreased. Furthermore, the GPIIb–IIIa complexes failed to bind fibrinogen when platelet extracts were electrophoresed through an agarose gel containing ^{125}I-labeled fibrinogen. The fact that the complexes were unusually sensitive to dissociation with EDTA, again suggests that they have a structural or organizational defect. Our hypothesis is that this defect affects the fibrinogen-binding determinant(s) on the complex. The relationship between this defect and that present in the platelets of the Guam family remains to be elucidated. It should be noted that with both types of variant, binding sites for both the RGDS and γ 400–411 receptors on fibrinogen appear to be affected. This may mean that expression of the binding sites for both peptides requires the same conformational change in GPIIb-IIIa.

Variant Paris I

This patient (R.P.) resembles a heterozygote in that crossed-immunoelectrophoresis revealed approximately 50% of the usual level of GPIIb-IIIa complexes in his platelets.[24] Again, a lack of platelet aggregation was associated with a defective fibrinogen binding to ADP-stimulated platelets. However, the platelets of this patient were distinguished by the presence of a normal storage pool of fibrinogen. This patient is important, for such a result suggests that platelet fibrinogen is of megakaryocyte origin. Neither SDS-PAGE nor crossed-immunoelectrophoresis revealed abnormalities of GPIIb or GPIIIa, and complex formation was normal. Furthermore, the complexes bound ^{125}I-labeled fibrinogen during crossed-immunoelectrophoresis, suggesting that the defect occurs in the mechanism of exposure of the fibrinogen-binding determinants on GPIIb-IIIa during platelet activation. Recent progress shows that intracellular mediators induce fibrinogen receptor expression on GPIIb-IIIa complexes after platelet stimulation.[131] Although speculatory, this patient could possess an abnormality of an activation pathway. Interestingly, the fact that his daughter possessed platelets with similar intermediate levels of GPIIb-IIIa, without having a functional platelet defect,* suggests that this variant may have a second abnormality other than that responsible for the reduced concentration of GPIIb-IIIa complexes.

Other Variants

It is now quite apparent that the aggregation defect in Glanzmann's thrombasthenia is associated with multiple allelic mutations at the GPIIb-IIIa locus. Apart from the variants considered in the preceding discussion, others are being described. For example, a preliminary report by Fitzgerald et al.[42] highlighted a patient with 30% of the normal amount of GPIIb-IIIa, in whom the residual GPIIIa had a faster-than-normal migration. In contrast, Jung et al.[71] have characterized a Japanese girl whose platelets contain a double population of GPIIb. Relative to the amount of GPIIb in normal platelets, she possessed 35% abnormal GPIIb and 20% normal GPIIb. The abnormality was contained within the GPIIb α chain, which migrated more slowly after disulfide reduction. Interestingly, the abnormal molecule was neither incorporated in GPIIb-IIIa complexes nor exposed on the platelet surface. The authors speculated that it was related to a precursor form of GPIIb. Although the residual complexes bound fibrinogen, they were present in insufficient amounts to support platelet aggregation. A similar, but less severe defect in the platelets of the patient's father showed the defect to be inherited. Finally, mention should be made of another Japanese girl, whose platelets contained normal amounts of GPIIb-IIIa complexes, but GPIIb and GPIIIa were abnormally glycosylated.[143] This seemed to involve mannose or glucose, or both, for the glycoproteins were less reactive with the lectin concanavalin A. Such results indicate that glycosylation changes may affect the expression of the active sites of the GPIIb-IIIa complex.

Other Platelet Function Abnormalities

As reviewed previously, thrombasthenic platelets exhibit a decreased reactivity with Ca^{2+}.[101] For example, Brass and Shattil[20] showed a 92% reduction in the high-affinity-binding sites and a 63% reduction in the number of low-affinity sites. Details of the distribution of Ca^{2+}-binding sites on GPIIb-IIIa complexes of normal platelets are given in Chapter 2. Such sites are important for GPIIb-IIIa complex formation and for the binding of adhesive proteins. Brass[19] suggested that GPIIb-IIIa complexes also played a role in the control of Ca^{2+} transport across the platelet membrane. However, Powling and Hardisty[123] showed that whereas monoclonal antibodies to GPIIb-IIIa complexes affect Ca^{2+} influx into agonist-stimulated control platelets, there was a normal influx into stimulated thrombasthenic platelets. This implies that GPIIb-IIIa complexes do not directly mediate agonist-induced Ca^{2+} uptake. Nonetheless, they remain a candidate for Ca^{2+} transport by unstimulated platelets.

Rosenstein et al.[125] noted that fibrin strands are thinner and less well-developed in clots made from thrombasthenic platelet-rich plasma. This may be related to the decrease in surface-expressed platelet procoagulant activities described in early studies on thrombasthenia (reviewed in Nurden[101]). A role for

*Nurden AT, Pidard D: Unpublished observations

GPIIb-IIIa complexes in the participation of platelets in fibrinolysis is implied from the results of Miles et al.[90] These authors showed that plasminogen interacts with normal human platelets through two distinct mechanisms. Whereas unstimulated platelets bind plasminogen through a GPIIb-IIIa-dependent mechanism, fibrin formation greatly enhances binding after platelet stimulation. Thus, both unstimulated and stimulated platelets from patients with classic thrombasthenia bound markedly reduced levels of plasminogen. Interestingly, unstimulated platelets from members of the Guam family variant bound plasminogen normally, showing that the binding determinant was expressed by this abnormal GPIIb-IIIa complex. The physiologic significance of the altered procoagulant and fibrinolytic properties of thrombasthenic platelets remains to be determined.

Normal human platelets express a specific receptor for IgE and, following receptor occupancy, platelets secrete a cytotoxic activity. This was first shown for patients infected with the parasite *Schistosoma mansoni*. Interestingly, Ameison et al.[4] showed that platelets of patients with type I and type II thrombasthenia failed to bind IgE, suggesting a role for GPIIb-IIIa complexes in the expression of IgE-binding sites on normal platelets. Monocytes from the same patients normally expressed IgE receptors. Platelets from the variant Paris I normally bound IgE, suggesting that the interaction was not mediated directly by the GPIIb-IIIa complexes. It should be noted that this interaction required no prior platelet activation. The clinical significance of these findings relative to the susceptibility of thrombasthenic patients to parasite infections is unknown. This remark also applies to their recently reported inability to react with certain strains of *Streptococcus sanguis*.[134]

It has been reported by Karpatkin et al.[73] that GPIIb-IIIa complexes may mediate platelet-tumor cell interactions and, in particular, metastasis formation. It would be interesting to know if thrombasthenic patients are protected from such events.

Megakaryocytes

To explore the basis of the genetic defect(s) in Glanzmann's thrombasthenia, we have looked for GPIIb-IIIa complexes in megakaryocytes isolated from the marrow of a type I and a type II patient.* It should be emphasized that in normal human megakaryocytes GPIIb and GPIIIa are synthesized and processed into GPIIb-IIIa complexes at an early stage of their development.[39] Thus, platelets normally appear in the circulation with GPIIb-IIIa complexes already embedded in the plasma membrane. Preliminary studies on the megakaryocytes of the type I patient were reported by Hourdillé et al.[64] The cells were examined by immunofluorescent or by immunocytochemical procedures. In the immunofluorescent studies, permeabilized megakaryocytes were identified in a double-staining procedure by their positive reaction with an antibody to VWF. The GPIIb-IIIa complexes were located by using the monoclonal antibody AP-2 (*see* Table 5-1) or the human alloantibody IgGL (*see* later section on perspectives). Results obtained with AP-2 are illustrated in Figure 5-9. Whereas mature megakaryocytes and their small precursor cells from normal individuals were strongly positive with AP-2 (and IgGL), most VWF-positive cells from the Glanzmann's thrombasthenia patient were negative. Nonetheless, as shown in Figure 5-9, an occasional cell exhibited a weak fluorescence. Four cells >20 um and six cells <20 um in diameter were weakly positive among 300 cells examined. Interestingly, a subsequent reexamination of platelets of the same patient by immunofluorescent procedures revealed the occasional AP-2-positive platelet.** Because the patient had received multiple blood transfusions (although none in the past year) a highly speculative suggestion is that AP-2-positive megakaryocytes are from colonies whose origin derive from transfused cells that survive the immune response.

A preliminary report by Solberg et al.[135] described how megakaryocyte colonies, grown in vitro from committed megakaryocytic progenitor cells present in the blood of a Glanzmann's patient, did not express GPIIb or GPIIIa. Taken together, these studies suggest that the glycoprotein defect in platelets in Glanzmann's thrombasthenia does indeed arise through an altered biosynthesis in megakaryocytes. They do not, however, establish the nature of the defect.

*Studies performed in collaboration with Dr. P. Hourdillé (Hôpital Cardiologique, Bordeaux, France) and Dr. M. Pico (Hospital Vall d'Hebron, Barcelona, Spain)
**Hourdillé P, Nurden A: Unpublished data

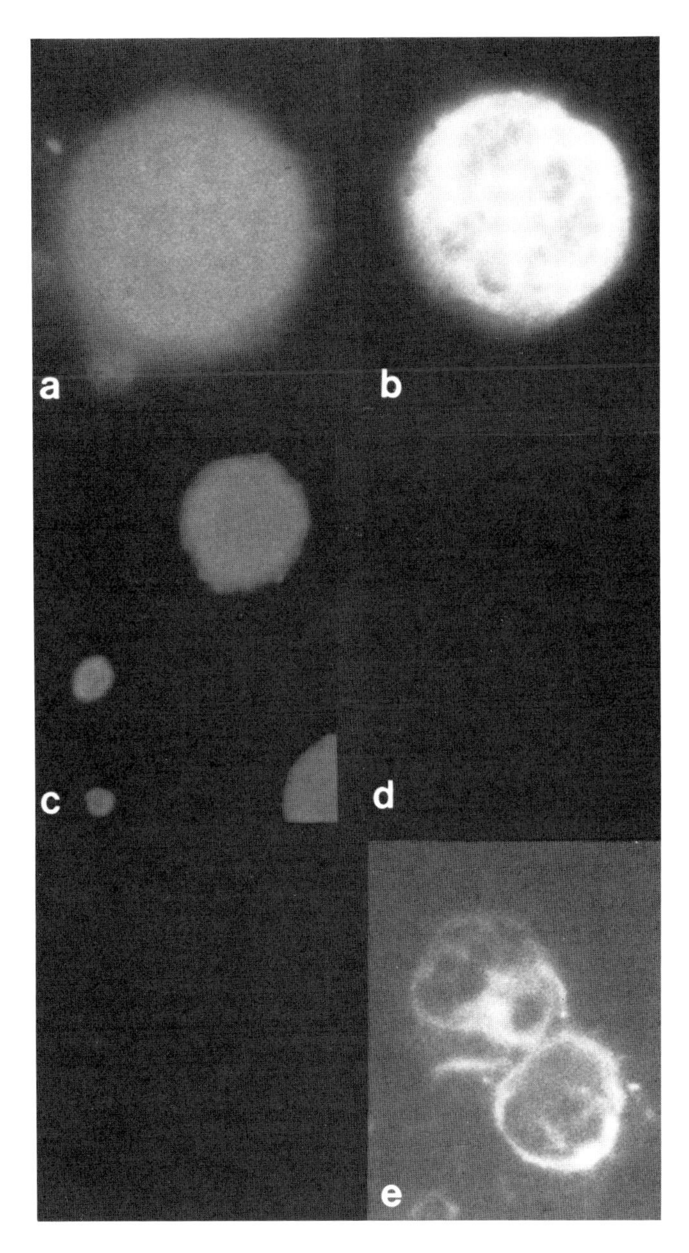

Figure 5-9. Location of GPIIb–IIIa complexes in acetone-permeabilized megakaryocytes and their precursors by immunofluorescence. Cells were double stained for VWF and GPIIb–IIIa with (1) tetramethylrhodamine (TRITC)-conjugated IgG of a goat anti-VWF antibody and (2) the monoclonal antibody AP-2 detected with fluorescein isothiocyanate (FITC)-conjugated F $(ab)'_2$ fragments of a rabbit antibody to mouse IgG. (*a*) A normal megakaryocyte recognized by anti-VWF antibody, (*b*) the same cell staining positively with AP-2, (*c*) binding of anti-VWF antibody to a mature and precursor megakaryocyte of a patient with type I Glanzmann's thrombasthenia, (*d*) the same cells failing to react with AP-2, and (*e*) weak labeling with AP-2 of an occasional megakaryocyte from the patient (Hourdillé et al.,[64] with permission).

Immunocytochemical studies combined with electron microscopy also confirmed the GPIIb–IIIa deficiency in thrombasthenic megakaryocytes.[64] Interestingly, the absence of GPIIb–IIIa complexes from demarcation membranes was not accompanied by alterations in megakaryocyte structure. Megakaryocyte maturation appears to proceed normally, suggesting that GPIIb–IIIa complexes do not play an essential role in the processes leading to platelet formation and release.

Although still at an early stage, our studies on the megakaryocytes of a type II patient suggest a general decrease in the GPIIb–IIIa content of the total population of cells.

Glycoprotein IIb–IIIa-like Analogues in Other Cells

The recent advances in our knowledge of the distribution of GPIIb–IIIa analogues in other blood cells and in various tissues has considerable implications for thrombasthenia. The reader is referred to Chapters 2, 9 and 13 for a full description of these related cell surface receptors.

Endothelial Cells

Glycoprotein IIb–IIIa-like complexes are a feature of normal endothelial cells. They have been suggested to mediate endothelial cell attachment to adhesive proteins in the extracellular matrix.[28] This receptor is both immunologically and biochemically related to the platelet GPIIb–IIIa complex. Molecular cloning and sequence data suggest that they share an identical β subunit (GPIIIa), but that the α subunit (GPIIb), although showing sequence homology, has distinct structural differences.[29,41,51] In fact, sequence data led Ginsberg et al.[51] to suggest that the GPIIb–IIIa-like complexes of endothelial cells may represent the previously identified vitronectin receptor of these cells. Recently, Giltay et al.[48] were able to culture endothelial cells from the umbilical cord vein of a newborn Glanzmann's thrombasthenia patient. This boy possessed platelets lacking GPIIb–IIIa complexes, and his mother had previously given birth to two thrombasthenic children. A monoclonal antibody, CLB-C17, directed against an epitope carried by both platelet and endothelial cell GPIIb–IIIa, bound normally to the cultured cells. Crossed-immunoelectrophoresis clearly showed that GPIIb–IIIa complexes were normally present, whereas immunoprecipitation experiments performed using lysates of metabolically—[^{35}S]methionine—labeled cells confirmed that the complex was being synthesized. Furthermore, GPIIIa of the patient's cells normally expressed the P1^{A1} antigen. These findings show that the platelet defect in Glanzmann's thrombasthenia is not automatically accompanied by an endothelial cell abnormality. Although this study needs to be repeated for other patients, a defective attachment of endothelial cells to the vessel wall would have dramatic consequences and would almost certainly be fatal.

Other Tissue Cells

There is evidence from functional testing that fibroblast-induced clot retraction is abnormal in thrombasthenia.[38] Furthermore, fibroblasts from a thrombasthenic patient have been shown to be less efficient in their ability to contract a collagen gel.[137] Although immunoprecipitation studies have shown the presence of GPIIb- and GPIIIa-related proteins in a fibroblastlike cell line,[29] it is unclear whether or not closely related glycoproteins to platelet GPIIb and GPIIIa are also present in fibroblasts of subendothelium, where the predominant receptor for the RGDS region of adhesive proteins has been characterized and is referred to as integrin.[66] Homologies are present between the α and the β subunits of fibroblast integrin and platelet GPIIb–IIIa, but they are less marked than those observed between the endothelial cell GPIIb–IIIa analogue and the platelet complex (*see* Hynes,[66] and also Chap. 13). Up to now, no studies have been reported on the membrane glycoproteins of fibroblasts of patients with Glanzmann's thrombasthenia. In view of the reported abnormalities of fibroblast function in this disorder, they would be interesting to perform.

Other Blood Cells

Initially, Gogstad et al.[54] reported that GPIIb–IIIa complexes were present in the surface membrane of normal monocytes and showed that they were deficient in monocytes isolated from patients with Glanzmann's disease. However, several authors subsequently showed that isolated monocytes were frequently contaminated with platelets or platelet fragments adsorbed to the monocyte surface (*see* Clemetson et al.[32] and discussion therein). Nonetheless, in addition to adsorbed platelet GPIIb–IIIa, it is apparent that white blood cells possess intrinsic GPIIb–IIIa related molecules in the same way as do endothelial and other tissue cells (discussed in Chap. 13). These include a set of three glycoproteins, known as LFA-1, Mac-1, and p150, 95, that are again noncovalently linked $\alpha:\beta$ heterodimers. These molecules mediate adhesion reactions of leukocytes, particularly those concerned with the inflammatory response. Being members of the same protein family, the glycoproteins have homologous α subunits and share a common β subunit. Sequence data first indicated that the α chains exhibit homologies with platelet GPIIb.[29,51] Parallel data obtained by cloning the β subunit then showed that it is also related by evolution to the β subunit of integrin and to GPIIIa.[74]

The absence of LFA-1, Mac-1, and p150,95 from leukocytes can affect several cell types and results in life-threatening bacterial infections and defects in virtually all adhesion-related functions of the cells.[40] In a preliminary report, we have described how the platelets of two such patients exhibited a normal platelet aggregation response and readily bound the monoclonal antibodies AP-2 (anti-GPIIb–IIIa) and Tab (anti-GPIIb).[119] Crossed-immunoelectrophoresis confirmed the presence of GPIIb–IIIa complexes, whereas SDS-PAGE showed a normal migration of GPIIb and GPIIIa. In the same study, monocytes from two patients with Glanzmann's thrombasthenia were shown to express LFA-1, Mac-1, and 150,95 on the surface of their lymphocytes, polymorphonuclear cells, or monocytes. Our results suggest that genetic deficiencies do not overlap between leukocyte and megakaryocyte lineages. Thus, even if GPIIb–IIIa-related analogues are coded for by a supergene family, their individual expression is under separate genetic control.

Despite the preceding findings, the situation of leukocyte abnormalities in thrombasthenia remains confused. Burns et al.[21] found that 25E11, a monoclonal antibody that binds to platelets, mononuclear cells, and neutrophils, immunoprecipitated glycoproteins of identical migration with GPIIb and GPIIIa from each type of cell. These glycoproteins were not expressed on mononuclear cells or neutrophils obtained from two thrombasthenic patients. In a parallel study, Altieri et al.[3] found that the monoclonal antibody 1OE5, which binds to platelet GPIIb–IIIa, also bound to monocytes. They further described that monocytes from two thrombasthenic patients did not bind the antibody, and that the abnormal monocytes failed to bind fibrinogen or express procoagulant activity after stimulation. Immunoprecipitation studies with [^{35}S]methionine-labeled normal monocytes showed a major band of M_r 92,000 and two other bands of M_r 116,000 and M_r 78,000 after disulfide reduction. Thus, the antigen shows clear structural differences to GPIIb–IIIa. Unfortunately, in both of the aforementioned studies the characterized antigens were not presented with respect to known leukocyte glycoproteins. Further clarification of the nature of the antigens under study is clearly required.

Clinically, I am not aware of manifestations of an altered monocyte function in Glanzmann's thrombasthenia, and most patients show no signs of an increased susceptibility to infection. Is it possible that phagocytic cells retain a capacity to synthesize platelet glycoproteins after platelet ingestion?

Acquired Thrombasthenia-like Defects

Although classic thrombasthenia is an inherited disorder, acquired defects can cause a thrombasthenia-like condition. For example, Di Minno et al.[37] described a patient with multiple myeloma and hemorrhagic tendency in whom a defective platelet aggregation resulted from the presence of a myeloma paraprotein with specificity for platelet GPIIIa. The paraprotein interfered with the binding of radiolabeled fibrinogen or VWF to stimulated normal platelets. Monoclonal paraproteins that induce hemostatic abnormalities have often been described in dysproteinemia. In another recent report, Niessner et al.[95] have described an otherwise healthy woman who developed a hemorrhagic diathesis with fluctuating clinical symptoms but without thrombocytopenia. When bleeding occurred, platelet function resembled that found in classic thrombasthenia, although platelet glycoprotein composition was normal. Although no antibody or platelet function inhibitor was evident in autologous plasma, an IgGl antibody was located bound to the patient's platelets. The eluted antibody immunoprecipitated GPIIb–IIIa complexes and inhibited ADP-induced fibrinogen binding to normal platelets. Because the patient's medical history made alloimmunization very unlikely, the hemorrhagic diathesis was interpreted as acquired thrombasthenia resulting from an anti-GPIIb–IIIa autoantibody.

The foregoing examples represent two individual cases of acquired thrombasthenia with an immunologic basis. Recently, we have located a different type of abnormality. The patient (R.D.)* had no history of bleeding until late in life when he acquired a persistent hemorrhagic condition during the development of a myeloproliferative syndrome. Platelet function-testing showed a lack of platelet aggregation with physiologic agonists, and biochemical studies revealed an absence of GPIIb–IIIa complexes and a severe decrease in platelet fibrinogen. No such modifications were noted among six family members tested. The myeloproliferative syndrome developed into acute leukemia, and the patient's death was recently reported. These modifications were associated with karyotype abnormalities of chromosome 17. An explanation for his condition is that these abnormalities affected the genes controlling the biosynthesis of GPIIb or GPIIIa, or both. Such an event would lead to a thrombasthenia-like condition. It is unknown if this has occurred in other leukemia patients.

Perspectives

I have shown how Glanzmann's thrombasthenia is a heterogeneous disorder and illustrated why it is such an interesting model for studies on cell–cell interaction. Part of this interest stems from the fact that two glycoproteins, GPIIb and GPIIIa are involved, and that thrombasthenia is one of the rare inherited disorders affecting genes of the family of adhesive protein receptors. The development of cDNA probes means that precise information concerning the genetic basis for thrombasthenia will soon be forthcoming. On the basis of the present information, gene deletions appear unlikely and, therefore, abnormalities in either the transcription of the genes for GPIIb and GPIIIa or in their postsynthetic processing are probable.

Gene therapy could be a potential treatment for the disease, for bone marrow transplantation will allow reincorporation of modified megakaryocytes. Allogeneic bone marrow transplantation has been successfully reported for one patient,[8] but it is a process full of risk. Transfusion of platelet concentrates remains the standard treatment, with the danger that the patient will develop antibodies against determinants on transfused GPIIb–IIIa complexes that are missing from his or her platelets. Such antibodies have been characterized and are useful probes of GPIIb–IIIa structure.[33,126]

BERNARD-SOULIER SYNDROME

As first described in 1948 by Bernard and Soulier,[12] the Bernard-Soulier syndrome (BSS) is a rare, hereditary disorder characterized by a prolonged bleeding time, thrombocytopenia, large platelets, defective prothrombin consumption, and severe hemorrhagic problems. The inheritance is autosomal and apparently recessive. Further information on the clinical background to the disease can be found in the reviews of Bellucci et al.[9] and George and Nurden.[44] This syndrome has become known as a disorder of platelet adhesion. As such, it is an important model for studying platelet function. At the same time, BSS has several other interesting features.

Platelet Morphology

The presence of enlarged platelets is a characteristic feature of this syndrome. They were first noted on stained peripheral blood smears. Because of their presence, BSS is often described as a "giant" platelet syndrome. Electron microscopy has confirmed the unusual platelet abnormality in BSS. For example, McGill et al.[87] collected blood directly into glutaraldehyde fixative and performed a quantitative morphometric analysis. Results showed that, on average, BSS platelets were much larger than normal and tended to be spherical. White et al.[150] described similar findings and also noted that the cells were much less resistant to deformation. Their increased deformability may contribute to the tendency of BSS platelets to spread readily on a foreign surface. Rendu et al.[124] used the mepacrine-labeling procedure to quantify the dense granule content of BSS platelets. Four patients were studied. Although a small population of normal-sized platelets was always located, each patient possessed a high proportion of cells with three or even four times the usual platelet content of dense granules (four to six granules per platelet). As reviewed by Bellucci et al.[8] and Nurden,[101] the BSS is just one of several platelet disorders in which "giant platelets" are characteristically present.

Platelet Function

Functional studies of platelets from BSS patients are often difficult to perform because thrombocytopenia is frequently severe. For example, for two patients regularly studied in Paris, typical whole blood platelet counts are 70,00 mm^2 and 30,000 mm^2, respectively (nor-

*Studies performed in collaboration with Dr. J. F. Quantara (Hôpital de Cimiez, Nice, France).

mal range 150,000–400,000 mm^2). The large platelets are also exceedingly difficult to isolate from red cells and leukocytes, and special procedures are required.[109,136]

Platelet Aggregation

The thrombocytopenia means that most studies are performed on washed platelets. The BSS platelets aggregate rapidly in response to ADP, collagen, and epinephrine, although light-transmission tracings in an aggregometer may be influenced by a reduced ability of the large platelets to contract within the aggregates. Furthermore, the more spheroid shape of many of the platelets may limit the formation of pseudopodia. Perhaps through facilitated contact, platelet aggregation may occur more rapidly than usual in this syndrome.[17] In line with a normal platelet aggregation mechanism, the binding of fibrinogen to ADP-stimulated platelets occurs normally.[114] Thus, BSS should be clearly distinguished from Glanzmann's thrombasthenia. An altered platelet reactivity with thrombin is a specific defect that will be discussed later.

As reviewed by George et al.[45] and by Nurden,[100] initial evidence for the presence of a specific platelet functional defect in BSS came from the findings that BSS platelets were not agglutinated by ristocetin, in the presence of human plasma, or by bovine VWF. This suggested a platelet membrane defect, and binding studies with ^{125}I-labeled VWF have confirmed an absent or decreased binding in the presence of ristocetin.[91,127] In contrast, and this should be clearly distinguished, the binding of VWF to thrombin-stimulated platelets and, therefore, to GPIIb–IIIa complexes, occurs normally.[129]

Interaction with Subendothelium

When blood from BSS patients is passed through a chamber containing everted de-endothelialized aorta, under conditions simulating normal blood flow, the platelets manifest decreased adhesion to the subendothelium. The defect is marked and resembles that observed in severe von Willebrands disease in which VWF is the abnormal protein (reviewed in George et al.[45] and Sixma[133]). The importance of VWF was confirmed by Olson et al.[112] who showed that, unlike normal platelets, those from BSS patients failed to bind to purified VWF coated onto a surface. Considerable evidence suggests that the defect in BSS principally involves the attachment of platelets to VWF bound in the vessel wall (reviewed in Sixma[133]). Recent studies have confirmed that the abnormal adhesion is observed at high and low shear rates and with citrated or nonanticoagulated blood.[130,148] The molecular basis of the defect is explained in the following section. Additionally, it should be noted that the thrombocytopenia may also be a contributory factor in bleeding; whereas an increased platelet size may affect transport of platelets toward the vessel wall.

Platelet Glycoprotein Analysis

After having discovered GPIIb and GPIIIa deficiencies in thrombasthenic platelets, it was logical to study patients with other functional platelet disorders. Thus, the BSS was an obvious choice and, in 1974, and again in Paris, I examined the membrane glycoproteins of two such patients. These studies pointed to a specific defect of GPI,[104] now known as GPIb. These and other early studies on membrane glycoproteins of BSS patients, have been reviewed elsewhere.[100,105]

Surface Labeling with Iodine-125

One consequence of the increased size of BSS platelets is a relative dilution of the surface membrane glycoproteins compared with intracellular α-granule and cytoplasmic proteins.[107] A typical single dimension SDS-PAGE analysis of ^{125}I-labeled BSS platelet glycoproteins is illustrated in Figure 5-10. Radiolabeling was performed under conditions designed to facilitate the detection of the membrane glycoproteins of the abnormal platelets. The pattern is additionally compared with that obtained for platelets of a patient with the May-Hegglin anomaly. In this inherited disorder, platelet size is increased similarly to that observed in the BSS, but platelet adhesion is not affected (reviewed in Nurden[101]). There is a specific absence of radiolabeling in the GPIb position of BSS platelets. This is typical of the result first reported by Nurden et al.[109] Platelet protein profiles are normal in BSS, indicating that the GPIb defect is not due to Ca^{2+}-activated pro-

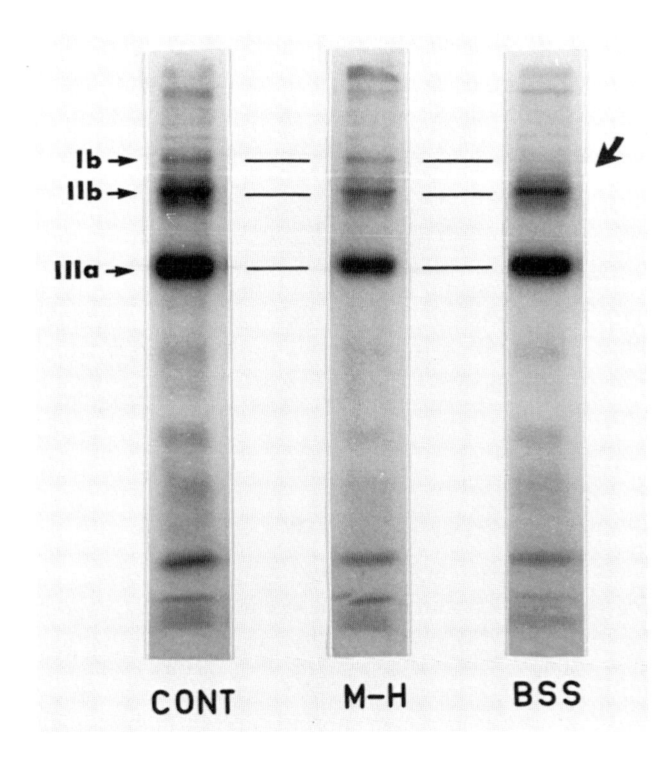

Figure 5-10. Single-dimension electrophoresis of the ^{125}I-labeled surface glycoproteins of BSS platelets. Washed normal human platelets and those from the BSS patient were isolated and their surface proteins radiolabeled as described by Nurden et al.[109] Platelets from a patient with another "giant" platelet syndrome, the May-Hegglin anomaly (M-H) were processed identically with BSS platelets. Platelets were solubilized with SDS and unreduced samples (100 μg protein) analyzed by electrophoresis on 7–12% gradient acrylamide slab gels. Autoradiographs of dried slab gels are illustrated (reproduced in part from Nurden et al.,[109] with copyright permission of the American Society for Clinical Investigation).

tease activity. It should be noted, however, that the presence of contaminating white cells in the BSS platelet suspension may lead to a substantial degradation of platelet glycoproteins by proteases released through cell lysis or after detergent solubilization.[132]

The specificity of the surface defect was confirmed by crossed-immunoelectrophoresis by which the failure to detect GPIb with immunological techniques and whole platelet lysates clearly pointed to an absence of the glycoprotein from BSS platelets.[57,79]

Surface Tritium Labeling

A major advance in our understanding of the nature of the lesion of BSS platelets resulted from the application of ^{3}H-labeling procedures to the study of platelet membrane glycoproteins. These methods involve the incorporation of ^{3}H into surface-exposed oligosaccharide chains of glycoproteins, whereas lactoperoxidase-catalyzed ^{125}I-labeling (see foregoing) incorporates ^{125}I into tyrosine or histidine residues. The ^{3}H-labeling procedure permitted the detection of previously unidentified glycoproteins. Clemetson et al.[31] analyzed ^{3}H-labeled platelets of three BSS patients using a high-resolution, two-dimensional gel electrophoresis procedure. These authors detected an absence or severe deficiency of GPIb α, GPIb β, GPV, and a low-molecular-mass glycoprotein, subsequently termed GPIX. Similar findings were reported for other patients by Nurden et al.[107] and by Berndt et al.[14] Figure 5-11 illustrates a typical pattern for BSS platelets as obtained after single-dimension SDS-PAGE. As described in Chapter 2, current evidence suggests that GPIb and GPIX exist in the normal platelet membrane as a noncovalent heterodimer complex. The organization of GPV relative to this complex remains undetermined.

Monoclonal Antibodies

The lack, or decreased concentration of GPIb–IX complexes in the surface membrane of BSS platelets means that they fail to bind monoclonal antibodies specific for epitopes carried by the complex (reviewed in Nurden[101]). The use

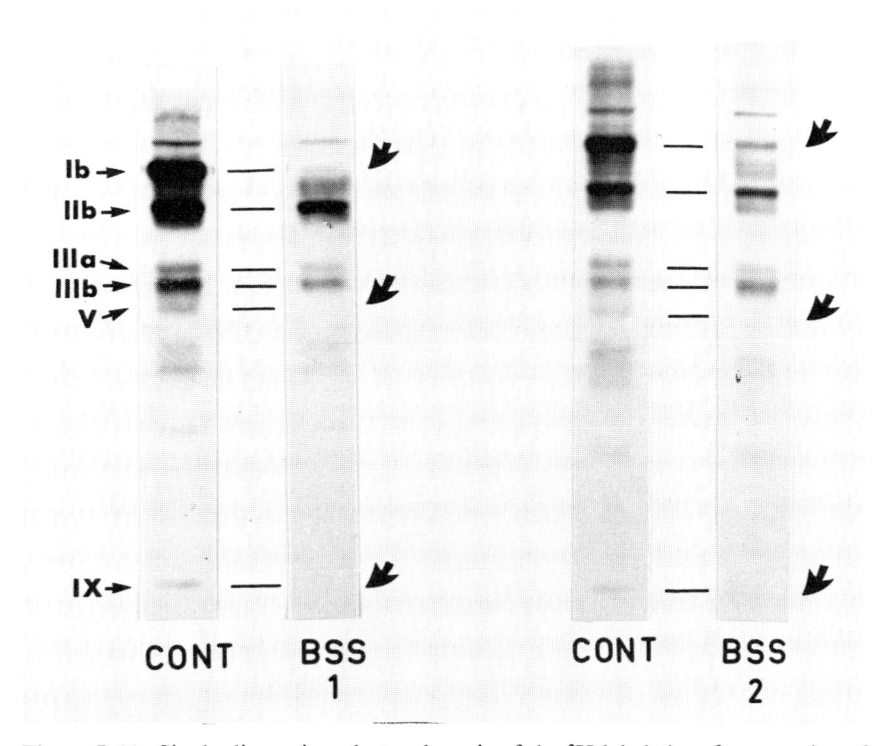

Figure 5-11. Single-dimension electrophoresis of the ^{3}H-labeled surface proteins of BSS platelets. Washed normal human platelets and those from two BSS patients were sequentially incubated with neuraminidase, galactose oxidase, and sodium [^{3}H]borohydride as described in Nurden et al.[107] Samples (100 μg protein) of the SDS-solubilized platelets were analyzed without disulfide reduction on 7–12% gradient acrylamide slab gels. The ^{3}H-labeled glycoproteins were located by fluorography. Traces of residual GPIb are revealed in the platelets of the second BSS patient.

of such antibodies in binding experiments permits the rapid diagnosis of the disorder.[92]

Functional Significance of the Glycoprotein Ib–IX Deficiency

The absence of GPIb–IX complexes, normally present as approximately 25,000 copies per platelet, constitutes a major lesion of the platelet membrane.

Receptor for von Willebrand Factor

As outlined in Chapter 2, current studies suggest that VWF binds to a determinant on the outer (40-kDa), poorly glycosylated segment of the GPIb α chain. It is the absence of this receptor that leads to the defective attachment of BSS platelets to VWF exposed in the injured vessel wall and to the failure of ristocetin to induce the agglutination of BSS platelets. In this way, the lesion is primarily responsible for the bleeding episodes experienced in this syndrome (*also see* section *Interaction with Subendothelium*).

Receptor for Thrombin

Although platelet aggregation occurs normally with most agonists in BSS (*see* section on platelet aggregation), the platelets show a reduced response to low concentrations of thrombin and exhibit a distinct lag phase before the onset of aggregation.[67] However, as illustrated in Nurden et al.,[110] it is clear that given sufficient thrombin, platelet aggregation can proceed rapidly and with a normal intensity. It is not known, as yet, how this decreased sensitivity relates to the glycoprotein lesion of BSS platelets. Jamieson and Okumura[67] showed that platelets from two BSS patients were deficient in both high- and low-affinity-binding sites for thrombin. There is general agreement that thrombin binds to at least one site on the outer part of the GPIb α chain (reviewed in Nurden[102]). This is close to, but different from, the binding determinant for VWF. This binding could be demonstrated for normal platelets by chemical cross-linking when a 200-240-kDa complex containing GPIb was located.[68,142] In both of these studies, no formation of the 200-240-kDa complex was seen when BSS platelets were used. This is important, for it reveals that even if low and previously undetected amounts of residual GPIb are present, binding of thrombin to this residual GPIb cannot be detected. As described by McGowan and Detwiler,[88] thrombin-induced platelet aggregation may involve at least two distinct activation mechanisms. The BSS platelets probably lack one of these mechanisms, and the absence of thrombin binding to GPIb could be responsible for the defective platelet aggregation response. Hydrolysis of GPV was initially thought to be a key step in the activation of human platelets by thrombin. However, as reviewed by Nurden,[101] recent evidence suggests that this is not an essential event. For example, anti-GPV antibodies block GPV hydrolysis without affecting platelet activation.[16] The significance of the absence of GPV from BSS platelets remains to be determined.

Altered Platelet Activation

In normal platelets, GPIb is thought to interact with actin-binding protein (ABP) located in the membrane cytoskeleton[43] and to have a phosphorylation site in its β subunit.[152] The significance of the absence of the interaction between GPIb and ABP in BSS platelets is unknown, but this absence may be a potential factor in determining the altered structure of the platelets. Studies on the composition and organization of the cytoskeleton in both nonactivated and activated BSS platelets would be interesting to perform. Phosphorylation of the GPIb β subunit has been shown to be stimulated when intraplatelet cyclic AMP levels are increased.[27] This phosphorylation was suggested to regulate Ca^{2+} transport across the membrane. Alternative explanations are that GPIb phosphorylation is involved in thrombin-induced platelet activation, or in controlling GPIb-ABP interactions.

Secreted Proteins

Unlike in Glanzmann's thrombasthenia (*see* earlier discussion on platelet fibrinogen content in this disorder), the absence of a membrane receptor is not associated with an α-granule protein deficiency. Thus, the secretable pool of VWF is normally present and GPIb is not involved in the targeting of this protein to α granules.[101]

Platelet Immunology

Initially, it was considered that GPIb was a platelet Fc receptor and that BSS platelets would, therefore, be deficient in this activity. However, Pfueller et al.[117] have clearly shown that BSS platelets normally express Fc receptors. Stricker et al.[141] claimed that heat-aggregated IgG bound to an M_r 210,000 glycoprotein and that this glycoprotein was missing from BSS platelets. Although high-molecular mass complexes containing GPIb have been detected after SDS-PAGE with normal platelets, a general deficiency of an M_r 210,000 glycoprotein in BSS platelets has yet to be confirmed. The significance of these observations therefore remains to be determined.

The detection of the P1[E1] alloantigen on GPIb (*see* Chap. 6) means that this alloantigen system is not expressed on BSS platelets. The platelets, however, normally express the Bak[a] and P1[A1] antigens, as would be expected from the presence of GPIIb-IIIa complexes. However, a particular feature of this syndrome is the abormal reactivity of platelets with drug-dependent antibodies. This defect is fully explained in Chapter 6. In brief, Kunicki et al.[78] were the first to show that platelets from BSS patients failed to express the antigen for quinidine- and quinine-dependent antibodies. Subsequently, the antigen was shown to be missing from BSS platelet lysates, thus suggesting that the antigen was GPIb.[81] A proposal that VWF was an additional cofactor for the formation of the immunogenic complex was made by Pfueller et al.,[116] but this has not been substantiated. In the light of recent advances, Chong et al.[30] demonstrated that a quinidine-dependent antibody specifically immunoprecipitated GPIb and GPIX from Triton X-100-soluble extracts of normal platelets. Furthermore, these authors showed that the epitope reacts with GPIX or with an epitope on GPIb that is sterically close to GPIX.[13,30] More recently, it has been claimed that GPV may also be a target antigen for such antibodies.[140]

Other Surface-Mediated Functions That Are Abnormal

In a comprehensive study of the surface properties of BSS platelets, Walsh et al.[147] reported abnormalities in the binding of coagulation factors V and VIII and found no platelet-associated factor XI activity. Intrinsic platelet coagulant activities, including platelet factor 3 (PF3), were normal or increased; yet collagen-induced coagulant activity was absent. Subsequent studies by Perret et al.[115] suggested an increased expression of phosphatidylethanolamine and phosphatidylserine on the surface of BSS platelets and the presence of a more generalized membrane perturbation. The relationship of these abnormalities, or of the GPIb-IX deficiency, to the altered prothrombin consumption, which is a characteristic of BSS, remains to be determined. Nonetheless, these findings may be of importance because Weiss et al.[149] have recently observed a much-decreased association of fibrin with those BSS platelets that remained in contact with subendothelium during perfusion experiments. This may be related to the deficiencies described here, to the decreased thrombin-binding capacity of the platelets, or to their defective binding of VWF; for VWF may react with polymerizing fibrin on the platelet surface.

Platelet Survival

As a result of their GPIb deficiency, BSS platelets have a pathologically low surface sialic acid density and decreased surface charge. For three patients studied by Grottum and Solum,[56] survival of their own platelets labeled with ^{51}Cr ranged from less than 24 hr to 2 to 3 days, instead of the 8 to 10 days that is normally observed for autologous platelets in normal subjects. This result is typical of those reported in early studies (reviewed in Bellucci et al.[9]). But, in recent studies by Heyns et al.,[61] platelet survival in four other BSS patients has been shown to vary with the degree of thrombocytopenia. One patient was extensively studied. In that case, the splenic platelet pool was normal and the intrasplenic platelet transit time prolonged. The spleen and the liver were the major sites of sequestration. Clearly, the factors controlling platelet survival in this syndrome need to be investigated further. Perhaps, as suggested by Nurden,[101] binding of antibodies to cryptic antigens may be an important factor. It should be said that interpretation of the studies of Heyns et al.[61] is handicapped by the absence of glycoprotein analysis, possibly the patient with a normal platelet count in this study was a variant of the disease.

Patient Heterogeneity

Less is known about patient heterogeneity in BSS than in Glanzmann's thrombasthenia, simply because fewer patients have been studied. For example, over a period of 10 years in Paris we have diagnosed 8 patients as compared with over 50 for thrombasthenia. Even so, results show that heterogeneity exists in the extent of the glycoprotein deletion. Thus, Clemetson et al.[31] described a patient whose platelets possessed 40% of the normal level of GPIb. Amounts of GPV and GPIX (then termed GP17) appeared similarly reduced. Low, but detectable, levels of GPIb associated with parallel deficiencies of GPV and GPIX were also described for other patients by Berndt et al.[14] and Nurden et al.[107] The presence of residual GPIb in the platelets of a BSS patient is illustrated in Figure 5-11. The functional state of the residual glycoproteins has not been investigated. Furthermore, it is not known if the detected glycoproteins are evenly distributed throughout the total platelet population. Flow cytofluorimetric analysis of the platelets of one patient studied by Johnston et al.[70] suggest that this may be the case.

Variants of the BSS with normal amounts of a functionally defective GPIb have yet to be detected. However, acquired BSS has been described. In a preliminary report, Berndt et al.[15] have described a BSS-like condition associated with a primary myelodysplastic disorder. Here, giant platelets were noted at the age of 8 and subsequent glycoprotein analysis revealed $<25\%$ of the normal amounts of the GPIb-IX complex. Marrow cytogenic studies showed the presence of monosamy 7 in all metaphases and an additional trisomy 21 in 10%. A patient with a lymphoproliferative disorder and a selective defect in ristocetin-induced platelet aggregation was reported by Stricker et al.[141] Here, an IgG antibody was characterized that bound to an M_r 210,000 protein of normal

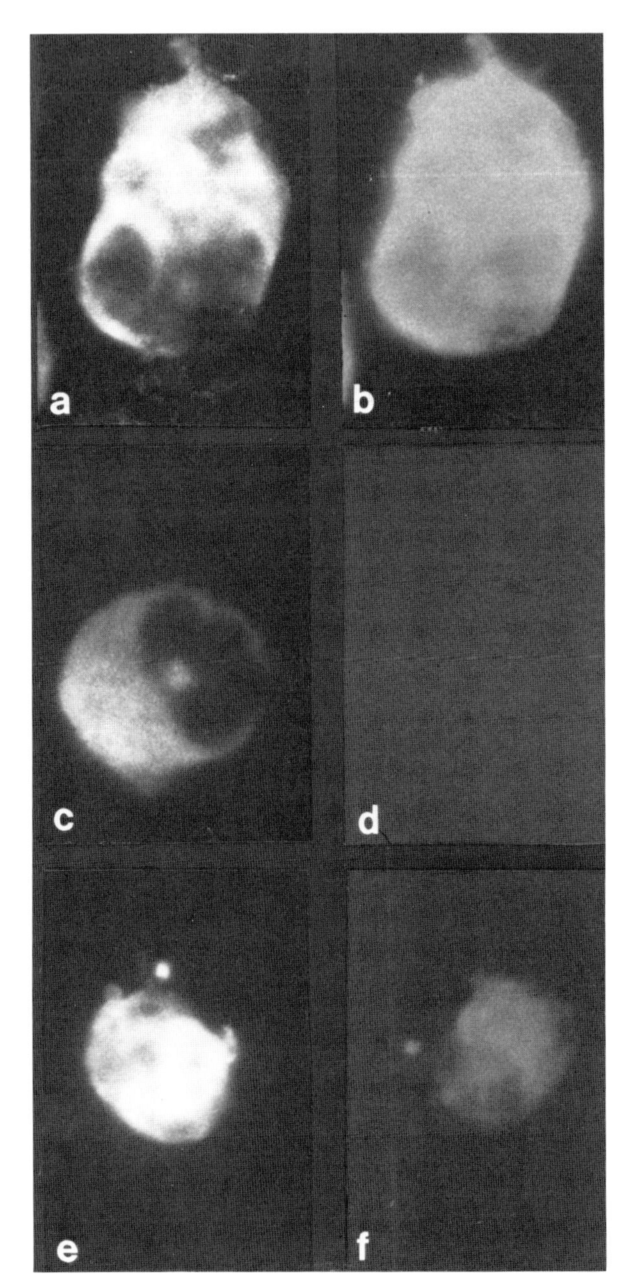

Figure 5-12. Detection of GPIb and GPIX in permeabilized megakaryocytes by immunofluorescence. Here, cells were double stained for fibrinogen and GPIb or GPIX using (1) FITC-conjugated IgG of a goat antifibrinogen antibody and (2) the murine monoclonal antibody AP-1 (anti-GPIb) or FMC 25 (anti-GPIX) detected using TRITC-conjugated F $(ab)'_2$ fragments of a rabbit antibody to mouse IgG. (*a*) A normal megakaryocyte recognized by antifibrinogen antibody, (*b*) the same cell staining positively with AP-1, (*c* and *e*) the binding of antifibrinogen antibody to megakaryocytes of a BSS patient, (*d*) the failure of BSS megakaryocytes to react with AP-1, and (*e*) the weak but positive reactivity of BSS megakaryocytes with FMC 25.

platelets that was missing in the BSS patient studied. The precise relationship of the M_r 210,000 protein with GPIb and its role in the interaction of platelets with VWF remains to be determined. Until the M_r 210,000 protein has been shown to be affected in other BSS patients, this result needs to be interpreted with caution.

Inheritance of the Defect

George et al.[46] studied two families with BSS, including four patients and three of their parents. None of the parents had experienced bleeding, and each had normal platelet counts and ristocetin-induced platelet aggregation. They possessed, however, a population of abnormally large platelets, and their platelets had intermediate levels of GPIb. Thus, both enlarged platelets and GPIb deficiency are inherited features of the disease, whereas intermediate levels of GPIb appear sufficient to support platelet adhesion. Subsequently, Berndt et al.[14] showed that obligate heterozygotes also possessed intermediate levels of GPIX; GPV was not studied.

Megakaryocytes

The megakaryocyte studies are of interest for two reasons: to explain the abnormal structure of BSS platelets; and the parallel deficiencies of three apparently structurally independent membrane glycoproteins. We have recently examined megakaryocytes obtained by sternal puncture from a typical BSS patient.* Standard electron microscopy revealed that the megakaryocytes were of normal size and had a normal granule distribution. However, a striking feature was an irregular distribution of the demarcation membranes, which often had a vacuolar appearance.[63] Similar findings were originally reported by Bernard et al.[11] We also sometimes observed large platelets fragmenting from the megakaryocytes, as if the latter were less stable than is usually observed. In immunofluorescent studies, permeabilized megakaryocytes were identified by their reactivity in a double-staining procedure with a polyclonal antibody to fibrinogen. Whereas megakaryocytes from normal individuals were strongly fluorescent with monoclonal antibodies AP-1 (anti-GPIb), AP-2 (anti-GPIIb-IIIa) and FMC 25 (anti-GPIX), those from the BSS patient were positive with AP-2, negative with AP-1, and weakly fluorescent with FMC 25. This finding is illustrated in Figure 5-12. Such preliminary results confirm a defective GPIb biosynthesis in the megakaryocytes of this BSS patient, but they also suggest that some GPIX synthesis does occur. It may be that in BSS a genetic defect of either GPIb or GPIX can account for the abnormal function, and that in the absence of one component of the complex the other glycoprotein may be degraded. As a further speculation, it is plausible that the GPIb-IX complex is necessary for the incorporation or retention of GPV in the membrane.

*Studies performed in collaboration with Dr. P. Hourdillé (Hôpital Cardiologique, Bordeaux, France) and Dr. M. Pico (Hospital Vall d'Hebron, Barcelona, Spain).

Perspectives

Unlike for GPIIb-IIIa complexes, little is known of the distribution of GPIb-like analogues in other cells, although its presence in endothelial cells has been reported.[5] For the moment, at least, BSS remains a disorder of platelets and megakaryocytes. Further studies with cDNA probes for GPIb, GPV, and GPIX will be necessary to increase our understanding of the nature of the defect. However, as with Glanzmann's thrombasthenia, there are strong indications that a variety of genetic defects can give rise to the BSS phenotype.

Transfusion of platelet concentrates remains the treatment of choice in the arrest of bleeding episodes. This provokes the risk of alloimmunization and the formation of antibodies against determinants of the GPIb-IX complex. One such antibody was characterized by Tobelem et al.[14] As with thrombasthenia, genetic engineering may hold some hope for the future. Although BSS remains a unique model for studying platelet adhesion, the rareness of the patients and the combination of a low platelet count associated with an abnormal platelet structure limit the number of studies that can be performed.

OTHER CONGENITAL DEFECTS OF PLATELET MEMBRANE GLYCOPROTEINS

It is not the purpose of this chapter to provide a comprehensive review of all inherited platelet disorders. For this the reader should consult Bellucci et al.,[9] George et al.,[45] or Nurden.[101] However, a recent discovery involving a membrane glycoprotein different from those implicated in the preceding disorders merits individual attention.

Glycoprotein Ia-Deficient Platelets

The interaction of platelets with collagen is generally considered to be of primary importance in the arrest of bleeding. Nieuwenhuis et al.[96] have recently described a patient whose platelets were totally refractory to collagen and that failed to express surface GPIa. The platelets responded normally to all other agonists tested. Collagen induced neither shape change nor aggregation in platelet-rich plasma or with washed platelets, and no breakdown of phosphatidylinositol followed the addition of this agonist. Subsequently, platelets of the same patient were confirmed to have a severe adhesion defect.[97] In particular, perfusion of the platelets across subendothelium or purified human collagen type III in an annular perfusion chamber revealed an anomaly at both low and high shear rates. Those platelets that adhered remained in the contact stage without subsequent spreading and aggregate formation. Addition of an antibody to VWF completely abolished residual adhesion at high shear rate. The results of this study point to a role for GPIa in platelet adhesion to collagen, especially that part of the mechanism which leads to platelet activation and spreading. Interest in these observations was further strengthened by the finding that GPIa is complexed with GPIIa in platelets and that the Ia-IIa complex corresponds to the VLA-2 heterodimer (VLA; very late activation antigen) present on lymphocytes and other cell types.[121] The distribution of GPIIa in the platelets of the aforementioned patient, and of the VLA-2 heterodimer in the lymphocytes of the same patient, remains to be determined.

CONCLUSIONS

Abnormalities of platelet adhesion to the subendothelium and of platelet aggregation are accompanied by a bleeding tendency. Historically, studies on the Bernard-Soulier syndrome and Glanzmann's thrombasthenia led to the identification of the key roles of GPIb and GPIIb-IIIa complexes in platelet adhesion and platelet aggregation, respectively. As a result, these disorders have come to the forefront of studies combining investigations into cell pathology and cell biology. The aim of this chapter has been to explain exactly why this is so.

REFERENCES

1. Aiken ML, Ginsberg MH, Plow EF: Identification of a new class of inducible receptors on platelets, thrombospondin interacts with platelets via a GPIIb-IIIa-independent mechanism. J Clin Invest 78:1713, 1986

2. Aiken ML, Ginsberg MM, Plow EF: Divalent cation-dependent and independent surface expression of thrombospondin on thrombin-stimulated human platelets. Blood 69:58, 1987

3. Altieri DC, Mannucci PM, Capitanio AM: Binding of fibrinogen to human monocytes. J Clin Invest 78:968, 1986

4. Ameisen JC, Joseph M, Caen JP, Kusnierz JP, Capron M, Boizard B, Wautier JL, Levy-Toledano S, Vorng H, Capron A: A role for glycoprotein IIb-IIIa complex in the binding of IgE to human platelets and platelet IgE-dependent cytotoxic functions. Br J Haematol 64:21, 1986

5. Asch AS, Fujimoto M, Adelman B, Nachman RL: An endothelial cell GP Ib-like molecule mediates von Willebrand factor binding (abstr). Circulation 74:232, 1986

6. Asch AS, Leung LLK, Polley MJ, Nachman RL: Platelet membrane topography: Colocalization of thrombospondin and fibrinogen with the glycoprotein IIb-IIIa complex. Blood 66:926, 1985

7. Belloc F, Heilmann E, Combrie R, Boisseau MR, Nurden AT: Protein synthesis and storage in human platelets: A defective storage of fibrinogen in platelets in Glanzmann's thrombasthenia. Biochim Biophys Acta 925:218, 1987

8. Bellucci S, Devergie AZ, Gluckman E, Tobelem G, Lethielleux P, Benbunan M, Schaison G, Boiron M: Complete correction of Glanzmann's thrombasthenia by allogenic bone-marrow transplantation. Br J Haematol 59:635, 1985

9. Bellucci S, Tobelem G, Caen JP: Inherited platelet disorders. Prog Hematol 131:223, 1983

10. Bennett JS, Vilaire G: Exposure of platelet fibrinogen receptors by ADP and epinephrine. J Clin Invest 64:1393, 1979

11. Bernard J, Caen J, Jeanneau C, Tichet M, Tobelem G: La dystrophie thrombocytaire hemorragipare. Acta Haematol 8:3, 1974

12. Bernard J, Soulier J-P: Sur une nouvelle variété de dystrophie thrombocytaire hémorragique congénitale. Semin Hôsp Paris 24:217, 1948

13. Berndt MC, Chong BH, Bull HA, Zola H, Castaldi PA: Molecular characterization of quinine/quinidine drug-dependent antibody platelet interaction using monoclonal antibodies. Blood 66:1292, 1985

14. Berndt MC, Gregory C, Chong BH, Zola H, Castaldi PA: Additional glycoprotein defects in Bernard-Soulier's syndrome: Confirmation of genetic basis by parental analysis. Blood 62:800, 1983

15. Berndt MC, Kabral A, Grimsley P, Watson N, Robertson TI, Bradstock KF: A variant of Ber-

nard-Soulier syndrome associated with juvenile myelodysplastic syndrome (abstr). Abstr Vol 21 Congress of the International Society of Haematology, 19 Congress of the International Society of Blood Transfusion, Sydney, Australia, p 321, 1986

16. Bienz D, Schnippering W, Clemetson KJ: Glycoprotein V is not the thrombin activation receptor on human blood platelets. Blood 68:720, 1986

17. Bithell TC, Parekh SJ, Strong RR: Platelet-function studies in the Bernard-Soulier syndrome. Ann NY Acad Sci 201:145, 1972

18. Boizard B, Wautier J-L: Lek[a], a new platelet antigen absent in Glanzmann's thrombasthenia. Vox Sang 46:47, 1984

19. Brass LF: Ca^{++} transport across the platelet plasma membrane: A role for membrane glycoprotein IIb and IIIa. J Biol Chem 260:2231, 1985

20. Brass LF, Shattil SJ: Identification and function of the high affinity binding sites for Ca^{2+} on the surface of platelets. J Clin Invest 73:626, 1984

21. Burns GF, Cosgrove L, Triglia T, Beall JA, Lopez AF, Werkmeister JA, Begley CG, Haddad AP, d'Apice AJF, Vadas MA, Cawley JC: The IIb-IIIa glycoprotein complex that mediates platelet aggregation is directly implicated in leukocyte adhesion. Cell 45:269, 1986

22. Burgess-Wilson ME, Cockbill S, Johnston GI, Heptinstall S: Platelet aggregation in whole blood from patients with Glanzmann's thrombasthenia. Blood 69:38, 1987

23. Caen JP: Glanzmann's thrombasthenia. Clin Haematol 1:383, 1972

24. Caen JP: Variant thrombasthénie Paris-I-Lariboisière. Trouble fonctionnel de l'agrégation des plaquettes humaines indépendant des glycoprotéines. CR Acad Sci Paris 300:417, 1985

25. Caen JP, Castaldi PA, Leclerc JC, Inceman S, Larrieu MJ, Probst M, Bernard J: Congenital bleeding disorders with long bleeding time and normal platelet count. I. Glanzmann's thrombasthenia (report of fifteen patients). Am J Med 41:4, 1966

26. Calvete JJ, McGregor JL, Rivas G, Gonzalez-Rodriguez J: Identification of a glycoprotein IIIa dimer in polyacrylamide gel separations of human platelet membranes. Thromb Haemostasis 58:694, 1987

27. Carroll RC: Oppositional regulation of platelet calcium flux by cAMP-mediated phosphorylation of glycoprotein Ib (abstr). Thromb Haemostasis 58:226, 1987

28. Charo IF, Bekeart LS, Phillips DR: Platelet glycoprotein IIb-IIIa-like proteins mediate endothelial cell attachment to adhesive proteins and the extracellular matrix. J Biol Chem 262:9935, 1987

29. Charo IF, Fitzgerald LA, Steiner B, Rall SC Jr, Bekeart LS, Phillips DR: Platelet glycoproteins IIb and IIIa: Evidence for a family of immunologically and structurally related glycoproteins in mammalian cells. Proc Natl Acad Sci USA 83:8351, 1986

30. Chong BH, Berndt MC, Koutts J, Castaldi PA: Quinidine-induced thrombocytopenia and leukopenia: Demonstration and characterization of distinct antiplatelet and antileukocyte antibodies. Blood 62:1218, 1983

31. Clemetson KJ, McGregor JL, James E, Dechavanne M, Luscher EF: Characterization of the platelet membrane glycoprotein abnormalities in Bernard-Soulier syndrome and comparison with normal by surface-labeling techniques and high-resolution two-dimensional gel electrophoresis. J Clin Invest 70:304, 1982

32. Clemetson KJ, McGregor JL, McEver RP, Jacques YV, Bainton DF, Domzig W, Baggiolini M: Absence of platelet membrane glycoproteins IIb/IIIa from monocytes. J Exp Med 161:972, 1985

33. Coller BS, Peerschke EI, Seligsohn U, Scudder LE, Nurden AT, Rosa JP: Studies on the binding of an alloimmune and two murine monoclonal antibodies to the platelet glycoprotein IIb-IIIa receptor. J Lab Clin Med 107:384, 1986

34. Coller BS, Seligsohn U, Little PA: Type I Glanzmann thrombasthenia patients from the Iraqi-Jewish and Arab populations in Israel can be differentiated by platelet glycoprotein IIIa immunoblot analysis. Blood 69:1696, 1987

35. Coller BS, Seligsohn U, Zivelin A, Zwang E, Lusky A, Modan M: Immunologic and biochemical characterization of homozygous and heterozygous Glanzmann thrombasthenia in the Iraqi-Jewish and Arab populations of Israel: Comparison of techniques for carrier detection. Br J Haematol 62:726, 1986

36. De Marco L, Girolami A, Zimmerman TS, Ruggeri ZM: Von Willebrand factor interaction with the glycoprotein IIb/IIIa complex. Its role in platelet function as demonstrated in patients with congenital afibrinogenemia. J Clin Invest 77:1272, 1986

37. Di Minno G, Coraggio F, Cerbone AM, Capitanio AM, Manzo C, Spina M, Scarpato P, Dattoli GMR, Mattioli PL, Mancini M: A myeloma paraprotein with specificity for platelet glycoprotein IIIa in a patient with a fatal bleeding disorder. J Clin Invest 77:157, 1986

38. Donati MB, Balconi G, Remuzzi G, Borgin R, Morasco L, de Gaetano G: Skin fibroblasts from a patient with Glanzmann's thrombasthenia do not induce fibrin clot retraction. Thromb Res 10:173, 1977

39. Duperray A, Berthier R, Chagnon E, Ryckewaert J-J, Ginsberg M, Plow E, Marguerie G: Bio-

synthesis and processing of platelet GPIIb–IIIa in human megakaryocytes. J Cell Biol 104:1665, 1987

40. Fischer A, Seger R, Durandy A, Grospierre B, Virelizier JL, Le Deist F, Griscelli C, Fischer E, Kazatchkine M, Bohler M-C, Descamps-Latscha B, Trung PH, Springer TA, Olive D, Mawas C: Deficiency of the adhesive protein complex lymphocyte function antigen 1, complement receptor type 3, glycoprotein p150,95 in a girl with recurrent bacterial infections. Effects on phagocytic cells and lymphocyte functions. J Clin Invest 76:2385, 1985

41. Fitzgerald LA, Charo IF, Phillips DR: Human and bovine endothelial cells synthesize membrane proteins similar to human platelet glycoproteins IIb and IIIa. J Biol Chem 260:10893, 1987

42. Fitzgerald LA, Chediak J, Jennings LK, Strother SV, Phillips DR: Identification of molecular variants of Glanzmann's thrombasthenia (abstr). Blood 66:289, 1985

43. Fox JEB: The platelet cytoskeleton. In Verstraete M, Vermylen J, Lijnen R, Arnout J (eds): Thrombosis and Haemostasis 1987, pp 175–225. Leuven, Leuven University Press, 1987

44. George JN, Nurden AT: Inherited disorders of the platelet membrane: Glanzmann's thrombasthenia and Bernard-Soulier syndrome. In Colman RW, Hirsh J, Marder VJ, Salzman EW (eds): Hemostasis and Thrombosis, pp 726–740, Philadelphia, JB Lippincott, 1987

45. George JN, Nurden AT, Phillips DR: Molecular defects in interactions of platelets with the vessel wall. N Engl J Med 311:1084, 1984

46. George JN, Reimann TA, Moake JL, Morgan RK, Cimo PL, Sears DA: Bernard-Soulier disease: A study of four patients and their parents. Br J Haematol 48:459, 1981

47. Giancotti FG, Languino LR, Zanetti A, Peri G, Tarone G, Dejana E: Platelets express a membrane protein complex immunologically related to the fibroblast fibronectin receptor and distinct from GP IIb/IIIa. Blood 69:1535, 1987

48. Giltay JC, Leeksma OC, Breederveld C, van Mourik JA: Normal synthesis and expression of endothelial IIb/IIIa in Glanzmann's thrombasthenia. Blood 69:809, 1987

49. Ginsberg MH, Forsyth J, Lightsey A, Chediak J, Plow EF: Reduced surface expression and binding of fibronectin by thrombin-stimulated thrombasthenic platelets. J Clin Invest 71:619, 1983

50. Ginsberg MH, Lightsey A, Kunicki TJ, Kaufmann A, Marguerie G, Plow EF: Divalent cation regulation of the surface orientation of platelet membrane glycoprotein IIb. Correlation with fibrinogen binding function and definition of a novel variant of Glanzmann's thrombasthenia. J Clin Invest 78:1103, 1986

51. Ginsberg MH, Loftus J, Ryckwaert J-J, Pierschbacher M, Pytela R, Ruoslahti E, Plow EF: Immunochemical and amino-terminal sequence comparison of two cytoadhesins indicates they contain similar or identical β subunits and distinct α subunits. J Biol Chem 262:5437, 1987

52. Glanzmann E: Hereditäre hämorrhagische thrombasthenie. Ein beitrag zür pathologie der blütplättchen. Jahr Kinderheilkd 88:113, 1918

53. Gogstad G, Hagen I, Korsmo R, Solum NO: Characterization of the proteins of isolated human platelet α-granules. Evidence for a separate α-granule pool of the glycoprotein IIb and IIIa. Biochim Biophys Acta 670:150, 1981

54. Gogstad G, Hetland O, Solum NO, Prydz H: Monocytes and platelets share the glycoproteins IIb and IIIa that are absent from both cells in Glanzmann's thrombasthenia type I. Biochem J 214:331, 1983

55. Gralnick HR, Williams SB, Coller BS: Asialo-von Willebrand factor interactions with platelets. Interdependence of glycoproteins Ib and IIb/IIIa for binding and aggregation. J Clin Invest 75:19, 1985

56. Grottum KA, Solum NO: Congenital thrombocytopenia with giant platelets: A defect in the platelet membrane. Br J Haematol 16:277, 1969

57. Hagen I, Nurden A, Bjerrum OJ, Solum NO, Caen JP: Immunochemical evidence for protein abnormalities in platelets from patients with Glanzmann's thrombasthenia and Bernard-Soulier syndrome. J Clin Invest 65:722, 1980

58. Hantgen RR, Taylor RG, Lewis JC: Platelets interact with fibrin only after activation. Blood 65:1299, 1985

59. Hardisty RM, Pannocchia A, Mahmood N, Nokes TJ, Pidard D, Bouillot C, Legrand C, Nurden AT: Partial platelet function defect in a variant of Glanzmann's thrombasthenia with intermediate levels of GP IIb/IIIa (abstr). Thromb Haemostasis 58:526, 1987

60. Hawiger J: Formation and regulation of platelet and fibrin hemostatic plug. Hum Pathol 18:111, 1987

61. Heyns A du P, Badenhorst PN, Wessels P, Pieters H, Lötter MG: Kinetics, in vivo redistribution and sites of sequestration of indium-111-labelled platelets in giant platelet syndromes. Br J Haematol 60:323, 1985

62. Herrmann FH, Meyer M, Gogstad GO, Solum NO: Glycoprotein IIb–IIIa complex in platelets of patients and heterozygotes of Glanzmann's thrombasthenia. Thromb Res 32:615, 1983

63. Hourdillé P, Belloc F, Heilmann E, Pico M, Nurden AT: Megakaryocytes from the marrow of a patient with Bernard-Soulier syndrome lacked GP

Ib and were deficient in GP IX (abstr). Thromb Haemostasis 58:476, 1987

64. Hourdillé P, Fialon P, Belloc F, Namur M, Boisseau MR, Nurden AT: Megakaryocytes from the marrow of a patient with Glanzmann's thrombasthenia lacked GP IIb-IIIa complexes. Thromb Haemostasis 56:66, 1986

65. Hourdillé P, Hasitz M, Belloc F, Nurden AT: Immunocytochemical study of the binding of fibrinogen and thrombospondin to ADP- and thrombin-stimulated human platelets. Blood 65:912, 1985

66. Hynes RO: Integrins: A family of cell surface receptors. Cell 48:549, 1987

67. Jamieson GA, Okumura T: Reduced thrombin binding and aggregation in Bernard-Soulier platelets. J Clin Invest 61:861, 1978

68. Jandrot-Perrus M, Didry D, Guillin MC, Nurden AT: Chemical cross-linking of human thrombin to platelet membrane glycoprotein Ib (abstr) Thromb Haemostasis 58:226, 1987

69. Jennings LK, Ashman RA, Wang WC, Dokter ME: Analysis of human platelet glycoproteins IIb-IIIa and Glanzmann's thrombasthenia in whole blood by flow cytometry. Blood 68:173, 1986

70. Johnston GI, Heptinstall S, Robins RA, Price MR: The expression of glycoproteins on single blood platelets from healthy individuals and from patients with congenital bleeding disorders. Biochem Biophys Res Commun 123:1091, 1984

71. Jung SM, Yoshida N, Aoki N, Tanoue K, Yamazaki H, Moroi M: Thrombasthenia with an abnormal platelet membrane GP IIb of different molecular weight. Blood 71:915, 1988

72. Karpatkin M, Howard L, Karpatkin S: Studies on the origin of platelet-associated fibrinogen. J Lab Clin Med 104:223, 1984

73. Karpatkin S, Pearlstein E, Ambrogio C, Coller BS: Role of adhesive proteins in platelet-tumor interactions in vitro and metastasis formation in vivo (abstr). Blood 68:319, 1986

74. Kishimoto TK, O'Connor K, Lee A, Roberts TM, Springer TA: Cloning of the β subunit of the leukocyte adhesion proteins: Homology to an extracellular matrix receptor defines a novel supergene family. Cell 48:681, 1987

75. Kornecki E, Niewiarowski S, Marinelli TA, Kloczewiak M: Effects of chymotrypsin and adenosine diphosphate on the exposure of fibrinogen receptors on normal human and Glanzmann's thrombasthenic platelets. J Biol Chem 256:5696, 1981

76. Kristopeit SM, Kunicki TJ: Quantitation of platelet membrane glycoproteins in Glanzmann's thrombasthenia and the Bernard-Soulier syndrome by electroimmunoassay. Throm Res 36:133, 1984

77. Kunicki TJ, Aster RH: Deletion of the platelet-specific alloantigen $P1^{A1}$ from platelets in Glanzmann's thrombasthenia. J Clin Invest 61:1225, 1978

78. Kunicki TJ, Johnson MM, Aster RH: Absence of the platelet receptor for drug-dependent antibodies in the Bernard-Soulier syndrome. J Clin Invest 62:716, 1978

79. Kunicki TJ, Nurden AT, Pidard D, Russell NR, Caen JP: Characterization of human platelet glycoprotein antigens giving rise to individual immunoprecipitates in crossed-immunoelectrophoresis. Blood 58:1190, 1981

80. Kunicki TJ, Pidard D, Cazenave JP, Nurden AT, Caen JP: Inheritance of the human platelet alloantigen $P1^{A1}$ in type I Glanzmann's thrombasthenia. J Clin Invest 67:717, 1981

81. Kunicki TJ, Russell N, Nurden AT, Aster RH, Caen JP: Further studies of the human platelet receptor for quinine- and quinidine-dependent antibodies. J Immunol 126:398, 1981

82. Lee H, Nurden AT, Thomaidis A, Caen JP: Relationship between fibrinogen binding and the platelet deficiencies in Glanzmann's thrombasthenia type I and type II. Br J Haematol 48:47, 1981

83. Legrand C, Nurden AT: Studies on platelets of patients with inherited platelet disorders suggest that collagen-induced fibrinogen binding to membrane receptors requires secreted ADP but not released α-granule proteins. Thromb Haemostasis 54:603, 1985

84. Leung LLK: Role of thrombospondin in platelet aggregation. J Clin Invest 74:1764, 1984

85. Lightsey AL, Plow EF, McMillan R, Ginsberg MH: Glanzmann's thrombasthenia in the absence of GP IIb and IIIa deficiency (abstr). Blood 58:199, 1981

86. McEver RP, Baenziger NL, Majerus PW: Isolation and quantitation of the platelet membrane glycoprotein deficient in thrombasthenia using a monoclonal antibody. J Clin Invest 66:1311, 1980

87. McGill M, Jamieson GA, Drouin J, Cho MS, Rock GA: Morphometric analysis of platelets in Bernard-Soulier syndrome. Size and configurations in patients and carriers. Thromb Haemostasis 52:37, 1984

88. McGowan EB, Detwiler TC: Modified platelet responses to thrombin. Evidence for two types of receptors or coupling mechanisms. J Biol Chem 261:739, 1986

89. McGregor JL, Clemetson KJ, James E, Greenland T, Lüscher EF, Dechavanne M: Studies on platelet glycoproteins of platelet membranes from Glanzmann's thrombasthenia. Eur J Biochem 116:379, 1984

90. Miles LA, Ginsberg MH, White JG, Plow EF: Plasminogen interacts with human platelets through

two distinct mechanisms. J Clin Invest 77:2001, 1986

91. Moake JL, Olson JD, Troll JH, Tang SS, Funicella T, Peterson DM: Binding of radioiodinated human von Willebrand factor to Bernard-Soulier, thrombasthenic and von Willebrand's disease platelets. Thromb Res 19:21, 1980

92. Montgomery RR, Kunicki TJ, Taves C, Pidard D, Corcoran M: Diagnosis of Bernard-Soulier syndrome and Glanzmann's thrombasthenia with a monoclonal assay on whole blood. J Clin Invest 71:385, 1983

93. Mosesson MW, Homandberg GA, Amrani DL: Human platelet fibrinogen gamma chain structure. Blood 63:990, 1984

94. Mustard JF, Kinlough-Rathbone RL, Packham MA, Perry DW, Harfenist EJ, Pai KRM: Comparison of fibrinogen association with normal and thrombasthenic platelets on exposure to ADP or chymotrypsin. Blood 54:987, 1979

95. Niessner H, Clemetson KJ, Panzer S, Mueller-Eckhardt C, Santoso S, Bettelheim P: Acquired thrombasthenia due to GP IIb/IIIa-specific platelet autoantibodies. Blood 68:571, 1986

96. Nieuwenhuis HK, Akkerman JWN, Houdijk WPM, Sixma JJ: Human blood platelets showing no response to collagen fail to express surface glycoprotein Ia. Nature 318:470, 1985

97. Nieuwenhuis HK, Sakariassen KS, Houdijk WPM, Nievelstein PFEM, Sixma JJ: Deficiency of platelet membrane glycoprotein Ia associated with a decreased platelet adhesion to subendothelium: A defect in platelet spreading. Blood 68:692, 1986

98. Niewiarowski S, Kornecki E Hershock D, Tuszynski GP, Bennett JS, Soria C, Soria J, Dunn F, Pidard D, Kieffer N, Nurden AT: Aggregation of chymotrypsin-treated thrombasthenic platelets is mediated by fibrinogen binding to glycoproteins IIb and IIIa. J Lab Clin Med 106:651, 1985

99. Nurden AT: Platelet macroglycopeptide. Nature 251:151, 1974

100. Nurden AT: Glycoprotein defects responsible for abnormal platelet function in inherited platelet disorders. In George JN, Nurden AT, Phillips DR (eds): Platelet Membrane Glycoproteins, pp 357-392. New York, Plenum Press, 1985

101. Nurden AT: Abnormalities of platelet glycoproteins in inherited disorders of platelet function. In MacIntyre E, Gordon J (eds): Platelets in Biology and Pathology III, pp 37-94. Amsterdam Elsevier, 1987

102. Nurden AT: Platelet membrane glycoproteins and their clinical aspects. In Verstraete M, Vermylen J, Lijnen R, Arnout J (eds): Thrombosis and Haemostasis 1987, pp 93-125, Leuven, Leuven University Press, 1987

103. Nurden AT, Caen JP: An abnormal glycoprotein pattern in three cases of Glanzmann's thrombasthenia. Br J Haematol 28:253, 1974

104. Nurden AT, Caen JP: Specific roles for platelet surface glycoproteins in platelet function. Nature 255:720, 1975

105. Nurden AT, Caen JP: The different glycoprotein abnormalities in thrombasthenic and Bernard-Soulier platelets. Semin Hematol 16:234, 1979

106. Nurden AT, Butcher PD, Hawkey CM: Comparative studies on the glycoprotein composition of mammalian platelets. Comp Biochem Physiol 56:407, 1977

107. Nurden AT, Didry D, Rosa JP: Molecular defects of platelets in Bernard-Soulier syndrome. Blood Cells 9:333, 1983

108. Nurden AT, Didry D, Kieffer N, McEver RP: Trace amounts of glycoproteins IIb and IIIa may be present in the platelets of most patients with Glanzmann's thrombasthenia. Blood 65:1021, 1985

109. Nurden AT, Dupuis D, Kunicki TJ, Caen JP: Analysis of the glycoprotein and protein composition of Bernard-Soulier platelets by single and two-dimensional SDS-polyacrylamide gel electrophoresis. J Clin Invest 67:1431, 1981

110. Nurden AT, George JN, Phillips DR: Human platelet membrane glycoproteins. In Shuman M, Phillips DR (eds): Biochemistry of the Platelet, pp 159-224, New York, Academic Press, 1986

111. Nurden AT, Rosa J-P, Fournier D, Legrand C, Didry D, Parquet A, Pidard D: A variant of Glanzmann's thrombasthenia with abnormal glycoprotein IIb-IIIa complexes in the platelet membrane. J Clin Invest 79:962, 1987

112. Olson JD, Moake JL, Collins MF, Michael BS: Adhesion of human platelets to purified solid-phase von Willebrand factor: Studies of normal and Bernard-Soulier platelets. Thromb Res 32:115, 1983

113. Peerschke EIB: The platelet fibrinogen receptor. Semin Hematol 22:241, 1985

114. Peerschke EIB, Zucker MB, Grant RA, Egan JJ, Johnson MM: Correlation between fibrinogen binding to human platelets and platelet aggregability. Blood 55:841, 1980

115. Perret B, Levy-Toledano S, Plantavid M, Bredoux R, Chap H, Tobelem G, Douste-Blazy L, Caen JP: Anbormal phospholipid organization in Bernard-Soulier platelets. Thromb Res 31:529, 1983

116. Pfueller SL, Hosseinzadeh PK, Firkin BG: Quinine- and quinidine-dependent antibodies. Requirement of factor VIII-related antigen for platelet damage and for in vitro transformation of lymphocytes from patients with drug-induced thrombocytopenia. J Clin Invest 67:907, 1981

117. Pfueller SL, Kerlero de Rosbo N, Bilston RA: Platelets deficient in glycoprotein I have normal Fc receptor expression. Br J Haematol 56:607, 1983

118. Pidard D, Didry D, Kunicki TJ, Nurden AT: Temperature-dependent effects of EDTA on the membrane glycoprotein IIb–IIIa complex and platelet aggreability. Blood 67:604, 1986

119. Pidard D, Fischer A, Bouillot C, Ledeist F, Nurden AT: Inherited deficiencies can affect separately the platelet membrane glycoprotein IIb–IIIa complex and the leukocyte LFA-1, Mac-1 and p150,95 complexes (abstr) Thromb Haemostasis 58:244, 1987

120. Piotrowicz RS, Yamada KM, Kunicki TJ: Human platelet glycoprotein Ic-IIa is an activation-independent fibronectin receptor (abstr). Thromb Haemostasis 58:304, 1987

121. Pischel KD, Bluestein HG, Woods VL Jr: Platelet glycoproteins Ia, Ic, and IIa are identical to the VLA adhesion related proteins of lymphocytes and other cell types. J Clin Invest 81:505, 1988

122. Plow EF, Ginsberg MH, Marguerie GA: Expression and function of adhesive proteins on the platelet surface. In Phillips DR, Shuman MA (eds): Biochemistry of Platelets, pp 225–256. New York, Academic Press, 1986

123. Powling MJ, Hardisty RM: Glycoprotein IIb–IIIa complex and Ca^{2+} influx into stimulated platelets. Blood 66:731, 1985

124. Rendu FR, Nurden AT, Lebret M, Caen JP: Further investigations on Bernard-Soulier platelet abnormalities: A study of 5-HT uptake and mepacrine fluorescence. J Lab Clin Med 92:689, 1981

125. Rosenstein R, Zacharski LR, Allen RD: Quantitation of human platelet transformation on siliconized glass: Comparison of "normal" and "abnormal" platelets. Thromb Haemostasis 46:521, 1981

126. Rosa J-P, Kieffer N, Didry D, Pidard D, Kunicki TJ, Nurden AT: The human platelet membrane glycoprotein complex GP IIb–IIIa expresses antigenic sites not exposed on the dissociated glycoproteins. Blood 64:1246, 1984

127. Ruan C, Tobelem G, Caen JP: Liaison du facteur VIII/Willebrand aux plaquettes de syndrome de Bernard-Soulier et de thrombasthénie de Glanzmann. Nouv Rev Fr Hématol 23:89, 1981

128. Ruggeri ZM, Bader R, De Marco L: Glanzmann thrombasthenia: Deficient binding of von Willebrand factor to thrombin-stimulated platelets. Proc Natl Acad Sci USA 79:6038, 1982

129. Ruggeri ZM, De Marco L, Gatti L, Bader R, Montgomery RR: Platelets have more than one binding site for von Willebrand factor. J Clin Invest 72:1, 1983

130. Sakariassen KB, Nievelstein FEM, Coller BS, Sixma JJ: The role of platelet membrane glycoproteins Ib and IIb–IIIa in platelet adherence to human artery subendothelium. Br J Haematol 63:681, 1986

131. Shattil SJ, Brass LF: Induction of the fibrinogen receptor on human platelets by intracellular mediators. J Biol Chem 262:992, 1987

132. Shulman S, Wiesner R, Troll W, Karpatkin S: Reevaluation of the presence of the major antigen Ca^{++} complex in Bernard-Soulier syndrome platelets. Thromb Res 30:61, 1983

133. Sixma JJ: Platelet adhesion in health and disease. In Verstraete M, Vermylen J, Lijnen R, Arnout J (eds): Thrombosis and Haemostasis 1987, pp 127–146. Leuven, Leuven University Press, 1987

134. Soberay AH, Herzberg MC, Rudney JD, Nieuwenhuis HK, Sixma JJ, Seligsohn U: Responses of platelets to strains of *Streptococcus sanguis*: Findings in healthy subjects, Bernard-Soulier, Glanzmann's and collagen-unresponsive patients. Thromb Haemostasis 57:222, 1987

135. Solberg LA, Oles KJ, Kaese SE, Gilchrist GS, Burgert EO, Mann KG, Nichols WL: Aberrant megakaryocytic/platelet antigen expression in congenital and acquired disorders (abstr). Thromb Haemostasis 54:278, 1985

136. Solum NO, Hagen I, Gjemdal T: Platelet membrane glycoproteins and the interaction between bovine factor VIII related protein and human platelets. Thromb Res 38:914, 1977

137. Steinberg BM, Smith K, Colozzo M, Pollack R: Establishment and transformation diminish the ability of fibroblasts to contract a native collagen gel. J Cell Biol 87:304, 1980

138. Stenberg PE, Shuman MA, Levine SP, Bainton DF: Redistribution of alpha granules and their contents in thrombin-stimulated platelets. J Cell Biol 98:748, 1984

139. Stormorken H, Gogstad GO, Solum NO, Pande M: Diagnosis of heterozygotes in Glanzmann's thrombasthenia. Thromb Haemostasis 48:217, 1982

140. Stricker RB, Shuman MA: Quinidine purpura: Evidence that glycoprotein V is a target platelet antigen. Blood 67:1377, 1986

141. Stricker RB, Wong D, Saks SR, Corash L, Shuman MA: Acquired Bernard-Soulier syndrome. Evidence for the role of a 210,000-molecular weight protein in the interaction of platelets with von Willebrand factor. J Clin Invest 76:1274, 1985

142. Takamatsu J, Horne MK III, Gralnick HR: Identification of the thrombin receptor on human platelets by chemical crosslinking. J Clin Invest 77:362, 1986

143. Tanoue K, Hasegawa S, Yamaguchi A, Yamamoto N, Yamazaki H: A new variant of thrombasthenia with abnormally glycosylated GP IIb/IIIa. Thromb Res 47:323, 1987

144. Tobelem G, Levy-Toledano S, Bredoux R, Michel H, Nurden A, Caen JP, Degos L: New approach to determination of specific functions of platelet membrane sites. Nature 263:427, 1976

145. Uzan G, Courtois G, Stanckovic Z, Crabtree GR, Marguerie G: Expression of the fibrinogen genes in rat megakaryocytes. Biochem Biophys Res Commun 140:543, 1986

146. von Leeuwen EF, von dem Borne AEG Kr, von Riesz LE, Nijenhuis LE, Engelfriet CP: Absence of platelet-specific alloantigens in Glanzmann's thrombasthenia. Blood 57:49, 1981

147. Walsh PN, Mills DCB, Pareti FI, Stewart GJ, Macfarlane DE, Johnson MM, Egan JJ: Hereditary giant platelet syndrome. Absence of collagen-induced coagulant activity and deficiency of factor XI binding to platelets. Br J Haematol 29:639, 1985

148. Weiss HJ, Turitto VT, Baumgartner HR: Platelet adhesion and thrombus formation on subendothelium in platelets deficient in glycoproteins IIb–IIIa, Ib and storage granules. Blood 67:322, 1986

149. Weiss HJ, Turitto VT, Baumgartner HR: Role of shear rate and platelets in promoting fibrin formation on rabbit subendothelium. Studies utilizing patients with quantitative and qualitative platelet defects. J Clin Invest 78:1072, 1986

150. White JG, Burris SM, Hasegawa D, Johnson M: Micropipette aspiration of human blood platelets. A defect in Bernard-Soulier's syndrome. Blood 63:1249, 1984

151. Woods VL, Wolff LE, Keller DM: Resting platelets contain a substantial centrally located pool of glycoprotein IIb–IIIa complex which may be accessible to some but not other extracellular proteins. J Biol Chem 261:15242, 1986

152. Wyler B, Bienz D, Clemetson KJ, Lüscher EF: Glycoprotein Ib is the only phosphorylated major membrane glycoprotein in human platelets. Biochem J 234:373, 1986

Part Three Antigenic Profile of the Platelet Plasma Membrane

6

Biochemistry of Platelet-Associated Isoantigens and Alloantigens

THOMAS J. KUNICKI

Platelet membrane glycoproteins play an important role in the immunology of the platelet both as specific immune receptors and as highly immunogenic targets. A comprehensive review of the biochemistry and physiology of these glycoproteins is provided in Chapters 2 and 5, and only salient aspects of their structure/function that are relevant to their immunogenicity will be summarized here.

The platelet membrane contains a number of highly disulfide-bonded glycoproteins (Table 6-1). These can be subdivided into two groups based upon gross structural characteristics. Members of the first group, including GPIb, GPIc and GPIIb, are composed of larger subunits, or α chains, that are disulfide-bonded to smaller subunits called β chains. Glycoproteins, such as GPIb, would be expected to dissociate upon reduction, generating two subunits whose relative molecular masses (M_r) are each smaller than the parent molecule. Members of the second group, represented by GPIa, GPIIa, and GPIIIa, are composed of a single polypeptide chain containing several intrachain disulfide bonds. The M_rs of these glycoproteins appear to increase after reduction, an effect caused by the decreased mobility of the then expanded and less compact, reduced polypeptide. In two-dimensional, nonreduced-reduced, sodium dodecyl sulfate-polyacrylamide gel electrophoresis (SDS-PAGE), these glycoproteins can be separated and unambiguously identified (Fig. 6-1). Three other glycoproteins, GPIIIb (also known as GPIV), GPV, and GPIX, apparently do not contain disulfide bonds, and their M_rs do not change upon reduction.

Antigenicity, ligand-binding capacity, and certain interactions with other proteins can be irreversibly lost as a result of denaturation in SDS. The introduction of crossed-immunoelectrophoresis (CIE) to the study of platelet glycoproteins by Hagen et al.[38,39] offered an important new alternative to platelet biochemistry and immunology. For example, CIE was the first method in which it was possible to demonstrate that GPIIb and GPIIIa exist in a calcium-dependent heterodimer complex (Fig. 6-2).[67] It has subsequently been determined that complex integrity is associated with, if not required for, the fibrinogen receptor activity of GPIIb-IIIa, which mediates platelet cohesion and is, thus, required for the proper hemostatic function of platelets.[32,59]

The intense interest in the GPIIb-IIIa complex that then ensued ultimately led to the realization that other glycoproteins also exist in the membrane of the intact platelet as noncovalent, functional complexes. A number of laboratories have generated data suggesting the existence of the heterodimeric complexes GPIc-IIa and GPIa-IIa.[35,65,66,92,93,112] Glycoprotein Ic-IIa functions as a receptor that mediates adhesion of nonactivated platelets to solid phase fibronectin,[92] whereas GPIa-IIa, sharing the same β subunit (GPIIa), is a recep-

Table 6-1
Major Membrane Glycoproteins

Glycoprotein	Molecular Mass (kDa) Intact Molecule	Large Subunit	Small Subunit	Biological Functions
GPIa	155/170*			Complexed to GPIIa Collagen receptor
GPIb	170	145	25	Complexed to GPIX Absent in Bernard-Soulier syndrome Receptor for Qn/Qd-dependent antibodies Receptor for vWF†
GPIc	150	125	25	Complexed to GPIIa Fibronectin receptor
GPIIa	130/145*			Complexed to GPIa or GPIc Common β subunit of certain adhesion receptors
GPIIb	145	125	25	Complexed to GPIIIa Absent in Glanzmann's thrombasthenia Activation-dependent receptor for fibrinogen, vWF†, fibronectin
GPIIIa	95/115*			Complexed to GPIIb Absent in Glanzmann's thrombasthenia Common β subunit of certain adhesion receptors
GPIIIb (GPIV)	95/95*			Receptor for thrombospondin
GPV	80/80*			Absent in Bernard-Soulier syndrome Thrombin substrate on intact platelet
GPIX	20/20*			Complexed to GPIb Absent in Bernard-Soulier syndrome

*Nonreduced/reduced.
†vWF, von Willebrand factor.

tor for solid-phase collagen.[66] Glycoprotein Ib is the larger component of another heterodimer complex, GPIb-IX,[3,18] and functions as a receptor for von Willebrand factor (VWF) that mediates platelet adhesion to the vessel wall.[85,101,135]

These heterodimer complexes, GPIIb-IIIa, GPIc-IIa, and GPIa-IIa, represent prototypes of a superfamily of cell adhesion receptors that share structural and antigenic homologies. Other members of this superfamily include the very late activation (VLA) antigens of T-lymphocytes,[44] the human fibroblast collagen receptor,[134] the human and avian fibroblast fibronectin receptors,[40,94] the human endothelial cell vitronectin receptor,[117] and lymphocyte-associated receptors, such as LFA-1, Mac-1, and p150,95.[102] On the basis of comparison of protein sequence homology, it is unlikely that GPIb-IX is related to this particular cell adhesion superfamily.[75,118]

A number of clinically relevant antigens have been localized to one of the major membrane glycoproteins, particularly GPIb, GPIIb, GPIIIa and, in two preliminary reports, to the GPIa-IIa complex and GPV. These antigens and the studies that led to their characterization will be discussed in detail. In addition to these platelet-specific antigens, platelets express alloantigens shared by other blood cells and tissues, namely histocompatibility antigens (HLA) and certain blood group antigens. This review will be concerned with the immunochemistry of platelet-specific glycoprotein antigens as well as HLA and blood group antigens associated with platelets.

PLATELET-SPECIFIC ISOANTIGENS

Inherited disorders of platelet function that are associated with specific glycoprotein deficiencies or abnormalities, reviewed in detail in Chapter 5, have provided a vehicle toward our

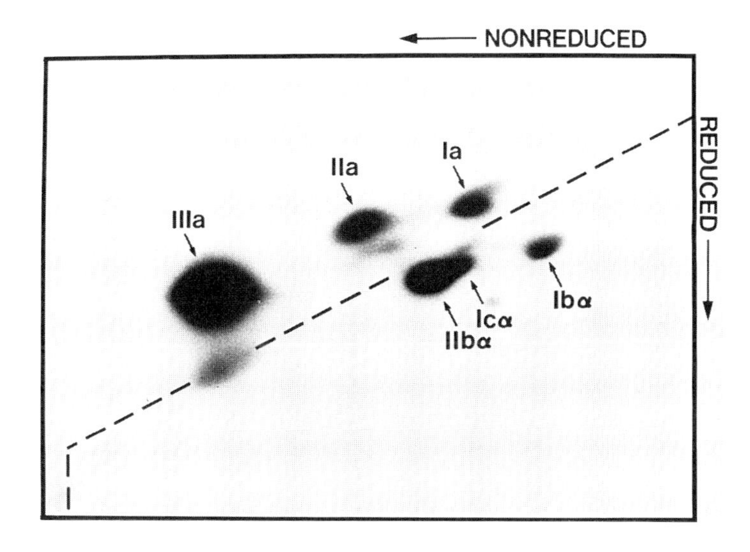

Figure 6-1. Two-dimensional, non-reduced-reduced SDS-PAGE. Platelets were radioiodinated using the lactoperoxidase-catalyzed method to label surface membrane proteins. Proteins solubilized in SDS were then subjected to electrophoresis under nonreduced conditions in 5% acrylamide cylinder gels (right to left). The separated proteins were then reduced in situ by incubation of the cylinder gel in buffer containing 5% 2-mercaptoethanol. The cylinder gel was then affixed to a second-dimension slab gel composed of 7% acrylamide, and the separated and reduced proteins were subjected to electrophoresis, from top to bottom. The resultant gel was fixed, stained, and subjected to autoradiography, and that section of the autoradiograph containing the major membrane glycoproteins is depicted. When the acrylamide gel is stained to visualize proteins, most proteins, because they do not contain disulfide bonds, are seen to migrate on a diagonal line. This is indicated on the autoradiograph by a dashed line. Those radiolabeled glycoprotein spots corresponding to GPIb α, GPIIb α, and GPIc α are seen to migrate below this diagonal, indicating that disulfide reduction caused a decrease in molecular size. Their corresponding β chains, with molecular masses ranging from 20 kDa to 25 kDa, do not migrate within the area encompassed by this figure. Radiolabeled spots corresponding to GPIa, GPIIa, and GPIIIa are located above the diagonal, indicating that disulfide reduction caused a decrease in electrophoretic mobility owing to the extended size of these molecules.

understanding of the function of these glycoproteins. These disorders also provide a setting for isoimmunization against platelet glycoproteins.

Thrombasthenic or Bernard-Soulier patients whose platelets are devoid of GPIIb-IIIa or GPIb-IX plus GPV, respectively, or whose platelets bear an altered form of these glycoprotein complexes, are at risk to develop antibodies against these glycoproteins presented on transfused normal platelets. A number of such instances have been reported, and these will be discussed individually. Empirically, the antibodies made by these patients do not distinguish allelic forms of the glycoproteins (such as Bak or P1^A alloantigens which will be discussed later in this chapter) but react with platelets of all normal individuals tested. Such antibodies are properly designated isoantibodies. The use of such human isoantibodies against GPIb, GPIIb, or GPIIIa helped to bridge the gap between our understanding of the functional defects inherent in these disorders and the glycoprotein defects associated with them.

The first isoantibody to be characterized was produced by a polytransfused thrombasthenic patient and designated IgG-L for the patient's surname initial.[15] Purified IgG-L, when mixed with normal platelets in vitro, induced all those dysfunctions associated with Glanzmann's thrombasthenia. By CIE, IgG-L was found to contain antibodies that recognize epitopes expressed on the complex of GPIIb-IIIa and antibodies that react with dissociated GPIIb. No reactivity with dissociated GPIIIa was apparent by CIE.[59] The presence of antibodies reactive with GPIIb but not GPIIIa was confirmed in an immunoblot assay.[100] It has not been determined whether the antibodies that react with free GPIIb in CIE or in the immunoblot assay are the same as those that react with complexed GPIIb in CIE. Alternatively, there may, in fact, be antibodies in IgG-L that react exclusively with the GPIIb contained in GPIIb–IIIa complexes, mimicking the specificities of subsequently characterized complex-specific murine monoclonal antibodies such as AP2.[90]

Another isoantibody produced by a thrombasthenic patient has recently been characterized.[64] This patient had previously been studied by White et al. in conjunction with an analysis of thrombin binding to thrombasthenic platelets.[136] At that time, and again several years thereafter, the patient became isoimmunized after a number of platelet transfusions. By an immunoblot assay (Fig. 6-3) and an antigen-capture ELISA (Fig. 6-4), this IgG isoantibody, OG, was found to bind to GPIIIa.[64] Like the GPIIb-specific isoantibody just described, OG also completely blocks aggregation induced by ADP (Fig. 6-6).

Coller et al. have described a third example of IgG isoantibodies, produced by a thrombasthenic patient, that completely blocked aggregation induced by 5-μM ADP and the binding of ^{125}I-labeled fibrinogen to platelets (50% inhibition at 0.5 mg/ml IgG).[8] The exact location of the epitope(s) in question was not determined but is assumed to be on GPIIb, GPIIIa, or both. This IgG antibody inhibited the binding of the murine monoclonal antibody 7E3, known to react with a component of the GPIIb–IIIa complex.[7]

Isoantibodies reactive with GPIb are less frequently encountered compared with those against GPIIb–IIIa, probably because the Bernard-Soulier syndrome (BSS) is less common than Glanzmann's thrombasthenia. However, Degos et al.[16] described such an IgG isoantibody that was specific for the larger, or α, subunit of GPIb. When mixed with normal platelets, this isoantibody induced platelet

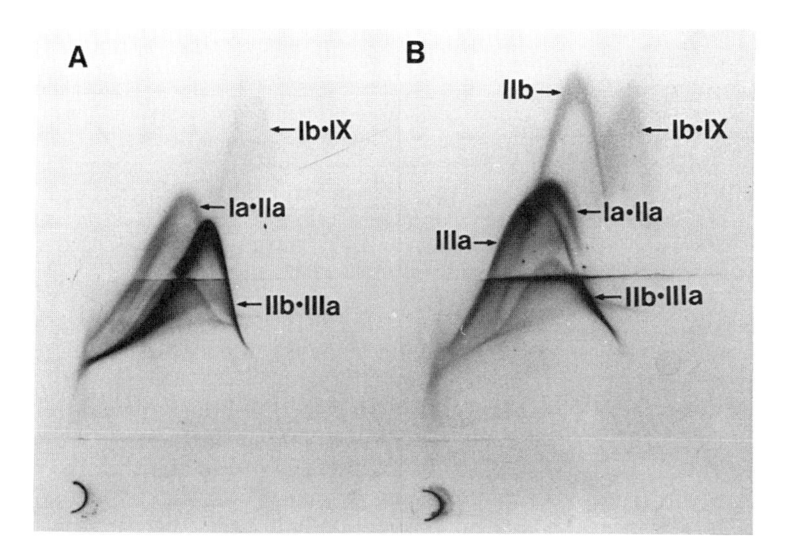

Figure 6-2. Crossed-immunoelectrophoresis. Platelet proteins radioiodinated as described in the legend to Figure 6-1 and solubilized in Triton X-100 in the presence of endogenous platelet calcium (*A*) or after addition of excess EDTA (*B*) were separated by agarose gel electrophoresis in the first dimension (left to right) then precipitated in a second dimension by electrophoresis (bottom to top) into agarose gel containing rabbit polyclonal antihuman platelet antibodies. The autoradiographs derived from these gels are depicted. In the presence of calcium (*A*), GPIIb and GPIIIa are complexed and, thus, coprecipitated in a single arc. When divalent cations are chelated by addition of excess EDTA (*B*), a reduction in the GPIIb–IIIa precipitin arc is seen with the appearance of two new precipitin arcs containing either free GPIIb or free GPIIIa. Those arcs containing these glycoproteins are indicated, as well as additional precipitin arcs containing GPIb–IX and GPIa–IIa.

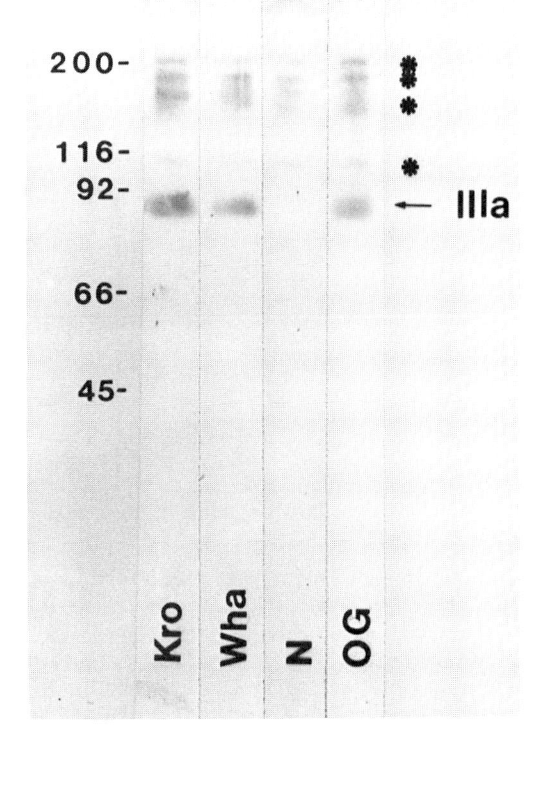

Figure 6-3. Immunoblot. Platelet proteins solubilized in SDS were separated by electrophoresis under nonreduced conditions in a 7% acrylamide slab gel and electrophoretically transferred to a nitrocellulose sheet. Individual strips from the nitrocellulose sheet were incubated with plasmas containing either anti-Pl^{A1} (*Kro* and *Wha*), no detectable platelet-specific antibody (*N*) or isoantibodies reactive with GPIIIa (*OG*). The position of molecular mass markers and the corresponding molecular mass in kilodaltons is shown at the left. The position of GPIIIa reactive with Kro, Wha, and OG plasmas is indicated. The remaining bands (*) represent nonspecific reactions typically seen with all plasmas tested, including control plasmas (*N*) and may represent endogenous platelet α-granule IgG that binds the detection reagent (goat antihuman IgG–alkaline phosphatase conjugate) (Kunicki TJ, et al.,[64] with permission).

dysfunction typical of BSS such that adhesion to subendothelium was impaired and the aggregation response in vitro to ristocetin or bovine factor VIII was inhibited.[119] No other isoantibodies specific for GPIb have since been described. One immunologic function of GPIb was also blocked by this isoantibody, namely, the binding of quinine- and quinidine-dependent human antibodies.[68] The capacity of platelets to be cleared from the circulation by antibody–drug complexes in sera of patients with drug-dependent immune thrombocytopenia had already been found to be a property of the GPIb complex, for BSS platelets failed to bind drug-dependent antibody in the presence of drug.[61]

The structural features of GPIb, GPIIb, or GPIIIa that are isoimmunogenic are currently unknown. A lack of adequate amounts of sera containing such antibodies precludes a definitive analysis of isoimmunogenicity of these glycoproteins. However, recent developments in the area of human hybridoma technology, discussed in detail in Chapter 14, may soon make available large amounts of monoclonal human isoantibodies, which would facilitate such studies.

PLATELET-SPECIFIC ALLOANTIGENS

Platelet-specific alloantigens have been implicated as immunogens in two clinical syndromes, neonatal alloimmune thrombocytopenic purpura (NATP) and posttransfusion purpura (PTP). Neonatal alloimmune thrombocytopenic purpura results from maternal sensitization to paternal alloantigens on fetal platelets and is a syndrome analogous to erythroblastosis fetalis (EF). However, in at least one-half of the reported cases of NATP, the affected infant has been a first-born child. Estimates of the incidence of NATP range from 1 : 2000 to 1 : 5000 live births. Many intriguing questions remain to be answered about NATP, including why only a few mothers who are negative for the platelet antigen in question deliver affected infants. In PTP, thrombocytopenia follows roughly 7 to 10 days after the immunogenic blood (platelet) transfusion. Unless fatal intracranial hemorrhage intervenes, the disappearance of cytolytic antibody parallels spontaneous recovery within 7 to 35 days. Persistence of noncytolytic antibody in the sera of recovered patients has been reported, albeit only in a few cases. Nearly all patients who

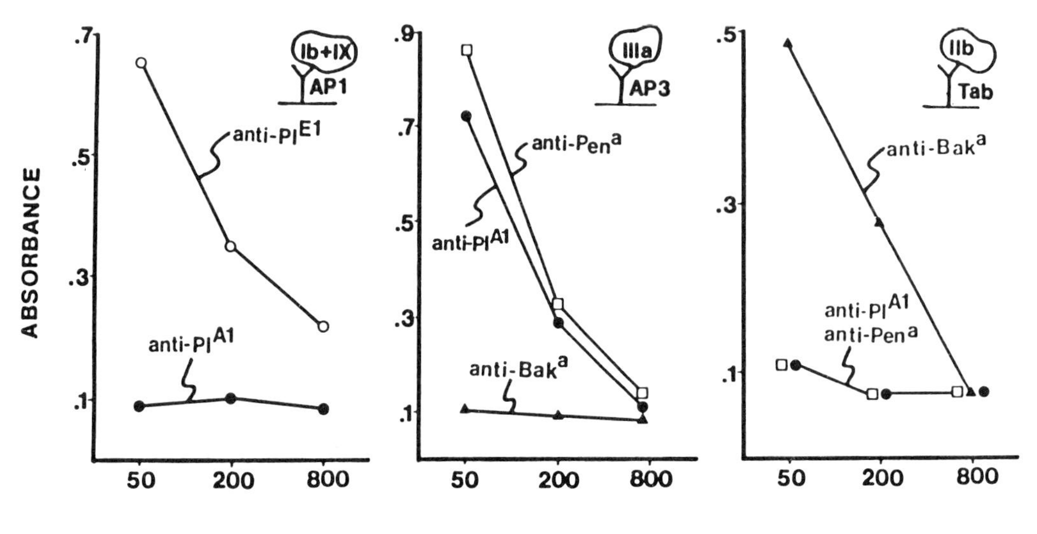

Figure 6-4. Antigen-capture ELISA. Murine monoclonal antibodies AP1 (anti-GPIb), AP3 (anti-GPIIIa), and Tab (anti-GPIIb), adsorbed to plastic microtiter trays, were used to immunopurify specific antigen from Triton X-100 lysates of washed human platelets. A lysate containing only dissociated GPIIb and GPIIIa was obtained by lysis in the presence of excess EDTA to dissociate most of GPIIb–IIIa and preclearing with AP2-Sepharose (anti-complex) to remove residual nondissociated GPIIb–IIIa. GPIb remains complexed to GPIX in such lysates and is indicated as such. Plasmas containing platelet-specific antibodies were then incubated in wells containing captured antigens, followed by (with appropriate intermittent washes and incubations) biotinylated murine monoclonal antihuman IgG (Fc), an avidin–biotin–alkaline phosphatase complex, and substrate (PNPP). The absorbance at 405 nm was then recorded and is indicated on the ordinate. The amount of human plasma tested per well is indicated on the abscissa as reciprocal antibody dilution. Note that anti-P1^{E1} bound specifically to GPIb, anti-P1^{A1} and anti-Pen^{a} reacted exclusively with GPIIIa, and anti-Bak^{a} bound to GPIIb. Normal human plasmas and plasmas containing high titers of HLA-specific antibodies never produced reactions above background (Kunicki TJ et al.,[64] with permission).

develop PTP are multiparous women who have never received a transfusion.

Reznikoff-Etievant et al.[98] were the first to demonstrate an increased frequency of HLA-B8 in mothers who become sensitized to P1^{A1} antigen on fetal platelets, and this finding has been confirmed by a number of laboratories.[81,115] In fact, the association of HLA-DR3 and production of anti-P1^{A1} in NATP is even stronger,[99] and HLA-DR3 has also been shown to be an immunogenetic risk factor in PTP.[17,83] These findings can only partially explain why selected individuals who are P1^{A1}-negative are at risk to develop anti-P1^{A1} upon exposure to transfused blood products or onset of pregnancy. Clearly, additional risk factors are brought into play. These will be discussed in more detail in Chapter 19.

As stated earlier, platelet-specific alloantigens are the causative immunogens in NATP and PTP. Sera from patients with PTP and mothers of infants with NATP have, thus, represented the major source of alloantibodies for the characterization of these antigens. In addition, sera of multitransfused individuals have also represented a source of platelet-specific alloantibodies. In the latter, platelet-specific antibodies are usually obscured by antibodies reactive with HLA antigens.

Eight platelet-specific alloantigen systems have now been reported in the literature, including DUZO,[80] P1^{A} (Zw),[109,124,127] P1^{E},[109]

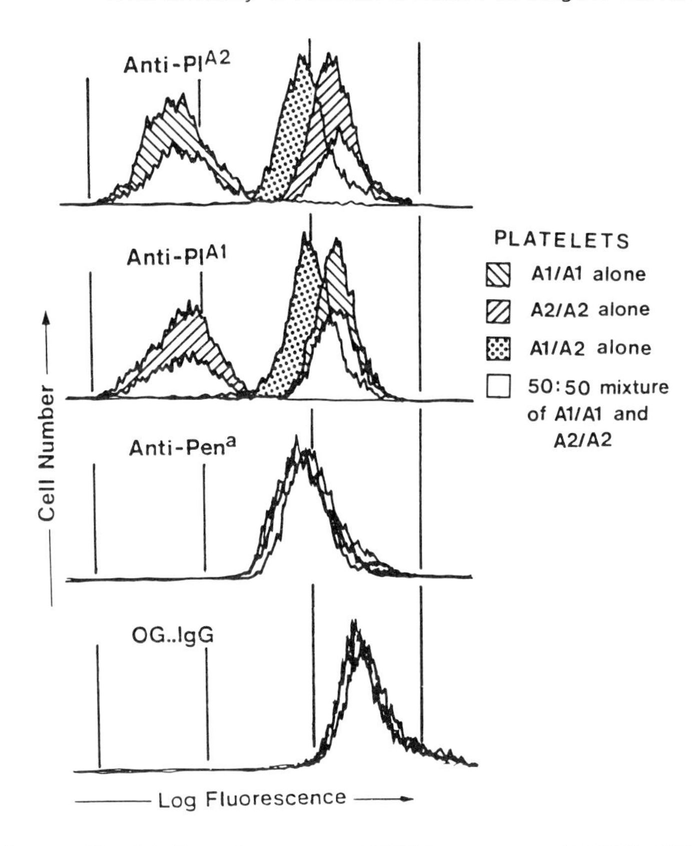

Figure 6-5. Cytofluorimetry. Platelets from donors typed P1^{A1}-homozygous (A1/A1), P1^{A1}-heterozygous (A1/A2), and P1^{A1}-negative (A2/A2), or a 50:50 mixture of A1/A1 and A2/A2 platelets were incubated with plasmas containing anti-P1^{A2}, anti-P1^{A1}, anti-Pen^{a}, or anti-GPIIIa (OG), washed and incubated with fluorescein-conjugated goat antihuman IgG + IgM. The amount of platelet-bound fluorescence was then determined by cytofluorimetry with a FACS II flow cytometer (Beckton-Dickinson, Mountain View, Calif.) The number of fluorescence-positive cells (ordinate) is plotted versus the log of the fluorescence recorded (abscissa). First, a reciprocal relationship between the binding of anti-P1^{A2} and anti-P1^{A1} is observed, as expected. Second, A1/A2 platelets clearly represent a homogeneous single population that binds one-half the maximum amount of anti-P1^{A1} and anti-P1^{A2}, in contrast to the mixture of A1/A1 and A2/A2 platelets that gave two equal populations, one maximally positive and one negative for the corresponding antibody. Third, the anti-GPIIIa isoantibody (OG) binds uniformly to all platelets tested, the amount bound equal to the maximum bindable anti-P1^{A1} or anti-P1^{A2}. Last, anti-Pen^{a} binds to one-half as many sites per platelet as anti-P1^{A1}, anti-P1^{A2}, or OG (Kunicki TJ et al.,[64] with permission).

Ko,[123] Bak,[51,54,131] Lek,[6] Pen,[29,110] and Yuk.[106,107] The DUZO system can no longer be legitimately analyzed because the proband has since deceased and no other antisera with this specificity have been identified. Comparative studies by a number of laboratories have determined that the Bak and Lek systems are the same,[51,129] such that Bak^{a} is identical with Lek^{a}, and Bak^{b} is identical with Lek^{b}. The newly defined Pen and Yuk systems have also been found to be the same.* Serologically, the Pen^{a} allele is the same as the Yuk^{b} allele, and the Pen^{b} allele is the same as the Yuk^{a} allele.

Given these developments, there remain five diallelic, platelet-specific alloantigen systems (Table 6-2). Two recently described alloantigens, P1^{T} and Br(a), which will be discussed later, are also listed in Table 6-2. P1^{A1} is, by far, the most immunogenic alloantigen and, thus, the most frequent cause of NATP or

*Aster, R. H. and Shibata, Y.: Personal communications.

Table 6-2
Platelet-Specific Alloantigen Systems

System	Alleles	Phenotype Frequency	Glycoprotein	References
Pl^{A}(Zw)	1(a)	98	IIIa	60,62,87,
	2(b)	28		109,124,127
Bak(Lek)	a	91	IIbα	6,51,54
	b	—		56,129,131
Pen(Yuk)	a(b)	>99	IIIa	29,31,105,106
	b(a)	1.7		107,108,110
Pl^{E}	1	>99	Ibα	30,109
	2	4		
Br	a	21	Ia–IIa	55
Pl^{T}	1	>99	V	2
Ko	a	15	?	123
	b	99		

PTP. Considering NATP alone, Pl^{A1} was determined to be the causitive immunogen in 29 of 38[130] and 45 of 88 cases,[63] whereas Bak^{a} was implicated in 2 cases,[131] Pl^{E2} in 1 case,[109] Pen^{a} in 2 cases,[29,107] and Pen^{b} in 2 cases.[106] Most patients with PTP have been Pl^{A1}-negative, and antibodies specific for Pl^{A1} have been detected in their sera during and shortly after the acute phase of thrombocytopenia. In one large study,[63] specificity for Pl^{A1} antigen was found in 43 of 56 cases (77%) in which platelet-reactive antibody was detected. The remaining alloantigens have been implicated in PTP, albeit less frequently: Pl^{A2} in 2 cases,[116] Bak^{a} in 2 cases,[6,51] Bak^{b} in 1 case,[54] and Pen^{a} in 1 case.[110]

Since well-characterized antisera recognizing Pl^{A1} have been available for several years, whereas those reactive with other antigens, particularly Bak and Pen (Yuk) antigens, are limited to only specialized laboratories, it is likely that estimates of the relative immunogenicity of the latter are slightly underestimated. Larger studies using antisera reactive with these antigens are currently in progress and should soon yield more accurate assessments of the importance in NATP of alloantigens other than Pl^{A1}. No data are available concerning the importance in NATP or PTP of Ko antigens and Pl^{E1}, because antibodies specific for these antigens have been found only in sera of individuals who had received multiple transfusions without the clinical picture of PTP.[109,123] Indeed, these individuals had reached a state of sensitization to blood products typical of individuals who today would be considered to have developed "refractoriness" to platelet transfusions, a condition associated with the development of high-titered, polyspecific, anti-HLA antibodies. This clinical situation will be discussed in more detail later. This is not meant to imply that antibodies reactive with platelet-specific antigens were not present in sera from those individuals. Although often obscured by the overwhelming response to HLA antigens, concomitant sensitization to platelet-specific antigens does routinely occur in such cases. Of note, the original description of antibody specific for Pl^{A2} (Zw^{b}) concerned not a case of NATP or PTP but a case of an individual who was sensitized by multiple transfusions.[124]

A comprehensive evaluation of the importance of IgG subclasses in immunization to platelet alloantigens has not yet been undertaken. However, limited studies have been performed. In the first association of Pl^{A2} in PTP,[116] antibodies of the IgG1 and IgG3 subclass were detected during the acute phase of thrombocytopenia, whereas the disappearance of IgG3 antibodies paralleled the onset of clinical improvement. Retrospective analysis of antisera from four other PTP patients uncovered the presence of both IgG1 and IgG3. These findings have led Taaning et al.[116] to postulate that the presence of antibodies of the IgG3 subclass may be relevant to the pathogenesis of thrombocytopenia in PTP.

Glycoprotein IIb–IIIa

The first indication that membrane glycoproteins express platelet alloantigens came from our laboratory[60] when we showed that platelets from five patients with Glanzmann's thrombasthenia (GT) expressed indetectable or substantially reduced levels of $P1^{A1}$ antigen. The level of $P1^{A1}$ paralleled the amount of GPIIb–IIIa present, the former quantitated by inhibition of ^{51}Cr release, the latter by scanning densitometry of glycoproteins separated on SDS-polyacrylamide gels. Given that the major molecular defect of GT platelets was an absence of, or deficiency in, GPIIb–IIIa and that those patients with residual GPIIb–IIIa expressed a similar residual amount of $P1^{A1}$, we postulated that $P1^{A1}$ must be associated with either, or both, GPIIb and GPIIIa. That suspicion was subsequently realized when we demonstrated that purified GPIIIa, but not GPIIb, expresses the $P1^{A1}$ alloantigen.[62] Shortly thereafter, the association of the $P1^{A}$ (Zw) alloantigen system with GPIIIa was confirmed by a number of laboratories using, at the time, the only antiserum reactive with $P1^{A2}$, the allelic counterpart of $P1^{A1}$, as well as other antisera reactive with $P1^{A1}$.[70,79,126]

Some insight into the structural nature of the $P1^{A}$ epitope on GPIIIa has been obtained. It is resistant to denaturation in SDS, extremes of *p*H (3 to 10), and moderate heating (56°C for 30 min), destroyed by disulfide bond reduction or boiling (100°C for 3 min), and unaffected by treatment of GPIIIa in protein mixtures with a combination of exo- and endoglycosidases sufficient to deglycosylate the molecule.[62,87] Taken together, these findings indicate that $P1^{A}$ epitopes consist of protein sequences held in a proper conformation by intact disulfide bonds and are independent of oligosaccharide content. As it is now appreciated that the GPIIIa molecule contains 56 cysteine residues, all of which are involved in disulfide bonds,[28] it is not difficult to understand why disulfide reduction would eliminate expression of a polypeptide antigen such as $P1^{A1}$. It now remains to be determined whether the epitope is combinatorial, consisting of a number of noncontiguous amino acids brought together in the tertiary structure of the molecule by the extensive disulfide bonding, or conformational, consisting of a contiguous amino acid sequence held in an antigenic tertiary conformation by intact disulfide bonding, or both.

In addition to the nonreduced GPIIIa monomer, $P1^{A1}$ can also be expressed on dimers and higher multimers of GPIIIa that are often produced during the processing of proteins for electrophoresis. The propensity of GPIIIa to form multimers may explain the observation that anti-$P1^{A1}$ will bind to proteins with relative molecular masses higher than GPIIIa, particularly in immunoblot assays.[79] When chymotrypsin is used to digest GPIIIa within the membrane of intact platelets, a peptide with an M_r under nonreduced conditions, reported to be 58 kDa in one study[56] and 66 kDa in another,[58] remains membrane-bound and retains expression of $P1^{A1}$. Anti-$P1^{A1}$ has also been shown to immunoprecipitate a combination of three peptides from a tryptic digest of soluble protein mixtures containing GPIIIa.[87] Under nonreduced conditions, these peptides have M_rs of 73 kDa, 68 kDa, and 17 kDa. Upon reduction of the immunoprecipitate, only a 17-kDa peptide is detected, indicating that the 73-kDa and 68-kDa species may be polymers of a 17-kDa fragment(s) that itself expresses the $P1^{A1}$ epitope under nonreduced conditions. By use of an immunoblot assay, others have confirmed that anti-$P1^{A1}$ antibodies bind to a low M_r (23-kDa) tryptic fragment derived by digestion of the purified GPIIb–IIIa complex.[122]

It is generally agreed that there are roughly 40,000 GPIIb–IIIa complexes accessible on the surface of nonactivated platelets. This estimate is based upon quantitative binding assays using a number of murine monoclonal antibodies specific for GPIIb, GPIIIa, or the complex, such as Tab, AP3, and AP2, respectively.[78,86,90] With a monoclonal antibody-based, indirect-binding assay to quantitate the number of anti-$P1^{A1}$ IgG molecules that bind to platelets at saturation, Janson et al.[46] determined that 34,000 to 43,000 molecules bind to platelets of individuals that are homozygous for $P1^{A1}$ (A1/A1), whereas roughly one-half that many, as expected, bind to platelets of individuals who are heterozygous (A1/A2). The finding of a maximum of roughly 40,000 $P1^{A1}$ epitopes per platelet agrees well with the aforementioned estimates of the number of GPIIb–IIIa heterodimer complexes available on the surface of nonactivated platelets. From these data, it is reasonable to conclude that there exists only one $P1^{A1}$ epitope per GPIIIa molecule.

During the course of the initial descriptions of the Bak (Lek) and Pen (Yuk) alloantigen systems, it became apparent that the alleles of both of these systems are not expressed on platelets of patients with GT.[6,29,106,131] Studies were immediately undertaken to confirm whether or not antigens of either system are associated with purified GPIIb–IIIa and, if that were the case, to determine which of the two glycoproteins bears the antigens.

By using both radioimmunoprecipitation and immunoblot assays, Kieffer et al. provided direct evidence that Bak^a is associated with the larger α subunit of GPIIb.[56] The Bak^a determinant is resistant to disulfide bond reduction and is still expressed on two major chymotryptic peptides (76 kDa and 60 kDa) derived from purified GPIIb. Further characterization of Bak antigens has not yet been reported. Additional evidence that Bak antigens are localized to GPIIb was derived from the study of Mulder et al.[84] In that study, immunoprecipitates derived with anti-P1^{A1} or anti-Bak^a contained both GPIIb and GPIIIa presumably because the protein preparation used as an antigen source contained predominantly free GPIIb and GPIIIa but also nondissociated GPIIb–IIIa complexes. Nonetheless, the amounts of the glycoproteins in the respective immunoprecipitates were not proportional, and the results could be interpreted to mean that anti-Bak^a antibodies preferentially precipitated GPIIb under conditions in which anti-P1^{A1} antibodies preferentially precipitated GPIIIa, as expected.

More recently, the Pen (Yuk) alloantigen system has been localized to GPIIIa, representing the second platelet-specific alloantigen system expressed on this glycoprotein.[31,105,108]

Quantitation, Surface Expression and Relationship Between Alloantigens Associated with Glycoprotein IIb–IIIa

The characterization of Pen and Bak antigens and a comparison of these with P1^A antigens has been assisted by a number of recent technical developments, including an antigen-capture ELISA developed by Furihata et al.,[31] an improved, quantitative antibody-binding assay devised by Lobuglio et al.,[74] and the general availability and application of cytofluorimetry.

In the antigen-capture ELISA,[31] murine monoclonal antibodies specific for platelet glycoproteins are coupled to a solid support and used to purify the glycoprotein antigen from a detergent solution containing a mixture of total platelet proteins. In this approach, which is patterned after the solid-phase radioimmunoassay of Woods et al.,[137] the adsorbed glycoprotein can then be used to screen for the presence of human antibodies in plasma or serum that react with antigens localized on that glycoprotein. One major advantage of this approach is that HLA antigens are not coadsorbed with the specific glycoprotein. Therefore, the presence of even high levels of broadly reactive anti-HLA antibodies in the test plasma (serum) will not interfere with the assay. By using this assay, one can clearly distinguish the specificity of platelet alloantibodies for captured glycoproteins, such as GPIb, GPIIb, or GPIIIa (*see* Fig. 6-4).

With the indirect binding assay described initially by LoBuglio et al.,[74] one can distinguish and quantitate the number of human antibody molecules bound to the surface of platelets through their specific interaction with antigen while obviating the requirement to use specific, purified human antibody. This assay uses a radiolabeled, murine monoclonal antibody specific for an epitope on the Fc region of human IgG as the detection reagent. With this assay, we have determined the average amount of anti-P1^{A1} and anti-Pen^a antibodies bound to human platelets at saturation, and these data are depicted in Table 6-3. The maximum number of anti-P1^{A1} IgG molecules bound by homozygous (A1/A1) platelets was found to be 40,600 to 51,000 (range: $n = 3$) per platelet. This figure agrees well with the estimated number of GPIIb–GPIIIa heterodimer complexes per platelet (40,000–50,000) based upon direct-binding assays that use murine monoclonal antibodies.[78,86,90] The number of anti-P1^{A1} molecules bound by heterozygous (A1/A2) platelets (14,600–28,500; $n = 5$) is, as expected, roughly one-half that amount bound by homozygous platelets. Residual IgG binding, reflected by the interaction of anti-P1^{A1} with P1^{A1}-negative (A2/A2) platelets, was 1200 to 2000 molecules per platelet. In the same assays, the number of anti-Pen^a IgG molecules bound per platelet (13,900–24,000; $n = 15$) was consistently one-half the number of GPIIb–IIIa complexes. This interesting discrepancy will be discussed in more detail later. Platelets of all donors tested did not react with anti-Pen^b by ELISA or indirect immunofluorescence and are, thereby, considered homozygous for Pen^a.

High-titered alloantisera with the lowest available levels of contaminating anti-HLA antibodies were selected for quantitation of anti-

Table 6-3
Quantitation of Alloantibodies Bound by Platelets

Antibody Tested	Platelet Type	Molecules of Antibody Bound Per Platelet*			
		N	*Mean*	*SD*	*Range*
Anti-P1^{A1}	A1/A1	3	46,553	5,520	40,596–51,495
	A1/A2	5	21,151	5,476	14,627–28,501
	A2/A2	3	1,508	441	1,234–2,016
Anti-Pen^{a}	a/a†	15	17,302	3,141	13,872–24,238

*According to the method of LoBuglio, et al.[74]
†Genotype based upon absence of reactivity with anti-Yuk^{a} (Pen^{b}) in the antigen capture ELISA described by Furihata et al.[31]

gens by cytofluorimetry. The anti-P1^{A2} antiserum used in these studies, still a relatively scarce resource, was that characterized by Slichter et al.[111] As is evident in Figure 6-5, anti-P1^{A1} and anti-P1^{A2} bind in a reciprocal fashion to platelets that are typed A1/A1, A1/A2, or A2/A2. The amount of anti-P1^{A1} bound by A1/A1 platelets is precisely double that bound by A1/A2 platelets, and one observes the same quantitative relationship when one compares the binding of anti-P1^{A2} to A2/A2 versus A1/A2 platelets. Of import to our understanding of this system is that, for heterozygous platelets (A1/A2), both alleles are expressed equally on each platelet. Thus, there is one population of platelets, all of which express both P1^{A1} and P1^{A2}. On the other hand, a 50:50 mixture of A1/A1 and A2/A2 platelets contains two populations when tested with anti-P1^{A1} or anti-P1^{A2}, one maximally positive and one negative for the respective allele. The quantitative difference observed between P1^{A1} and Pen^{a} in the indirect monoclonal antibody binding assay was also observed by cytofluorimetry. The amount of anti-Pen^{a} bound to Pen^{a} homozgous platelets was equivalent to one-half the maximum bindable anti-P1^{A1}, anti-P1^{A2}, or GPIIIa-specific isoantibody (OG; *see* Fig. 6-5).

Effect of Glycoprotein IIb–IIIa-Specific Alloantibodies on Platelet Function

Although certain other alloantibodies, such as those specific for HLA or blood group antigens, may induce aggregation,[42,45] anti-P1^{A1} will normally inhibit aggregation by virtue of its ability to block the binding of fibrinogen.[19,125] Anti-P1^{A1} will also inhibit fibrinogen binding and aggregation induced by physiologic agonists, such as ADP, provided that one uses P1^{A1}-positive platelets as targets.[125] The requirement for complete saturation of available GPIIb–IIIa molecules by anti-P1^{A1} is demonstrated by our comparison of the effect of anti-P1^{A1} on ADP-induced aggregation of A1/A1 versus A1/A2 and A2/A2 platelets (Fig. 6-6). In our hands, anti-P1^{A1} will completely inhibit the aggregation of A1/A1 platelets, but the aggregation of A1/A2 platelets is only delayed or partially inhibited at equivalent or greater levels of antibody. As expected, aggregation of A2/A2 platelets is unaffected by the addition of anti-P1^{A1}. Thus, it would appear that blocking of only one-half of the available GPIIb–IIIa molecules on A1/A2 platelets by anti-P1^{A1} is insufficient to completely inhibit fibrinogen binding and aggregation. Bearing this in mind, it was somewhat surprising to find, in the same assays, that platelets saturated with anti-Pen^{a} (and thus bearing a maximum of roughly 20,000 anti-Pen^{a} IgG per platelet) do not aggregate in response to ADP. Thus, not only is the fibrinogen-binding site on GPIIb–IIIa apparently blocked by the binding of both anti-Pen^{a} IgG and anti-P1^{A1} IgG, but complete inhibition of aggregation of identical platelet preparations can be effected by the binding of only 20,000 molecules of the former while requiring the binding of 40,000 molecules of the latter.

We can offer at least two explanations for this intriguing discrepancy, both of which can be tested. First, it is possible that anti-Pen^{a} IgG normally binds bivalently, such that a single IgG molecule bridges two GPIIIa molecules on adjacent GPIIb–IIIa complexes, whereas anti-

*Furihata K, Kunicki TJ: Unpublished observations

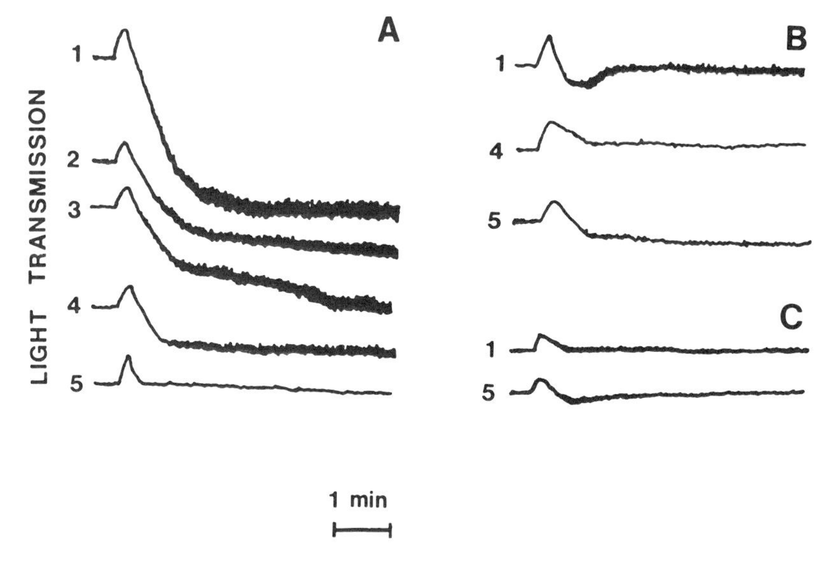

Figure 6-6. Inhibition of platelet aggregation by allo- and isoantibodies. Aggregation of citrated platelet-rich plasma (PRP) was induced at 37°C by addition of 5 μM ADP. To test for inhibition, PRP was preincubated for 30 min at 37°C with an appropriate dilution of plasma containing specific antibody. All of the donors used in this study were homozygous for Pen² (a/a), but differed in expression of $P1^{A1}$. Note that anti-$P1^{A1}$ (*panel A*) failed to inhibit aggregation of $P1^{A1}$-negative (A2/A2) platelets (*1*), inhibited only partially the aggregation of $P1^{A1}$-heterozygous (A1/A2) platelets (*2, 3,* and *4*), and inhibited completely the aggregation of $P1^{A1}$-homozygous (A1/A1) platelets (*5*). On the other hand, anti-Pen^a (*panel B*) and anti-GPIIIa (OG; *panel C*) completely inhibited aggregation of platelets from every donor tested regardless of $P1^{A1}$ phenotype (Kunicki TJ et al.,[64] with permission).

$P1^{A1}$ normally binds monovalently. Alternatively, there may exist two distinct but quantitatively equal populations of GPIIIa on the platelet surface, one that expresses both $P1^A$ and Pen epitopes and another that expresses only $P1^A$ epitopes. If the alternative explanation is correct, then the latter GPIIIa population that expresses only $P1^A$ epitopes is probably not important in the aggregation process because it would be unblocked by anti-Pen^a under conditions in which aggregation does not occur. Studies are currently in progress to assess these alternative explanations for this phenomenon.

Another platelet function that is consistently inhibited by anti-$P1^{A1}$ antibodies is clot retraction.[109] Anti-Pen^a antibodies, on the other hand, do not inhibit clot retraction.* To our knowledge, the effect of anti-Bak antibodies on this function has not been investigated.

The tissue distribution of platelet alloantigens will be discussed in detail in Chapters 9 and 13. Given the recent finding that the human umbilical vein endothelial cell (HUVE) GPIIIa analogue expresses the $P1^{A1}$[50,71] and Pen^a epitopes,[50] although HUVE are negative for Bak(Lek),[50,71] the potential impact of antibodies reactive with $P1^A$ or Pen antigens upon endothelial cell function and vascular homeostasis in vivo warrants further investigation.

Additional Considerations

Murine hybridoma technology has advanced to a point where the production of murine monoclonal antibodies specific for platelet glycoproteins is a straightforward matter. One laboratory has reported the characterization of two monoclonal antibodies specific for GPIIIa, Gi4, and Gi6, that can distinguish the $P1^{A1}$ epitope.[43,103] This conclusion is based upon the observations that the binding of Gi4 and Gi6 is competed for by serum containing anti-$P1^{A1}$ from the mother of a child affected with NATP; and Gi6 was observed to be a potent inhibitor of the aggregation of $P1^{A1}$-positive, but not $P1^{A1}$-negative, platelets induced by all physiologic agonists tested, except collagen. Whether Gi4 and Gi6 actually bind at, or simply close to, the $P1^{A1}$ epitope remains to be determined.

It should be noted that, with the exception of the descriptions of Yuk antigens which originated in Japan, surveys of the gene frequencies of platelet alloantigens were performed in white populations of various ethnic backgrounds and have thus produced quite similar results. Two recent reports shed some light upon the frequency of $P1^{A1}$ in nonwhite populations, and indicate, not surprisingly, that the frequencies of platelet alloantigens in blacks or Orientals relative to whites is different. In the first comparative study, the phenotype frequency of $P1^{A1}$ in American blacks was found to be 99.6%, whereas that in American whites (96.8%) was similar to previously reported values.[96] A preliminary study of the $P1^{A1}$ phenotype frequency in the Japanese has also produced results different from those observed in Caucasian populations.[106] All of 300 Japanese blood donors tested were found to be positive for $P1^{A1}$, whereas one would expect to identify at least six $P1^{A1}$ negative individuals in an equivalent number of Caucasian blood donors.

The ontogeny of platelet-specific antigens is an area that remains to be systematically investigated. In what probably represent the first reports on this subject, $P1^{A1}$ and Bak^a antigens were shown to be expressed on fetal platelets as early as 16 weeks of gestation in one study, and $P1^{A1}$ was detected on fetal platelets at 22 weeks gestation in another study.[37,49] Although it has been known for some time that human megakaryocytes express membrane IIb–IIIa,[95,121] it has only recently been demonstrated that the $P1^{A1}$ alloantigen is expressed on the GPIIIa molecule of cultured human megakaryocytes.[20]

A number of recent reports have suggested that $P1^{A1}$-negative platelets can adsorb soluble $P1^{A1}$ antigen present in transfused blood products and, thereby, be rendered passively $P1^{A1}$-positive.[11,53,132] This finding is thought to provide a basis for the development of thrombocytopenia by $P1^{A1}$-negative individuals who produce anti-$P1^{A1}$ antibodies in PTP. Although $P1^{A1}$ antigen can still be detected in platelet-poor plasma that has been subjected to ultracentrifugation, as described in the preceding studies, filtration through microfilters (e.g., 0.22-μm pore size), in our hands, will eliminate all traces of such "soluble" $P1^{A1}$ antigen.* Because filtration in this manner is unlikely to eliminate soluble $P1^{A1}$ (GPIIIa), it is more likely that the suspected passive transfer of $P1^{A1}$ antigen from $P1^{A1}$-positive platelet-poor (but not platelet-free) plasma to $P1^{A1}$-negative platelet suspensions is mediated by the adsorption of or coisolation of either platelet membrane vesicles or platelet membrane debris. Nonetheless, the presence of platelet membrane fragments in $P1^{A1}$-positive transfused blood products, which can become adsorbed onto the $P1^{A1}$-negative platelets of the recipient, still represents an important clinical complication of transfusion therapy and a potentially critical factor in the etiology of PTP. The existence of platelet membrane fragments or platelet microparticles in fresh-frozen plasma and cryoprecipitate and their accumulation in stored platelet concentrates has been documented.[33,34] These membrane microparticles were demonstrated using a monoclonal antibody to GPIIb and, therefore, likely retain the GPIIb–IIIa complex and the $P1^{A1}$ antigen.[33]

*Warejcka D, Kunicki TJ: Unpublished results

The approximate locations of platelet-specific alloantigens associated with GPIIb–IIIa are depicted schematically in Figure 6-7.

Glycoprotein Ib–IX (and V)

The diallelic alloantigen system $P1^E$ was established through the characterization of sera from the proband, a polytransfused patient with longstanding thrombocytopenia who developed antibody reactive with the phenotypically predominant allele $P1^{E1}$;[109] and the

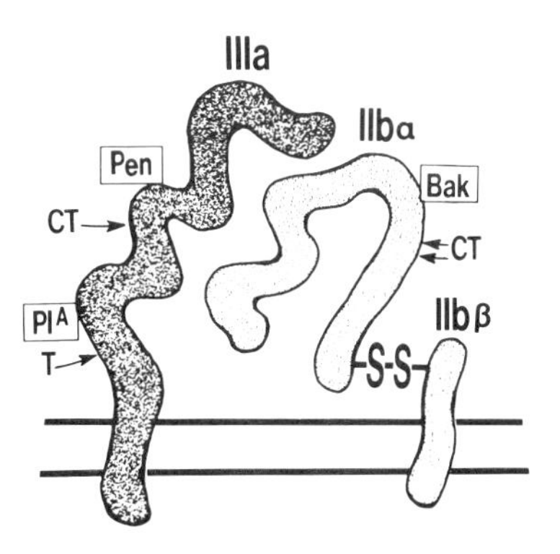

Figure 6-7. Glycoprotein IIb–IIIa. The approximate locations of epitopes defining the alloantigen systems, $P1^A$, Pen, and Bak, are indicated as are sites of cleavage by trypsin (*T*) and chymotrypsin (*CT*).

mother of an infant with NATP, herself $P1^{E1}$-positive, who developed antibody specific for the corresponding allele, $P1^{E2}$. That antibody, anti-$P1^{E2}$, failed to react with platelets of the proband.[109] Whereas all of the previously characterized alloantigen systems have been localized to one of the components of the highly immunogenic GPIIb-IIIa complex, $P1^{E}$ appears to be associated with GPIb and is, thus, the first alloantigen system to be localized to this glycoprotein.[30] In a recent report, we obtained several lines of evidence that anti-$P1^{E1}$ in the sera of the proband binds to an epitope(s) on the larger α subunit of GPIb:[30] First, in the antibody-specific, complement-dependent, ^{51}Cr-release assay, platelets from two BSS patients (lacking GPIb, GPIX, and GPV; and HLA-A2-negative) did not react with anti-$P1^{E1}$ antisera, whereas platelets of a third BSS patient that were HLA-A2-positive, were probably lysed by high-titered anti-HLA-A2 antibodies (still reactive in lymphocytotoxicity assays at $>1:1000$ dilution) present in these same sera. Second, in the antigen-capture ELISA (*see* Fig. 6-4), an assay unaffected by the presence of anti-HLA, anti-$P1^{E1}$ IgG bound specifically to GPIb-IX held by AP1 but not to GPIIb-GPIIIa held by AP2. Third, in an ELISA employing solid-phase purified glycoproteins, anti-$P1^{E1}$ IgG bound to glycocalicin, the NH_2-terminal proteolytic fragment produced from GPIb α by calpain. Fourth, anti-$P1^{E1}$ antisera consistently precipitated, almost exclusively, GPIb-IX complexes from lysates containing all of the tritium-labeled membrane glycoproteins, the only contaminant being trace amounts of HLA antigen. Finally, anti-$P1^{E1}$ antisera routinely inhibit ristocetin-induced platelet agglutination, a property of platelets mediated by GPIb (*see* Chap. 2), but have no effect upon platelet aggregation mediated by GPIIb-IIIa.

Given these findings, it is logical to conclude that the $P1^{E1}$ antigen is associated with GPIb α. Unfortunately, no additional examples of anti-$P1^{E1}$ antibodies have been identified since the case history of the proband, who is now deceased, was reported in 1964, and sera containing anti-$P1^{E2}$ are no longer available. We are, thus, precluded from a further characterization of the $P1^{E1}$ epitope.

In the initial report, a newly defined alloantigen, $P1^{T}$, has been assigned to GPV by Beardsley et al.[2] The alloantigen in question was implicated as the cause of a single case of NATP and has thus far been found on platelets from all of 50 normal donors. No reactivity was observed with Bernard-Soulier platelets known to lack GPV.

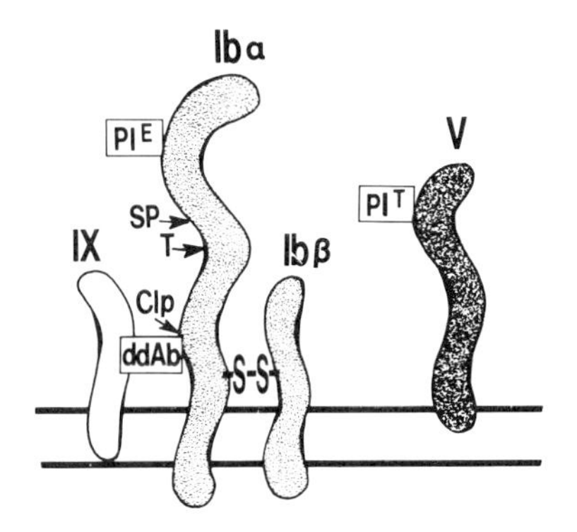

Figure 6-8. Glycoproteins Ib-IX and V. The approximate locations of epitopes defining the $P1^{E}$ and $P1^{T}$ alloantigen systems are indicated along with sites of cleavage by serratia protease (*SP*), trypsin (*T*), and platelet calpain (*Clp*). The location of antigen(s) on GPIb-IX recognized by drug-dependent antibodies (*ddAb*) (discussed in detail in Chap. 8) is also depicted in this figure.

Figure 6-8 depicts schematically the locations of alloantigens associated with GPIb-IX and GPV.

Glycoprotein Ia-IIa

As discussed in the beginning of this review, it is now known that GPIa-IIa is a heterodimer that functions as a specific receptor for adhesion of platelets to collagen.[66] In a timely report, Kiefel et al.[55] have defined a new platelet-specific alloantigen, Br(a), which is associated with GPIa-IIa. Serum from the mother of an infant affected with NATP contained the antibody specific for Br(a), which has a phenotypic frequency in the German population of 21%. Subsequently, three additional cases of NATP resulting from sensitization to Br(a) were identified by the same laboratory. From lysates of surface-iodinated platelets, anti-Br(a) coprecipitates two glycoproteins whose relative molecular masses, under either nonreduced or reduced conditions in single-dimension acrylamide gels, correspond to GPIa and GPIIa.

HLA

Refractoriness to platelet transfusions is an important clinical situation that has long been known to be caused predominantly, if not exclusively, by sensitization to HLA antigens. From the standpoint of transfusion therapy, then, HLA remains the most important alloantigen system of platelets.

The major histocompatibility complex (MHC) is a set of linked genes that encodes polymorphic cell surface glycoproteins that play various functional roles in the immune system.[12,57] In humans, MHC genes have been divided into three classes: Class I genes encode the heavy chains of a group of cell surface antigens that include the major transplantation antigens, HLA-A, HLA-B, and HLA-C; class II genes direct synthesis of both subunits of the cell surface, immune response-related antigens, including DR, DQ, and DP; and class III genes encode certain components of the complement system.

The presence of HLA antigens on platelets had been established by a number of laboratories long before the distinction was made between class I and class II antigens.[82,109,113] It is now appreciated that class I antigens are expressed on human platelets but class II antigens are not. There is every indication that HLA class I molecules of the platelet are identical with those of other cell systems, consisting of a larger, glycosylated subunit (or heavy chain) noncovalently associated with a smaller subunit, now known to be β-2-microglobulin. Given the relative ease of obtaining large numbers of platelets for antigen purification, early investigations of the structure of HLA molecules largely used human platelets as a source of the antigen.[4,13,14,36,89,91,120,128]

In contrast to the uniformity of HLA expression reported for human lymphocytes,[73] platelet expression of both HLA-A and HLA-B antigens can vary two- to threefold. Some of the variation in expression of these antigens is now known to be genetically directed. For HLA-B antigens, the expression of "public" determinants, such as Bw4 and Bw6, is genetically related to the expression of "private" determinants carried by the same HLA-B molecule.[73,114]

It has been reported that HLA antigens can be passively absorbed onto platelets from plasma, raising the intriguing suggestion that most, if not all, of platelet HLA antigens are plasma derived.[69] The fact that HLA antigens can apparently be eluted from platelets after their incubation in chloroquine, whereas other intrinsic antigens, such as $P1^{A1}$, are not is used by some to argue that this hypothesis is correct.[5,48,88]

Although much of this work has been qualitative, the amount of HLA antigen on platelets before and after chloroquine stripping has been quantitated.[48] Using the framework-specific monoclonal antibody W6/32 to measure platelet-associated HLA antigens, roughly 60,000 to 120,000 molecules of W6/32 were found to bind per platelet before chloroquine stripping, and roughly 80% of that amount was bound subsequently to chloroquine stripping.[48] This observation would suggest that most of the platelet-associated HLA antigen is intrinsic, but that a significant portion (20%) is passively acquired from plasma. The results of other studies differ in two respects: first, the total amount of HLA antigen was found to be substantially less; and second, the contribution of adsorbed HLA antigen to the total antigen pool was not as substantial.[46,104] For example, it has been reported that the average number of HLA-A2, Bw4, and Bw6 molecules expressed on platelets is roughly 6400, 3600, and 3800, respectively.[46] Santoso et al. contend that the amount of HLA antigen adsorbed onto platelets is insufficient to alter the HLA specificity of platelets in vitro.[104] To test that hypothesis in vivo, HLA-A2-negative donor platelets were infused into HLA-A2-positive recipients with severe thrombocytopenia. Donor platelets failed to adsorb recipient HLA-A2 antigen even after 18 hr of circulation in vivo.[104] The recent finding that HLA antigens can be phosphorylated on intact platelets also argues for a transmembrane, and therefore intrinsic, orientation of substantial amounts of the total platelet-associated HLA antigen.[27]

Kao[47] has reported that the chloroquine-elutable platelet HLA concentration and plasma HLA concentration for a given individual do not correlate. Given this finding, he contends that it is unlikely that chloroquine-elutable platelet HLA molecules are derived from plasma.

Our understanding of the effect of HLA antibodies upon platelet function is somewhat fragmented. In the presence of fibrinogen and calcium, HLA antibodies will induce rapid aggregation and release, and this response is inhibited by apyrase and aspirin, the former a scavenger of released platelet ADP, the latter a specific inhibitor of the platelet release reaction.[42,45] On the other hand, a monoclonal antibody reactive with β-2-microglobulin has been shown to inhibit the second (release-dependent) wave of platelet aggregation induced by ADP or epinephrine and to completely inhibit aggregation induced by arachidonate or thromboxane A_2.[10] From these findings, one can argue that platelet HLA molecules are closely associated in an as yet undetermined manner with receptors that mediate platelet cohesion, such as GPIIb-IIIa.

BLOOD GROUP ANTIGENS

Of the major blood group antigens, ABH, P, Ii, and Le^a antigens have been shown to be carried by human platelets, whereas other common antigens systems, such as Rh, Duffy, Kell, Kidd, and Lutheran, are not.[22-26]

The biochemistry of the ABH structural determinants is well known. Carbohydrate determinants that specify ABH antigens are attached to oligosaccharide core moieties on glycoproteins or glycolipids by specific transferases.[9,97,133] Terminal sugars that confer A antigen activity (*N*-acetylgalactosamine) or B antigen activity (D-galactose) are linked β (1-3) to the H determinant (-*N*-acetylglucosamine-β-D-galactose-L-fucose). The attachment of *N*-acetylglucosamine to β-D-galactose can be one of two forms: a β(1-3) linkage designated type 1 chain or a β(1-4) linkage designated type 2 chain. The major portion of erythrocyte A or B antigen is composed of type 2 glycolipids. However, because soluble plasma A and B glycolipid is composed almost entirely of type 1 glycolipid, then it follows that passively adsorbed erythrocyte A and B antigen consists of type 1 glycolipid. This difference provides a convenient method to distinguish intrinsic from adsorbed A and B antigen on blood cells.

The intrinsic ABO antigens of the platelet membrane are carried by glycolipids possessing type 2H chains.[133] Additional ABO antigens on platelets reside on glycolipid molecules possessing the type 1H chain and are thought to be largely passively adsorbed from plasma.[1,26,52,72,76]

By fluorescence flow cytometry, Dunstan and Simpson have shown that oligosaccharide blood group antigens, including ABH, Ii, Le^a, and P antigens, exhibit a greater variability in the number of sites per platelet when compared with antigens with a more homogeneous distribution, such as P1^{A1}, Bak^a, and HLA.[22] This finding was considered a possible explanation for the biphasic survival of ABO-incompatible platelets when transfused in vivo. Were this hypothesis correct, then rapid clearance of a subpopulation with high antigen density would be followed by the normal clearance rate those platelets bearing comparatively less antigen. Immune-mediated clearance resulting from sensitization to P1^{A1} or HLA, on the other hand, would more closely approximate a single exponential curve because these antigens are more uniformly distributed over the entire platelet population.

ABO-compatibility figures significantly in the outcome of matched platelet transfusions in refractory patients.[41,72,77] Variability in response to ABO-matched platelets probably reflects both differences in the titer of anti-A or anti-B in the plasma of the recipient, as well as the wide distribution of ABO antigens on platelets alluded to previously.

Roughly 50% to 55% of ABH antigens on human platelets are represented by type 2 chains and, hence, are probably intrinsic antigens.[26] The remainder are represented by type 1 chains and presumably adsorbed. Group O platelets can adsorb substantial amounts of either A or B substance and that adsorption is quantitatively affected by the Lewis and secretor type of the donor plasma. For example, the amount of A antigen adsorption by group O platelets decreases as follows: Le(a−b−)Se > Le(a−b+)Se > Le(a+b−)se>Le(a−b−)se.[1,26] Once reincubated in autologous plasma, group O platelets rapidly lose adsorbed A or B antigen by passive elution. Group A or group B platelets adsorb and elute an amount of A or B antigen that never represents more than one-half of the total, the remainder representing intrinsic antigen.[26]

There is an indication that heterogeneity in density of ABH antigen on platelets may actually be predetermined at the level of the megakaryocyte. Measuring the distribution of platelet antigens on cultured human megakaryocytes by indirect immunofluorescence, Dunstan has found that, in contrast to the homogeneous labeling observed with anti-P1^{A1}, the labeling with human polyclonal or mouse monoclonal antibodies specific for blood group A antigen or type 2H carbohydrate residues is very heterogeneous.[20] The expression of A antigen was uniform within individual megakaryocyte colonies, but antigen density between colonies differed markedly. The progeny of individual megakaryocytes all retained the same level of A antigen expression as the parent cell.

Like HLA antigens, ABH antigens associated with platelets can be adsorbed from plasma, as described in the literature cited previously. Additional evidence for the presence and stability of intrinsic platelet HLA and ABH antigens is derived from a comparison of antigen expression on fresh versus blood bank-stored platelets. When platelet concentrates are stored under accepted blood bank conditions, e.g., in 50 ml to 60 ml of citrate–phosphate–dextrose–adenine (CPDA-1) plasma in polyolefin (Fenwall PL 732) bags at 22°C with continuous cartwheel agitation, it has been shown, by radioimmunoassay, that during a 10-day period of storage, there is no significant reduction in the amount of platelet-associated Pl^{A1}, blood group A or B antigen, and HLA antigens.[21] This result indicates that optimum storage conditions now employed by most blood banks are unlikely to alter the immunogenicity of platelets, at least for these antigens.

CONCLUSION

Since the initial description of platelet-specific antigens, noteable progress has been made both in our understanding of their structure and in our appreciation of their importance in clinical medicine. The application of molecular biology techniques to the study of platelet membrane glycoproteins and advancements in human hybridoma technology represent two areas that are likely to contribute enormously to future accomplishments in the study of human platelet glycoprotein immunogenicity.

This work was supported, in part, by National Heart, Lung and Blood Institute grant HL 37471 and American Heart Association Established Investigator Award 83-186.

REFERENCES

1. Aster RH: Effect of anticoagulant and ABO compatibility on recovery of transfused human platelets. Blood 26:732, 1965

2. Beardsley DS, Ho JS, Moulton T: Pl^{T}: A new platelet specific antigen on glycoprotein V (abstr). Blood 70 (Suppl 1):347a, 1987

3. Berndt M, Gregory C, Kabral A, Zola H, Fournier D, Castaldi PA: Purification and preliminary characterization of the glycoprotein Ib complex in the human platelet membrane. Eur J Biochem 151:637, 1985

4. Bernier I, Dautigny A, Colombani J, Jolles P: Detergent-solubilized HL-A antigens from human platelets: A comparative study of various purification techniques. Biochim Biophys Acta 356:82, 1974

5. Blumberg N, Masel D, Mayer T, Horan P, Heal J: Removal of HLA-A,B antigens from platelets. Blood 63:448, 1984

6. Boizard B, Wautier J-L: Lek^{a}, a new platelet antigen absent in Glanzmann's thrombasthenia. Vox Sang 46:47, 1984

7. Coller BS: A new murine monoclonal antibody reports an activation-dependent change in the conformation and/or microenvironment of the platelet GPIIb/IIIa complex. J Clin Invest 76:101, 1985

8. Coller BS, Peerschke EI, Seligsohn U, Scudder LE, Nurden AT, Rosa J-P: Studies on the binding of an alloimmune and two murine monoclonal antibodies to the platelet glycoprotein IIb–IIIa receptor. J Lab Clin Med 107:384, 1986

9. Crookston MC: Blood group antigens acquired from the plasma. In Sandler SG, Nusbacher J, Schanfield MS (eds): Immunobiology of the Erythrocyte, p 99. New York, AR Liss, 1980

10. Curry RA, Messner RP, Johnson GJ: Inhibition of platelet aggregation by monoclonal antibody reactive with beta-2-microglobulin chain of HLA complex. Science 224:509, 1984

11. Dancis A, Ehmann C, Ferziger R, Demopoulos B, Karpatkin S: Studies on the mechanism of Pl^{A1} post-transfusion purpura (PTP). Blood 68(Suppl 1):106, 1986

12. Dausset J: The major histocompatibility complex in man. Science 213:1469, 1981

13. Dautigny A, Bernier I, Colombani J, Jolles P: Purification and characterization of HL-A antigens from human platelets, solubilized by the non-ionic detergent NP-40. Biochim Biophys Acta 298:783, 1973

14. Dautigny A, Bernier I, Colombani J, Jolles P: Human platelets as a source of HL-A antigens: A study of various solubilization techniques. Biochimie 57:1197, 1975

15. Degos L, Dautigny A, Brouet JC, Colombani M, Ardaillou N, Caen JP, Colombani J: A molecular defect in thrombasthenic platelets. J Clin Invest 56:236, 1975

16. Degos L, Tobelem G, Lethielleux P, Levy-Toledano S, Caen J, Colombani J: Molecular defect in platelets from patients with Bernard-Soulier syndrome. Blood 50:899, 1977

17. De Waal LP, van Dalen CM, Engelfriet CP, von dem Borne AEG Kr: Alloimmunization against the platelet-specific Zw[a] antigen, resulting in neonatal alloimmune thrombocytopenia or post-transfusion purpura, is associated with the supertypic Drw52 antigen including DR3 and DRw6. Hum Immunol 17:45, 1986

18. Du X, Beutler L, Ruan C, Castaldi PA, Berndt MC: Glycoprotein Ib and IX are fully complexed in the intact platelet membrane. Blood 69:1524, 1987

19. Duncan JR, Rosse WF: Alloantibody-induced platelet serotonin release is blocked by antibody to the platelet P1[A1] antigen. Br J Haematol 64:331, 1986

20. Dunstan RA: The expression of ABH antigens during in vitro megakaryocyte maturation: Origin of heterogeneity of antigen density. Br J Haematol 62:587, 1986

21. Dunstan RA, Simpson MB: Stability of platelet surface antigens during storage. Transfusion 25:563, 1985

22. Dunstan RA, Simpson MB: Heterogeneous distribution of antigens on human platelets demonstrated by fluorescence flow cytometry. Br J Haematol 61:603, 1985

23. Dunstan RA, Simpson MB, Rosse WF: Erythrocyte antigens on human platelets. Absence of Rh, Duffy, Kell, Kidd and Lutheran antigens. Transfusion 24:243, 1984

24. Dunstan RA, Simpson MB, Rosse WF: Le[a] blood group antigen on human platelets. Am J Clin Pathol 83:90, 1985

25. Dunstan RA, Simpson MB, Rosse WF: Presence of P blood group antigens on human platelets. Am J Clin Pathol 83:731, 1985

26. Dunstan RA, Simpson MB, Knowles RW, Rosse WF: The origin of ABH antigens on human platelets. Blood 65:615, 1985

27. Feuerstein N, Monos DS, Cooper HL: Phorbol ester effect in platelets, lymphocytes, and leukemic cells (HL-60) is associated with enhanced phosphorylation of class I HLA antigens. Biochem Biophys Res Commun 126:206, 1985

28. Fitzgerald LA, Steiner B, Rall SC, Lo S, Phillips DR: Protein sequence of endothelial glycoprotein IIIa from a cDNA clone. Identity to platelet glycoprotein IIIa and similarity to "integrin." J Biol Chem 262:3936, 1987

29. Friedman JM, Aster RH: Neonatal alloimmune thrombocytopenic purpura and congenital porencephaly in two siblings associated with a "new" maternal antiplatelet antibody. Blood 65:1412, 1985

30. Furihata K, Hunter J, Aster RH, Koewing G, Shulman NR, Kunicki TJ: Human anti-P1[E1] antibody recognizes epitopes associated with the alpha subunit of platelet glycoprotein Ib. Br J Haematol 68:103, 1988

31. Furihata K, Nugent DJ, Bissonette A, Aster RH, Kunicki TJ: On the association of the platelet-specific alloantigen, Pen[a], with glycoprotein IIIa. Evidence for heterogeneity of glycoprotein IIIa. J Clin Invest 80:1624, 1987

32. George JN, Nurden AT, Phillips DR: Molecular defects in interactions of platelets with the vessel wall. N Engl J Med 311:1084, 1984

33. George JN, Pickett EB, Heinz R: Platelet membrane glycoprotein changes during the preparation and storage of platelet concentrates. Transfusion (in press) 1988

34. George JN, Pickett EB, Heinz R: Platelet membrane microparticles in blood bank fresh frozen plasma and cryoprecipitate. Blood 68:307, 1987

35. Giancotti FG, Lanfuino LR, Zanetti A, Peri G, Tarone G, Dejana E: Platelets express a membrane protein complex immunologically related to the fibroblast fibronectin receptor and distinct from GPIIb/IIIa. Blood 69:1535, 1987

36. Gockerman JP, Jacob W: Purification and characterization of papain-solubilized HLA antigens from human platelets. Blood 53:838, 1979

37. Gruel Y, Boizard B, Daffos F, Forestier F, Caen J, Wautier J-L: Determination of platelet antigens and glycoproteins in the human fetus. Blood 68:488, 1986

38. Hagen I, Bjerrum OJ, Solum NO: Characterization of human platelet proteins solubilized with Triton X-100 and examined by crossed immunoelectrophoresis. Reference patterns of extracts from whole platelets and isolated membranes. Eur J Biochem 99:9, 1979

39. Hagen I, Nurden AT, Bjerrum OJ, Solum NO, Caen J: Immunochemical evidence for protein abnormalities in platelets from patients with Glanzmann's thrombasthenia and Bernard-Soulier syndrome. J Clin Invest 65:722, 1980

40. Hasegawa SR, Hasegawa E, Chen W-T, Yamada KM: Characterization of a membrane-associated glycoprotein implicated in cell adhesion to fibronectin. J Cell Biochem 28:307, 1985

41. Heal JM, Blumberg N, Masel D: An evaluation of crossmatching, HLA and ABO matching for platelet transfusions to refractory patients. Blood 70:23, 1987

42. Heinrich D, Stephinger U, Mueller-Eckhardt C: Specific interaction of HLA antibodies (eluates) with washed platelets. Br J Haematol 35:441, 1977

43. Heinrich D, Scharf T, Santoso S, Clemetson KJ, Mueller-Eckhardt C: Monoclonal antibodies against human platelet membrane glycoproteins IIb-IIIa. II. Different effects on platelet function. Thromb Res 38:547, 1985

44. Hemler ME, Huang C, Schwarz L: The VLA protein family. Characterization of five distinct cell surface heterodimers each with a common 130,000 molecular weight beta subunit. J Biol Chem 262:3300, 1987

45. Holmlund G, Thlikainen A, Penttinen K: The effect of HLA antibodies on platelet aggregation. Scand J Immunol 6:157, 1977

46. Janson M, McFarland J, Aster RH: Quantitative determination of platelet surface alloantigens using a monoclonal probe. Hum Immunol 15:251, 1986

47. Kao KJ: Plasma and platelet HLA in normal individuals: Quantitation by competitive enzyme-linked immunoassay. Blood 70:282, 1987

48. Kao KJ, Cook DJ, Scornik JC: Quantitative analysis of platelet surface HLA by W6/32 anti-HLA monoclonal antibody. Blood 68:627, 1986

49. Kaplan C, Patereau C, Reznikoff-Etievant MF, Muller JY, Dumez Y, Kesseler A: Antenatal $P1^{A1}$ typing and detection of GPIIb-IIIa complex. Br J Haematol 60:586, 1985

50. Kawai Y, Newman PJ, Furihata K, Kunicki TJ, Montgomery RR: The $P1^{A1}$ alloantigen is expressed on human endothelial cells (abstr). Clin Res 34:2, 1986

51. Keimowitz R, Collins J, Davis K, Aster R: Post-transfusion purpura associated with alloimmunization against the platelet-specific antigen, Bak^a Am J Hematol 21:79, 1986

52. Kelton JG, Hamid C, Aker S, Blajchman MA: The amount of blood group A substance on platelets is proportional to the amount in the plasma. Blood 59:980, 1982

53. Kickler TS, Ness PM, Herman JH, Bell WR: Studies on the pathophysiology of post-transfusion purpura. Blood 68:347, 1986

54. Kickler TS, Furihata K, Kunicki TJ, Herman JH, Aster RH: A new platelet alloantigen allelic to Bak^a and its association with post-transfusion purpura (abstr). Blood 68(Suppl 1):111a, 1986

55. Kiefel V, Santoso S, Katzmann B, Mueller-Eckhardt C: Neonatal alloimmune thrombocytopenia (NAIT) caused by a new platelet specific alloantibody Br(a) (abstr). Blood 70 (Suppl 1):340a, 1987

56. Kieffer N, Boizard B, Didry D, Wautier J: Immunochemical characterization of the platelet-specific alloantigen Lek^a. A comparative study with the $P1^{A1}$ alloantigen. Blood 64:1212, 1984

57. Klein J: The major histocompatibility complex of the mouse. Science 203:516, 1979

58. Kornecki E, Chung S-Y, Holt JC, Cierniewski CS, Tuszynski GP, Niewiarowski S: Identification of $P1^{A1}$ alloantigen domain on a 66 kDa protein derived from glycoprotein IIIa of human platelets. Biochim Biophys Acta 818:285, 1985

59. Kunicki TJ: Organization of glycoproteins within the platelet plasma membrane. In George JN, Nurden AT, Phillips DR (eds): Platelet Membrane Glycoproteins. New York, Plenum Press, 1985

60. Kunicki TJ, Aster RH: Deletion of the platelet-specific alloantigen $P1^{A1}$ from platelets in Glanzmann's thrombasthenia. J Clin Invest 61:1225, 1978

61. Kunicki TJ, Aster RH: Absence of the platelet receptor for drug dependent antibodies in the Bernard-Soulier syndrome. J Clin Invest 62:716, 1978

62. Kunicki TJ, Aster RH: Isolation and immunologic characterization of the human platelet alloantigen, $P1^{A1}$. Mol Immunol 16:353, 1979

63. Kunicki T, Aster RH: Qualitative and quantitative tests for platelet alloantibodies and drug-dependent antibodies. In McMillan R (ed): Methods in Hematology: Immune Cytopenias. New York, Churchill-Livingstone, 1983

64. Kunicki TJ, Furihata K, Bull B, Nugent D: The immunogenicity of platelet membrane glycoproteins. Transfusion Med Rev 1:21, 1987

65. Kunicki TJ, Nurden AT, Pidard D, Russell NR, Caen JP: Characterization of human platelet glycoprotein antigens giving rise to individual immunoprecipitates in crossed immunoelectrophoresis. Blood 58:1190, 1981

66. Kunicki TJ, Nugent DJ, Staats S, Orchekowski RP, Wayner EA, Carter WG: The human fibroblast class II extracellular matrix receptor mediates platelet adhesion to collagen and is identical to the platelet glycoprotein Ia-IIa complex. J Biol Chem 263:4516, 1988

67. Kunicki TJ, Pidard D, Rosa J-P, Nurden AT: The formation of calcium dependent complexes of platelet membrane glycoproteins IIb and IIIa in solution as determined by crossed immunoelectrophoresis. Blood 58:268, 1981

68. Kunicki TJ, Russell N, Nurden AT, Aster RH, Caen JP: Further studies of the human platelet receptor for quinine- and quinidine-dependent antibodies. J Immunol 126:398, 1981

69. Lalezari P, Driscoll AM: Ability of thrombocytes to acquire HLA specificity from plasma. Blood 59:167, 1982

70. Lane J, Brown M, Bernstein I, Wilcox PK, Slichter SJ, Nowinski RC: Serological and biochem-

ical analysis of the P1^{A1} alloantigen of human platelets. Br J Haematol 50:351, 1982

71. Leeksma OC, Giltay JC, Zandbergen-Spaargaren J, Modderman PW, van Mourik JA, von dem Borne AEG Kr: The platelet alloantigen Zw^a or P1^{A1} is expressed by cultured endothelial cells. Br J Haematol 66:369, 1987

72. Lewis JH, Draude J, Kuhns WJ: Coating of "O" platelets with A and B group substances. Vox Sang 5:434, 1968

73. Liebert M, Aster RH: Expression of HLA-B12 on platelets, on lymphocytes and in serum: A quantitative study. Tissue Antigens 9:199, 1977

74. LoBuglio AF, Court WS, Vincour L, Maglott G, Shaw GM: Immune thrombocytopenic purpura. Use of a ^{125}I-labeled anti-human IgG monoclonal antibody to quantify platelet-bound IgG. N Engl J Med 309:459, 1983

75. Lopez JA, Chung DW, Fujikawa K, Hagen FS, Papayannopoulou T, Roth GJ: Cloning of the alpha chain of human platelet glycoprotein Ib: A transmembrane protein with homology to leucinerich alpha-2-glycoprotein. Proc Natl Acad Sci USA 84:5615, 1987

76. Majsky A: Antigenicity of blood platelets. Curr Top Microbiol Immunol 58:138, 1969

77. McElligott MC, McFarland JG, Anderson AJ, Menitove JE: ABO incompatibility in HLA-matched platelet transfusions. Blood 64(Suppl):228, 1984 (abstract)

78. McEver RP, Bennett EM, Martin MN: Identification of two structurally and functionally distinct sites on human platelet membrane glycoprotein IIb–IIIa using monoclonal antibodies. J Biol Chem 258:5269, 1983

79. McMillan R, Mason D, Tani P, Schmidt GM: Evaluation of platelet surface antigens: Localization of the P1^{A1} alloantigen. Br J Haematol 51:297, 1982

80. Moulinier J: Iso-immunization maternelle anti-plaquettaire et purpura neonatal. Le system de group plaquettaire 'Duzo'. Proceedings of the Sixth Congress of the European Society of Haematology, Copenhagen, 1957

81. Mueller-Eckhardt C: HLA-B8 antigen and anti-P1^{A1} allo-immunization. Tissue Antigens 19:154, 1982

82. Mueller-Eckhardt C, Heinrich D, Mersch-Baumert K, Czitrom A, Walker P: A critical evaluation of HL-A phenotype and genotype frequencies in a large German population determined by platelet complement fixation and lymphocytotoxicity. Humangenetik 24:319, 1974

83. Mueller-Eckhardt C, Kiefel V, Mueller-Eckhardt G, Bambauer R, Baur J, Behringhoff B, Duess U, Heinrich D, Klein HO, Lechner K: Post-transfusion purpura. A survey of thirteen cases. Klin Wochenschr 64:1198, 1986

84. Mulder A, van Leeuwen EF, Veenboer GJM, Tetteroo PAT, von dem Borne AEG Kr: Immunochemical characterization of platelet-specific alloantigens. Scand J Haematol 33:267, 1984

85. Nachman RL, Jaffe EA, Weksler BW: Immunoinhibition of ristocetin induced platelet aggregation. J Clin Invest 59:143, 1977

86. Newman PJ, Allen RW, Kahn RA, Kunicki TJ: Quantitation of membrane glycoprotein IIIa on intact human platelets using the monoclonal antibody, AP3. Blood 65:227, 1985

87. Newman P, Martin L, Knipp M, Kahn R: Studies on the nature of the human platelet alloantigen, P1^{A1}: Localization to a 17,000 dalton polypeptide. Mol Immunol 22:719, 1985

88. Nordhagen R, Flaathen ST: Chloroquine removal of HLA antigens from platelets for the platelet immunofluorescence test. Vox Sang 48:156, 1985

89. Pellegrino MA, Ferrone S, Pellegrino AG, Oh SK, Reisfeld RA: Evaluation of two sources of soluble HL-A antigens: Platelets and serum. Eur J Immunol 4:250, 1974

90. Pidard D, Montgomery RR, Bennett JS, Kunicki TJ: Interaction of AP2, a monoclonal antibody specific for the human platelet glycoprotein IIb–IIIa complex, with intact platelets. J Biol Chem 258:12582, 1983

91. Pincus JH, Kahan BD, Mittal KK: A role for cAMP in the preparation of human platelets for the extraction of histocompatibility antigens. Immunochemistry 13:565, 1976

92. Piotrowicz RS, Orchekowski RP, Nugent DJ, Yamada KM, Kunicki TJ: Human platelet glycoprotein Ic–IIa functions as an activation-independent fibronectin receptor. J Cell Biol 106:1359, 1988

93. Pischel KD, Hemler ME, Huang C, Bluestein HG, Woods VL: Use of the monoclonal antibody 12F1 to characterize the differentiation antigen VLA-2. J Immunol 138:226, 1987

94. Pytela R, Pierschbacher MD, Ginsberg MH, Plow EF, Ruoslahti E: Platelet membrane glycoprotein IIb/IIIa: Member of a family of Arg-Gly-Asp-specific adhesion receptors. Science 231;1559, 1986

95. Rabellino EM, Levene RB, Leung LLK, Nachman RL: Human megakaryocytes. II. Expression of platelet proteins in early marrow megakaryocytes. J Exp Med 154:88, 1981

96. Ramsey G, Salamon DJ: Frequency of P1^{A1} in blacks. Transfusion 26:531, 1986

97. Rege VP, Painter TJ, Watkins WM, Morgan WTJ: Isolation of serologically active fucose-con-

taining oligosaccharides from human blood group H substance. Nature 203:360, 1964

98. Reznikoff-Etievant MF, Dangu C, Lobet R: HLA-B8 antigen and anti-P1^{A1} allo-immunization. Tissue Antigens 18:66, 1981

99. Reznikoff-Etievant MF, Muller JY, Julien F, Patereau C: An immune response gene linked to MHC in man. Tissue Antigens 22:312, 1983

100. Rosa J-P, Kieffer N, Didry D, Pidard D, Kunicki TJ, Nurden AT: The human platelet membrane glycoprotein complex GPIIb-IIIa expresses antigenic sites not exposed on the dissociated glycoproteins. Blood 64:1246, 1984

101. Ruan C, Tobelem G, McMichael AJ, Drouet L, Legrand Y, Degos L, Kieffer N, Lee H, Caen JP: Monoclonal antibody to human platelet glycoprotein I. Br J Haematol 49:511, 1981

102. Sanchez-Madrid F, Nagy J, Robbins E, Simon P, Springer TA: A human leukocyte differentiation antigen family with distinct alpha subunits and a common beta subunit: The lymphocyte function-associated (LFA-1), the C3bi complement receptor (OKM1/Mac-1), and the p150,95 molecule. J Exp Med 158:1786, 1983

103. Santoso S, Lohmeyer J, Rennich H, Clemetson KJ, Mueller-Eckhardt C: Platelet surface antigens: Analysis by monoclonal antibodies. I. Immunological and biochemical studies. Blut 48:161, 1984

104. Santoso S, Mueller-Eckhardt G, Santoso S, Kiefel V, Mueller-Eckhardt C: HLA antigens on platelet membranes. In vitro and in vivo studies. Vox Sang 51:327, 1986

105. Santoso S, Shibata Y, Kiefel V, Mueller-Eckhardt C: Identification of Yuk(b) alloantigen on platelet glycoprotein IIIa (abstr). Thromb Haemostasis 58:197, 1987

106. Shibata Y, Matsuda I, Miyaji T, Ichikawa Y: Yuk^{a}, a new platelet antigen involved in two cases of neonatal alloimmune thrombocytopenia. Vox Sang 50:177, 1986

107. Shibata Y, Miyaji T, Ichikawa Y, Matsuda I: A new platelet antigen system Yuk^{a}/Yuk^{b}. Vox Sang 51:334, 1986

108. Shibata Y, Mori H: A new platelet-specific alloantigen system, Yuk^{a}/Yuk^{b} is located on platelet membrane glycoprotein IIIa. Proc Jpn Acad 63:36, 1987

109. Shulman NR, Marder V, Hiller M, Collier E: Platelet and leukocyte isoantigens and their antibodies: Serologic, physiologic and clinical studies. Prog Hematol 4:222, 1964

110. Simon T, Collins J, Kunicki T, Furihata K, Smith K, Aster R: Post-transfusion purpura with antiplatelet antibody specific for the platelet antigen Pen^{a} (abstr). Blood 68(Suppl 1):117a, 1986

111. Slichter SJ, Ballem P, Teramura G: Characteristics of P1^{A1} antibodies produced in neonatal thrombocytopenia (NAT) versus post-transfusion purpura (PTP) (abstr). Blood 62(Suppl 1):247a, 1983

112. Sonnenberg A, Janssen H, Hogervorst F, Calafat J, Hilgers J: A complex of platelet glycoproteins Ic and IIa identified by a rat monoclonal antibody. J Biol Chem 262:10376, 1987

113. Svejgaard A: Iso-antigenic systems of human blood platelets—a survey. Ser Haematol 2:1, 1969

114. Szatkowski NS, Aster RH: HLA antigens of platelets. IV. Influence of "private" HLA-B locus specificities on the expression of Bw4 and Bw6 on human platelets. Tissue Antigens 15:361, 1980

115. Taaning E, Antonsen H, Petersen S, Svejgaard A, Thomsen M: HLA antigens and maternal antibodies in antibodies in allo-immune neonatal thrombocytopenia. Tissue Antigens 21:351, 1983

116. Taaning E, Killmann S-A, Morling N, Ovesen H, Svejgaard A: Post-transfusion purpura (PTP) due to anti-Zw^{b} ($-$P1^{A2}): The significance of IgG3 antibodies in PTP. Br J Haematol 64:217, 1986

117. Thiagarajan P, Shapiro SS, Levine E, DeMarco L, Yalcin A: A monoclonal antibody to human platelet glycoprotein IIIa detects a related protein in cultured human endothelial cells. J Clin Invest 75:896, 1985

118. Titani K, Takio K, Handa M, Ruggeri ZM: Amino acid sequence of the von Willebrand factor-binding domain of platelet membrane glycoprotein Ib. Proc Natl Acad Sci USA 84:5610, 1987

119. Tobelem G, Levy-Toledano S, Bredoux R, Michel H, Nurden A, Caen JP: New approach to determination of specific functions of platelet membrane sites. Nature 263:427, 1976

120. Tragardh L, Klareskog L, Curman B, Rask L, Peterson PA: Isolation and properties of detergent-solubilized HLA antigens obtained from platelets. Scand J Immunol 9:303, 1979

121. Vainchenker W, Deschamps JF, Bastin JM, Guichard J, Titeux GM, Breton-Gorius J, McMichael AJ: Two monoclonal antiplatelet antibodies as markers of human megakaryocyte maturation: Immunofluorescent staining and platelet peroxidase detection in megakaryocyte colonies and in in vivo cells from normal and leukemic patients. Blood 59:514, 1982

122. van der Schoot CE, Wester M, von dem Borne AEG Kr, Huisman HG: Characterization of platelet-specific alloantigens by immunoblotting: Localization of Zw and Bak antigens. Br J Haematol 64:715, 1986

123. van der Weerdt C: The platelet agglutination test in platelet grouping. In Histocompatibility Testing, Vol II. Copenhagen, Munksgaard, 1965

124. van der Weerdt C, Veenhoven-von Riesz L, Nijenhuis L, van Loghem J: The Zw blood group system in platelets. Vox Sang 8:513, 1963

125. van Leeuwen E, Leeksma O, van Mourik J, Engelfriet C, von dem Borne A: Effect of the binding of anti-Zw[a] antibodies on platelet function. Vox Sang 47:280, 1984

126. van Leeuwen EF, von dem Borne AEG Kr, von Riesz LE, Nijenhuis LE, Engelfriet CP: Absence of platelet-specific alloantigens in Glanzmann's thrombasthenia. Blood 57:49, 1981

127. van Loghem J, Dorfmeijer H, van der Hart M: Serological and genetical studies on a platelet antigen (Zw). Vox Sang 4:161, 1959

128. Voigtmann R, Uhlenbruck G, Pardoe GI, Rogers K: The preparation and purification of HL-A monospecific antigens using platelets and various lymphoid sources. Eur J Immunol 4:674, 1974

129. von dem Borne A, van der Plas-van Dalen CM: Bak[a] and Lek[a] are identical antigens. Br J Haematol 62:404, 1986

130. von dem Borne A, van Leeuwen E, von Riesz L, van Boxtel C, Engelfriet C: Neonatal alloimmune thrombocytopenia: Detection and characterization of the responsible antibodies by the platelet immunofluorescence test. Blood 57:649, 1981

131. von dem Borne A, von Riesz E, Verheugt F, ten Cate J, Koppe J, Engelfriet C, Nijenhuis L: Bak[a], a new platelet-specific antigen involved in neonatal alloimmune thrombocytopenia. Vox Sang 39:113, 1980

132. Warejcka D, Janson M, Aster RH: Pl^{A1} antigen but not HLA antigens can be acquired by platelets from plasma. Blood 66(Suppl 1):321, 1985

133. Watkins WM: Biochemistry and genetics of the ABO, Lewis and P blood group systems. Adv Hum Genet 10:1, 1980

134. Wayner EA, Carter WG: Identification of multiple cell adhesion receptors for collagen and fibronectin in human fibrosarcoma cells possessing unique α and common β subunits. J Cell Biol 105:1873, 1987

135. Weiss H, Hoyer L, Rickles FR, Varma A, Rogers J: Quantitative assay of a plasma factor deficient in von Willebrand's disease that is necessary for platelet aggregation. Relationship to factor VIII procoagulant activity and antigen content. J Clin Invest 52:2708, 1973

136. White GC, Workman EF, Lunblad RL: Thrombin binding to thrombasthenic platelets. J Lab Clin Med 91:76, 1978

137. Woods VL, Oh EH, Mason D, McMillan R: Autoantibodies against the platelet glycoprotein IIb/IIIa complex in patients with chronic ITP. Blood 63:368, 1984

7

Platelet Autoantigens

DIANA S. BEARDSLEY

IDIOPATHIC (OR IMMUNE) THROMBOCYTOPENIC PURPURA

Overview of Clinical Syndrome

The syndrome of spontaneous bruising, petechiae, and purpura caused by acquired destruction of platelets, which has been recognized for more than 200 years, has been termed "idiopathic" thrombocytopenic purpura (ITP) reflecting the enigmatic character of this condition. In the 1950s Harrington et al.[18] discovered the immunologic cause of the platelet destruction in this disease. He found that plasma from ITP patients could cause a dramatic thrombocytopenia when infused into normal recipients and that this activity was specifically associated with the globulin fraction of the plasma. The platelet destructive component was shown by Shulman et al.[44] to be a 7S globulin, presumably an antiplatelet antibody. More recently, McMillan et al.[33] and Karpatkin et al.[22] have demonstrated in vitro synthesis of antiplatelet antibody by splenic lymphocytes from ITP patients. Furthermore, $F(ab')_2$ fragments of splenic lymphocyte supernatants were found to bind specifically to platelet antigens.[36] As the autoimmune basis of platelet destruction has been known for more than 10 years, it has been suggested that the terminology for this syndrome be changed from *idiopathic* to *autoimmune* thrombocytopenic purpura. This nomenclature has gained acceptance in the recent literature.[20]

As biochemical understanding of the clinical syndrome advances, however, it is likely that other mechanisms will be found to play a role. Although most cases of ITP may be caused by autoantibody production, a subset may be due to circulating immune complexes[61] or even cell-mediated immune phenomena.[4] In this chapter, we will refer to the clinical syndrome as ITP (idiopathic or immune thrombocytopenia) and specify autoimmune thrombocytopenia when there is clear evidence for the involvement of antiplatelet autoantibodies.

The clinical features of ITP vary from patient to patient, falling into two general categories—acute and chronic (Table 7-1). Acute ITP typically affects children, often appearing suddenly after a viral illness or immunization. Males and females are affected with equal frequency, and the disease usually remits spontaneously after a few weeks or months.[37] The chronic designation generally connotes disease lasting more than 6 to 12 months and is the common form of ITP in adults. Adult women are three times more likely than men to develop chronic ITP, and the presence of other associated autoimmune phenomena is not uncommon.[31] The striking differences in the clinical features of acute and chronic ITP syndromes have led some investigators to hypothesize different pathogenic mechanisms for acute and chronic ITP. However, recent studies, discussed later in this chapter, have determined that autoantibodies are often present in patients with both acute and chronic ITP.

Table 7-1
Comparison of Typical Clinical Features of Acute and Chronic ITP

Acute	Chronic
Peak age 2–6 yr	Predominately adults
Male/female = 1 : 1	Male/female = 1 : 3
Abrupt onset	Insidious onset
Thrombocytopenia often severe, but resolves within 6–12 mo	Duration > 1 yr
Preceding viral illness in two-thirds of cases	Often incidental diagnosis

Antiplatelet Antibody in Idiopathic Thrombocytopenic Purpura

The demonstration of antibody involvement in the pathogenesis of ITP prompted attempts to charactcrizc the responsible antiplatelet antibodies. The goal of much of this work was to find a method for detecting the presumed antiplatelet autoantibodies on the platelet surface by analogy with the erythrocyte Coombs' test, the expectation being that such an assay would be diagnostic for autoimmune platelet destruction.

Indirect serum assays for antiplatelet antibody generally cannot differentiate between alloantibodies and autoantibodies, and the early agglutination tests were also plagued by spontaneous platelet aggregation and the presence of nonspecific immunoglobulin receptors on the platelet surface.[20] Direct assays involve quantitation of platelet-associated immunoglobulin (PAIgG) by a large number of different techniques, usually employing an antiglobulin reagent. The various approaches have been reviewed recently by Kelton,[23] McMillan,[32] and Karpatkin[20] and are discussed in detail in Chapter 16. Although the quantities of PAIgG found on normal platelets vary depending upon the precise technique and antiglobulin reagent used, approximately 90% of patients who have the clinical syndrome of ITP will have a significant elevation of PAIgG. In spite of the remarkable sensitivity of these tests, their clinical value as diagnostic criteria is limited by the fact that PAIgG is elevated in many other clinical situations, including malignancy, sepsis, toxemia of pregnancy, and immune complex disease.[23] In a prospective study, Kelton found that elevated PAIgG had a specificity of less then 50% in diagnosing ITP.[24] A major limitation of the antiglobulin assays for probing the biochemical details of the immunologic interactions in ITP has been that only a small fraction of the total PAIgG is actually the pathogenic autoantibody of interest. George et al.[15] have reported that the normal, nonimmune PAIgG is actually an α-granule protein, probably taken up by megakaryocytes at the time platelets are produced.[16,17] They suggested that this PAIgG decreases during the lifetime of the cells. An elevated PAIgG, then, may simply reflect a shift in the average age of the platelet population; thus, it may be more akin to the erythrocyte reticulocyte count rather than the Coombs' test.

IDENTIFICATION OF PLATELET AUTOANTIGENS

Background

Attempts to characterize platelet autoantigens have employed several techniques including differential antiglobulin reactivity with platelets congenitally deficient in particular surface glycoproteins, immunoprecipitation, immunoblotting, and isolation or immobilization of potential target antigenic proteins with murine monoclonal antibodies. An underlying feature of most successful approaches is physical separation of the targets for the antiplatelet autoantibodies from the more abundant, ubiquitous, nonimmune platelet-associated IgG.

Identification of the Antigenic Platelet Proteins

Glycoproteins IIb and IIIa

The antigenic targets for the autoantibodies important in ITP are generally thought to be "public" antigens present on most normal platelets. However, the actual identification of the antigenic surface proteins was not accomplished until the 1980s. The various platelet proteins that have been reported to contain target antigens for platelet autoantibodies are listed in Table 7-2. With use of a platelet suspension immunofluorescent test, van Leeuwen et al. found that antibodies from 35 of 42 ITP patients were reactive with platelets from eight normal donors, but failed to bind to platelets from a patient with type I Glanzmann's thrombasthenia.[56] The latter platelets are se-

Table 7-2
Autoantigens Identified as the Targets of Antibodies in ITP

Antigenic Protein	Method of Identification	Source of Antibody	Ref
GPIIb–IIIa	Differential immunofluorescence using platelets deficient in GPIIb–IIIa	Sera eluated from platelets	56
GPIIb or GPIIb–IIIa	Impaired binding of anti-GPIIb monoclonal antibody to ITP platelets	Patients' platelets	58
GPIIb–IIIa; GPIb	Binding to proteins immunobolized by monoclonal antibody	Plasma/serum	62,63
GPIIIa	Immunoblotting	Sera eluted from control platelets	6
>200 kDa, 130 kDa, 105 kDa, 45 kDa	Immunoblotting	Splenic culture supernatant eluted from control platelets	30
50 kDa–240 kDa multiple antigenic bands	Immunoblotting	Serum	29
210-kDa glycoprotein	Immunoblotting	Serum	48
66 kDa	Immunoblotting	Serum	49
GPIb	Different immunofluorescence; immunoprecipitation	Plasma	51
GPIb	Crossed-immuno-electrophoresis; immunoblotting	Human hybridoma; serum	40
25 kDa	Immunoblotting	Serum	46
GPV	Immunoblotting	Serum	5
GPV	Immunoblotting	Serum	47
66 kDa, 108 kDa (cytoplasm)	Immunoblotting	Serum	19
GPIIIa (cryptic antigens)	Immunoblotting	Serum	60
GPIIIa (neoantigen)	Immunoblotting; ELISA; crossed-im-munoelectrophoresis	Human hybridoma; serum	41
GPIIb	Immunoblotting	Serum	52

verely deficient in GPIIb and GPIIIa. This suggested that antigenic sites were contained on the GPIIb–IIIa complex. Varon and Karpatkin raised an antiplatelet murine monoclonal antibody, 3B2, directed against GPIIb, which had decreased reactivity with platelets from 15 of 16 patients with ITP.[58] Reactivity was normal with platelets from the same patients during remission. These authors recognized the limitations of their methodology, pointing out that the antiplatelet autoantibodies in these patients might be directed against antigenic determinants either on GPIIb, the GPIIb–IIIa complex, or at any other site that could secondarily inhibit subsequent binding of 3B2. Other groups have documented that glycoproteins IIb and IIIa frequently contain autoantigens in ITP (*see* Tables 7-2 and 7-3), and the target epitopes for a number of these antibodies have been specifically localized to the GPIIIa portion of the GPIIb–IIIa complex.[6,41]

The technique of immunoblotting has been used to identify the antigens present on GPIIIa and a number of other platelet glycoproteins (*see* Table 7-2). Platelet membranes or whole platelets are solubilized in sodium dodecyl sul-

Table 7-3
Identification of Autoantigens in Series of at Least 20 Patients with ITP

Clinical Setting		Antigen	Frequency	Ref
ITP	$N = 108$	GPIb	3/108	62
ITP	$N = 108$	GPIIb–IIIa	5/108	63
ITP	$N = 48$	GPIIIa and others	36/48	7
ITP	$N = 23$	Multiple bands	21/23	29
Chronic ITP	$N = 59$	GPIb or IIb–IIIa	34/59 30 IIb–IIIa 11 Ib 2 both	35
ITP	$N = 74$	GPIb	23/74	40
ITP	$N = 40$	GPIIb and others	11/40	52

fate (SDS), separated according to their relative molecular masses (M_r) by polyacrylamide gel electrophoresis (PAGE), and then transferred to nitrocellulose paper. Immobilized on the nitrocellulose, the individual proteins are accessible for reaction with the potential autoantibody (in serum, plasma, or eluates from platelets), followed by localization with an antihuman globulin reagent. The antigenic protein bands can be visualized by autoradiography with use of an ^{125}I-labeled antiglobulin probe or by a color reaction catalyzed by an enzyme linked to the antiglobulin probe.[3] The nonimmune platelet immunoglobulin appears at an M_r of approximately 200 kDa (nonreduced) using Laemmli discontinuous SDS gel electrophoresis conditions. Most of the major surface glycoproteins migrate far enough from this region to achieve a physical separation of the nonimmune IgG from the protein targets of antiplatelet autoantibodies. Figure 7-1 shows results of immunoblotting experiments indicating that GPIIIa contains the target antigen for the antiplatelet autoantibodies found in sera from 7 of 13 chronic ITP patients studied. Identification of the antigenic protein was based upon its comigration with GPIIIa in both reduced and nonreduced SDS-PAGE and the absence of the antigen from type 1 Glanzmann's thrombasthenic platelets, known to be severely deficient in both GPIIb and GPIIIa. It should be noted that, because immunoblotting requires the denaturation of platelet proteins by the SDS detergent, it is probable that some platelet autoantigens may become altered during this process and may not be identified. On the other hand, the antiserum being tested could contain alloantibodies against antigens present on the control platelets used as a source for the electrophoretically separated platelet proteins. True autoantibodies must be distinguished from alloantibodies by comparing the reactivity with that of autologous platelets. For example, to prove that GPIIIa could be the target of antiplatelet autoantibodies, the immunoblot reactivity was confirmed by using the patients' own platelets during remission and by demonstrating that $F(ab')_2$ fragments bound to the same protein band.[6] The detailed investigations, such as the preceding summarized immunoblotting studies, have helped to establish the presence of anti-GPIIIa autoantibodies in some cases of ITP and are likely to be of value for further characterization of the epitopes involved. Although such extensive studies are not applicable as a routine diagnostic test for autoimmune thrombocytopenia, they may aid in the development of other assays for clinical use.

Autoantigens of Functional Significance

The glycoprotein IIb–IIIa complex is necessary for fibrinogen binding during normal platelet aggregation (*see* Chap. 2). Not all anti-GPIIb–IIIa or anti-GPIIIa platelet autoantibodies have the same target epitope. A subset of these autoantibodies has been shown to interfere with normal platelet aggregation. Neissner et al.[39] and Balduini et al.[1] have reported patients with an acquired syndrome indistinguishable from Glanzmann's thrombasthenia caused by anti-GPIIb–IIIa autoantibodies. Two ITP patients studied by Beardsley et al.[5] had anti-GPIIIa autoantibodies that interfered with binding of ^{125}I-labeled fibrinogen to stimulated platelets in a concentration-dependent manner. Although a functional defect

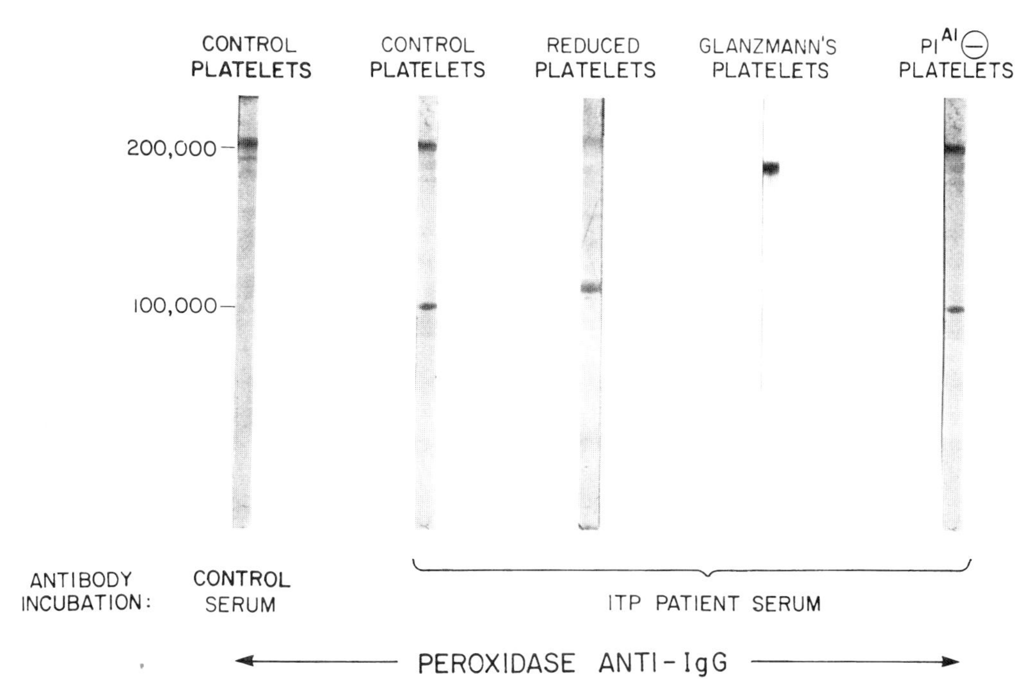

Figure 7-1. Chronic ITP. Photographs of nitrocellulose transfers of platelet proteins incubated with ITP serum or control serum as indicated, followed by biotinylated goat antihuman IgG, avidin, and biotinylated horseradish peroxidase. Colored bands appeared after addition of chloronaphthol. Note the specific 100,000-M_r protein which binds IgG. This protein is absent from Glanzmann's thrombasthenic platelets and is converted to an M_r of 110,000 upon reduction of disulfide bonds.

could not be detected in these two patients with routine platelet aggregation tests, they had prolonged bleeding times and significant hemorrhagic manifestations, although they were only mildly thrombocytopenic. Target epitopes close to the fibrinogen-binding site on GPIIb-IIIa may explain these observations and account for a clinical course characterized by more bleeding than anticipated from the degree of thrombocytopenia. Other investigators have previously hypothesized that such autoantibodies, even in the absence of thrombocytopenia, could be a frequent cause of symptomatic mild platelet dysfunction.[25,26,64]

Platelets in the congenital Bernard-Soulier syndrome have an inherited platelet disorder characterized by a deficiency of the GPIb-IX complex as well as GPV. These platelets fail to agglutinate in the presence of ristocetin and have defective adhesion to subendothelium (*see* Chap. 5). Two cases of acquired Bernard-Soulier syndrome have been reported in patients with autoantibodies that inhibit ristocetin-induced platelet agglutination.[11,48] In one case the autoantibody was shown by immunoprecipitation to react with GPIb.[11] Sugiyama and coworkers[49] studied a patient with defective collagen-induced platelet aggregation in association with an antiplatelet antibody reactive with a 62-kDa protein as demonstrated by immunoprecipitation.

Acute Postviral Idiopathic Thrombocytopenic Purpura

Because the clinical course of acute ITP in childhood is different from that of chronic ITP in adults (*see* Table 7-1), different pathogenic mechanisms had been suggested for the two syndromes. Proposed etiologic factors for acute postviral ITP have included viral interference with megakaryocyte maturation, cross-reactive antigens on virus and platelets, viral-antiviral immune complexes binding to platelets, viral-induced disseminated intravascular coagulation, and true autoantibody production. Lightsey et al.[28] found that IgG produced by splenic lymphocytes from two children with acute ITP bound specifically to platelets. A group of four children with acute varicella-associated thrombocytopenia studied by Beardsley et al. were found to have true autoantibodies directed against an 85-kDa platelet surface protein that was thrombin-sensitive and, therefore, might be GPV.[5] Stricker et al. also reported that in six of seven cases of acute postviral ITP in children anti-GPV autoantibodies were present.[47] Probably many cases of acute ITP in childhood will also be associated with circulating platelet autoantibodies. Study of larger groups of patients, such as Nugent's idiotypic characterization,[40] will determine which target antigens are important in ITP and whether or not antigenic differences will aid in identifying which cases of ITP are destined to become chronic.

Autoantigens on Glycoprotein Ib

Antiplatelet autoantibodies directed against GPIb have been well documented (*see* Table 7-2) and may be associated with a particularly severe form of ITP. By the monoclonal antibody target antigen-capture technique anti-GPIb antibodies were found in only 3 of 108 patients.[62] Szatkowski et al. documented the anti-GPIb specificity of a complement fixing autoantibody in plasma from an ITP patient using lysis inhibition, immunoprecipitation, crossed-immunoelectrophoresis, and differential immunofluorescence with Bernard-Soulier, Glanzmann's thrombasthenic, and normal platelets.[51] Nugent et al.[40] reported a case with remarkably similar clinical features to Szatkowski's patient[51] and found anti-GPIb reactivity in this patient's plasma by immunoblotting. They used the patient's splenic lymphocytes to make a human hybridoma cell line that produces a monoclonal antibody with this same reactivity.[40] Severe thrombocytopenia, complement-fixing antibody, and poor response to steroids, intravenous IgG, or splenectomy, were also features of one of Woods and McMillan's cases with an anti-GPIb antibody.[62] These are unusual in ITP; recently, Lehman et al.[27] reported a similar case, but the target antigen was not identified in their patient.

Santoso and associates[42] recently showed that anti-GPIIb–IIIa antibodies can be cleared from the platelet surface by capping and internalization of antigen–antibody complexes, whereas anti-GPIb antibodies could not be removed through membrane redistribution. It is tempting to speculate that GPIb antigenic targets might be related to the severe form of platelet lysis described earlier[40,51] and that the presence of anti-GPIb autoantibodies in future cases of ITP may also lead to complement fixation and poor response to the usual therapeutic modalities. If confirmed, one could then predict the clinical course of this unusual form of ITP on the basis of the identification of a particular target antigen or detection of a specific IgG idiotype in patient plasma.

Unique Platelet Autoantigens

Antigenic Proteins in the Platelet Cytoplasm

Immune platelet destruction often occurs in patients known to have other autoimmune diseases, particularly systemic lupus erythematosus (SLE). Because circulating immune complexes are often present in SLE, they have been implicated in the immune platelet destruction,[12,32] but autoantibody production has also been reported.[43] Kaplan and colleagues could demonstrate autoantibodies against platelet proteins of 66 kDa or 108 kDa in just three of nine SLE patients studied.[19] In these cases they found that the target antigens were present in the cytoplasmic rather than the membrane fraction of the platelets. The precise role of these antibodies in the pathogenesis of the thrombocytopenia is open to further investigation.

Cryptic Platelet Autoantigens

Particularly puzzling antibodies sometimes occur against platelet autoantigens that are "cryptic" in vivo, but appear after treatment of platelets with EDTA or formalin. Von dem Borne has shown that the in vitro platelet agglutination phenomenon, known as *pseudothrombocytopenia* is caused by IgG antibodies directed against cryptic antigens that are revealed in the presence of EDTA. Also identified were antibodies against cryptic antigens present on formalin or paraformaldehyde fixed platelets.[60] The target antigens of these antibodies are thought to reside on GPIIb–IIIa, based upon the observation that agglutination did not occur with Glanzmann's thrombasthenic platelets. Because these antibodies do not appear to cause platelet destruction in vivo, their clinical significance remains to be assessed. It is conceivable that certain in vivo conditions may induce changes in the conformation or exposure of GPIIb-IIIa mimicking those caused by EDTA. In vitro, the presence of these antibodies can make it more difficult to interpret the results of serologic assays. The origin of these antibodies is not known, but one possibility is that they arise during a period of platelet damage such as sepsis.[55,60]

Platelet "Senescence" Neoantigens

A novel platelet neoantigen or senescence antigen has been characterized by Nugent et al. who created a human monoclonal cell line using Epstein-Barr virus transformation of ITP splenic lymphocytes.[41] Antibody 5E5 binds to the GPIIb-IIIa complex as shown by enzyme-linked immunosorbent assay (ELISA) and crossed-immunoelectrophoresis and to GPIIIa as demonstrated by immunoblotting. Binding of 5E5 to intact platelets increases as the platelets are stored in vitro. The investigators hypothesize that this neoantigen may serve as a marker for the clearance of older patients from the circulation.

Variety of Autoantigens in Idiopathic Thrombocytopenic Purpura

There clearly is heterogeneity among the autoantigens found in ITP. Table 7-2 lists those proteins that have been implicated, to date, as targets for ITP antibodies. Lynch and Howe studied 23 ITP patients by immunoblotting and found reactivity with at least one protein in 21 cases.[29] Because most sera bound to more than one band, and adsorption studies suggested that the antigens were on the platelet surface, these authors concurred with other investigators that multiple platelet autoantibodies may coexist in ATP.[7,30] However, in immunoblotting studies there is always the possibility that the additional reactive bands result from degradation of the principal antigenic protein. The action of proteolytic enzymes, released during cell lysis, may convert target glycoproteins into one or more smaller fragments that still contain the antibody-reactive epitope.

Another target antigenic protein that has been noted has an M_r of 100 kDa under both reduced and nonreduced conditions. Because it is present on thrombasthenic platelets, this protein is believed to be different from GPIIIa.[7] However, its actual identity is not clear. Recently, serum antibodies against glycosphingolipids have also been reported in ITP.[57] Circulating autoantibodies reacting with a 25-kDa protein have been noted in 29 of 30 with acquired immunodeficiency syndrome by Stricker and coworkers.[46] The identity of the antigen was unknown, and it was not clear that it was related to the immune platelet destruction because essentially all HIV-positive individuals tested had this antibody whether they were thrombocytopenic or not. Other investigators have found that the autoantibodies in HIV-related ITP have similar characteristics to those found in chronic autoimmune thrombocytopenia in that they reacted with normal platelets but not with Glanzmann's thrombasthenic platelets.[54]

Specific Assays: Study of Larger Series of Patients

Woods and McMillan developed the first specific assays for antibodies directed against the major platelet surface glycoproteins, GPIIb-IIIa and GPIb.[62,63] They used monoclonal antibodies specific for either the GPIIb-IIIa complex or GPIb in microtiter wells to immobilize these particular proteins from a nonionic detergent solution. Plasma from ITP patients was then incubated with the proteins, and bound antibodies against these specific proteins were detected with antiglobulin. As with immunoblotting, immunofluorescence, and immunoprecipitation, this method does not differentiate between alloantibodies and autoantibodies; however, it has been useful as a direct way to determine whether a patient has circulating anti-GPIb or anti-GPII-IIIa antibodies.

With an updated technique, McMillan recently found anti-GPIIb-IIIa or anti-GPIb antibodies in plasma samples from 34 of 59 patients with ITP.[35] This method offers the advantage of using intact platelets to interact with a potential autoantibody before solubilization. Antigen-antibody complexes are recovered with antiglobulin, and the target antigen is then determined with a radiolabeled monoclonal antibody specific for GPIb or

GPIIb-IIIa. Antibodies identified by this assay would be those directed against platelet surface epitopes on the protein of interest. Specific assays such as this approach and other antigen-capture techniques,[14] probably offer the best promise to date as a routine clinical diagnostic test for antiplatelet antibodies in ITP.

When modified by using allotype specific platelet proteins, the antigen-capture approach can be used to study alloimmune platelet destruction.[35] Another clever method to detect antibodies against platelets uses intact platelets reacted simultaneously with patient serum and a specific murine monoclonal antiplatelet antibody[38] (*see* Chap. 20). Complexes reactive with both the murine and human antibodies are then isolated after platelet solubilization. Initially, this approach was used to decipher anti-HLA and platelet-specific alloantibodies present in the same sample, but preliminary results suggest that the approach might also be applicable to the identification of platelet autoantigens in ITP.

Further Characterization of Platelet Autoantigens

Are Platelet Autoantigens Really "Public" Antigens?

Infusion of platelets into patients with autoimmune thrombocytopenia often results in rapid clearance of the transfused platelets; however, a recent report documented that in 7 of 11 ITP patients transfused with random donor platelets, there was an increase in platelet count.[9] These results raise the question of whether or not all normal platelets contain the target antigens against which ITP antibodies are directed. Van Leeuwen et al. found that eluates from platelets of 42 patients with ITP reacted equally well with platelets from at least eight normal donors regardless of Zw^a ($P1^{A1}$), Bak^a (Lek), or Ko phenotype, although 35 of these antibodies failed to react with thrombasthenic platelets.[56] Harrington's infusions of ITP plasma caused thrombocytopenia in only 65% of his normal recipients, suggesting that there might be some variation in the platelets' susceptibility to destruction by ITP antibodies.[18] However, nearly all the recipients had a decrease in the number of circulating platelets, even if the count remained in the normal range.

The anti-GPIIIa autoantigens identified by immunoblotting studies were shown by Beardsley et al.[6] to be equally reactive with both $P1^{A1}$-positive and $P1^{A1}$-negative platelets. Evidence to date, then, suggests that ITP autoantigens are common to most normal platelets and are different from the $P1^A$ (Zw^a), Bak^a (Lek), and Ko alloantigen systems. Comparisons with the Pen (or Yuk), or $P1^E$ alloantigens have not yet been reported.

Antigenic Comparison of Megakaryocytes and Platelets

Megakaryocyte number is usually increased in patients with ITP, and the megakaryocytes present in the bone marrow are often described as "young." This observation raises the question of whether or not the target antigens for ITP autoantibodies are present on these platelet precursors and, if they are, why do the megakaryocytes survive? That there may be significant cross-reactivity between platelcts and megakaryocytes has been demonstrated by using a rabbit antiserum raised against human platelets.[59] Monoclonal antibodies directed specifically against the GPIIb-IIIa complex are reactive with >90% of the megakaryocytes, suggesting that these proteins appear in the plasma membrane early in thrombopoiesis.[10,53] However, the detection of GPIb on megakaryocytes is variable.[53]

Little is known about the presence of particular autoantigens on human megakaryocytes. McKenna and Pisciotta demonstrated fluorescent staining of megakaryocytes using ITP serum.[30a] With use of IgG, purified from serum or produced by cultured lymphocytes of two ITP patients, McMillan et al. showed that the antibody had specificity for both platelets and megakaryocytes.[34] Ballem et al. have studied in vivo platelet clearance rates and thrombopoietic responses in 38 patients with chronic ITP.[2] In spite of increased megakaryocyte cycle activity, a number of their patients were found to have decreased or ineffective platelet production possibly because of antibody interference with late thrombopoiesis or because of destruction of platelets before they leave the marrow. Recently, Stahl and coworkers have reported electron microscopic studies of megakaryocytes from four ITP patients.[45] Although most megakaryocytes showed ultrastructural evidence for damage, the younger-appearing megakaryocytes (25-50% of the total) were intact. Because the healthy cells had not yet begun active megakaryopoeisis, the results suggest that this population did not share full immunologic cross-reactivity with platelets. Further studies that use particular platelet autoantibodies are clearly needed to address this important question.

POSSIBLE CLINICAL VALUE OF PLATELET AUTOANTIGEN CHARACTERIZATION

Over the past 5 years, the target antigens of a number of platelet autoantibodies have been identified. Antigenic epitopes on the GPIIb-IIIa complex have been observed most frequently (*see* Table 7-2), but a number of other proteins including GPIb and GPV on the platelet surface are occasionally the targets of autoantibodies. Assays designed to detect autoantibodies against particular antigens offer promise for confirming the diagnosis of true autoimmune thrombocytopenia. Next, one must ask whether or not target antigen identification will lead to information of value in understanding and managing the clinical syndrome of ITP. Current results suggest the cautiously optimistic view that these results will indeed be useful.

The presence of autoantibodies in plasma and on platelets has been clearly documented in some cases of both acute and chronic ITP, and there is preliminary evidence that particular antigens will be implicated more frequently in acute ITP and others in chronic ITP. For example, anti-GPIIIa antibodies have been reported most frequently in chronic ITP and anti-GPV antibodies in the acute syndrome. The occurrence of anti-GPIb antibodies in several patients with an unusually severe form of ITP, resistant to the usual therapeutic modalities, is also intriguing. It remains to be seen whether or not these findings will be supported in studies involving larger groups of patients.

Among the anti-GPIIIa autoantibodies, a subset has been identified that interferes with the normal fibrinogen-binding function of the GPIIb-IIIa complex. Patients with these antibodies have impaired platelet function, hence, identification of these epitopes appears to have clinical relevance in helping to predict the "safe" platelet count for a particular patient. Determination of autoantigen specificity, then, offers the promise of being a laboratory assay diagnostic for autoimmune thrombocytopenia. It may also indicate that a particular patient is likely to have a chronic course of disease, have an increased hemorrhagic tendency, or be resistant to certain types of therapy. Future work in the area will determine just how informative autoantigen identification will be.

This work was suppported, in part, by National Heart, Lung, and Blood Institute grant HL01485.

REFERENCES

1. Balduini CL, Grignani G, Sinigaglia F, Bisio A, Pacchiarini L, Rota D, Calabring S, Baldini C, Mauri C, Ascari E: Severe platelet dysfunction in a patient with autoantibodies against membrane glycoproteins IIb/IIIa. Haemostasis 1:98, 1987

2. Ballem PJ, Segal GM, Stratton JR, Gersheimer T, Adamson JW, Slichter SJ: Mechanisms of thrombocytopenia in chronic autoimmune thrombocytopenic purpura. Evidence of both impaired platelet production and increased platelet clearance. J Clin Invest 80:33, 1987

3. Beardsley DJS: Identification of platelet membrane targets for human antibodies by immunoblotting. In Hawiger J (ed): Methods in Enzymology. New York, Academic Press 1988 (in press)

4. Beardsley DJS, Anderson KC, Ezekowitz A: T cell mediated platelet destruction in immune thrombocytopenic purpura. Blood 68:103a, 1986

5. Beardsley DJS, Ho J, Beyer EC: Varicella associated thrombocytopenia: Antibodies against an 85 kD thrombin sensitive protein (?GPV). Blood 66:1030a, 1985

6. Beardsley DJS, Spiegel JE, Jacobs MM, Handin RI, Lux SE: Platelet membrane glycoprotein IIIa contains target antigens that bind anti-platelet antibodies in immune thrombocytopenias. J Clin Invest 74:1701, 1984

7. Beardsley DJS, Taatjes H, Lux SE: Target antigens in immune thrombocytopenic purpura. Clin Res 32:494a, 1984

8. Beardsley DJS, Timmons S, Bobeck H, Hawiger J: Human antiplatelet antibodies which interfere with fibrinogen binding. Blood 64:845a, 1984

9. Carr JM, Kruskall MS, Kaye JA, Robinson SH: Efficacy of platelet transfusions in immune thrombocytopenia. Am J Med 80:1051, 1986

10. Coller BS, Peerschke EI, Scudder LE, Sullivan CA: A murine monoclonal antibody that completely blocks the binding of fibrinogen to platelets produces a thrombasthenic-like state in normal

platelets and binds to glycoprotein IIb and/or IIIa. J Clin Invest 72:325, 1983

11. Devine DV, Currie MS, Rosse WF, Greenberg CS: Pseudo-Bernard-Soulier syndrome—thrombocytopenia caused by autoantibody to platelet glycoprotein Ib. Blood 70:428, 1987

12. Dixon RH, Rosse WF: Platelet antibody in autoimmune thrombocytopenia. Br J Haematol 31:129, 1975

13. Donnell RL, McMillan R, Yelonosky RJ, Longmire RL, Lightsey AL: Different antiplatelet antibody specificity in immune thrombocytopenic purpura. Br J Haematol 34:147, 1976

14. Furihata K, Nugent DJ, Bissonette A, Aster RH, Kunicki TJ: On the association of the platelet-specific alloantigen, Pen[a], with glycoprotein IIIa. J Clin Invest 80:1624, 1987

15. George JN, Saucerman S, Levine SP, Knieriem LK, Bainton DF: Immunoglobulin G is a platelet alpha granule-secreted protein. J Clin Invest 76:2020, 1985

16. Handagama PJ, George JN, Shuman MA, McEver RP, Bainton DF: Incorporation of a circulating protein into megakaryocyte and platelet granules. Proc Natl Acad Sci USA 84:861, 1987

17. Handagama PJ, Shuman MA, Bainton DF: Uptake of circulating albumin, immunoglobulin G, and fibrinogen by guinea pig megakaryocytes in vivo (abstr). Blood 70:154a, 1987

18. Harrington WJ, Minnich V, Hollingsworth JW, Moore CV: Demonstration of a thrombocytopenic factor in the blood of patients with thrombocytopenic purpura. J Lab Clin Med 38:1, 1951

19. Kaplan C, Champeix, Blanchard D, Muller JY, Cartron JP: Platelet antibodies in systemic lupus erythematosis. Br J Haematol 67:89, 1987

20. Karpatkin S: Autoimmune thrombocytopenic purpura. Sem Hematol 22:260, 1985

21. Karpatkin S, Siskind GW: Studies on the specificity of antiplatelet autoantibodies. Proc Soc Exp Biol Med 147:715, 1974

22. Karpatkin S, Strick N, Siskind GW: Detection of splenic antiplatelet antibody synthesis in idiopathic autoimmune thrombocytopenic purpura (ATP). Br J Haematol 23:167, 1972

23. Kelton JG: The measurement of platelet-bound immunoglobulins: An overview of the methods and the biological relevance of platelet-associated IgG. Prog Hematol 13:163, 1983

24. Kelton JG, Powers, PJ, Carter CJ: A prospective study of the usefulness of the measurement of platelet-associated IgG for the diagnosis of idiopathic thrombocytopenic purpura. Blood 60:1050, 1982

25. Lackner H, Karpatkin S: On the "easy bruising" syndrome with normal platelet count. A study of 75 patients. Ann Intern Med 83:190, 1975

26. Karpatkin S, Lackner H: Association of antiplatelet antibody with functional platelet disorders. Am J Med 59:599, 1975

27. Lehman HA, Lehman LO, Rustagi K, Rustagi RN, Plunkett RW, Farolino DL, Conway J, Logue GL: Complement-mediated autoimmune thrombocytopenia: Monoclonal IgM antiplatelet antibody associated with lymphorecticular malignant disease. N Engl J Med 316:194, 1987

28. Lightsey AL, McMillan R, Koenig HM, Schanberger JE, Lang JE: In vitro production of platelet-binding IgG in childhood idiopathic thrombocytopenic purpura. J Pediatr 88:414, 1976

29. Lynch DM, Howe SE: Antigenic determinants in idiopathic thrombocytopenic purpura. Br J Haematol 63:301, 1986

30. Mason D, McMillan R: Platelet antigens in chronic idiopathic thrombocytopenic purpura. Br J Haematol 56:529, 1984

30a. McKenna JL, Pisciotta A: Fluorescence of megakaryocytes in idiopathic thrombocytopenic purpura (ITP) stained with fluorescent antiglobulin serum. Blood 19:664, 1962

31. McMillan R: Chronic idiopathic thrombocytopenic purpura. N Engl J Med 304:1135, 1981

32. McMillan R: Immune thrombocytopenia. Clin Haematol 12:69, 1983

33. McMillan R, Longmire RL, Yelenosky R, Smith RS, Craddock, CG: Immunoglobulin synthesis in vitro by splenic tissue in idiopathic thrombocytopenic purpura. N Engl J Med 286:681, 1972

34. McMillan R, Luiken GA, Levy R, Yelenosky R, Longmire RL: Antibody against megakaryocytes in idiopathic thrombocytopenic purpura. J Am Med Assoc 239:2460, 1978

35. McMillan R, Tani P, Millard F, Berchtold P: Platelet associated and plasma anti-glycoprotein autoantibodies in chronic ITP. Blood 70:1040, 1987

36. McMillan R, Tani P, Mason D: The demonstration of antibody binding to platelet-associated antigens in patients with immune thrombocytopenic purpura. Blood 56:993, 1980

37. McWilliams NB, Maurer HM: Acute idiopathic thrombocytopenic purpura in children. Am J Hematol 7:87, 1979

38. Kieffel V, Santoso S, Weisheit M, Mueller-Eckhardt C: Monoclonal antibody-specific immobilization of platelet antigens (MAIPA). A new tool for the identification of platelet-reactive antibodies. Blood 70:1722, 1987

39. Niessner H, Clemetson KJ, Panzer S, Mueller-Eckhardt, Santoso S, Bettelheim P: Acquired thrombasthenia due to GPIIb/IIIa-specific platelet autoantibodies. Blood 68:571, 1986

40. Nugent DJ: Identification of antiplatelet antibody idiotypes associated with glycoprotein Ib specificity, present in ITP plasma and produced by

human hybridomas from ITP spleen cell fusions. Thromb Haemostasis 58a:531, 1987

41. Nugent DJ, Kunicki TJ, Berglund C, Bernstein ID: A human monoclonal antibody recognizes a neoantigen on glycoprotein IIIa expressed on stored and activated platelets. Blood 70:16, 1987

42. Santoso S, Kiefel V, Mueller-Eckhardt C: Redistribution of platelet glycoproteins induced by allo- and autoantibodies. Thromb Haemostasis 58:866, 1987

43. Shoenfeld Y, Hsu-Lin SC, Gabriels JE, Silberstein LE, Furie BC, Furie B, Stollar BD, Schwartz RS: Production of autoantibodies by human-human hybridomas. J Clin Invest 70:205, 1982

44. Shulman NR, Marder VJ, Weinrach RS: Similarities between known anti-platelet antibodies and the factor responsible for thrombocytopenia in idiopathic purpura. Physiologic, serologic and isotopic studies. Ann NY Acad Sci 124:499, 1965

45. Stahl CP, Zucker-Franklin D, McDonald TP: Incomplete antigenic cross-reactivity between platelets and megakaryocytes: Relevance to ITP. Blood 67:421, 1986

46. Stricker RB, Abrams DI, Corash L, Shuman MA: Target platelet antigen in homosexual men with immune thrombocytopenia. N Engl J Med 313:1375, 1985

47. Stricker RB, Koerper MA, Bussel J, Shuman MA: Target platelet antigens in childhood immune thrombocytopenic purpura. Blood 68:118a, 1986

48. Stricker RB, Wong D, Saks SR, Corash L, Shuman MA: Acquired Bernard Soulier syndrome. J Clin Invest 76:1274, 1985

49. Sugiyama T, Okuma M, Ushikubi F, Sensaki S, Kanaji K, Uchino H: A novel platelet aggregating factor found in a patient with defective collagen-induced platelet aggregation and autoimmune thrombocytopenia. Blood 69:1712, 1987

50. Szatkowski NS, Aster RH: Idiopathic (autoimmune) thrombocytopenic purpura associated with a complement-fixing autoantibody and response to plasma exchange. Scand J Haematol 35:525, 1985

51. Szatkowski NS, Kunicki TJ, Aster RH: Identification of glycoprotein Ib as a target for autoantibody in idiopathic (autoimmune) thrombocytopenic purpura. Blood 67:310, 1986

52. Tomiyama Y, Kurata Y, Mizutani H, Kanakura Y, Tsukakio T, Yonezawa T, Tarui S: Platelet glycoprotein IIb as a target antigen in two patients with chronic idiopathic thrombocytopenic purpura. Br J Haematol 66:535, 1987

53. Vainchenker W, Deschamps JF, Bastin JM, Guichard J, Titeux M, Breton-Gorius J, McMichael AJ: Two monoclonal antiplatelet antibodies as markers of human megakaryocyte maturation. Immunofluorescent staining platelet peroxidase detection in megakaryocyte colonies and in in vivo cells from normal and leukemic patients. Blood 59:514, 1982

54. van der Lelie J, Lange JMA, Vos JJE, van Dalen CM, Kanner SA, von dem Borne AEGKr: Autoimmunity against blood cells in human immunodeficiency virus (HIV) infection. Br J Haematol 67:109, 1987

55. van der Lelie J, van der Plas-van Dalen CM, von dem Borne AEGKr: Platelet autoantibodies in septicemia. Br J Haematol 58:755, 1984

56. van Leeuwen EF, van der Ven JThM, Engelfriet CP, von dem Borne AEGKr: Specificity of autoantibodies in autoimmune thrombocytopenia. Blood 59:23, 1982

57. van Vliet HHDM, Kappers-Klunne MC, van der Hel JWB, Abels J: Antibodies against glycosphingolipids in sera of patients with idiopathic thrombocytopenic purpura. Br J Haematol 67:103, 1987

58. Varon D, Karpatkin S: A monoclonal antiplatelet antibody with decreased reactivity for autoimmune thrombocytopenic platelets. Proc Natl Acad Sci USA 80:6992, 1983

59. Vasquez JJ, Lewis JH: Immunocytochemical studies on platelets. The demonstration of a common antigen in human platelets and megakaryocytes. Blood 16:968, 1960

60. von dem Borne AEGKr, van der Lelie H, Vos JJE, van der Plan-van Dalen CM, Risseeuw-Bogaert NJ, Ticheler MDA, Pegels HG: Antibodies against cryptantigens of platelets. Curr Stud Hematol Blood Transfusion 52:33, 1986

61. Walsh CM, Nardi MA, Karpatkin S: On the mechanism of thrombocytopenic purpura in sexually active homosexual men. N Engl J Med 311:635, 1984

62. Woods VL, Kurata Y, Montgomery RR, Tani P, Mason D, Oh EH, McMillan R: Autoantibodies against platelet glycoprotein Ib in patients with chronic immune thrombocytopenic purpura. Blood 64:156, 1984

63. Woods VL Jr, Oh EH, Mason D, McMillan R: Autoantibodies against the platelet glycoprotein IIb/IIIa complex in patients with chronic idiopathic thrombocytopenic purpura. Blood 63:368, 1984

64. Zahavi J, Marder VJ: Acquired "storage pool disease" of platelets associated with circulating antiplatelet antibodies. Am J Med 56:883, 1974

8

Biochemistry of Drug-Dependent Platelet Autoantigens

MICHAEL C. BERNDT · BENG H. CHONG · ROBERT K. ANDREWS

Thrombocytopenia is a frequent and occasionally insidious complication associated with the therapeutic use of drugs. Drug-induced thrombocytopenia can occur by either *nonimmune* or *immune* mechanisms. Nonimmune drug-induced thrombocytopenia is associated with drugs that either directly suppress the bone marrow production of platelets (e.g., chemotherapeutic agents) or accelerate the clearance rate of circulating platelets (e.g., ristocetin).[38] In contrast, immune drug-induced thrombocytopenia is associated with the development of a drug-dependent antibody that causes platelet clearance. This review is concerned with the immune form of thrombocytopenia, in particular that induced by the drugs quinine, quinidine and heparin, and will consider possible mechanisms for the interaction of drug and antibody with platelets.

Two general pathways have been proposed for the induction of immune drug-induced thrombocytopenia. Ackroyd[1] suggested that a complex of drug and the platelet membrane acts as an antigen for antibody production. Several potential mechanisms consistent with this basic pathway are shown in Figure 8-1. An alternative pathway was postulated by Miescher[53] and by Shulman,[66] who suggested that a drug–antibody complex is nonspecifically absorbed onto the platelets resulting in their destruction as innocent bystanders, e.g., a mechanism involving drug–antibody immune complex binding to platelet Fc receptor(s) (Fig. 8-2).

QUININE/QUINIDINE DRUG-DEPENDENT ANTIBODY

General Characteristics of Quinine/Quinidine Drug-Dependent Antibody Interaction with Platelets

Although more than 50 drugs have been shown to cause drug-induced immune thrombocytopenia, the phenomenon most frequently occurs as a clinical entity with two drugs, quinine and its stereoisomer, quinidine.[38] Quinine/quinidine drug-dependent antibodies are usually of the IgG1 subclass[73] and occur in plasma at concentrations as high as ≈ 25 μg/ml.[19] The coexistence of IgG3 and IgM drug-dependent antibodies has also been reported, but this is a less frequent occurrence.[73] Thrombocytopenia caused by quinine or quinidine is seldom an insidious disorder, usually presenting with purpura, bruising, and mucosal bleeding. The degree of thrombocytopenia is frequently severe with a platelet nadir of 10,000 to 20,000 platelets per microliter.[42] The thrombocytopenia is often of sudden onset and frequently occurs after previous intermittent or prolonged exposure to quinine or quinidine without incident. As discussed by Kelton et al.,[42] a patient can be considered to have drug-induced thrombocytopenia if all of four criteria are fulfilled: (1) the patient is not thrombocytopenic before ingestion of the drug; (2) the thrombocytopenia develops during drug treatment and resolves on cessation of the drug; (3)

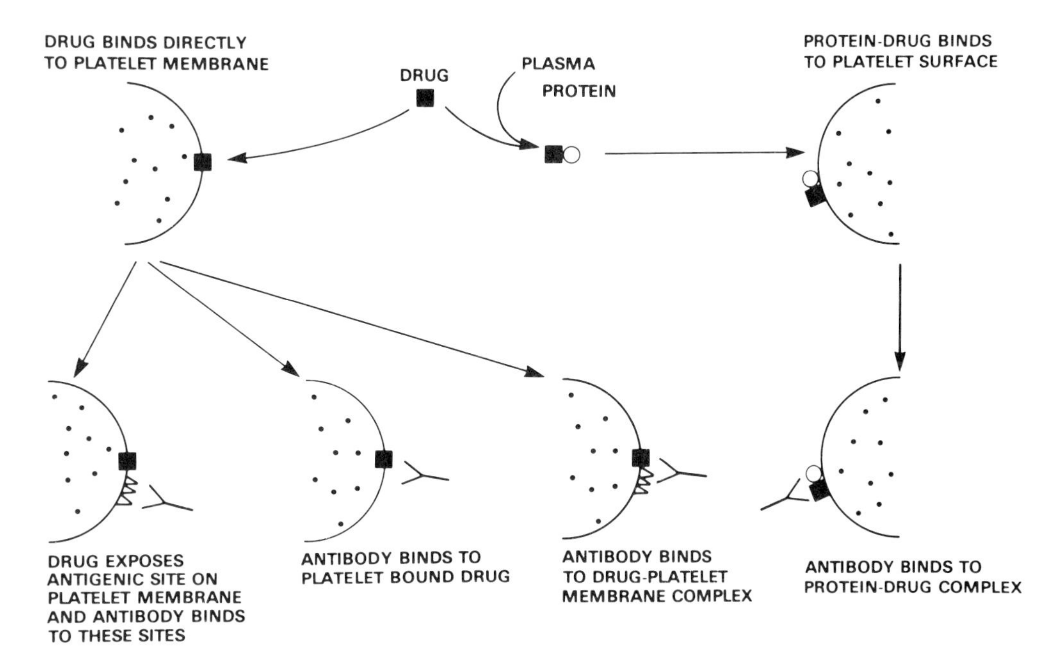

Figure 8-1. Potential mechanisms for binding of drug-dependent antibody to platelets by the Fab region of the drug-dependent antibody (Hackett T et al.,[38] by permission of the copyright owners, Thieme-Stratton, Inc., New York).

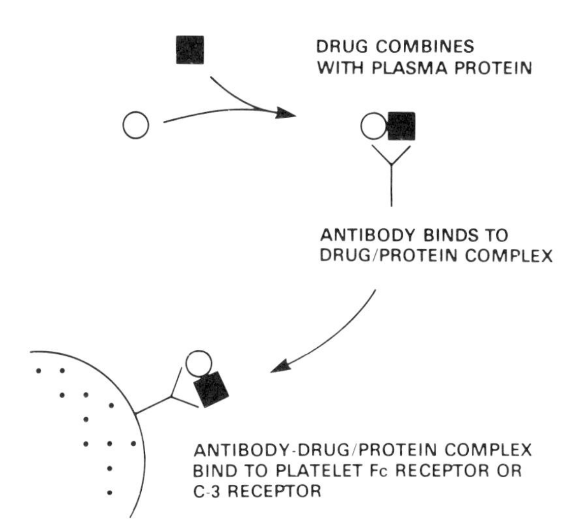

Figure 8-2. Potential mechanism for binding of drug-dependent antibody to platelets by the Fc region of the drug-dependent antibody (Hackett T et al.,[38] by permission of the copyright owners, Thieme-Stratton, Inc., New York).

the thrombocytopenia does not recur after cessation of drug treatment; and (4) there is no evidence for another cause of thrombocytopenia. The clinical diagnosis of quinine/quinidine drug-induced thrombocytopenia requires, if possible, a positive in vitro test for the presence of drug-dependent antibody in the patient's plasma or serum. An acceptable in vitro test should demonstrate that the patient's plasma or serum produces a measurable platelet effect in the presence of drug, that this effect does not occur or occurs less readily in the absence of drug, and that control plasma or serum plus drug do not produce this effect.[38] Quinine/quinidine drug-dependent antibodies are commonly assayed in vitro by the direct measurement of the drug-dependent binding of patient IgG to platelets or by measuring the complement-mediated lysis of platelets after binding of drug-dependent antibody (Table 8-1).

There is considerable variation in the platelet binding characteristics of quinine/quinidine drug-dependent antibodies. In five patients with quinidine-induced immune thrombocytopenia, Kelton et al.[42] found between 60,000 and 240,000 copies of IgG per platelet at a quinidine concentration of 1 mM, whereas essentially no binding of IgG occurred at a quinidine concentration of 27 μM. With two quinine and two quinidine patient sera, Christie and Aster[19] found 36,000 to 161,000 drug-dependent IgG binding sites per platelet at satura-

Table 8-1
In Vitro Tests for Quinine/Quinidine Drug-Dependent Antibody

Test	Basis of Test	Ref
Platelet suspension immunofluorescent test	Platelet-bound antibody detected with fluorescently tagged second antibody	73,76
Radioimmunoassay	Platelet-bound antibody detected with radiolabeled protein A	26,30
Radioimmunoassay	Platelet-bound antibody detected with radiolabeled murine monoclonal antihuman IgG	27,62
Platelet aggregometry	Complement-mediated lysis measured by platelet aggregometry	28
Chromium lysis assay	Complement-mediated release of ^{51}Cr from ^{51}Cr-labeled platelets	46,47

tion with a K_d for the interaction of 38 nM to 340 nM. With individual serum, half-maximal binding of drug-dependent antibody occurred at drug concentrations between 2 μM and 60 μM. Smith et al.[67] studied three individuals with quinine- or quinidine-induced thrombocytopenia and reported 40,000 to 100,000 IgG-binding sites per platelet with a K_d for binding of 10 nM to 100 nM. In a separate study, Christie et al.[22] studied 16 patients with quinine- or quinidine-induced thrombocytopenia and examined in detail the structural features of quinine and quinidine necessary for the binding of drug-induced antibodies to platelets. The patient sera fell into three distinct groups: 8/16 reacted only with the sensitizing drug or with its dihydro or desmethoxy derivatives (Fig. 8-3); 3/16 had similar reactivity, except that they were less reactive with the desmethoxy derivative; and 5/16 had broad specificity reacting with sensitizing drug, its stereoisomer, and one or more derivatives including at least one C-9 derivative. The combined data from the foregoing studies demonstrate that there is considerable heterogeneity between individual quinine/quinidine drug-dependent antibodies in the amount of drug required to promote binding to platelets, the number of platelet-binding sites recognized, the binding affinities of the antibodies, and the structural features of quinine or quinidine required for optimal platelet binding. This apparent heterogeneity is further reflected in studies evaluating the mechanism of drug-dependent antibody interaction with platelets (*see under* section on binding mechanisms) and in studies concerning the nature of the receptor/antigen recognized by quinine/quinidine drug-dependent antibodies (discussed later).

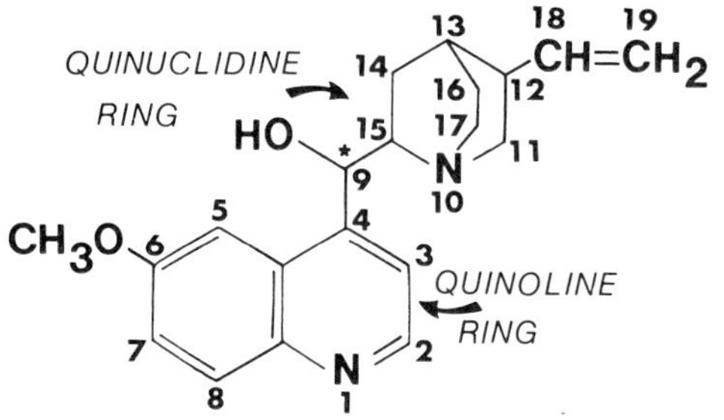

Figure 8-3. Structure of the optical isomers, quinine and quinidine. The asterisk marks the site of the C-9 asymmetric center. The dihydro derivatives of quinine and quinidine have a single bond between carbons 18 and 19. The desmethoxy derivatives of quinine and quinidine are missing the methoxy group at carbon 6 (modified from Berndt MC, Castaldi PA: Blood Rev 1:111, 1987, by permission of the copyright owners, Churchill Livingstone, Edinburgh).

Mechanism of Binding of Quinine/Quinidine Drug-Dependent Antibodies to Platelets

In an elegant series of experiments, Christie and Aster[19] examined in detail the role of drug in the binding of drug-dependent antibodies to platelets. Platelets incubated with 0.4 mM [^{3}H]quinine and washed twice were found to have ≃ 600,000 drug molecules bound per platelet. These platelets, however, failed to bind quinine-dependent antibody unless excess soluble drug was also present. When quinine-dependent patient serum was incubated with platelets in the presence of 90 μM [^{3}H]quinine, more quinine was associated with the platelets after six washing steps than with equivalent controls using normal serum. These results suggest that either a quinine-antibody complex binds to platelets (compatible with an Fc-receptor mechanism) or that the complex formed between drug and platelet membrane constituent is labile but is stabilized by the binding of the patient antibody.

The results of two studies have been published that apparently support an Fc-receptor mechanism for the binding of drug-dependent antibody to platelets. Van Leeuwen et al., who used the IgG fraction isolated from the serum of a patient with quinidine-dependent antibodies, prepared $(Fab')_2$ fragments by pepsin digestion and showed that they no longer bound to platelets in the presence of drug.[73] Similar results were obtained by Lerner et al. for a single patient with quinidine-induced thrombocytopenia.[49] If the Fc region and not the $(Fab')_2$ region of the patient IgG is essential for the binding of drug-dependent antibody to platelets, one would predict that the $(Fab')_2$ fragments would compete with intact antibody for the binding of drug and, hence, inhibit the binding of intact antibody to platelets. Unfortunately, this experiment was not performed in either study. Therefore, an alternative explanation for these results—that the Fab region of the patient IgG is destroyed by pepsin digestion—cannot be excluded.

In contrast to the aforementioned results, most of the available evidence strongly supports an Fc receptor-independent mechanism for the binding of drug-dependent antibodies to platelets that directly involves the Fab region of the antibody. First, Shulman was unable to demonstrate the direct binding of drug by drug-dependent antibody.[66] Similarly, van Leeuwen et al. were unable to detect immune complexes in antibody-containing serum after the addition of drug.[73] Second, most investigators have found that platelets from patients with Bernard-Soulier syndrome are unreactive with quinine/quinidine drug-dependent antibodies, yet Bernard-Soulier platelets have normal levels of platelet Fc-receptor expression.[58] Third, we have described an antiplatelet monoclonal antibody, FMC 25, that either as intact IgG or as $(Fab')_2$ fragments, blocks the binding of quinine and quinidine drug-dependent antibodies to platelets.[6] The FMC 25 $(Fab')_2$ fragments were found not to inhibit the aggregation of washed platelets by acetone-aggregated IgG, an Fc receptor-mediated platelet stimulus. Control experiments established that the acetone-aggregated IgG did not cause the dissociation of the platelet-bound FMC 25 $(Fab')_2$ fragments, strongly suggesting that drug-dependent antibody binds to platelets by an Fc receptor-independent mechanism. The results are in agreement with those of Kunicki et al., who found that heat-aggregated IgG did not inhibit the lysis of ^{51}Cr-labeled platelets by drug-dependent antibodies.[48] A fourth line of evidence lies in the report of Chong et al., who studied a patient who had developed concomitant quinidine-induced thrombocytopenia and leukopenia.[14] The patient's serum had two distinct quinidine-dependent antibodies, as the antibody eluted off sensitized platelets reacted only with platelets, and that eluted off sensitized granulocytes reacted only with granulocytes. With this patient, the presence of cell-specific and distinct drug-dependent antibodies would appear to be incompatible with a mechanism that involves binding of drug-antibody complex to cellular Fc receptors. Fifth, in contrast to the results of van Leeuwen et al.[73] and Lerner et al.,[49] Smith et al.[67] reported that the $(Fab')_2$ fragments of each of three drug-dependent antiplatelet antibodies bound to platelets in a drug-dependent manner, approaching saturation levels similar to those of the corresponding intact IgG. The $(Fab')_2$ fragments, but not the Fc fragments, competed for drug-dependent platelet binding of radiolabeled patient IgG at approximately the same molar ratio as unlabeled IgG. Finally, Christie et al.[21] demonstrated that platelets coated with drug-dependent antibody rosetted protein-A-Sepharose beads and that normal platelets rosetted protein-A-Sepharose beads coated with drug-dependent antibody. Both of these reactions occurred only in the presence of the sensitizing drug. The rosetting of protein-A-Sepharose beads by drug-dependent antibody-coated platelets was inhibited by the $(Fab')_2$ fragments of a goat antibody directed against human IgG Fc fragments. Conversely, the rosetting by normal platelets of protein-A-Sepharose beads, coated with drug-dependent antibody, was inhibited by the $(Fab')_2$ fragments of a goat antibody directed against human IgG $(Fab')_2$ fragments. Because protein A binds the Fc region of human IgG, these results strongly indicate that drug-dependent antibody binds to platelets through its Fab domain.

Role of the Glycoprotein Ib–IX Complex as the Platelet Receptor/ Antigen Recognized by Quinine/ Quinidine Drug-Dependent Antibodies

In 1978, Kunicki and coworkers[47] made the key observation that platelets from patients with the Bernard-Soulier syndrome failed to react with quinine/quinidine drug-dependent antibodies, a result subsequently confirmed by a number of laboratories.[14,19,48] The Bernard-Soulier syndrome is an autosomal-recessive, platelet bleeding abnormality characterized by giant platelets, thrombocytopenia, and the absence of platelet agglutination with human von Willebrand factor and ristocetin or with bovine von Willebrand factor.[5] Bernard-Soulier syndrome platelets are deficient in several membrane glycoproteins (GP), the GPIb–IX complex,[8,25] GPV,[8,25,69] and a protein of molecular mass (M_r), 210,000,[70] suggesting that one or more of these deficient glycoproteins may be the target platelet antigen(s) recognized by quinine/quinidine drug-dependent antibodies. There is now convincing evidence that most patients with quinine/quinidine-induced purpura have a serum antibody or antibodies that react with a specific-binding domain(s) on the human platelet GPIb–IX complex.

Glycoprotein Ib and GPIX exist as a heterodimer complex in the intact platelet membrane[29] and remain tightly associated following detergent solubilization[6,9] (Fig. 8-4). Glycoprotein Ib has an apparent molecular mass on sodium dodecyl sulfate (SDS)-polyacrylamide gels of 170,000 and consists of two disulfide-linked subunits, $GPIb_\alpha$ (M_r, 135,000) and $GPIb_\beta$ (M_r, 25,000). Glycoprotein IX has an

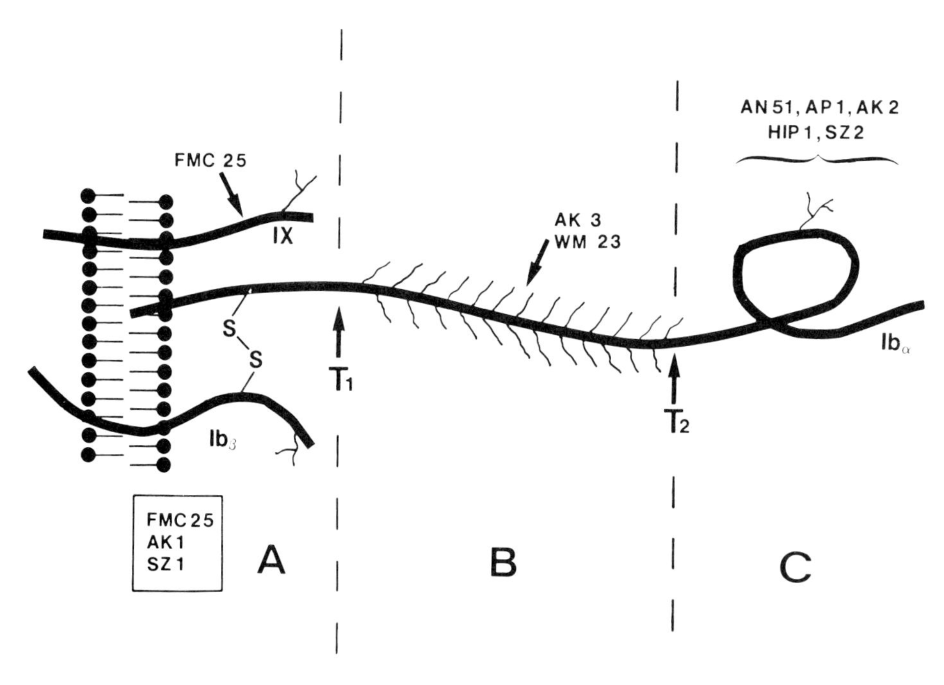

Figure 8-4. Structure of the human platelet membrane GPIb–IX complex. The α chain contains a central macroglycopeptide core. Either side of this region is a proteolytically sensitive domain, T_1 and T_2. Cleavage at both these sites splits the complex into three domains: a membrane-associated region (A), macroglycopeptide (B), and a peptide tail region (C). Epitope-mapped monoclonal antibodies, as defined by our laboratory, are indicated for each domain. FMC 25 is directed against GPIX. AK 1 and SZ 1 are directed against complex-specific epitopes in region A.[29] AK 3 and WM 23 are directed against epitopes in the macroglycopeptide domain, B, whereas the remaining five antibodies are directed against the peptide tail region, C. The membrane-associated region (A) contains the binding site(s) for quinine/quinidine drug-dependent antibodies.

apparent molecular mass of 22,000 under both nonreducing and reducing conditions.[9] The α chain of GPIb contains a central macroglycopeptide core[39,77] with an apparent molecular mass of 118,000.[55] At each end of the macroglycopeptide core is a proteolytically sensitive domain[39] (cleavage sites T_1 and T_2, Fig. 8-4). Cleavage at both sites generates an approximately 45,000-M_r peptide tail region (C, Fig. 8-4), macroglycopeptide (B, Fig. 8-4), and an approximately 25,000-M_r fragment that remains membrane-associated, disulfide-linked to the β subunit, and complexed with GPIX (A, Fig. 8-4).[6,39,77] Platelets contain an intracellular calcium-dependent protease, calpain, that specifically cleaves at T_1 to yield a water-soluble proteolytic fragment of the α chain of GPIb, termed *glycocalicin* (regions $B + C$, Fig. 8-4).[6]

In 1983, we obtained the first direct evidence that quinine/quinidine drug-dependent antibodies bind to the human platelet GPIb-IX complex.[14] A quinidine-dependent antibody from a patient with simultaneous drug-induced thrombocytopenia and leukopenia immunoprecipitated GPIb and GPIX from Triton-solubilized, periodate-labeled platelets. Similar results have subsequently been reported by us and by others with different patient sera.[6,27] Previously, Kunicki and coworkers[48] had shown that semipurified GPIb and a putative, copurified 210,000-M_r "analogue" of GPIb had receptor activity for quinine/quinidine drug-dependent antibodies. Purified glycocalicin, however, had no receptor activity, suggesting that the membrane-associated region of the GPIb-IX complex (A, Fig. 8-4) contained the epitope or epitopes for quinine/quinidine drug-dependent antibodies. Direct support for this view was obtained in studies from our laboratory that examined the effect of specific anti-GPIb-IX complex monoclonal antibodies on the interaction between quinine/quinidine drug-dependent antibodies and platelets.[6] Comparable results were obtained with six patient sera; three sera from patients with quinine-induced thrombocytopenia and three sera from patients with quinine-induced thrombocytopenia. A murine monoclonal antibody, FMC 25, directed against an epitope on GPIX, had no effect on platelet aggregation induced by collagen or ADP or on ristocetin-induced platelet agglutination. FMC 25 and its $(Fab')_2$ fragments, however, were potent inhibitors of drug-dependent, antibody-induced platelet lysis and blocked binding of drug-dependent antibodies to platelets as assessed by indirect platelet immunofluorescence. In contrast, a second murine monoclonal antibody, AN 51, directed against an epitope on the glycocalicin region of GPIb, had the reciprocal effect on platelet function. AN 51 blocked ristocetin-induced platelet agglutination but not drug-dependent, antibody-induced platelet lysis or the binding of drug-dependent antibody to platelets. Selective proteolytic removal of most of the α subunit of GPIb (glycocalicin) from platelets with calpain did not affect binding of drug-dependent antibody to platelets. Furthermore, a quinidine-dependent platelet antibody immunoprecipitated purified GPIb-IX complex, GPIb-IX complex from normal platelets, and the membrane-associated proteolytic remnant of the GPIb-IX complex from calpain-treated platelets. This result suggests that if the role of drug in the recognition of platelets by drug-dependent antibody involves the binding of drug to the platelet membrane and formation of a neoantigen, then the drug-binding site(s) must be on the membrane-associated region of the GPIb-IX complex. Platelet antigen for quinine/quinidine, drug-dependent antibodies could not be detected by Western blot analysis on either GPIb or GPIX, a result confirmed by Stricker and Shuman.[69] Preincubation of drug-dependent antibody with purified GPIb-IX complex inhibited the subsequent binding of antibody to platelets, but the separated components, GPIb and GPIX were both ineffective. The combined results suggest that quinine/quinidine, drug-dependent antibodies recognize a conformational epitope(s) present primarily when GPIX is associated with GPIb (or a proteolytic remnant of GPIb, *see* Fig. 8-4).

Recently, we have confirmed these observations using a much larger series of epitope-mapped monoclonal antibodies directed against the GPIb-IX complex[7] (*see* Fig. 8-4). Five of the monoclonal antibodies, AK 2, AN 51, AP 1, SZ 2, and HIP 1, are directed against the 45,000-peptide tail region of GPIb; two antibodies, AK 3 and WM 23, are directed against the macroglycopeptide core; and the remaining three antibodies, FMC 25, AK 1, and SZ 1, are directed against the membrane-associated region of the GPIb-IX complex. AK 1 and SZ 1 are both directed against complex-specific epitopes on the GPIb-IX complex.[29] Monoclonal antibodies directed against the peptide tail and macroglycopeptide regions of GPIb had little, if any, effect on the complement-mediated lysis of platelets by drug-dependent antibodies. In contrast, all three antibodies directed against the membrane-associated region of the GPIb-IX complex strongly inhibited this reaction. Cross-blocking studies indicate that AK 1 and SZ 1 are directed against a very similar or identical epitope and that these two antibodies only partially cross-block FMC 25.[29] These results confirm the importance of the membrane-associated region of the GPIb-IX complex in the binding of quinine/quinidine, drug-dependent antibodies. Because there are approximately 25,000 copies of the GPIb-IX complex per platelet[29] and up to 200,000 apparent drug-dependent antibody-binding sites per platelet (*see under* preceding section on general characteristics), there must be multiple drug-dependent antibody epitopes present in the membrane-associated region of the GPIb-IX complex. Pfueller et al.[56] using a more sensitive immunogold Western blotting technique, have demonstrated with individual patient serum the presence of drug-dependent epitopes on both GPIb and GPIX. In addition, with some patient sera, there may be drug-dependent epitopes present on membrane glycoproteins other than the GPIb-IX complex (*see* following section). Alternatively, there may only be 20,000 to 30,000 drug-dependent, antibody-binding sites per platelet. Higher apparent numbers of drug-dependent, antibody-binding sites could arise from aggregated IgG carried onto platelets by drug-dependent antibody, from exposure of platelet Fc receptors, or from secretion and rebinding of α-granule IgG.

Drug-Dependent Antibody Binding to Platelets Independent of the Glycoprotein Ib-IX Complex

In 1982, van Leeuwen et al. reported that 3 of 14 sera from patients with quinine/quinidine-induced thrombocytopenia showed some reactivity with Bernard-Soulier syndrome platelets as judged by indirect platelet immunofluorescence.[73] One quinidine-dependent patient serum reacted with Bernard-Soulier platelets but much less strongly than with normal platelets. By absorption experiments, two quinine-dependent sera were found to be two- to fourfold less reactive toward Bernard-Soulier syndrome platelets than toward normal platelets, if account is made of the increased surface membrane of the Bernard-Soulier syndrome platelets. None of these three patient sera caused drug-dependent lysis of Bernard-Soulier syndrome platelets, suggesting that only drug-dependent antibody directed against the GPIb-IX complex is capable of fixing complement and causing the pathophysiology of drug-dependent, antibody-induced thrombocytopenia. All 14 patient sera were reported to react normally with Glanzmann's thrombasthenic platelets, which are deficient in the platelet membrane GPIIb-IIIa complex.[5] In contrast, Christie and Mullen have described a patient whose serum gave drug-dependent immunoprecipitation of both GPIb-IX complex and GPIIb-IIIa complex.[20] In an elegant series of experiments, Pfueller et al.[56] have examined the antigen specificity of antibodies in quinine- and quinidine-induced thrombocytopenia using immunogold Western blot analysis. Glycoprotein assignments were confirmed by Western blot analysis of Bernard-Soulier syndrome and Glanzmann's thrombasthenic platelets. Two quinine-dependent sera showed drug-dependent binding to GPIb and GPIIIa. A third quinine-dependent serum bound to GPIb, GPIIb, GPIIIa, and a 57,000-M_r protein that was absent in Bernard-Soulier syndrome platelets (possibly the calpain remnant of the α chain of GPIb disulfide-linked to $GPIb_\beta$). A fourth quinine-dependent serum and a quinidine-dependent serum bound to GPIb and GPIX. Binding to GPIb varied with different normal platelet donors. Absorption of one quinine-dependent serum with Glanzmann's thrombasthenic platelets indicated that there were distinct populations of antibodies with different antigen specificities. It would, therefore, appear that a substantial number of patients with quinine/quinidine-induced thrombocytopenia have drug-dependent antibodies directed against the GPIIb-IIIa complex in addition to drug-dependent antibodies directed against the GPIb-IX complex.

Drug-Independent Autoantibody in Patients with Quinine/Quinidine-Induced Thrombocytopenia

In a study of eight patients with quinine/quinidine-induced thrombocytopenia, Kelton et al.[42] made the interesting observation that in two patients, the time to recovery after cessation of drug was greater than 4 weeks, that is, the thrombocytopenia persisted well after the drug was cleared from the blood. This observation is consistent with the presence of drug-*independent* antibody in these patients. Hackett et al. suggested that persistent immune thrombocytopenia after drug cessation could be explained by a protein–drug complex acting as the initial determinant for antibody production.[38] With time, the specificity of the antibodies widens, and drug would no longer be necessary for antigen identification. There have been several recent reports characterizing the presence of drug-independent antibodies associated with quinidine-induced thrombocytopenia.[33,49,69,71] The binding of these antibodies to platelets appears to involve the Fab-binding region of IgG.[49] An interesting patient described by Szatkowski,[71] after receiving quinidine for 2 months, developed a drug-independent, complement-fixing autoantibody that reacted with normal platelets but not with Bernard-Soulier syndrome platelets. Similarly to the quinine/quinidine, drug-dependent antibodies (discussed earlier), the patient autoantibody recognized a determinant(s) in the membrane-associated region of the GPIb–IX complex. Stricker and Shuman showed that six of six sera from patients with quinidine-induced thrombocytopenia had a drug-independent antibody that recognized platelet membrane glycoprotein V.[69]

HEPARIN-INDUCED DRUG-DEPENDENT ANTIBODY

Heparin-Induced Thrombocytopenia: Clinical Aspects

Thrombocytopenia is a well recognized complication of heparin therapy. The reported incidence varies considerably from 1% to 30%, but the true incidence is probably about 5%.[13b] There appears to be two distinct types of heparin-induced thrombocytopenia. According to the nomenclature described in a previous review,[13b] type I is a mild thrombocytopenia of early onset and type II is a severe delayed-onset thrombocytopenia. Type I is more common than type II (Table 8-2).

The patients with heparin-associated thrombocytopenia type I are usually asymptomatic. The mechanism is probably nonimmune, as the onset is early (usually on day 1 or 2 of heparin therapy), even in those patients with no prior exposure to the drug. The thrombocytopenia may resolve despite continuation of heparin and may not recur upon rechallenge with heparin after the platelet count has returned to normal.[13b] The thrombocytopenia in type I is probably due to the platelet proaggregating effect of heparin itself.[15,63]

On the other hand, there are several lines of evidence to suggest that the mechanism of type II heparin-induced thrombocytopenia is immunologic. First, the time lag between the administration of heparin and the onset of

Table 8-2
Heparin-Induced Thrombocytopenia: Characteristics of Two Clinical Types of Disease

Characteristic	Type I	Type II
Frequency for patients receiving heparin	≈5%*	≈0.6%†
Etiology	Probably nonimmune	Immune
Thrombocytopenia	Mild (>100,000 platelets/μl)	Usually severe (<100,000 platelets/μl)
Onset of thrombocytopenia	<7 days	>7 days‡
Associated thromboembolic complications	Absent	Present

*Estimate based on a review of most of the published clinical prospective studies.[13b]
†Estimate based on a retrospective study.[41]
‡With prior exposure to heparin the onset may be early.

thrombocytopenia (usually 7–12 days) is consistent with an immune response. Second, patients with heparin-induced thrombocytopenia have elevated levels of platelet-associated IgG during the thrombocytopenic phase of their illness.[23,43] Third, several investigators have demonstrated in patients' sera the presence of a factor that induces heparin-dependent platelet aggregation, [^{14}C]serotonin release, and thromboxane synthesis.[15,32] This factor was located in the IgG fraction.[18,23,72] The heparin-dependent antibody described in this review refers specifically to the antibody isolated from patients with heparin-induced thrombocytopenia type II.

The clinical importance of type II is the occurrence of associated thrombotic complications which often has serious sequalae.[18,41] About 30% of these patients die, and a further 20% develop arterial occlusion, resulting in gangrene that requires subsequent amputation.

Heparin-Dependent Antiplatelet Antibody

The antibody in most of the patients with heparin-induced thrombocytopenia is IgG, which may occur alone or in combination with IgM antibody. Occasionally, patients may have antibody of only the IgM class. Cines et al. found that 17 of 27 patients studied had only IgG antibody, six had both IgG and IgM antibodies, and four had only IgM antibody.[24] Although the heparin-dependent antibody fixes complement on target platelets, it does not cause platelet lysis,[16,23] suggesting that the complement sequence does not proceed to completion and that the terminal lytic components are not activated. However, fixation of complement on platelets appears to be a prerequisite for platelet activation by the antibody. Without an intact complement pathway, antibody-induced [^{14}C]serotonin release and platelet aggregation do not occur.[16,23]

The heparin-dependent antibody usually has a strong platelet aggregating property, which is uncommon with other human antiplatelet autoantibodies. Many laboratories have taken advantage of this platelet aggregating activity for detecting the antibody. Although other antibodies (such as the quinine/quinidine antibodies) may be detected by using an aggregometer, the decrease in optical density induced by these antibodies is primarily due to platelet lysis, rather than to aggregation.[13a,28] Another characteristic of the heparin-dependent antibody is the ability to induce the production of a large amount of thromboxane A_2 following its reaction with platelets.[10,18] Other human antiplatelet antibodies, such as the autoantibodies in idiopathic thrombocytopenic purpura and anti-P1^{A1} antibodies in posttransfusion purpura, produce no detectable thromboxane A_2 when they are incubated with platelets.[13a*] The heparin-dependent antibody also induces the heparin-dependent release of platelet granule constituents such as serotonin[32] and increases the availability of platelet factor 3.[3,16]

The ability of the heparin-dependent antibody to mediate the release/production of platelet proaggregating and procoagulant moieties, particularly thromboxane A_2, may be an important factor contributing to the development of thrombotic complications in patients with heparin-induced thrombocytopenia. In these patients, the elaboration of these moieties following heparin–antibody–platelet interaction may lead to the formation of circulating platelet aggregates. Because these platelet aggregates are not lysed by activated complement, they may persist in circulation as microemboli or act as nidus for thrombus formation. In comparison, the interaction in vitro of other human antiplatelet antibodies with platelets usually does not result in platelet aggregation. Where aggregates are formed, they are rapidly lysed by activated complement, as with quinine/quinidine-dependent antibodies.[13a,28]

Heparin-Independent Antiplatelet Antibody

Although the antiplatelet antibody in most patients with heparin-induced thrombocytopenia requires exogenous heparin for its reaction with platelets, several investigators have recently described a heparin-independent antiplatelet antibody in some patients. The sera of four patients reported by Lynch and Howe[51] contained an antibody that bound to platelets without exogenous heparin, although the binding of antibody markedly increased when heparin was added. Sandler et al.[64] found that the serum of a patient with heparin-induced thrombocytopenia could induce platelet aggre-

*Chong BH: Unpublished observations.

gation of normal platelets without added heparin, although the reaction was more rapid in the presence of exogenous heparin. Pfueller and David[57] showed that sera of their patients could induce aggregation of normal platelets in the absence of exogenous heparin if epinephrine, in subaggregating concentrations, was also added. There are several possible explanations for this phenomenon. One possibility is that the antibody in these patients recognizes a complex formed by heparin and a platelet membrane component as the normal antigen, but it also cross-reacts with, and binds less avidly to, the platelet membrane component alone. Alternatively, as heparin-induced thrombocytopenia is not a monoclonal disorder, several polyclonal antibodies may be present, and each could recognize a different epitope on the heparin-platelet antigenic complex. Some of these antibodies may recognize an epitope(s) that is present on the platelet membrane component in its native state, but other antibodies may have specificity for epitopes that are formed or become exposed only after the formation of the heparin–platelet complex. Without exogenous heparin, only the former type of antibodies would bind to platelets, but in the presence of heparin, both types of antibodies would bind and, therefore, facilitate the aggregation of platelets. A third possibility suggested by Pfueller and David is that the antibody recognizes platelet antigens that are expressed after platelet activation by heparin or by epinephrine.[57] This mechanism would explain their finding of platelet aggregation caused by patient sera in the presence of subthreshold concentrations of epinephrine but in the absence of exogenous heparin. The possible involvement of endogenous heparin secreted by platelets on activation by either epinephrine or adhesion[74] has not been ruled out. Regardless of the mechanism of antibody–platelet interaction, the clinical significance of this heparin-independent antibody is uncertain because the thrombocytopenia and thrombosis in patients with heparin-induced thrombocytopenia resolves after cessation of heparin treatment.

Different Preparations and Molecular Fractions of Heparin and Heparinoid Recognized by the Antibody

It is now widely accepted that the thrombocytopenia that develops during heparin therapy is due to heparin itself and not to a contaminant in the heparin preparation. Heparin from different animal sources, and possibly different lots of heparin from the same source, may have different capacities to induce thrombocytopenia. Several clinical studies have shown a higher incidence of thrombocytopenia with bovine lung heparin preparation.[4,61] Stead et al. recently reported five patients who developed thrombocytopenia when given one particular lot of bovine heparin.[68] However, the antibody produced appears to have a broad specificity. It usually reacts with heparin from a different lot or different animal source from that which the patient was given and even with low-molecular-weight heparin fractions.[10,52,72] Messmore et al. found that the antibody in most of their patients reacted with several commercial preparations of low-molecular-weight heparin, in addition to standard heparin.[52] However, Leroy et al. observed a lower cross-reactivity rate (44%) with one preparation of low-molecular-weight heparin, C5216 (Choay).[50] Chong and coworkers have tested 17 patients for cross-reactivity with a new low-molecular-weight heparinoid, Org 10172, and only the plasma of three patients showed cross-reaction with heparin and heparinoid.[17] The divergence of results in different studies may be due to heterogeneity of such antibodies. This may also account for the variability in response to treatment of heparin-induced thrombocytopenia with low-molecular-weight heparins and heparinoid.[40,50,75]

Heparin-Dependent Antibody Interaction with Endothelial Cells

Cines and coworkers recently demonstrated that antibody in the sera of patients with heparin-induced thrombocytopenia could bind to endothelial cells and cause the cell-surface expression of tissue factor.[24] They found that incubation of patient sera with endothelial cells led to the deposition of increased amounts of either IgG alone or IgG and IgM immunoglobulins, and in a few instances, IgM or IgA alone. Bound antibody activated complement and caused the increased binding of complement component C3 to endothelial cells. The antibody that bound to endothelial cells was probably identical with that which reacted with platelets because the former antibody could be absorbed by platelets previously exposed to heparin. However, unlike the reaction of the antibody with platelets, which required heparin, antibody could bind to endothelial cells in the absence of added heparin, although antibody-binding was markedly increased in its presence. The explanation for the heparin-independent antibody binding to endothelial cells may be the presence of cell-bound heparin or related glycosaminoglycans.

Cines et al. postulated that the antibody recognizes an antigenic complex that is, at least partly, composed of heparin or heparan.[24] They provided two lines of evidence for this hypothesis. First, patient sera deposited less immunoglobulin on endothelial cells that had been preincubated with heparinase to remove cell-bound heparan. Second, decreased amounts of IgG became bound to endothelial cells when the patient sera had been previously incubated either with platelets exposed to heparin or with heparin/heparan-Sepharose beads. Binding of the antibody to endothelial cells also resulted in the elaboration of a procoagulant activity indistinguishable functionally and antigenically from tissue factor. The antibody-induced production of tissue factor by endothelial cells was enhanced by the presence of platelets.

Cines et al. suggested that the endothelial cell immunoinjury and the concomitant production of tissue factor mediated by the antibody may contribute to the development of thromboembolic complications in patients with heparin-induced thrombocytopenia.[24] However, in these patients the risk of development of thrombosis rapidly decreases after heparin withdrawal, even though the heparin-dependent antiplatelet antibody is known to persist for several weeks. The major determining factor is probably heparin-dependent antibody–platelet interaction with consequential elaboration of platelet proaggregating and procoagulant materials and the formation of platelet aggregates and microemboli.

Antibody–Heparin–Platelet Interaction: Fc-Mediated Mechanism

The initial step in an Fc-mediated mechanism is the binding of heparin to the antibody to form an immune complex. Cines and coworkers have provided experimental data in support of this proposal.[23] They found increased amounts of radiolabeled heparin within the 7S (IgG) fraction with patient IgG, compared with control IgG, when they incubated each with [^{3}H]heparin before analysis by sucrose-density gradient centrifugation. In contrast, Green et al. were unable to demonstrate heparin binding to the heparin-dependent antibody.[37] They incubated [^{35}S]heparin with patient and control plasma and separated antibody-bound from unbound heparin by precipitation of the immune complexes with antihuman IgG antibody. Similarly, Sandler and his coworkers could not demonstrate binding of heparin-dependent antibody to heparin when they attempted to absorb out the platelet aggregating activity from a patient serum using heparin–Sepharose CL-6B affinity chromatography.[64]

Assuming that heparin does bind to antibody, the next step in this mechanism would be the binding of the heparin-antibody complex to platelets by the Fc portion of the antibody molecule. Kelton et al.[44] have recently reported results consistent with this mechanism. They found that both Fc and $(Fab')_2$ fragments of patient IgG and the Fc fragment of control IgG inhibited platelet [^{14}C]serotonin release stimulated by patient serum and heparin. Control $(Fab')_2$ fragments had no effect. These results are consistent with the hypothesis that the $(Fab')_2$ region of the antibody is required for the recognition and binding of heparin and that the Fc region of the antibody is needed for attachment of the immune complex to a platelet Fc receptor. This view is further supported by the results of Castaldi and coworkers.[11] These investigators found that purified rabbit IgG, which is known to bind to the platelet Fc receptor, blocked heparin-dependent antibody-mediated platelet aggregation. The inhibitory activity of the rabbit IgG was located in the Fc portion of the molecule. In contrast, Pfueller and David[57] were unable to demonstrate inhibition of heparin-dependent antibody-induced aggregation of washed platelets with high concentrations of human IgG. Furthermore, the heparin-dependent antibody-induced aggregation in platelet-rich plasma was not abolished by heat-aggregated IgG which, under these conditions, binds to platelets but does not cause aggregation.[59] The reason for the divergence of results of the latter study from those of the preceding two is unclear.

Antibody–Heparin–Platelet Interaction: Fc-Independent Mechanism

An alternate mechanism for the attachment of heparin-dependent antibody to platelets is by an Fc-independent process whereby the antibody recognizes an antigenic complex formed between heparin and platelets. Although Shanberger and his colleagues have shown that heparin binds to platelets,[65] it is not clear whether or not heparin and platelets form a tightly bound complex that is capable of acting as an immunogen. Green and coworkers showed that the heparin-dependent, platelet-aggregating activity in their patient's plasma could be entirely removed by incubating it with platelets previously exposed to heparin.[37] Although this finding is compatible with an Fc-independent mechanism, no study has yet demonstrated binding of the Fab fragment of the antibody to a heparin–platelet complex.

Platelet Antigen/Receptor for Heparin-Dependent Antibody

There are a number of platelet proteins that have affinity for heparin and may potentially form a heparin–platelet antigenic complex for the attachment of the heparin-dependent antiplatelet antibody. Gogstad and his coworkers[35] were able to identify six such proteins by using crossed-affinity immunoelectrophoresis. They were GPIb, antigens 17 and 25 (which may represent the GPIa–IIa complex and GPIV, respectively), platelet factor 4, thrombospondin, and an unidentified α-granule protein termed G4. The first three of these are surface membrane proteins and the latter three are α-granule proteins that may be expressed on the platelet surface following their release. In addition to GPIb, Wolf and Wick isolated another heparin-binding platelet protein that has a M_r of 207 kDa (nonreduced) and 57 kDa (reduced).[78]

The identity of the putative platelet antigen for heparin-dependent antiplatelet antibody is still controversial. There is some indirect evidence to suggest that GPIb is the platelet antigen. First, GPIb has been shown to have affinity for heparin.[35] Second, Adelman and coworkers showed that heparin-dependent antibody-induced platelet aggregation could be inhibited by an anti-GPIb monoclonal antibody, 6D1, and by a 52/48-kDa tryptic fragment of von Willebrand factor.[2] This tryptic fragment binds to GPIb in the absence of ristocetin and blocks von Willebrand factor-dependent platelet agglutination. However, Chong and Castaldi[15] and Castaldi and coworkers[11] found that the sera/plasma of patients with heparin-induced thrombocytopenia caused heparin-dependent aggregation of Bernard-Soulier syndrome platelets, which genetically lack GPIb. Taken together, it would, therefore, appear that the antibody-binding site is in close proximity to, rather than directly on, GPIb.

Lynch and Howe have examined the binding specificity of the antibody using Western blot analysis. They found increased immunoglobulin binding in the presence of heparin to three proteins with M_rs of 180 kDa, 124 kDa, and 82 kDa (nonreduced).[51] Radiolabeled heparin also bound to the same three proteins. It was suggested that the 180-kDa, 124-kDa, and 82-kDa proteins might be thrombospondin, its digestive product, and GPV, respectively. However, the molecular mass of thrombospondin under the nonreducing conditions used in their Western blot studies would be $\simeq$ 450 kDa. Furthermore, Bernard-Soulier syndrome platelets, which lack GPV, aggregate normally in response to heparin-dependent antibody.[11,15]

Cheng and Hawiger have isolated a Fc fragment-binding protein from human platelets with an M_r of 255 kDa.[12] On reduction, the protein dissociated into subunits with an M_r of 50 kDa. This platelet Fc receptor has similar molecular mass characteristics to those of the heparin-binding platelet protein isolated by Wolf and Wick, which had M_rs of 207 kDa (nonreduced) and 50 kDa (reduced).[78] The latter protein was also shown to bind heparin-dependent antibody. The human platelet Fc receptor is thought to be closely associated with GPIb[54] as is the heparin-dependent antibody-binding site on platelets.[2] Given the variability of molecular mass estimation by different laboratories, the molecular mass of the heparin-dependent antibody-binding protein and that of the Fc receptor are sufficiently similar to suggest that the two proteins are identical. This conclusion, together with the findings of Kelton et al.[44] and Castaldi and coworkers,[11] strongly supports the concept that the heparin-dependent antibody binds to platelets through a platelet Fc receptor (discussed earlier).

CONCLUSIONS

There is considerable heterogeneity in the mechanisms whereby quinine/quinidine drug-dependent antibodies bind to platelets and in the nature of the epitopes recognized by these antibodies. For most patients with quinine/quinidine-induced thrombocytopenia, it is probable that drug binds to the membrane-associated region of the GPIb-IX complex, resulting in the formation of neoantigen(s). The patient responds to this antigenic stimulus by developing an antibody that recognizes the drug-dependent neoantigen(s) on the GPIb-IX complex. In a few patients, the neoantigen(s) formed between drug and the GPIIb-IIIa complex also elicits the formation of drug-dependent antibodies. It is also possible that in a small number of patients, drug mediates the formation of an antibody that binds to platelets by an undefined Fc receptor-dependent mechanism. Patients receiving quinidine may also develop a drug-independent autoantibody that reacts with the GPIb-IX complex, GPV, or other components of the human platelet membrane.

There are still considerable gaps in our understanding of the molecular interaction between heparin, platelets, and the heparin-dependent antibody. Although several studies have provided data concerning the nature of the antibody, the platelet antigen/immune receptor and some aspects of heparin-platelet-antibody interaction, the precise mechanism of antibody binding to platelets (whether through a Fc-dependent or a Fc-independent mechanism) is still uncertain, and the exact identity of the platelet antigen/immune receptor is still to be established. The kinetics of the binding of the antibody to platelets, the binding of heparin to the antibody, and the binding of heparin to platelets are unknown.

Within the last few years, there has been an explosion in our understanding of the biochemistry of platelet membrane surface proteins. This has arisen largely as a result of the purification or cloning of the major platelet membrane glycoproteins. It can be reasonably anticipated that these advances will directly translate into the inevitable resolution of the complete mechanism of the interaction of drug-dependent antibodies with platelets.

This work was supported by National Health and Medical Research Council of Australia grants 6K14443 and 860271. Michael C. Berndt is the recipient of a Wellcome Australian Senior Research Fellowship.

REFERENCES

1. Ackroyd JF: The role of Sedormid in the immunological reaction that results in platelet lysis in Sedormid purpura. Clin Sci 13:409,1954

2. Adelman B, Sobel M, Fujimura Y, Ruggeri ZM, Zimmerman TS: Platelet glycoprotein Ib is a binding site that participates in platelet aggregation in heparin-associated thrombocytopenia (abstr). Clin Res 34:449A, 1986

3. Babcock RB, Dumper CW, Scharfman WB: Heparin-induced immune thrombocytopenia. N Engl J Med 295:237, 1976

4. Bell WR, Royall RM: Heparin-associated thrombocytopenia: A comparison of three heparin preparations. N Engl J Med 303:902, 1980

5. Berndt MC, Caen JP: Platelet glycoproteins. In Spaet T (ed): Progress in Hemostasis and Thrombosis, Vol 7, p 111. Orlando, Grune & Stratton, 1984

6. Berndt MC, Chong BH, Bull HA, Zola H, Castaldi PA: Molecular characterization of quinine/quinidine drug-dependent antibody platelet interaction using monoclonal antibodies. Blood 66:1292, 1985

7. Berndt MC, Du X, Beutler L, Booth WJ, Castaldi PA: Localization of functional domains on human platelet GPIb-IX complex by eiptope analysis with monoclonal antibodies (abstr). Thromb Haemostasis 58:34, 1987

8. Berndt MC, Gregory C, Chong BH, Zola H, Castaldi PA: Additional glycoprotein defects in Bernard-Soulier's syndrome: Confirmation of genetic basis by parental analysis. Blood 62:800, 1983

9. Berndt MC, Gregory C, Kabral A, Zola H, Fournier D, Castaldi PA: Purification and preliminary characterization of the glycoprotein Ib complex in the human platelet membrane. Eur J Biochem 151:637, 1985

10. Blockmans D, Beaunameaux H, Vermylen J, Verstraete M: Heparin-induced thrombocytopenia: Platelet aggregation studies in the presence of heparin fractions or semi-synthetic analogues of various molecular weights and anticoagulant activities. Thromb Haemostasis 55:90, 1986

11. Castaldi PA, Davies PH, Berndt MC: Antiplatelet heparin-dependent antibody interacts with

the platelet Fc-receptor (abstr). Thromb Haemostasis 54:61, 1985

12. Cheng CM, Hawiger J: Affinity isolation and characterization of immunoglobulin G Fc fragment-binding glycoprotein from human blood platelets. J Biol Chem 254:2165, 1979

13a. Chong BH: Drug-induced thrombocytopenia: A study of the mechanism of thrombocytopenia caused by heparin and quinidine (Doctoral thesis). Sydney, N.S.W.: University of Sydney, 1985

13b. Chong BH: Heparin-induced thrombocytopenia. Blood Rev. 2:108, 1988

14. Chong BH, Berndt MC, Koutts J, Castaldi PA: Quinidine-induced thrombocytopenia and leukopenia; demonstration and characterization of distinct antiplatelet and antileukocyte antibodies. Blood 62:1218, 1983

15. Chong BH, Castaldi PA: Platelet proaggregating effect of heparin: Possible mechanism for non-immune heparin-associated thrombocytopenia. Aust NZ J Med 16:715, 1986

16. Chong BH, Grace CS, Rozenberg MC: Heparin-induced thrombocytopenia: Effect of heparin platelet antibody on platelets. Br J Haematol 49:531, 1981

17. Chong BH, Ismail F, Cade J, Gallus AS, Gordon S, Chesterman CN: Heparin-induced thrombocytopenia: In vitro studies with low molecular weight heparinoid, Org 10172 (abstr). Thromb Haemostasis 58:308, 1987

18. Chong BH, Pitney WR, Castaldi PA: Heparin-induced thrombocytopenia: Association of thrombotic complications with heparin-dependent IgG antibody that induces thromboxane synthesis and platelet aggregation. Lancet 2:1246, 1982

19. Christie DJ, Aster RH: Drug–antibody–platelet interaction in quinine- and quinidine-induced thrombocytopenia. J Clin Invest 70:989, 1982

20. Christie DJ, Mullen PC: Binding of drug-dependent antibodies to Bernard-Soulier platelets (abstr). Thromb Haemostasis 54:173, 1985

21. Christie DJ, Mullen PC, Aster RH: Fab-mediated binding of drug-dependent antibodies to platelets in quinidine- and quinine-induced thrombocytopenia. J Clin Invest 75:310, 1984

22. Christie DJ, Weber RW, Mullen PC, Cook JM, Aster RH: Structural features of the quinidine and quinine molecules necessary for binding of drug-induced antibodies to human platelets. J Lab Clin Med 104:730, 1984

23. Cines DB, Kaywin P, Bina M, Tomaski A, Schreiber AD: Heparin-associated thrombocytopenia. N Engl J Med 303:788, 1980

24. Cines DB, Tomaski A, Tannenbaum S: Immune endothelial cell injury in heparin-associated thrombocytopenia. N Engl J Med 316:581, 1986

25. Clemetson KJ, McGregor JL, James E, Dechavanne M, Luscher EF: Characterization of the platelet membrane glycoprotein abnormalities in Bernard-Soulier syndrome and comparison with normal by surface-labeling techniques and high-resolution two-dimensional gel electrophoresis. J Clin Invest 70:304, 1982

26. Connellan JM, Quinn M, Wiley JS: The use of ^{125}I labelled staphylococcal protein A in the diagnosis of autoimmune thrombocytopenic purpura and other immune mediated thrombocytopenias. Pathology 18:111, 1986

27. Devine DV, Rosse WF: Identification of platelet proteins that bind alloantibodies and autoantibodies. Blood 64:1240, 1984

28. Deykin D, Hellerstein LJ: The assessment of drug-dependent and isoimmune antiplatelet antibodies by the use of platelet aggregometry. J Clin Invest 51:3142, 1972

29. Du X, Beutler L, Ruan C, Castaldi PA, Berndt MC: Glycoprotein Ib and glycoprotein IX are fully associated in the intact platelet membrane. Blood 69:1524, 1987

30. Faig D, Karpatkin S: Cumulative experience with a simplified solid-phase radioimmunoassay for the detection of bound antiplatelet IgG, serum auto-, allo-, and drug-dependent antibodies. Blood 60:807, 1982

31. Follea G, Hamandjian I, Trzeciak MC, Nedey C, Streichenberger R, Dechavanne M: Pentosane polysulphate associated thrombocytopenia. Thromb Res 42:413, 1986

32. Fratantoni JC, Pollat R, Gralnick H: Heparin-induced thrombocytopenia—Confirmation of diagnosis with in vitro methods. Blood 45:395, 1975

33. Garty M, Illfeld D, Kelton JG: Correlation of a quinidine-induced platelet-specific antibody with development of thrombocytopenia. Am J Med 79:253, 1985

34. George JN, Onofre AR: Human platelet surface binding of endogenous secreted factor VIII/von Willebrand factor and platelet factor 4. Blood 59:194, 1982

35. Gogstad GO, Solum NO, Krutnes MB: Heparin-binding platelet proteins demonstrated by crossed affinity immunoelectrophoresis. Br J Haematol 53:563, 1983

36. Gouault-Heilmann M, Payen D, Contant G, Intrator L, Huet Y, Schaeffer A: Thrombocytopenia related to synthetic heparin analogue therapy. Thromb Haemostasis 54:557, 1985

37. Green D, Harris K, Reynolds N, Roberts M, Patterson R: Heparin immune thrombocytopenia

—Evidence for a heparin–platelet complex as the antigenic determinent. J Lab Clin Med 91:167, 1978

38. Hackett T, Kelton JG, Powers P: Drug-induced platelet destruction. Semin Thromb Hemost 8:116, 1982

39. Handa M, Titani K, Holland LZ, Roberts JR, Ruggeri ZM: The von Willebrand factor-binding domain of platelet membrane glycoprotein Ib. Characterization by monoclonal antibodies and partial amino acid sequence analysis of proteolytic fragments. J Biol Chem 261:12579, 1986

40. Horellon MH, Conrad J, Lecrubier C, Samana M, Roque-D'Orbcastelo de Fenoyl O, Di Maria G, Bernadou A: Persistent heparin-induced thrombocytopenia, therapy with low molecular weight heparin. Thromb Haemostasis 51:134, 1984

41. Kapsch D, Silver D: Heparin-induced thrombocytopenia with thrombosis and hemorrhage. Arch Surg 116:1423, 1981

42. Kelton JG, Meltzer D, Moore J, Giles AR, Wilson WE, Barr R, Hirsch J, Neame PB, Powers PJ, Walker I, Bianchi F, Carter CJ: Drug-induced thrombocytopenia is associated with increased binding of IgG to platelets both in vivo and in vitro. Blood 58:524, 1981

43. Kelton JG, Sheridan D, Brain H, Powers PJ, Turpie AG, Carter CJ: Clinical usefulness of testing for a heparin-dependent platelet aggregating factor in patients with suspected heparin-associatedthrombocytopenia. J Lab Clin Med 103:606, 1984

44. Kelton JG, Sheridan DP, Santos AV, Moore JC: The pathophysiology of heparin-induced thrombocytopenia (abstr). Blood 66:290a, 1985

45. King DJ, Kelton JG: Heparin-associated thrombocytopenia. Ann Intern Med 100:535, 1984

46. Kunicki TJ, Aster RH: Deletion of the platelet-specific alloantigen $P1^{A1}$ from platelets in Glanzmann's thrombasthenia. J Clin Invest 61:1225, 1978

47. Kunicki TJ, Johnson MM, Aster RH: Absence of the platelet receptor for drug-dependent antibodies in the Bernard-Soulier syndrome. J Clin Invest 62:716, 1978

48. Kunicki TJ, Russell N, Nurden AT, Aster RH, Caen JP: Further studies of the human platelet receptor for quinine- and quinidine-dependent antibodies. J Immunol 126:398, 1981

49. Lerner W, Caruso R, Faig D, Karpatkin S: Drug-dependent and non–drug-dependent antiplatelet antibody drug-induced immunologic thrombocytopenic purpura. Blood 66:306, 1985

50. Leroy J, Leclerc MH, Delahousse B, Guerois C, Foloppe P, Gruel Y, Toulemonde F: Treatment of heparin-associated thrombocytopenia and thrombosis with low molecular weight heparin (CY216). Semin Thromb Hemost 11:326, 1985

51. Lynch DM, Howe SE: Heparin-associated thrombocytopenia antibody binding specificity to platelet antigens. Blood 66:1176, 1985

52. Messmore HL, Fareed J, Corey J, Griffin B, Miller A, Zuckerman L, Parvez Z, Seghatchian J, Choay J: In vitro assessment of low molecular weight heparin in patients with thrombocytopenia induced by standard heparin (abstr). Blood 64:238a, 1984

53. Miescher PA, Miescher A: Die Sedormid-anaphylaxie. Schweiz Med Wochenschr 82:1279, 1952

54. Moore A, Ross GD, Nachman RL: Interaction of platelet membrane receptor with von Willebrand factor, ristocetin, and the Fc region of immunoglobulin G. J Clin Invest 62:1053, 1978

55. Okumura T, Lombart C, Jamieson GA: Platelet glycocalicin. II. Purification and characterization. J Biol Chem 251:5950, 1976

56. Pfueller SL, Bilston RA, Logan D, Firkin BG: Heterogeneity of drug-dependent platelet antigens and their antibodies in quinine- and quinidine-induced thrombocytopenia: Involvement of glycoproteins Ib, IIb, IIIa and IX shown by blotting with immunogold. (submitted for publication) 1988

57. Pfueller SL, David R: Different platelet specificities of heparin-dependent platelet aggregating factors in heparin-associated immune thrombocytopenia. Br J Haematol 64:149, 1986

58. Pfueller SL, de Rosbo NK, Bilston RA: Platelets deficient in glycoprotein I have normal Fc receptor expression. Br J Haematol 56:607, 1984

59. Pfueller SL, Weber S, Luscher EF: Studies of the mechanism of the human platelet release reaction induced by immunologic stimuli. III. Relationship between the binding of soluble IgG aggregates to the Fc receptor and cell response in the presence and absence of plasma. J Immunol 118:514, 1977

60. Phillips DR, Jennings LK, Prasanna HR: Calcium-mediated association of glycoprotein G (thrombin-sensitive protein, thrombospondin) with human platelets. J Biol Chem 255:11629, 1980

61. Powers PJ, Kelton JG, Carter CJ: Studies on the frequency of heparin-associated thrombocytopenia. Thromb Res 33:439, 1984

62. Rosse WF, Devine DV, Ware R: The reactions of IgG-binding ligands with platelets and platelet-associated IgG. J Clin Invest 73:489, 1984

63. Salzman EW, Rosenberg RD, Smith MH, Lindon JN, Favreau L: Effect of heparin and heparin fractions on platelet aggregation. J Clin Invest 65:64, 1980

64. Sandler RM, Seifer DB, Morgan K, Pockros PJ, Wypych J, Weiss LM, Schiffman S: Heparin-induced thrombocytopenia and thrombosis; Detection and specificity of a platelet-aggregating IgG. Am J Clin Pathol 83:760, 1985

65. Shanberger JN, Kambayashi J, Nakagawa M: The interaction of platelets with a tritium-labeled heparin. Thromb Res 9:595, 1976

66. Shulman NR: Immunoreactions involving platelets: I. A steric and kinetic model for formation of a complex from a human antibody, quinidine as a haptene, and platelets; and for fixation of complement by the complex. J Exp Med 107:665, 1958

67. Smith ME, Jordan JV Jr, Reid DM, Jones CE, Shulman NR: Drug-antibody binding to platelets is mediated by the Fab domain and is not Fc-dependent (abstr). Blood 64:274A, 1984

68. Stead RB, Schafer AI, Rosenberg RD, Handin RI, Josa M, Khuri SF: Heterogeneity of heparin lots associated with thrombocytopenia and thromboembolism. Am J Med 77:185, 1984

69. Stricker RB, Shuman MA: Quinidine purpura: Evidence that glycoprotein V is a target platelet antigen. Blood 67:1377, 1986

70. Stricker RB, Wong D, Saks SR, Corash L, Shuman MA: Acquired Bernard-Soulier syndrome. J Clin Invest 76:1274, 1985

71. Szatkowski NS, Kunicki TJ, Aster RH: Identification of glycoprotein Ib as a target for antibody in idiopathic (autoimmune) thrombocytopenic purpura. Blood 67:310, 1986

72. Trowbridge AA, Caraveo J, Green JB, Amaral B, Stone MJ: Heparin-related immune thrombocytopenia. Studies of antibody-heparin specificity. Am J Med 65:277, 1978

73. van Leeuwen EF, Engelfriet CP, von dem Borne AEGKr: Studies on quinine- and quinidine-dependent antibodies against platelets and their reaction with platelets in the Bernard-Soulier syndrome. Br J Haematol 51:551, 1982

74. Vannucchi S, Fibbi G, Pasquali F, Rosso MD, Cappelletti R, Chiarugi V: Adhesion-dependent heparin production by platelets. Nature 296:352, 1982

75. Vitoux JF, Mathieu JF, Roncato M, Fiessinger JN, Aiach M: Heparin-associated thrombocytopenia: Treatment with low molecular weight heparin. Thromb Haemostasis 55:37, 1980

76. von dem Borne AEGKr, Helmerhorst FM, van Leeuwen EF, Pegels HG, von Riesz E, Engelfriet CP: Autoimmune thrombocytopenia: Detection of platelet autoantibodies with the suspension immunofluorescence test. Br J Haematol 45:319, 1980

77. Wicki AN, Clemetson KJ: Structure and function of platelet membrane glycoproteins Ib and V. Effects of leukocyte elastase and other proteases on platelet response to von Willebrand factor and thrombin. Eur J Biochem 153:1, 1985

78. Wolf H, Wick G: Antibodies interacting with, and corresponding binding site for, heparin on human thrombocytes. Lancet 2:222, 1986

9

Phylogeny and Tissue Distribution of Platelet Antigens

PETER J. NEWMAN

Although human platelet membrane glycoprotein structure and function has been a topic of intensive laboratory investigation for over 15 years, the realization that platelet proteins have relatives that may play equally important roles in other tissues throughout the human body has only very recently come to our attention. Publications dealing with the identification of platelet glycoprotein analogues in "nonrelated" hemopoietic cells, vascular endothelium, cells of the immune system, bone marrow osteoclasts, fibroblasts, and smooth-muscle cells have been as numerous as those dealing strictly with platelet structure and function, and the information derived from these studies has led to unanticipated insights concerning the normal role of these molecules on the cell surface. Moreover, comparative phylogenetic studies have demonstrated the presence of platelet antigens throughout the animal kingdom, ranging from mammalian to avian species. Collectively, these observations have led to important new opportunities in defining the molecular mechanisms involved in mediating cell surface interactions, including those that take place during hemostasis. This chapter summarizes recent work that has augmented our knowledge of the phylogeny and tissue distribution of platelet membrane glycoproteins, deriving data both from my laboratory and from the many other investigators in this rapidly growing field.

GLYCOPROTEIN Ib

Introduction and Properties

Human platelet glycoprotein (GP) Ib is a major integral membrane protein that mediates, in large part, the von Willebrand factor (VWF)-dependent adhesion of platelets to exposed vascular endothelium.[8,62] Glycoprotein has a molecular mass (M_r) of 170 kilodaltons (kDa), and is composed of a 145-kDa α chain disulfide-linked to a 25-kDa β chain.[76] The α chain may be proteolytically split, yielding a major fragment of 130 kDa, termed *glycocalicin,* that has been shown to contain 60% carbohydrate by weight.[72] Approximately 80% of the carbohydrate of glycocalicin is *O*-linked, and the structures of the major *O*-linked residues have been identified by gas chromatography–mass spectroscopy.[109] Wyler et al[114] have shown that the β-chain can be phosphorylated. Glycoprotein Ib exists complexed 1:1 with GPIX (M_r, 20,000), both in detergent solution[13] and in the intact platelet membrane.[27] Both of these membrane glycoproteins are missing from the platelets of individuals with the Bernard-Soulier syndrome.[24] Studies performed by Okita et al.[71] and Fox et al.[30] indicate that GPIb is linked to the platelet cytoskeleton by actin-binding protein and may thus play a role in regulating platelet deformability[111] and in maintaining normal cell shape.

Human Cells

There are two reports that GPIb-like molecules are present in human umbilical vein endothelial cells as well as in human platelets. Asch et al. described a 210-kDa endothelial cell polypeptide that was metabolically labeled and then immunoprecipitated by the anti-GPIb monoclonal antibody, JA1.[4] This antibody also blocked ristocetin-supported VWF binding to, and the subsequent agglutination of, endothelial cells. Sprandio and colleagues[95] reported that the GPIb-specific monoclonal antibody, AP1, bound approximately 75,000 saturable sites on the endothelial cell surface. After surface radioiodination, AP1 was able to immunoprecipitate endothelial cell proteins of 150 kDa, 130 kDa, 110 kDa, and 95 kDa. Neither of the foregoing studies could exclude simple immunologic cross-reactivity as the basis for their observations; therefore, validation of their results must await further comparison of the endothelial cell products with platelet GPIb by peptide mapping, amino acid composition, or sequence analysis.

Human Transformed Cell Lines

Because platelets are not capable of appreciable protein synthesis, it would be useful to identify an actively growing nucleated cell to serve as a resource for studying the synthesis and expression of GPIb and GPIX. Tabilio and coworkers[101] reported that a human erythroleukemia cell line, HEL, Specifically bound the monoclonal antibody AN 51, which has been shown to be specific for GPIb.[61] Kieffer et al. have isolated the AN 51-reactive protein from HEL cells[47] and found it to be a 60-kDa polypeptide. In addition to its reactivity with AN 51, the 60-kDa polypeptide was shown to react specifically with one polyclonal and five other monoclonal antibodies, each directed against epitopes on platelet GPIb. They were unable to demonstrate, however, an association of this polypeptide with either $GPIb_\beta$ or a GPIX-like molecule.

The K562 cell line, obtained from a patient in blast crisis of chronic myeloid leukemia, has also been shown to express a number of erythroid, myeloid, and megakaryocytic markers, including platelet GPIIIa (see later section on Human Transformed Cell Lines). Glycoprotein Ib, however, was not detected on K562 cells by cytofluorimetry employing AN 51.[100]

Nonhuman Cells

In 1977, Nurden et al. examined the glycoprotein composition of 13 different mammalian species by one-dimensional sodium dodecyl sulfate-polyacrylamide gel electrophoresis (SDS-PAGE) and periodate-Schiff (PSA) reagent[69] and found evidence for the presence of glycoproteins related to human GPI, GPII, and GPIII, as they were referred to at that time, in monkeys, dogs, bears, deer, rabbits, cats, and lions, to name a few. Biochemical techniques for examining glycoprotein content were of comparatively low resolution at that time, however, so these studies are interesting mainly from a historical perspective. Recently, Kupinsky and Miller have shown that guinea pig platelets possess a functional receptor for VWF that has many features characteristic of GPIb.[52,53] This study employed a monoclonal antibody, designated PG-1, that was produced by immunization with guinea pig platelets. PG-1 selectively inhibits ristocetin-induced agglutination and ristocetin-supported ^{125}I-labeled VWf binding, but it has no effect on ADP-induced platelet aggregation. PG-1 recognizes a two-chain glycoprotein composed of an *M*r, 143,000 polypeptide disulfide linked to a smaller 25,000-Da chain, nearly identical in size with the human platelet GPIb α and β chains. Guinea pig platelet GPIb was also shown to be synthesized by guinea pig megakaryocytes, thus these megakaryocytes may represent a useful source for further study of this important platelet membrane receptor.

GLYCOPROTEIN IIa

Introduction and Properties

Glycoprotein IIa was first identified as a platelet membrane component by Phillips and Agin[76] over 10 years ago. It is characterized by an upward shift in mobility on SDS-PAGE gels following disulfide bond reduction, a property that is attributed to the presence of intrachain disulfide bridges. Glycoprotein IIa has a M_r of 138,000 nonreduced, and 157,000 reduced, and is readily radiolabeled by both ^{125}I and sodium metaperiodate/[^{3}H]$NaBH_4$ techniques.[23]

Human and Nonhuman Cells

Glycoprotein IIa has recently been shown to be identical with the β chain of the fibronectin receptor and with the shared β subunit of the five known very late activation (VLA) antigens[44] that are present on lymphocytes, platelets, and certain other human tissues. By using the monoclonal antibody A-1A5, which is specific for the VLA β chain, Pischel et al.[81] were able to immunoprecipitate from platelets surface-labeled components corresponding to $GPIc_\alpha$, GPIa, and GPIIa. They further identified platelet GPIIa as the shared VLA β chain and showed that it was present in the membrane of platelets complexed with GPIa to form VLA-2.[82] Platelets may also express small amounts of VLA-3,[82] which is thought to be composed of GPIc complexed with GPIIa. Relevant to these studies are the recent findings of Takada et al.[102] that VLA-3 and VLA-5 are equivalent to the avian and human fibronectin receptors, respectively. The authors further demonstrated that the β chain of the fibronectin receptor is identical with VLA_β. Thus, although the GPIIb-IIIa complex has been reported to be the receptor for fibronectin following platelet activation (see the following section), it is possible that the small amount of VLA-3 found on platelets by Pischel et al.[82] may serve as another fibronectin receptor. Evidence that this is indeed so has recently been provided by the report of Piotrowicz et al.,[80] which indicated that GPIIa and GPIc exist in a complex in the membrane of platelets and that this complex actually functions as an activation-independent platelet receptor for fibronectin. Moreover, Giancotti et al.[36] have identified a GP168-138-kDa membrane glycoprotein complex on the surface of human platelets, distinct from the GPIIb-IIIa complex and similar in mobility to GPIc-IIa, that is precipitated by antibodies specific for the β chain of the murine fibroblast fibronectin receptor. Thus, as GPIIa represents the β subunit of both the VLA and fibronectin families of heterodimers, it is likely to be very broadly distributed. Evidence that this is true has been provided by Pischel et al.,[82] who showed that the monoclonal antibody A-1A5 (originally described as anti-VLA_β) reacts with nearly all human tissues tested. The reported expression of GPIIa on endothelial cells[110] and the erythroleukemia cell line K562[35] can now be better understood in light of the foregoing findings.

GLYCOPROTEINS IIb AND IIIa

Introduction and Properties

The plasma membrane heterodimer protein complex composed of glycoproteins IIb and IIIa is central to the role of platelet-subendothelial and platelet-platelet interactions. This glycoprotein complex functions in platelets as a receptor for fibrinogen,[6,11] for VWF in the absence of fibrinogen,[90] and for fibronectin[32,84] and vitronectin.[87] The binding of these ligands to the GPIIb-IIIa complex is mediated, at least in part, by an ArG-Gly-Asp recognition sequence that is present on each of these ligands.[32,33,43,85,87] The GPIIb-IIIa complex also serves as the transmembrane link to the platelet cytoskeleton.[77] Previous work by many investigators has established that GPIIb (nonreduced M_r, 136,000) is composed of a heavy-chain ($GPIIb_\alpha$, M_r, 125,000) disulfide-linked to a light-chain ($GPIIb_\beta$, M_r, 21,000), whereas GPIIIa contains numerous intrachain disulfide bonds[76] that, upon reduction, result in an increase in M_r during SDS-PAGE (nonreduced M_r, 90,000; reduced M_r 105,000). The genes encoding both of these glycoproteins have recently been cloned and sequenced; the GPIIIa gene from endothelial cells[28] and the GPIIb gene from HEL cells.[86] The detailed structures of both of these glycoproteins are extensively covered in Chapter 2 of this volume; therefore, the present discussion will be limited to those details necessary for comparison with analogues of these proteins found in various other human and animal tissues.

Glycoprotein IIIa is composed of 762 amino acids (AA) in its mature form and contains an additional 26 AA signal sequence in its preform.[28] Mature GPIIIa contains approximately 16% carbohydrate by weight,[60] which include both *O*- and *N*-linked side chains.[68] The structures of both the high mannose and complex *N*-linked chains have been solved by Tsuji and Osawa.[108] Two different alloantigenic determinants, Pl^{A1} [49] and Pen,[31] are associated with GPIIIa; Pl^{A1} alloantigenic determinant has been further localized to a 17-kDa polypeptide fragment of this molecule.[68] The structural details of these and other platelet-specific alloantigens are reviewed in Chapter 6.

The structure of GPIIb is quite different from that of GPIIIa. Bray and coworkers showed that the α and β subunits of GPIIb are derived from a single polypeptide precursor,[15] i.e., a single mRNA species encoded both chains. This data was recently confirmed and extended by Poncz et al.,[86] who sequenced a single 3.3-kb cDNA that encodes a large GPIIb precursor polypeptide comprised of 1039 amino acids which, in order from the amino-terminus, code for a singal sequence (30 AA), the α subunit (871 AA), and finally the $GPII_\beta$ chain (137 AA). After synthesis, both the signal peptide and the β chain are cleaved, with the α and β chains remaining associated through disulfide bonds. The only obvious transmembrane domain was found within the smaller β subunit, suggesting that the entire GPIIb molecule may be anchored to the membrane by this chain. Like GPIIIa, the structures of the major *N*-linked sugar residues for GPIIb have been solved.[108] The Lek (Bak) alloantigenic determinant is associated with GPIIb,[46] but it has not yet been localized to a specific region of the molecule.

That GPIIb-GPIIIa exists as a calcium-dependent complex in detergent solution was first shown by Kunicki et al.,[51] who demonstrated that a single precipitin arc formed during crossed-immunoelectrophoresis (CIE) of Triton-solubilized platelets contained both GPIIb and GPIIIa. When platelet lysates were treated with EDTA, however, this arc disappeared, with the concomitant appearance of two new precipitin arcs, each containing only one of the glycoproteins. Glycoproteins IIb and IIIa were later shown to exist as a complex in the membrane of intact platelets by Pidard et al., who used the complex-specific murine monoclonal antibody, AP2,[78] which bound approximately 50,000 sites on the surface of unactivated platelets. Because this figure is very similar to that obtained by Scatchard analysis, using both a GPIIb-specific[59] and GPIIIa-specific[64] monoclonal antibody, each of which recognizes its respective antigens in either the free or complexed state, it appears that no free GPIIb or GPIIIa exists on the platelet surface.

Human Cells

Evidence has been accumulating over the last several years that GPIIb-IIIa, or molecules that are immunologically cross-reactive with IIb-IIIa, may be present on the surfaces of human cells other than platelets. It is now apparent that the GPIIb-IIIa complex is merely one member of a superfamily of structurally related receptors involved in mediating the attachment of cells to each other or to the extracellular matrix. Thus, the real issue to be addressed when dealing with the presence of platelet GPIIb-IIIa on other human cells is: Which cells, if any, contain molecules identical with GPIIb and GPIIIa, and which cells express glycoproteins that are phylogenetically related, i.e., a member of the superfamily of cytoadhesive receptors that may share one or more immunologically cross-reactive or structurally similar domains? This somewhat complicated issue can be illustrated by examining the literature pertaining to the question of whether or not human monocytes contain GPIIb and GPIIIa or related molecules.

Monocytes

In 1982, Burckhardt et al.[18] reported that a monoclonal antibody made against human monocytes specifically immunoprecipitated a surface-labeled bimolecular complex of 93,000 and 135,000 Da from both monocytes and platelets, and designated this shared component as the monocyte-platelet antigen (MPA). The two molecules exhibited mobility changes during reduced and nonreduced SDS-PAGE characteristic of GPIIb-IIIa. Immunofluorescent staining of monocytes by this monoclonal antibody persisted when adherent platelets were removed by washing in 0.5M EDTA. To further preclude the possibility that the observed monocyte staining may have been due to adherent platelets or platelet fragments, the authors demonstrated reexpression of MPA on the surface of monocytes 18 hr after pronase treatment. The monocytes were allowed to recover, however, in culture medium that contained serum (see later discussion). In support of their findings, we reported[65] that the monoclonal anti-GPIIIa antibody, AP3, bound to monocytes and neutrophils, but it did not bind to lymphocytes, as assessed by cytofluorometry (Fig. 9-1). Gogstad et al.[40] and Bai et al.[5] also published evidence that monocytes express GPIIb and GPIIIa.

None of the foregoing studies demonstrated actual synthesis (i.e., by metabolic incorporation of radiolabeled amino acids) of GPIIb or GPIIIa by monocytes and, therefore, it could not be ruled out that each of the observations made in these studies were actually due to contamination with platelets[74] or with platelet membrane fragments (which are known to occur in serum[34]), bound to the surface of monocytes. Thus, in challenge of these observations, Clemetson et al,[23] using monocytes purified by centrifugal elutriation, were unable to detect IIb or IIIa in monocytes by using the

PLATELETS

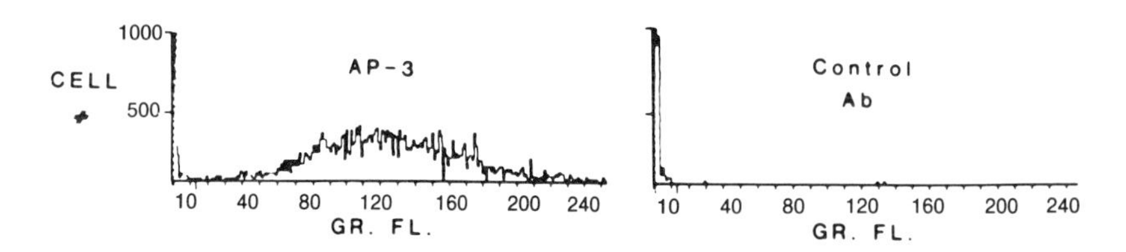

MONOCYTES

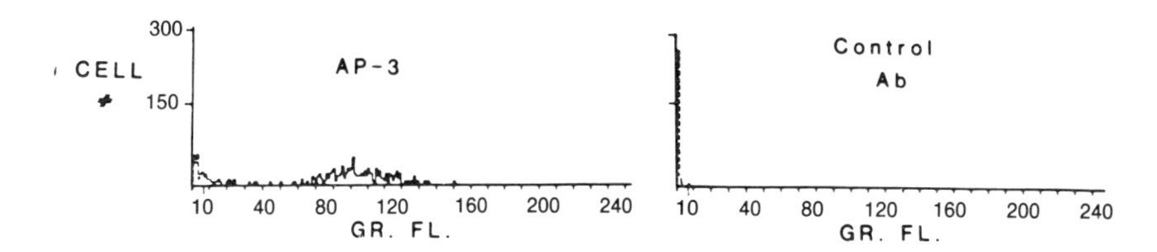

GRANULOCYTES

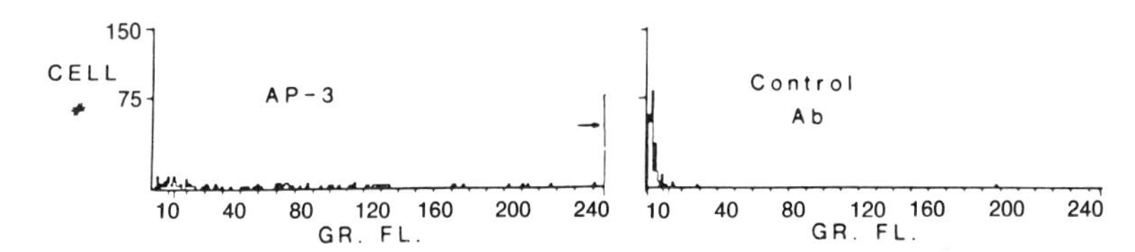

LYMPHOCYTES

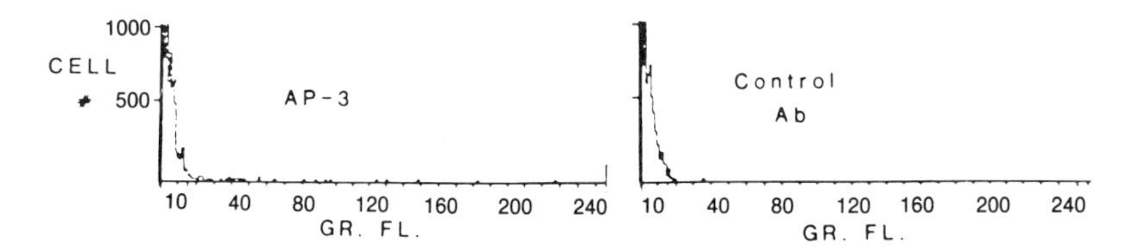

Figure 9-1. Cytofluorographic analysis of AP3 binding to red cell-depleted whole blood. Binding is represented as the number of cells (*y*-axis) plotted as a function of the amount of green fluorescence (antibody bound) per cell. The *right panels* show the binding of an irrelevant murine monoclonal antibody of the same subclass as AP3 (IgG1). Note that the AP3 epitope appears on platelets, monocytes, granulocytes (note arrow at far right = intense staining of a subpopulation of neutrophils), but not at all on lymphocytes.

anti-GPIIb–GPIIIa monoclonal antibodies T10 and P4, as well as a polyclonal antibody rabbit antiplatelet reagent. Levene and Rabellino[57] pulse-labeled monocytes with [^{35}S] methionine and showed that rabbit polyclonal antisera specific for GPIIb and GPIIIa, as well as a IIb–IIIa complex-specific monoclonal antibody, PC-1, were all unreactive with any monocyte protein that could be metabolically labeled. As pointed out by Altieri et al.,[2] however, the negative results obtained by both Clemetson et al. and Levene and Rabellino, could be explained if the monocyte molecules are not identical with, but merely related to, platelet GPIIb and GPIIIa. If only a few epitopes are shared, some (anti-MPA;[18] P140, P112, J15;[5] AP3;[64,65] 10E5[2]), but not all (T10, P4;[22] and PC-1[57]) antiplatelet monoclonal antibodies might be cross-reactive, and polyclonal reagents, because of their lower specificity, might be unable to identify a shared monocyte surface component. Given these findings, it is reasonable to conclude here that monocytes, which seem to have a special affinity for platelets and platelet membrane fragments, do not actually express platelet GPIIb or GPIIIa molecules per se. It is probable, however, that they do synthesize antigens that are phylogenetically related to GPIIb-IIIa (discussed later) and, thus, express a number of cross-reactive epitopes that are recognizable by particular antiplatelet monoclonal antibodies. In this light, it might be more accurate to interpret data concerning the tissue distribution of platelet antigens in the context of the distribution of particular epitopes, rather than of the whole protein.

Relationship to the Fibronectin and Vitronectin Receptors

Glycoprotein IIb and GPIIIa are now known to be members of a family of receptors, each of which plays a role in mediating the attachment of cells either to each other or to the extracellular matrix. Each of these receptors has a common α-β chain configuration, and many, including GPIIb-IIIa, recognize the amino acid sequence Arg-Gly-Asp (one-letter amino acid abbreviation, RGD) on the ligand to which they bind. Thus, Pytela et al.[88] coupled the 12-kDa cell-attachment domain of fibronectin,[79] which contains the biologically active peptide sequence RGDS,[79,115] to Sepharose and used this affinity support to purify the fibronectin receptor (FNR) from human MG-63 osteosarcoma cells. A heterodimer complex having M_rs of 140 and 120 kDa was eluted with the synthetic peptide G*RGD*SP. Similar fibronectin receptor complexes have been isolated from chick embryo fibroblasts,[1,42,45] mouse[37] and hamster[17] fibroblasts, human adherent cell lines,[16] and human platelets,[81] although the avian form may be composed of a trimolecular, rather than bimolecular, complex. With a similar approach, Pytela et al.[89] were able to affinity isolate the receptor for vitronectin (VNR) from human osteosarcoma cells by using either vitronectin-Sepharose or G*RGD*SP-Sepharose and found that the receptor was composed of two subunits have reduced M_rs of 125 and 115 kDa. Thus, platelet GPIIb-IIIa, the VNR, and the FNR are functionally related, in that they each recognize RGD-containing ligands, and are structurally related insofar as they are each composed of α and β subunits of similar sizes.

Endothelial Cells

The structural and functional relatedness between members of the cytoadhesin family has provided crucial insight to the expression of platelet GPIIb- and GPIIIa-like proteins on human endothelial cells. Thiagarajan et al.[106] first reported that the GPIIIa-specific murine monoclonal antibody, B2.12, reacted with a similar protein on endothelial cells. The two molecules appeared similar, rather than identical, however, as they were of slightly different relative molecular masses, and a second antiplatelet GPIIIa monoclonal antibody, B59.2, did not bind the endothelial cell form. Within 18 months, five other laboratories[9,29,56,67,83] confirmed the presence of a GPIIIa-like molecule on endothelial cells and extended the observation to include a structurally and immunologically related GPIIb-like molecule on endothelial cells as well. Not until amino acid and nucleotide sequence data became available, however, was it possible to precisely determine the relationship between platelet GPIIb-IIIa and these two endothelial cell proteins. In retrospect, it now appears that the endothelial cell analogues of GPIIb and GPIIIa are more closely related to, if not identical with, the human vitronectin receptor. Evidence for this comes from several independent sources and will be discussed one subunit at a time. Suzuki et al.[99] purified the VNR α chain from human placenta and directly sequenced the first 11 NH_2-terminal amino acids. Charo et al.[20] reported the amino acid sequence of the NH_2-terminus of platelet $GPIIb_{\alpha}$, and Poncz et al. have sequenced the entire GPIIb molecule.[86] The VNR_{α} and IIb_{α} NH_2-termini are compared below, and as shown, represent distinct, but somewhat related polypeptides (34% sequence similarity over the entire 636 AA of the partial VNR sequence.)[86]

VNR_{α}: NH_2-FNLDVDSPAEY

IIb_{α}: NH_2-LNLDPVQLYFY

Each of these NH_2-terminal sequences has been confirmed by Ginsberg et al.,[39] who additionally showed that a polyclonal anti-VNR antibody precipitated from endothelial cells two proteins having M_rs identical with the purified VNR α and β subunits, but different from platelet IIb–IIIa. Additionally, we[67] and others[9,29,56,83,106] have shown that the endothelial cell proteins identified with antiplatelet IIb–IIIa antibodies have relative molecular masses different from platelet GPIIb and GPIIIa. Thus, by size criteria alone, the endothelial cell cytoadhesin α subunit appears more closely related to VNR_α than to GPIIb. Moreover, both a polyclonal and monoclonal antiplatelet GPIIb antibody failed to react with the VNR α subunit,[39] and we have shown that the monoclonal antibody PMI-1, which is directed against platelet GPIIb,[92] does not react with the endothelial cell GPIIb-like molecule.* Further indirect evidence that the endothelial cell α chain is VNR_α recently has been provided by Cheresh,[21] who isolated a heterodimer complex of 135 kDa and 115 kDa from human endothelial cells by G*RGD*SPK-Sepharose affinity chromatography. Two monoclonal antibodies specific for the α chain of the human VNR, and unreactive with platelet GPIIb, reacted specifically with the 135-kDa subunit. Thus, taken together, it would appear the endothelial cell α chain is actually VNR_α, rather than $GPIIb_\alpha$, although this has not yet been directly demonstrated (i.e., by isolating the endothelial cell protein and comparing its amino-terminal sequence with either one of those shown earlier).

Although the endothelial cell cytoadhesin α subunit appears to be distinct from GPIIb, there is considerable evidence that the β subunit shares the same primary sequence with GPIIIa. Fitzgerald et al. reported that the amino acid sequence of endothelial cell GPIIIa is identical with platelet GPIIIa.[28] As Ginsberg et al. have shown that GPIIIa and VNR_β have identical amino-termini,[39] it is probable that VNR_β=GPIIIa. Thus, although endothelial cells were previously thought to contain platelet GPIIIa, it is more likely that they rather have the VNR and that the amino acid sequence of "GPIIIa" was actually obtained by sequencing the endothelial cell cDNA coding for VNR_β.

*Doers, M. and Newman, P.: Unpublished observations.

Interestingly, Giltay et al.[38] recently reported the normal synthesis and expression of endothelial cell (EC) "GPIIb and GPIIIa" in a patient with type I Glanzmann's thrombasthenia. Because foregoing observations strongly indicate that ECIIb and ECIII are actually the VNR α and β subunits, it is reasonable to conclude that thrombasthenics are deficient only in platelet GPIIb–IIIa and that the expression of the vitronectin receptor is unaffected by the disorder. Because the β subunits of the VNR and the IIb–IIIa complex are identical, and the β chain is normal in thrombasthenic endothelial cells, it is inviting to speculate that thrombasthenia is most often due to genetic defects of platelet GPIIb and not of GPIIIa. Whether or not GPIIb defects are responsible for all thrombasthenic phenotypes awaits further analysis, i.e., probing of their genomic DNAs with GPIIb- and GPIIIa-specific cDNA probes.

Leukocyte Adhesion Molecules

Independently of the investigators studying the glycoproteins involved in the adhesive reactions of platelets and fibroblasts, a number of laboratories have been actively studying the structure and function of accessory molecules involved in T- and B-lumphocyte function. Because cell surface interactions between lymphocytes, monocytes, and granulocytes are of fundamental importance in antigen presentation and subsequent elicitation of an immune response, it is not surprising that specialized molecules have evolved to mediate these important interactions. These cellular adhesive reactions are mediated, in part, by another family of structurally related membrane glycoprotein receptors, consisting of the LFA-1, Mac-1 (also called CR3), and p150,95 leukocyte cell surface receptors. Like the GPIIb-IIIa/VNR/FNR family, each of the receptors in the leukocyte adhesion molecule (LAM) family is composed of noncovalently linked α–β heterodimers. The α subunits of LFA-1, Mac-1, and p150,95 are distinct,[91] but related[103] polypeptides having M_rs of 180kDa, 170kDa, and 150kDa, respectively, whereas the β subunit is an identical 95-kDa glycoprotein common to all three proteins.[91] LFA-1 is expressed on T and B cells, granulocytes, and monocytes, and plays an accessory role in antigen-specific helper and cytolytic T-cell function.[96] Mac-1 and p150,95 are expressed on the surface of monocytes and neutrophils, and mediate adhesive reactions between these cells and the endothelium during inflammatory reactions.[97,107] Mac-1 and p150,95 also bind the iC3b fragment of complement.[10,63,112]

That the LFA-1/Mac-1/p150,95 LAM family is functionally related to the GPIIb–IIIa/VNR/FNR family is indicated by two recent observations. Wright et al.[113] have shown that the Mac-1 antigen binds to a region of C3 containing the sequence Arg-Gly-Asp. Structural relatedness between these two families, beyond that of the common $\alpha-\beta$ heterodimer subunit configuration, has also been demonstrated recently in a number of laboratories. Tamkun et al.[104] determined the primary structure of the avian fibronectin receptor β subunit, and both Kishimoto et al.[48] and Law et al.[55] have sequenced the common β subunit of LFA-1, Mac-1, and p150/95. Comparison of these two β-chain sequences with that of VNR_β (=GPIIIa) is shown in Figure 9-2, and as can be seen, each of the β chains share short (10–20 amino acids) stretches of significant (>80%) amino acid sequence similarity, with 45% to 50% overall sequence similarity between each of the chains over the entire length of the molecules. Comparison between the α subunits of the LAM α chains with those published for GPIIb, FNR_α, and VNR_α has so far been limited to the amino termini[103] and, also, reveals a significant degree of sequence similarity. Thus, it is clear from the data reviewed that these two families of cell adhesion receptors are phylogenetically related and are members of a still larger superfamily of broadly distributed molecules involved in mediating basic cell–cell communication and interaction of cells with each other and their extracellular environment.

Osteoclasts, Smooth-Muscle Cells, and Fibroblasts

In an immunohistochemical study of bone marrow biopsy specimens, Beckstead et al.[9] reported that both a polyclonal and monoclonal (AP3) antibody specific for platelet GPIIIa strongly stained osteoclast plasma membranes. Antibodies specific for the GPIIb–IIIa complex were negative, however, suggesting that the cell surface molecule present on osteoclasts may contain a GPIIIa-like β chain, together with a non-GPIIb α subunit. This complex may have functions different from that of the platelet fibrinogen receptor. In support of this notion, two groups studying bone marrow osteoclast differentiation and function have reported that these cells contain a glycoprotein complex that may be structurally and immunologically related to GPIIb–GPIIIa. Davies et al.,[26] using a monoclonal antibody against osteoclasts that inhibits bone resorption, described an osteoclast functional antigen (OFA) composed of a 95–105-kDa glycosylated heterodimer. Rat antiserum raised against the 95-kDa component of the OFA stained a 95-kDa band in platelets by immunoblotting, and the larger 105-kDa OFA band was shown to release a smaller peptide upon reduction, similar to that of $GPIIb_\beta$. Baron and coworkers[7] have shown that a similar OFA is highly enriched in chick and dog kidney osteoclasts, with as many as 1×10^7 molecules per cell. They further showed that this complex is the major (Na^+, K^+) ATPase in these cells, and suggested that its function may be coupled to calcium or to proton transport during the process of bone resorption. Molecular cloning and amino acid sequence analysis of the OFA components, currently underway in these two laboratories, should clarify the proposed similarity of OFA with the GPIIb–IIIa complex.

Molecules structurally and immunologically related to GPIIb and GPIIIa have also been found in human smooth-muscle cells,[20] human fibroblast cell lines,[20,83] large- and small-vessel endothelial cells, the epithelial and dendritic cells of lymph nodes, and the vitamin A-storing cells of the liver (Table 9-1).[19] In light of current information regarding immunologic cross-reactivity between members of the cytoadhesin family, the precise relationship between these molecules and GPIIb–IIIa, the VNR, and the FNR must await primary structure determination.

Human Transformed Cell Lines

The first report of GPIIb- or GPIIIa-like molecules on a culturable human cell line was made by Gewirtz et al.,[35] who suggested that the K562 cell line, obtained from a patient in blast crisis of chronic myeloid leukemia, constitutively expressed platelet GPIIa (discussed earlier) and GPIIIa. They did not examine the K562 cells for the presence of GPIIb. Later, Tabilio and coworkers[100] demonstrated that phorbol myristate acetate (PMA) induction of K562 cells resulted in a greater than 50-fold increase in GPIIIa expression, whereas an antibody directed against the GPIIb–IIIa complex was

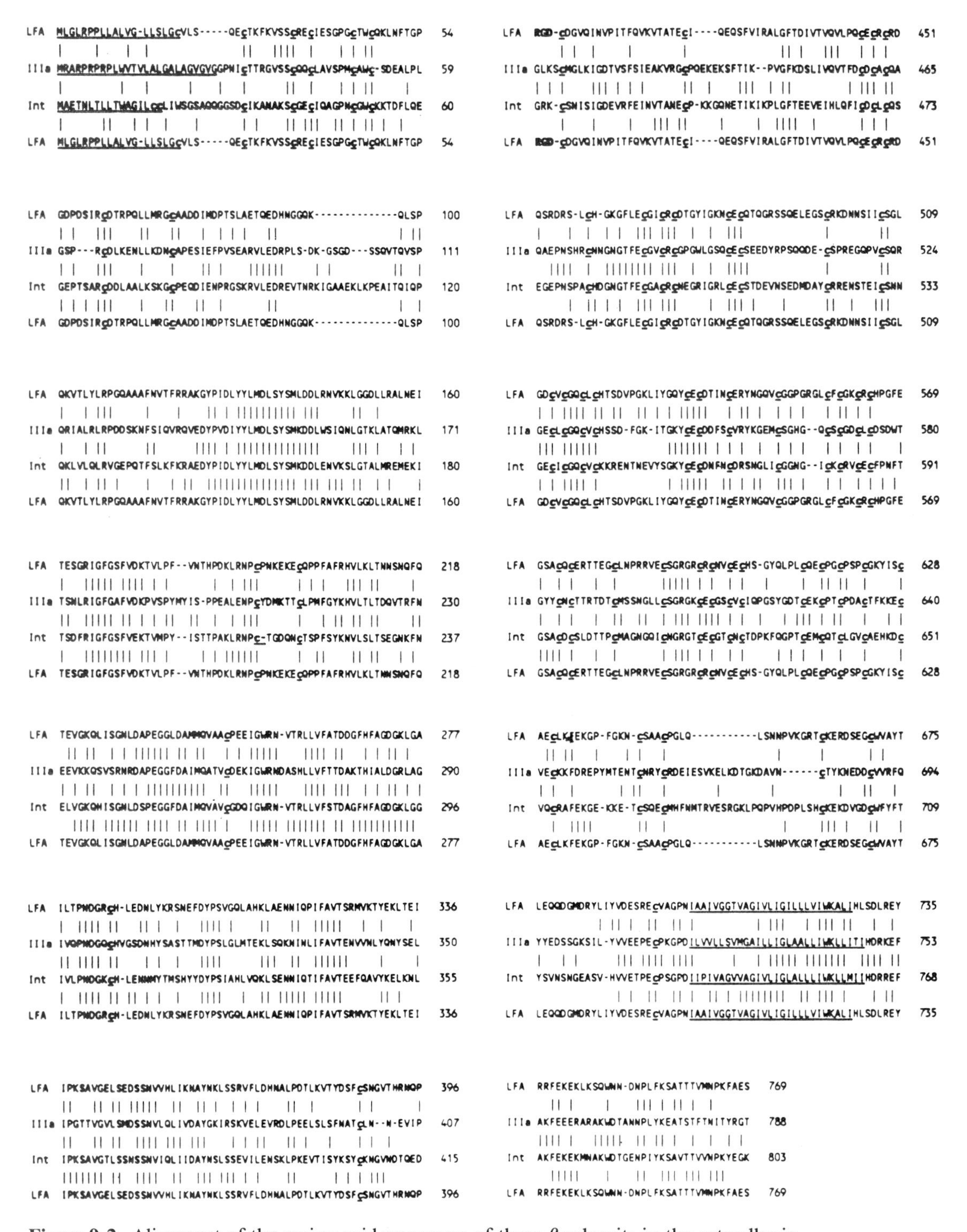

Figure 9-2. Alignment of the amino acid sequences of three β subunits in the cytoadhesin family: human GPIIIa (IIIa), chicken integrin band 3 (Int), and the β chain of LFA-1 = Mac-1 = p150,95 (LFA). LFA_β is displayed at both the top and bottom to facilitate comparison with GPIIIa and integrin. Cysteines are in register (adapted from Fitzgerald LA et al: J Biol Chem 262:10893, 1987;[29] Kishimoto TK et al: Cell 48:681, 1987,[48] Tamkun JW et al: Cell 46:271, 1986[104]).

Table 9-1
GPIIb–IIIa and Related Antigens on Human and Nonhuman Cells

Cell Type	References
Human Cells	
Endothelial cells	9,29,38,39,56,67,83,106
Fibroblasts	20,83,89
Monocytes	2,5,18,23,40,57,65
Neutrophils	65
Osteocytes	7,9,26
Placenta	99
Smooth muscle	20
Transformed Cells	
HEL	15,19,83,94,101
K562	35,94,100
MEG-01	70
Melanoma	D. Cheresh, unpublished
U937	83
Nonhuman Cells	
Primate platelets	41,50,69,93
Dog platelets	25,50,54,73,93
Bovine endothelium, platelets	20,29
Bovine smooth muscle	20
Rat platelets	19,50
Rabbit platelets	93
Guinea pig platelets	52,53
Chicken thrombocytes	50

unreactive with both uninduced and PMA-induced K562 cells. More recently, Silver et al.[94] directly showed that K562 cells expressed GPIIIa, but not GPIIb, when stimulated with PMA. They further showed that RNA from K562 cells directed the synthesis of a GPIIIa precursor polypeptide, but a similar precursor molecule for GPIIb could not be detected. All of these results might be explained if K562 cells possessed the VNR, rather than GPIIb–IIIa, because GPIIIa = VNR_{β}. This should now be easy to test by reacting K562 cells with polyclonal and monoclonal reagents that have been raised against the VNR α chain. A second transformed cell line, which has been useful for both biochemical and molecular genetic studies of GPIIb and GPIIIa, is the human erythroleukemia (HEL) hemopoietic cell line. Originally described by Martin and Papayannopoulou,[58] these cells have been shown to synthesize both GPIIb and GPIIIa.[15,19,83,101] Additionally, both GPIIb[86] and GPIIIa* have been cloned out of HEL cell cDNA expression libraries. These cells have also been useful in studying the cellular biosynthesis and processing of these two glycoproteins.[15,94]

Several other cell lines have been established and shown to express GPIIb or GPIIIa analogues. Plow and coworkers demonstrated that the promyeloid cell line U937 could be induced with PMA to synthesize and express GPIIb–IIIa-related molecules on their cell surface.[83] Ogura et al[70] established a human megakaryocytic cell line, MEG-10, from the bone marrow of a patient in blast crisis of chronic myelogenous leukemia and showed that it contained not only GPIIb–IIIa, but a number of other platelet antigens as well, including GPIb, VWF, and platelet peroxidase. Finally, Cheresh and colleagues have demonstrated that human melanoma cells synthesize and express GPIIIa, which probably functions as the β subunit of a VNR in these cells.†

*Poncz, M.: Personal communication.

†Cheresh, D.: Personal communication.

Nonhuman Cells

In addition to its intrinsic importance from a strictly phylogenetic standpoint, there are a number of other good reasons to study the expression of human platelet antigens in animal cells, not the least of which is the establishment of model systems for the in vivo study of platelet disorders of clinical importance. Early serologic work by Shulman et al.[93] demonstrated the interesting finding that the human platelet alloantigen, Pl^{A1}, which is located on GPIIIa, is strongly expressed on the platelets of nonhuman primates, dogs, and rabbits, but it is absent in guinea pigs and rats (Table 9-2). Lane et al.[54] extended these observations somewhat by directly immunoprecipitating GPIIIa from dog platelets with a human anti-Pl^{A1} alloantiserum. Thus, the Pl^{A1} alloantigenic determinant has been conserved as part of the structure of GPIIIa at least as far back as dogs, and probably to rabbits.

Kunicki and Newman[50] have shown additionally that molecules structurally and immunologically related to GPIIb–IIIa go even as far back phylogenetically as the chicken. As shown in Figure 9-3, glycoproteins having electrophoretic mobilities on nonreduced/reduced two-dimensional gels diagnostic for GPIIb and GPIIIa have also been found in baboons, dogs, and rats. It is likely, however, that the number of antigenic determinants shared with human GPIIb–IIIa would decrease with the divergence of the species from *Homo sapiens*. Thus, baboon platelets bind not only Pl^{A1} antibodies, but they also react well with the GPIIb–IIIa complex-specific monoclonal antibody, AP2.[41] Dog platelets have been shown to be highly reactive with anti-Pl^{A1} antibodies,[93] AP2,[73] and 7E3, a murine monoclonal antibody that shows an increased affinity for human GPIIb–IIIa following platelet activation.[25] On the other hand, rat and guinea pig platelets, although having been shown to contain GPIIb–IIIa-related molecules[19,52,53] do not contain the Pl^{A1} structural epitope,[93] and rat platelets are unreactive with the monoclonal anti-GPIIIa antibody, AP3.*

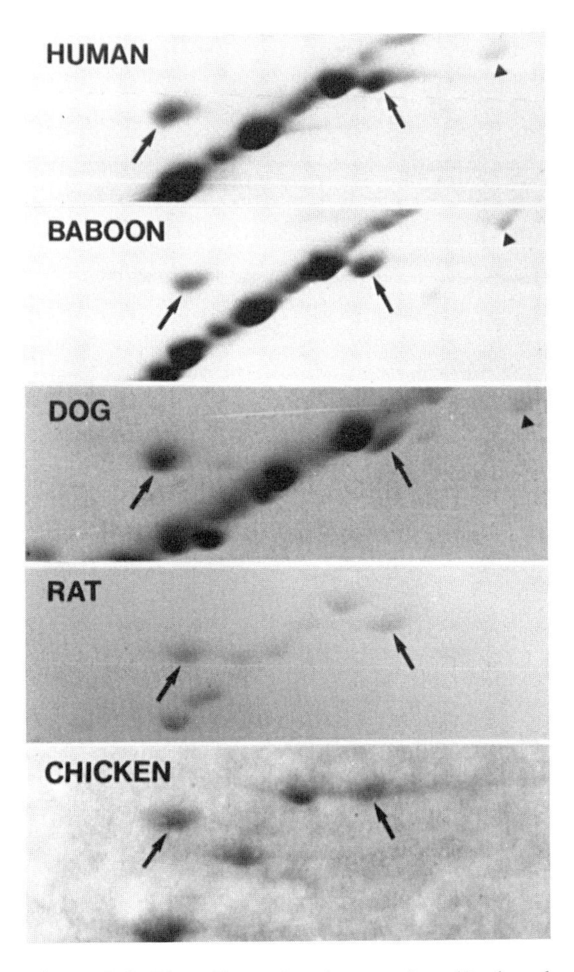

Figure 9-3. Two-dimensional nonreduced/reduced SDS–PAGE analysis of platelet/thrombocyte proteins from a variety of species. Arrow to the right depicts GPIIIa (above the diagonal); arrow to the left, GPIIb. Gels shown were stained with Coomassie Blue (Kunicki TJ, Newman PJ: Proc Natl Acad Sci USA 82:7319, 1987,[50] with permission of the authors).

Table 9-2
Phylogeny of Pl^{A1} Alloantigen Expression

Species	GPIIb–IIIa	Pl^{A1}
Human	Yes	Yes
Baboon	Yes	Yes
Dog	Yes	Yes
Rabbits	Yes	Some
Guinea pig	Yes	No
Rat	Yes	No
Chicken	Yes	No

*Doers, M. and Newman, P.: Unpublished observations.

GLYCOPROTEIN IV

Introduction and Properties

Glycoprotein IV, also termed GPIIIb, is the smallest of the major membrane glycoproteins, with a M_r in the range of 88,000–97,000. Under nonreducing conditions, GPIV comigrates with GPIIIa during SDS–PAGE. Unlike GPIIIa, however, the mobility of GPIV does not change upon addition of β-mercaptoethanol, suggesting that it does not contain an appreciable number of intrachain disulfide bonds. Thus, as shown in Figure 9-4, GPIV migrates on the diagonal of a two-dimensional nonreduced/reduced gel,[76] whereas GPIIIa migrates above the diagonal.

Until recently, little was known of the function and tissue distribution of GPIV. Over 10 years ago, Phillips and Agin[75] reported that of all the surface-labeled glycoproteins of intact platelets examined, only GPIV was resistant to hydrolysis by chymotrypsin and trypsin, which suggests that the protein may be highly glycosylated. At about the same time, Bolin et al.[14] showed that the amount of GPIV was significantly increased in the platelets of patients with myoproliferative disease. Neither of these observations, however, provided further insight into the possible role of GPIV in platelet physiology.

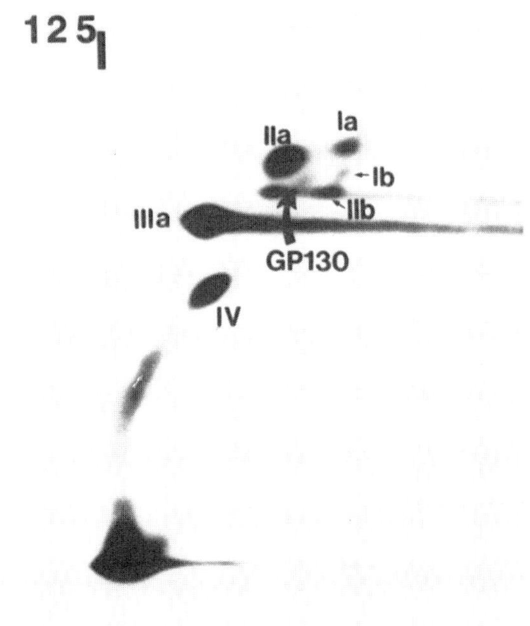

Human and Nonhuman Cells

Lately, two laboratories have assigned possible functions to GPIV. Tandon et al.[105] reported that the murine monoclonal antibody OKM-5, raised against monocytes, reacted with platelet GPIV by enzyme-linked immunosorbent assay (ELISA), and inhibited platelet aggregation induced by collagen, and suggested that GPIV may, therefore, play a major role in collagen-induced platelet aggregation. Contrary to this report, Asch et al.[3] showed that OKM-5 blocked the binding of thrombospondin to an 88-kDa platelet membrane protein and suggested that GPIV was the thrombospondin receptor. The 88-kDa membrane glycoprotein was also identified in endothelial cells, monocytes, and a variety of human tumor cell lines,[3] thus GPIV, like the GPIIb–IIIa complex, may be more widely distributed than previously realized.

Figure 9-4. Two-dimensional nonreduced/reduced gel of radioiodinated human platelet membrane proteins.

OTHER PLATELET ANTIGENS

A 140-kDa membrane glycoprotein that is expressed on the surface of platelets, only after activation, has been described by two laboratories. Termed GMP-140[98] or PADGEM,[113] this antigen has been localized to the α granules of unstimulated platelets. After stimulation with thrombin, α granules fuse with the surface-connected open canalicular system, resulting in the redistribution of GMP-140 to the platelet surface. Appearance of this antigen on the platelet surface appears to require secretion, as platelets stimulated with low-dose ADP express little GMP-140. Although the function of GMP-140 is not known, it was found in granules of bone marrow megakaryocytes and, interestingly, in some marrow endothelial cells.[9] The implications of the latter finding remain unexplored, but leave open the possibility of molecular cloning of GMP-140 from currently available endothelial cell cDNA libraries.

Recently, we have identified another surface antigen that appears to be shared by platelets and endothelial cells and is also synthesized by the human erythroleukemia (HEL) cell line.[6] This antigen, which is present in thrombasthenic platelets, is characterized by an M_r of 130,000 Da under both reducing and nonreducing conditions, can be surface-labeled with radioiodine or $[^3H]NaBH_4$, and is removed from the platelet surface with trypsin. We have tentatively named this membrane glycoprotein GP-130, and have isolated a number of cDNA clones from an endothelial cell expression library that encode it. Comparison of limited nucleotide sequence of GP-130 with both the NIH Genebank and the European Molecular Biology Laboratory EMBL nucleotide sequence data library has thus far (October, 1987) revealed no homology with previously characterized proteins. The electrophoretic migration of GP-130 relative to that of other known platelet membrane proteins is shown in Figure 9-4. Its hemostatic function is as yet unknown.

CONCLUSIONS

The last several years has seen a virtual explosion in the number of articles detailing the presence of "platelet-specific" antigens on other cell types, both human and nonhuman. One of the more illuminating features of these discoveries has been the realization that many of the functions carried out by platelets, including adhesion to extracellular matrix components, self-association (aggregation), secretion, and spreading, are likely to be reproduced in some form by many other cell types during the process of development, wound healing, and general "housekeeping." Of the more than 40 spots seen in a two-dimensional SDS gel of platelet proteins, still only a handful have names and assigned functions. Most of these have been elucidated first only because they were associated with a particular platelet disorder. It could be argued that the remaining uncharacterized antigens have equally important roles because nonfunctional examples of these do not exist in nature, possibly because they result in lethal mutations. With the application of molecular-cloning techniques, the next several years should yield important new information about many of these previously unstudied platelet proteins. No doubt, most of these will be found to have interesting functions on nonplatelet cell types as well.

This work was supported in part by the National Heart, Lung, and Blood Institute grant HL 38166 and a Grant-in-Aid from the American Heart Association (85-730) with funds contributed in part by the American Heart Association of Wisconsin. I am grateful to Drs. Mortimer Poncz, University of Pennsylvania, and David Cheresh, Research Foundation of Scripps Clinic, for sharing their data prior to publication. I also thank Dr. Stanford Roodman, St. Louis University, for his help in performing the cytofluorometry studies shown in Figure 1.

REFERENCES

1. Akiyama SK, Yamada S, Yamada KM: Characterization of a 140-kD avian cell surface antigen as a fibronectin-binding molecule. J Cell Biol 102:442, 1986

2. Altieri DC, Mannucci PM, Capitanio AM: Binding of fibrinogen to human monocytes. J Clin Invest 78:968, 1986

3. Asch AS, Barnwell J, Silverstein RL, Nachman RL: Isolation of the thrombospondin membrane receptor. J Clin Invest 79:1054, 1987

4. Asch AS, Adelman B, Fujimoto M, Nachman RL: Identification and isolation of a platelet GPIb-like protein in human umbilical vein endothelial cells and bovine aortic smooth muscle cells. J Clin Invest 81:1600, 1988

5. Bai Y, Durbin H, Hogg N: Monoclonal antibodies specific for platelet glycoproteins react with human monocytes. Blood 64:139, 1984

6. Baldassare JJ, Kahn RA, Knipp MA, Newman PJ: Reconstitution of platelet proteins into phospholipid vesicles. Functional proteoliposomes. J Clin Invest 75:35, 1985

7. Baron R, Neff L, Roy C, Boisvert A, Caplan M: Evidence for a high and specific concentration of (Na^+, K^+)ATPase in the plasma membrane of the osteoclast. Cell 46:311, 1986

8. Baumgartner HR, Tschopp TB, Weiss HJ: Platelet interaction with collagen fibrils in flowing blood. II. Impaired adhesion-aggregation in bleeding disorders: A comparison with subendothelium. Thromb Hemostasis 37:17, 1977

9. Beckstead JH, Stenberg PE, McEver RP, Shuman MA, Bainton DF: Immunohistochemical localization of membrane and α-granule proteins in human megacaryocytes: Application to plastic-embedded bone marrow biopsy specimans. Blood 67:285, 1986

10. Beller DI, Springer TA, Schreiber RD: Anti-Mac-1 selectively inhibits the mouse and human type three complement receptor. J Exp Med 156:1000, 1982

11. Bennett JS, Vilaire G: Exposure of fibrinogen receptors by ADP and epinephrine. J Clin Invest 64:1393, 1979

12. Berman CL, Yeo EL, Wencel-Drake JD, Furie BC, Ginsberg MH, Furie B: A platelet alpha granule membrane protein that is associated with the plasma membrane after activation. Characterization and subcellular localization of platelet activation-dependent granule-external membrane protein. J Clin Invest 78:130, 1986

13. Berndt M, Gregory C, Kabral A, Zola H, Fournier D, Castaldi PA: Purification and preliminary characterization of the glycoprotein Ib complex in the human platelet membrane. Eur J Biochem 151:637, 1985

14. Bolin RB, Okumura T, Jamieson GA: Changes in distribution of platelet membrane glycoproteins in patients with myeloproliferative disorders. Am J Hematol 3:63, 1977

15. Bray PF, Rosa J-P, Lingappa VR, Kan YW, McEver RP, Shuman MA: Biogenesis of the platelet receptor for fibrinogen: Evidence for separate precursors for the glycoproteins IIb and IIIa. Proc Natl Acad Sci USA 83:1480, 1986

16. Brown PJ, Juliano RL: Expression and function of a putative cell surface receptor for fibronectin in hamster and human cell lines. J Cell Biol 103:1595, 1986

17. Brown PJ, Juliano RL: Selective inhibition of fibronectin-mediated cell adhesion by monoclonal antibodies to a cell-surface glycoprotein. Science 228:1448, 1985

18. Burckhardt JJ, Kerr Anderson WH, Kearney JF, Cooper MD: Human blood monocytes and platelets share a common component. Blood 60:767, 1982

19. Charo IF, Boyles J, Zoellner C, Phillips DR: Distribution and localization of platelet GPIIb- and GPIIIa-like molecules on cells of human and rat tissue (abstr). Blood 68:314a, 1986

20. Charo IF, Fitzgerald LA, Steiner B, Rall Jr SC, Bekeart LS, Phillips DR: Platelet glycoproteins IIb and IIIa: Evidence for a family of immunologically and structurally related glycoproteins in mammalian cells. Proc Natl Acad Sci USA 83:8351, 1986

21. Cheresh DA: Human endothelial cells synthesize and express an Arg-Gly-Asp-directed adhesion receptor involved in attachment to fibrinogen and von Willebrand factor. Proc Natl Acad Sci USA 84:6471, 1987

22. Clemetson KJ: Glycoproteins of the platelet plasma membrane. In George JN, Nurden AT, Phillips DR (eds): Platelet Membrane Glycoproteins. New York, Plenum Press, 1985

23. Clemetson KJ, McGregor JL, McEver RP, Jacques YV, Bainton DF, Domzig W, Baggiolini M: Absence of platelet membrane glycoproteins IIb/IIIa from monocytes. J Exp Med 161:972, 1985

24. Clemetson KL, McGregor JL, James E, Dechavanne M, Luscher EF: Characterization of the platelet membrane glycoprotein abnormalities in Bernard-Soulier syndrome and comparison with normal platelets by surface labeling techniques and high-resolution two-dimensional gel electrophoresis. J Clin Invest 70:304, 1982

25. Coller BS, Scudder LE: Inhibition of dog platelet function by in vivo infusion of $F(ab')_2$ fragments of a monoclonal antibody to the platelet glycoprotein IIb/IIIa receptor. Blood 66:1456, 1985

26. Davies J, Warwick J, Rimmer E, Horton M: Molecular characterization of the osteoclast (abstr). J Bone Miner Res 2:372a, 1987

27. Du X, Beutler L, Ruan C, Castaldi PA, Berndt MC: Glycoprotein Ib and IX are fully complexed in the intact platelet membrane. Blood 69:1524, 1987

28. Fitzgerald LA, Steiner B, Rall SC, Lo SS, Phillips DR: Protein sequence of endothelial glycoprotein IIIa derived from a cDNA clone. Identity with platelet glycoprotein IIIa and similarity to "integrin." J Biol Chem 262:3936, 1987

29. Fitzgerald LA, Charo IF, Phillips DR: Human and bovine endothelial cells synthesize membrane proteins similar to human platelet glycoproteins IIb and IIIa. J Biol Chem 260:10893, 1985

30. Fox JEB: Linkage of a membrane skeleton to integral membrane glycoproteins in human platelets. Identification of one of the glycoproteins as glycoprotein Ib. J Clin Invest 76:1673, 1985

31. Furihata K, Nugent DJ, Bissonette A, Aster RH, Kunicki TJ: On the association of the platelet-specific alloantigen, Pen^a, with glycoprotein IIIa. Evidence for heterogeneity of glycoprotein IIIa. J Clin Invest 80:1624, 1987

32. Gardner JM, Hynes RO: Interaction of fibronectin with its receptor on platelets. Cell 42:439, 1985

33. Gartner TK, Bennett JS: The tetrapeptide analogue of the cell attachment site of fibronectin inhibits platelet aggregation and fibrinogen binding to activated platelets. J Biol Chem 260:11891, 1985

34. George JN, Thoi LL, McManus LM, Reimann TA: Isolation of human platelet membrane microparticles from plasma and serum. Blood 60:834, 1982

35. Gewirtz AM, Burger D, Rado TA, Benz EJ, Jr, Hoffman R: Constitutive expression of platelet glycoproteins by the human leukemia cell line K562. Blood 60:785, 1982

36. Giancotti FG, Lanfuino LR, Zanetti A, Peri G, Tarone G, Dejana E: Platelets express a membrane protein complex immunologically realted to the fibroblast fibronectin receptor and distinct from GPIIb/IIIa. Blood 69:1535, 1987

37. Giancotti FG, Tarone G, Knudsen K, Damsky C, Comoglio PM: Cleavage of a 135 kD cell

surface glycoprotein correlates with loss of fibroblast adhesion to fibronectin. Exp Cell Res 156:182, 1985

38. Giltay JC, Leeksma OC, Breederveld C, van Mourik JA: Normal synthesis and expression of endothelial cell IIb/IIIa in Glanzmann's thrombasthenia. Blood 69:809, 1987

39. Ginsberg MH, Loftus J, Ryckwaert J-J, Pierschbacher M, Pytela R, Ruoslahti E, Plow EF: Immunochemical and amino-terminal comparison of two cytoadhesins indicates they contain similar or identical β subunits and distinct α subunits. J Biol Chem 262:5437, 1987

40. Gogstad G, Hetland Ø, Solum NO, Prydz H: Monocytes and platelets share the glycoproteins IIb and IIIa that are absent from both cells in Glanzmann's thrombasthenia type 1. Biochem J 214:331, 1983

41. Hanson SR, Pareti FI, Ruggeri ZM, Marzec UM, Kunicki TJ, Montgomery RR, Zimmerman TS, Harker LA: Effects of monoclonal antibodies against the platelet glycoprotein IIb/IIIa complex on thrombosis and hemostasis in the baboon. J Clin Invest 81:149, 1988

42. Hasegawa T, Hasegawa E, Chen W-T, Yamada KM: Characterization of a membrane-associated glycoprotein implicated in cell adhesion to fibronectin. J Cell Biochem 28:307, 1985

43. Haverstick DM, Cowan JF, Yamada KM, Santoro SA: Inhibition of platelet adhesion to fibronectin, fibrinogen, and von Willebrand factor substrates by a synthetic tetrapeptide derived from the cell-binding domain of fibronectin. Blood 66:946, 1985

44. Hemler ME, Huang C, Schwarz L: The VLA protein family. Characterization of five distinct cell surface heterodimers each with a common 130,000 molecular weight β subunit. J Biol Chem 262:3300, 1987

45. Horwitz A, Duggan K, Greggs R, Decker C, Buck C: the cell substrate attachment (CSAT) antigen has properties of a receptor for laminin and fibronectin. J Cell Biol 101:2134, 1985

46. Kieffer N, Boizard B, Didry D, Wautier J: Immunochemical characterization of the platelet-specific alloantigen Lek^{a}. A comparative study with the Pl^{A1} alloantigen. Blood 64:1212, 1984

47. Kieffer N, Debili N, Wicki A, Titeux M, Henri A, Mishna Z, Brenton-Gorius J, Vainchenker W, Clemetson KJ: Expression of platelet glycoprotein Ibα in HEL cells. J Biol Chem 261:15854, 1986

48. Kishimoto TK, O'Conner K, Lee A, Roberts TM, Springer TA: Cloning of the β subunit of the leukocyte adhesion proteins: Homology to an extracellular matrix receptor defines a novel supergene family. Cell 48:681, 1987

49. Kunicki TJ, Aster RH: Isolation and immunologic characterization of the human platelet alloantigen, Pl^{A1}. Mol Immunol 16:353, 1979

50. Kunicki TJ, Newman PJ: Synthesis of analogs of human platelet membrane glycoprotein IIb–IIIa complex by chicken peripheral blood thrombocytes. Proc Natl Acad Sci USA 82:7319, 1987

51. Kunicki TJ, Pidard D, Rosa J-P, Nurden AT: The formation of Ca^{++}-dependent complexes of platelet membrane glycoproteins IIb and IIIa in solution as determined by crossed immunoelectrophoresis. Blood 58:268, 1981

52. Kupinski J, Miller JL: Synthesis by guinea pig megakaryocytes of platelet glycoprotein receptors for fibrinogen and von Willebrand factor. Thromb Res 43:345, 1986

53. Kupinski JM, Miller JL: Identification of receptors for fibrinogen and von Willebrand factor mediating aggregation in guinea pig platelets. Thromb Res 43:335, 1986

54. Lane J, Brown M, Bernstein I, Wilcox PK, Slichter SJ, Nowinski RC: Serological and biochemical analysis of the Pl^{A1} alloantigen of human platelets. Br J Haematol 50:351, 1892

55. Law SKA, Gagnon J, Hildreth JEK, Wells CE, Willis AC, Wong AJ: The primary structure of the β-subunit of the cell surface adhesion glycoproteins LFA-1, CR3, and p150,95 and its relationship to the fibronectin receptor. EMBO J 6:915, 1987

56. Leeksma OC, Zandbergan-Spaargaren J, Giltay JC, van Mourik JA: Cultured human endothelial cells synthesize a plasma membrane protein complex immunologically related to the platelet glycoprotein IIb/IIIa complex. Blood 67:1176, 1986

57. Levene RB, Rabellino EM: Platelet glycoproteins IIb and IIIa associated with blood monocytes are derived from platelets. Blood 67:207, 1986

58. Martin P, Papayannopoulou T: HEL cells: A new human erythroleukemia cell line with spontaneous and induced globin expression. Science 216:1233, 1982

59. McEver RP, Baenziger NL, Majerus PW: Isolation and quantitation of the platelet membrane glycoprotein deficient in thrombasthenia using a monoclonal hybridoma antibody. J Clin Invest 66:1311, 1980

60. McEver RP, Baenziger JU, Majerus PW: Isolation and characterization of the polypeptide subunits of membrane glycoprotein IIb–IIIa from human platelets. Blood 59:80, 1982

61. McMichael AJ, Rust NA, Pilch JR, Sochynsky R, Morton J, Mason DY, Ruan C, Tobelem G, Caen JP: Monoclonal antibody to human platelet glycoprotein I. Immunological studies. Br J Haematol 49:501, 1981

62. Meyer D, Baumgartner HR: Role of von Willebrand factor in platelet adhesion to the subendothelium. Br J Haematol 54:1, 1983

63. Micklem KJ, Sim RB: Isolation of the com-

plement-fragment-iC3b-binding proteins by affinity chromatography. Biochem J 231:233, 1985

64. Newman PJ, Allen RW, Kahn RA, Kunicki TJ: Quantitation of platelet membrane glycoprotein IIIa on intact human platelets using the monoclonal antibody, AP3. Blood 65:227, 1985

65. Newman PJ, Allen RW, Roodman ST, Kunicki TJ, Kahn RA: A monoclonal antibody specific for human platelet membrane glycoprotein IIIa binds to monocytes and neutrophils (abstr). Blood 62(suppl. 5):263, 1983

66. Newman PJ, Doers MP, Gorski J: Molecular cloning of a 130 kD membrane protein expressed on human platelets, umbilical vein endothelial cells, and human erythroleukemia (HEL) cells (abstr). J Cell Biol 105:53a, 1987

67. Newman PJ, Kawai Y, Montgomery RR, Kunicki TJ: Synthesis by cultured human umbilical vein endothelial cells of two proteins structurally and immunologically related to platelet membrane glycoproteins IIb and IIIa. J Cell Biol 103:81, 1986

68. Newman PJ, Martin LS, Knipp MA, Kahn RA: Studies on the nature of the human platelet alloantigen, Pl^{A1}: Localization to a 17,000 dalton polypeptide. Mol Immunol 22:719, 1985

69. Nurden AT, Butcher PD, Hawkey CM: Comparative studies on the glycoprotein composition of mammalian platelets. Comp Biochem Physiol 56B:407, 1977

70. Ogura M, Morishima Y, Ohno R, Kato Y, Hirabayashi N, Nagura H, Saito H: Establishment of a novel human megakaryoblastic cell line, MEG-01, with positive Philadelphia chromosome. Blood 66:1384, 1985

71. Okita JR, Pidard D, Newman PJ, Montgomery RR, Kunicki TJ: On the association of glycoprotein Ib and actin-binding protein in human platelets. J Cell Biol 100:317, 1985

72. Okumura T, Lombart C, Jamieson GA: Platelet glycocalicin. II. Purification and characterization. J Biol Chem 251:5950, 1976

73. Patterson WR, Kunicki TJ, Bell TG: Two-dimensional electrophoretic studies of platelets from dogs affected with basset hound heriditary thrombopathy: A thrombasthenia-like defect. Thromb Res 42:195, 1986

74. Perussia B, Jankiewicz J, Trinchieri G: Binding of platelets to human monocytes: A source of artifacts in the study of the specificity of antileukocyte antibodies. J Immunol Methods 50:269, 1982

75. Phillips DR, Agin PP: Platelet plasma membrane glycoproteins: Identification of a proteolytic substrate for thrombin. Biochem Biophys Res Commun 75:940, 1977

76. Phillips DR, Agin PP: Platelet plasma membrane glycoproteins: Evidence for the presence of nonequivalent disulfide bonds using nonreduced-reduced two-dimensional gel electrophoresis. J Biol Chem 252:2121, 1977

77. Phillips DR, Jennings LK, Edwards HH: Identification of membrane proteins mediating the interaction of human platelets. J Cell Biol 86:77, 1980

78. Pidard D, Montgomery RR, Bennett JS, Kunicki TJ: Interaction of AP-2, a monoclonal antibody specific for the human platelet glycoprotein IIb-IIIa complex, with intact platelets. J Biol Chem 258:12582, 1983

79. Pierschbacher MD, Ruoslahti E: Cell attachment activity of fibronectin can be duplicated by small synthetic fragments of the molecule. Nature 309:30, 1984

80. Piotrowicz RS, Orchekowski RP, Nugent DJ, Yamada KY, Kunicki TJ: Glycoprotein Ic-IIa functions as an activation-independent fibronectin receptor on human platelets. J Cell Biol 106:1359, 1988

81. Pischel KD, Bluestein HG, Woods VL: Lymphocytes bear molecules that are antigenically and structurally similar to platelet GPIa, $GPIc_{\alpha}$, and GPIIa (abstr.). Blood 66:311a, 1985

82. Pischel KD, Hemler ME, Huang C, Bluestein HG, Woods VL: Use of the monoclonal antibody 12F1 to characterize the differentiation antigen VLA-2. J Immunol 138:226, 1987

83. Plow EF, Loftus JC, Levin EG, Fair DS, Dixon D, Forsyth J, Ginsberg MH: Immunologic relationship between platelet membrane glycoprotein GPIIb/IIIa and cell surface molecules expressed by a variety of cells. Proc Natl Acad Sci USA 83:6002, 1986

84. Plow EF, McEver RP, Coller BS, Woods VL, Marguerie GA, Ginsberg MH: Related binding mechanisms for fibrinogen, fibronectin, von Willebrand factor, and thrombospondin on thrombin-stimulated platelets. Blood 66:724, 1985

85. Plow EF, Pierschbacher MD, Ruoslahti E, Marguerie GA: The effect of Arg-Gly-Asp-containing peptides on fibrinogen and von Willebrand factor binding to platelets. Proc Natl Acad Sci USA 82:8057, 1985

86. Poncz M, Eisman R, Heidenreich R, Silver S, Vilaire G, Surrey S, Schwartz, Bennett JS: Structure of platelet membrane glycoprotein IIb. Homology to the α subunits of the vitronectin and fibronectin membrane receptors. J Biol Chem 262:8476, 1987

87. Pytela R, Pierschbacher MD, Ginsberg MH, Plow EF, Ruoslahti E: Platelet membrane glycoprotein IIb/IIIa: Member of a family of Arg-Gly-Asp-specific adhesion receptors. Science 231:1559, 1986

88. Pytela R, Pierschbacher MD, Ruoslahti E: Identificationa nd isolation of a 140 kd cell surface glycoprotein with properties expected of a fibronectin receptor. Cell 40:191, 1985

89. Pytela R, Pierschbacher MD, Ruoslahti E: A 125/115 kDa cell surface receptor specific for vitronectin interacts with the arginine-glycine-aspartic acid adhesion sequence derived from fibronectin. Proc Natl Acad Sci USA 82:5766, 1985

90. Ruggeri ZM, DeMarco L, Gatti L, Badeer R, Montgomery RR: Platelets have more than one binding site for von Willebrand factor. J Clin Invest 72:1, 1983

91. Sanchez-Madrid F, Nagy J, Robbins E, Simon P, Springer TA: A human leukocyte differentiation antigen family with distinct alpha subunits and a common beta subunit: The lymphocyte function-associated (LFA-1), the C3bi complement receptor (OKM1/Mac-1), and the p150,95 molecule. J Exp Med 158:1786, 1983

92. Shadle PJ, Ginsberg MH, Plow EF, Barondes SH: Platelet-collagen adhesion: Inhibited by a monoclonal antibody that binds glycoprotein IIb. J Cell Biol 99:2056, 1984

93. Shulman NR, Marder VJ, Hiller MC, Collier EM: Platelet and leukocyte isoantigens and their antibodies: Serologic, physiologic and clinical studies. Prog Hematol 4:222, 1964

94. Silver SM, McDonough MM, Vilaire G, Bennett JS: The in vitro synthesis of polypeptides for the platelet membrane glycoproteins IIb and IIIa. Blood 69:1031, 1987

95. Sprando JD, Shapiro SS, Thiagarajan P, McCord S: Cultured human umbilical vein endothelial cells contain a membrane glycoprotein immunologically related to platelet glycoprotein Ib. Blood 71:234, 1988

96. Springer TA, Davignon D, Ho MK, Kurzinger K, Martz E, Snachez-Madrid F: LFA-1 and Lyt-2,3 molecules associated with T lymphocyte killing; and Mac-1, an LFA-1 homologue associated with complement receptor function. Immunol Rev 68:111, 1982

97. Springer TA, Thompson WS, Miller LJ, Schmalstieg FC, Anderson DC: Inherited deficiency of the Mac-1, LFA-1, p150,95 glycoprotein family and its molecular basis. J Exp Med 160:1901, 1984

98. Stenberg PE, McEver RP, Shuman MA, Jacques YV, Bainton DF: A platelet alpha-granule membrane protein (GMP-140) is expressed on the plasma membrane after activation. J Cell Biol 101:880, 1985

99. Suzuki S, Argraves WS, Pytela R, Arai H, Krusius T, Pierschbacher MD, Ruoslahti E: cDNA and amino acid sequences of the cell adhesion protein receptor recognizing vitronectin reveal a transmembrane domain and homologies with other adhesion protein receptors. Proc Natl Acad Sci USA 83:8614, 1986

100. Tabilio A, Pelicci PG, Vinci G, Mannoni P, Civin CI, Vainchenker W, Testa U, Lipinski M, Rochant H, Brenton-Gorius J: Myeloid and megakaryocytic properties of K-562 cell lines. Cancer Res 43:4569, 1983

101. Tabilio A, Rosa J-P, Testa U, Kieffer N, Nurden AT, Del Canizo MC, Brenton-Gorius J, Vainchenker W: Expression of platelet membrane glycoproteins and α-granule proteins by a human erythroleukemia cell line (HEL). EMBO J 3:453, 1984

102. Takada Y, Huang C, Hemler ME: Fibronectin receptor structures in the VLA family of heterodimers. Nature 326:607, 1987

103. Takada Y, Strominger JL, and Hemler ME: The very late antigen family of heterodimers is part of a superfamily of molecules involved in adhesion and embryogenesis. Proc Natl Acad Sci USA 84:3239, 1987

104. Tamkun JW, DeSimone DW, Fonda D, Patel RS, Buck C, Horwitz AF, Hynes RO: Structure of integrin, a glycoprotein involved in transmembrane linkage between fibronectin and actin. Cell 46:271, 1986

105. Tandon NN, Hines A, Jamieson GA: Role for platelet glycoprotein IV in collagen-induced platelet aggregation (abstr). Blood 66:1148a, 1985

106. Thiagarajan P, Shapiro SS, Levine E, DeMarco L, Yalcin A: A monoclonal antibody to human platelet glycoprotein IIIa detects a related protein in cultured human endothelial cells. J Clin Invest 75:896, 1985

107. Todd RF III, Arnaout MA, Rosin RE, Crowley CA, Peters WA, Babior BM: Subcellular localization of the large subunit of Mo1 (Mo1 alpha; formally gp110), a surface glycoprotein associated with neutrophil adhesion. J Clin Invest 74:1280, 1984

108. Tsuji T, Osawa T: Structures of the carbohydrate chains of membrane glycoproteins IIb and IIIa of human platelets. J Biochem 100:1387, 1986

109. Tsuji T, Tsunehisa S, Watanabe Y, Yamamoto K, Tohyana H, Osawa T: The carbohydrate moiety of human platelet glycocalicin. The structure of the major ser/thr-linked sugar chain. J Biol Chem 258:6335, 1983

110. van Mourik JA, Leeksma OC, Reinders JH, de Groot PG, Zandbergen-Spaargaren J: Vascular endothelial cells synthesize a plasma membrane protein indistinguishable from the platelet membrane glycoprotein IIa. J Biol Chem 260:11300, 1985

111. White JG, Burris SM, Tukey D, Smith C, Clawson CC: Micropipette aspiration of human platelets: Influence of microtubules and actin filaments on deformability. Blood 64:210, 1984

112. Wright SD, Rao PE, Van Voorhis WC, Craigmyle LS, Iida K, Talle MA, Westberg EF,

Goldstein G, Silverstein SC: Identification of the C3bi receptor of human monocytes and macrophages by using monoclonal antibodies. Proc Natl Acad Sci USA 80:5699, 1983

113. Wright SD, Reddy PA, Jong MT, Erickson BW: C3bi receptor (complement receptor type 3) recognizes a region of complement protein C3 containing the sequence Arg-Gly-Asp. Proc Natl Acad Sci USA 84:1965, 1987

114. Wyler B, Bienz D, Clemetson KJ, Luscher EF: Glycoprotein Ib_{β} is the only phosphorylated major membrane glycoprotein in human platelets. Biochem J 234:373, 1986

115. Yamada KM, and Kennedy DW: Dualistic nature of adhesive protein function: Fibronectin and its biologically active peptide fragments can autoinhibit fibrinogen function. J Cell Biol 99:29, 1984

10

Activation-Specific Platelet Antigens

BARRY S. COLLER

The activation-specific platelet antigens discussed in this review belong to three different categories: (1) membrane antigens that are present on unactivated platelets, but undergo an alteration in conformation or in microenvironment upon activation; (2) antigens that are not present on the membrane of unactivated platelets, but that become expressed on the surface of activated platelets; and (3) antigens that appear to be linked to one or more platelet activation/transduction mechanisms, as judged by the ability of antibodies directed against them to induce platelet activation. The platelet glycoprotein IIb–IIIa (GPIIb–IIIa) complex is the prototype of the first category and the changes in its structure with activation will be discussed in detail. Glycoprotein Ib probably is also in this category. The antigens in the second category are of two types: those like the α-granule integral membrane protein of a relative molecular mass (M_r) 140,000 that join the plasma membrane when α-granule membranes fuse with the plasma membrane after the release reaction is stimulated, and those like thrombospondin, platelet factor 4, and von Willebrand factor, that are not integral membrane proteins but become expressed on the platelet surface after activation because of their high affinity for receptors in α-granule membranes or on the platelet surface. In the third category are one or more interesting antigens with an M_r ~21,000–26,000 that can induce platelet activation when specific monoclonal antibodies bind to them.

At the outset it is important to emphasize that the word *activation* is often used in a vague manner to encompass numerous different phenomena, including, platelet shape change; induction of platelet GPIIb–IIIa receptor exposure or the exposure of other receptors; elevation of cytosolic calcium; induction of arachidonic acid metabolism; activation of protein kinase C by generation of diacylglycerol and inositol trisphosphate; release of α granule, dense body, or lysosomal contents; induction of platelet coagulant activity; and initiation of platelet aggregation. In addition, the term activation is often used without specifying the agonist, and this leads to further confusion, because agonists show considerable specificity in the processes they initiate. Furthermore, a single agonist can show a dose-dependent variation in initiating these different phenomena. Finally, the platelet preparation (platelet-rich plasma, washed platelets, gel-filtered platelets, and so on), its milieu, and the technical details of the experiment (pH, stirring, and the like) may all have dramatic effects on the observed activation responses. Thus, a precise description of an activated platelet requires information on the platelet preparation, the agonist, the dose, the experimental conditions, and the phenomena activated. Although these criteria can be met in well-defined in vitro systems, we know very little about which of the agonists that potentially exist in vivo actually operate, alone or in combination, in different physiologic and pathologic states. Until these data are available, extrapolation from the in vitro to the in vivo condition will remain speculative.

RECENT ADVANCES IN UNDERSTANDING ANTIBODY–ANTIGEN INTERACTIONS

As all of the data to be described in this review rely upon the recognition of an antigen by an antibody, it is useful to review the assumptions upon which this technique is based and the constraints that the technique imposes. Although a full discussion of this subject is not possible in this brief review, several emerging concepts are worthy of note.

1. Antibody recognition sites on native proteins injected into the commonly employed animal species probably include discontinuous regions of the linear amino acid sequence. This conclusion follows from the data suggesting that the antigen recognition zone of the well-studied enzyme, lysozyme, is ~20 × 25 Å, whereas the likelihood of an area that size on lysozyme being occupied exclusively by a continuous array of amino acids is nearly zero.[3,5,139] Of course, the data from this single antigen–antibody reaction will require confirmation, but additional support for this view comes from studies employing exhaustive depletion of antibodies with peptides encompassing the entire protein, in which a significant percentage of the antibodies could not be removed.[11]
2. Many antibodies have been prepared against large proteins by immunizing with just small polypeptides containing as few as six or seven amino acids known to be present in the protein, even though these peptides cannot have the tertiary structure present in the native protein. By using overlapping peptide sequences from proteins, one can demonstrate that often virtually all regions of a given protein are potentially immunogenic.[75,93]
3. When animals are immunized with a native protein, however, not all regions of the protein are equally immunogenic. Several hypotheses have been advanced to explain this phenomenon and to predict the immunogenic regions. Regions with hydrophilic amino acids and regions with the greatest segmental or atomic mobility (loops, turns) have been proposed as the most immunogenic because these regions are most likely to be present on the exterior of the molecule with a "continuous" (linearly arranged) organization.[142] However, because the peptide studies indicate that virtually the entire protein is potentially immunogenic, it may be that the selection of particular regions as antigenic is more a function of the host's immune system and the evolutionary differences between the immunogen and the host's analogous protein, than of the intrinsic physico-chemical properties of the antigen.[11] Determination of the regions with the greatest segmental or atomic mobility may still be important because peptides taken from these regions appear to be able to induce those antibodies with the greatest likelihood of cross-reacting with the native protein.[11,139]
4. Proteins are probably always undergoing a large number of rapid conformational changes. For example, a molecular dynamic simulation of myoglobin at 300° K indicated that approximately 2000 minima (conformations) would be thermally accessible in the neighborhood of the native structure and these could be sampled in just 300 psec.[33] Moreover, there is evidence that at least some antigens undergo conformational changes as a result of antibody binding.[26]
5. Immunoglobulins, themselves, have considerable molecular flexibility in the antigen-binding site, and this may be crucial in molding the final fit of the antigen into the antibody-combining site and in the effector functions of the immunoglobulin.[26,44,96]

A reasonable summary of the current view, then, is that protein loops and turns, along with the carboxyl- and amino-termini often are the most immunogenic regions of native molecules, and antibodies against short peptides from these regions often react well with the native protein. However, the highest-affinity antibodies made against the native protein (i.e., those that probably have large contact areas) almost always recognize a discontinuous amino acid region on the antigen. Moreover, the antigens are in constant motion, assuming different conformations that may affect both their functional and antigenic properties. Finally, the antibodies themselves probably benefit from molecular flexibility in making the final fit with the antigen. Thus, it is probably best to discard the older, rigid lock-and-key analogy for a more sinuous one—a "handshake" has been proposed.[26]

ACTIVATION-DEPENDENT ANTIGENS

Membrane Antigens Present on the Surface of Unactivated Platelets That Are Altered by Platelet Activation

The Glycoprotein IIb–IIIa Complex

There is compelling evidence that the GPIIb–IIIa complex acts as a receptor for fibrinogen, von Willebrand factor, and fibronectin when platelets are stimulated with different agonists.[9,16,104,115] The binding of one or more of these ligands is crucial for platelet function, as evidenced by the severe hemorrhagic diathesis that accompanies a congenital absence of the receptor in Glanzmann's thrombasthenia. In fact, this interaction appears to be required for platelet aggregation to be induced by all of the agonists that are thought to operate in vivo, namely ADP, epinephrine, collagen, thrombin, and thromboxane A_2. The mechanism by which this receptor becomes "exposed"—that is, its conversion from a low affinity for the ligands to a high affinity—remains poorly understood.[17] Exquisite control over this mechanism is crucial because inappropriate exposure could lead to fatal thrombosis, and failure of exposure could lead to fatal hemorrhage.

Biochemical and molecular biologic analyses have led to important discoveries about the basic structures of GPIIb and GPIIIa and how they are complexed in the platelet membrane. These approaches, however, usually require significant perturbation of the system, and so it is difficult to obtain information about the receptors in their native environment during activation. Immunologic approaches, although limited by the availability of specific probes, have the powerful advantage of being able to analyze specific conformations of the glycoproteins on platelets as they exist on the hydrated surface, before, during, and after activation. The information obtained from such analyses can thus be a powerful complement to the biochemical studies.

The biochemistry and molecular biology of GPIIb and GPIIIa are described in detail in Chapter 2. These glycoproteins are part of a broad family of glycoprotein receptors, each of which is composed of a complex of two different glycoproteins (designated α and β subunits) that are involved in adhesive functions in different tissues and different species (reviewed in detail in Chapter 2).[14,45,77,112,114,118] Emerging data suggest that most, if not all, of the α subunits share amino acid homologies, as do the β subunits. In addition, each of the β subunits can combine with more than one α subunit.

Members of this class include the vitronectin receptor (a unique α subunit, but the β subunit is identical with platelet GPIIIa), the fibronectin receptor, the leukocyte antigens LFA-1, Mac-1, p150,95, and the very late activation (VLA) class of lymphocyte antigens.[112,118,119,125,134,138] Phylogenetically, this class of glycoprotein receptors extends at least to the chicken embryo and probably to *Drosophila* species.[87,135] In fact, a GPIIb–IIIa-like molecule has been identified on avian thrombocytes by a monoclonal antibody raised against human platelet GPIIb–IIIa.[69] The platelet also appears to have two additional glycoprotein complexes that may well be in this same family; GPIc and GPIIa probably function as a fibronectin receptor and GPIa and GPIIa may function as a collagen receptor.[25a,45,67,89]

Glycoprotein IIb–IIIa is one of the receptors that recognizes peptides containing the tripeptide sequence Arg-Gly-Asp (RGD).[39,111,116,118] All three ligands that bind to GPIIb–IIIa contain regions with that sequence, and small peptides containing the sequence can inhibit the binding of all three ligands to the platelet surface.[54,143] Moreover, fragmentation studies indicate that the regions of fibronectin and von Willebrand factor that bind to GPIIb–IIIa are the ones that contain the RGD sequence.[38,48] The binding of fibrinogen is more complex because the carboxylterminal dodecapeptide of the γ chain (HHLGGAKQAGDV) binds to platelets, even though it does not contain an RGD sequence, and it can also block the binding of all three ligands.[63,117] Additional support for the importance of the γ-chain peptide comes from the observation that fibrinogen that contains a variant γ chain in which there is deletion of the terminal four amino acids and introduction of a new 20-amino acid segment as a result of alternative splicing of mRNA, bound less well to platelets.[104] There are two regions of the Aα chain that do contain RGD sequences; one is in the coiled coil region and the other is in the more mobile carboxyl-terminal region.[140] The latter is presumably a better candidate for a functional binding site because of its greater flexibility and strategic location at the end of the molecule. However, fibrinogen species that lack the terminal RGD sequence are still able to bind to platelets and cause their aggregation.[106] Moreover, some animals whose platelets aggregate well in response to stimulation have fibrinogen molecules that lack this RGD sequence.[106] Although the RGD sequence in the coiled coil region of the Aα chain may be involved in binding to platelets, its greater constraint and more central location make it a theoretically less attractive candidate region.

As both RGD-containing peptides and the γ-chain peptide both bind to platelets, there has been interest in defining the relationship, if any, between their binding sites. On the basis of differences in the effect of RGD-containing peptides and the γ-chain peptide on both fibrinogen binding and the binding of a monoclonal antibody to GPIIb-IIIa, it was suggested that the RGD and γ-chain peptides bind to different sites.[40] The opposite conclusion was reached by another group of investigators who showed that the γ-chain peptide inhibited the binding of RGD-containing peptides in what appeared to be a competitive manner; that the γ-chain peptides could elute GPIIb-IIIa bound to an immobilized RGD-containing peptide; and that RGD-containing peptides could elute GPIIb-IIIa from an immobilized γ-chain peptide.[72] Further support for the peptides sharing the same binding site comes from a study showing that RGD-containing peptides could inhibit the platelet binding of fibrinogen fragments that did not have the carboxyl-terminal RGD sequence.[105]

Definitive conclusions about the relationship between the binding sites for these peptides must be tempered, however, because it remains possible that there are two different receptors and that occupancy of one allosterically alters the other so that it has a reduced affinity for the other peptide sequence. There are, in fact, data showing that the binding of RGD-containing peptides to the GPIIb-IIIa complex alters the conformation of other regions of the molecule and may even lead to gross changes in the distribution of GPIIb-IIIa receptors on the platelet surface.[36,59,71,99] One interesting possibility to explain how RGD-containing peptides and the γ-chain peptide could share the same binding site is that a region of the γ-chain peptide may mimic an RGD sequence, as it is organized in three-dimensional space perhaps with the positively charged lysine substituting for the positively charged arginine by orienting near the GD sequence. In fact, when an R (arginine) was substituted for the A (alanine) in the γ-chain peptide AGDV sequence, the resulting peptide had high affinity for platelets, especially when additional arginine residues were placed on the amino-terminal end.[122]

Other peptides may also have high affinity for GPIIb-IIIa. For example, a casein-derived peptide was shown to have high affinity for GPIIb-IIIa and to be able to block the binding of the ligands.[61] The rationale for searching for such a peptide was that milk curdling resembles blood coagulation. Before one overemphasizes the meaning of such observations, however, it may be worthwhile to insert a reservation about the potential for nonspecific phenomena with small peptides. For example, it has been reported that small peptides taken from portions of the myoglobin sequence bound to antibodies against myoglobin, suggesting their specificity. However, these same peptides also bound to antibodies made against an unrelated protein (staphylococcal nuclease) nearly as well. The antimyoglobin antibodies, in fact, bound to other unrelated peptides, suggesting that the interactions relied on the presence of lysine and aromatic residues, rather than on a unique linear sequence.[8] Most recently, trigramin, a peptide of M_r ~9000 from the snake venom of *Trimeresurus gramineus*, was shown to bind to GPIIb-IIIa and inhibit platelet aggregation[58]; its binding to platelets was also inhibited by RGDS-containing peptides and γ-chain peptide.

It is reasonable to conclude from the preceding analysis that GPIIb-IIIa has a site, or sites, that recognize RGD-containing peptides and the fibrinogen γ-chain peptide. The binding affinities of both of these peptides is considerably below that of the native ligands, however, indicating that there must be additional interactions that stabilize the binding. Synthetic peptide alterations like the one previously described have successfully increased the affinity of such peptides so that they approximate the affinities of the ligands.[123] Such peptides offer considerable promise in deciphering the structure of the binding site, and they may even be useful clinically as inhibitors of platelet function. The major caveats concerning the latter include the high concentrations required to achieve inhibition; the short in vivo survival times given their small size and likely clearance by the kidney; concerns about specificity, since the RGD recognition site seems to be involved in many different adhesive protein systems; and the potential immunogenicity of peptides that may have to be designed with larger numbers of amino acids to achieve the requisite affinity and specificity.

Studies conducted over the past decade have provided the basic information about the organization of the GPIIb-IIIa complex in the platelet membrane and the phenomenologic changes that occur with activation. These have recently been reviewed, and can be summarized as follows:[17]

- At least a portion of both GPIIb and GPIIIa is available on the external surface of unactivated platelets, as judged by radiolabeling studies.
- Glycoprotein IIb-IIIa exists as a calcium-dependent heterodimer complex on both unactivated and activated platelets.[68] Although it was attractive to consider the hypothesis that GPIIb and GPIIIa are separated in unactivated platelets and come together as a result of the release of calcium in response to platelet activation, there is considerable biochemical evidence against this idea.[17,68] Immunologic data also support their being complexed in unactivated platelets, and this will be reviewed in greater detail later.
- The GPIIb-IIIa complex is present on the platelet surface at very high density. In fact, it has been estimated from the number of receptors per platelet (~40,000-60,000) and the molecular dimensions of the complex that as much as 50% of the surface area of unactivated platelets is occupied by GPIIb-IIIa complexes.[86]
- Events that occur after fibrinogen binds to platelets are likely to be crucial for platelet aggregation. These events probably include clustering of receptors, with the latter furnishing a geometric advantage in permitting the fibrinogen molecules to span between platelets. For example, a lowering of the temperature of the platelet suspension below the point at which receptors move freely in the lateral direction interferes with aggregation, even though fibrinogen can bind.[107] Moreover, a combination of monoclonal antibodies directed at the GPIIb-IIIa receptor that do not interfere with fibrinogen binding can inhibit platelet aggregation, presumably by altering the postbinding phenomena.[88] Another potential reflection of these alterations is the time-dependent irreversibility of fibrinogen binding, with less and less of the bound fibrinogen being displaceable with cold fibrinogen or EDTA treatment.[103]
- Complexes of GPIIb-IIIa extracted from platelets with nonionic detergents can bind fibrinogen and fibronectin, even in the absence of platelet activating agents.[17,98] This suggests that at least a fraction of the GPIIb-IIIa molecules on platelets is probably present in a conformation(s) that can bind fibrinogen. Moreover, one might also infer that the activation mechanism does not result from an allosteric effect of the agonists in binding directly to GPIIb-IIIa. More recent evidence showing that solubilized GPIIb-IIIa can be purified on affinity columns containing immobilized RGD- and γ-chaining-containing peptides reinforces these conclusions.[118]
- Proteolytic enzymes, such as chymotrypsin, can alter the platelet surface so that fibrinogen binds to GPIIb-IIIa even in the absence of agonists that activate platelets.[65,90,103] Although early experiments suggested that fibrinogen binding coincided with the proteolysis of GPIIIa to a M_r ~66,000 fragment, other studies suggested that such proteolysis was not a necessary precondition for fibrinogen binding.[66,103] It remains possible that more subtle proteolytic alterations occur.[91,109] Alternatively, it is possible that these enzymes induce changes in the proteins that surround the GPIIb-IIIa complexes, rather than altering the complex itself. Here, the microenvironmental changes may affect the binding of fibrinogen to the platelet surface.

Monoclonal and polyclonal antibodies to the GPIIb-IIIa receptor have provided vital information in the analysis of the structural and functional properties of the glycoproteins.

Heterologous polyclonal antibodies have been used to study the glycoproteins in two-dimensional immunoelectrophoresis, and these studies helped demonstrate the calcium dependence of the complex and the ability of the isolated complex to bind fibrinogen and its fragments.[53,68] Moreover, the subtlety of the receptor's fibrinogen-binding site was amply demonstrated by the failure of any combination of antibodies prepared against the purified, but denatured, glycoproteins to inhibit fibrinogen binding to the complex.[76]

Monoclonal antibodies, by virtue of their single epitope specificity and homogeneity, have proved to be exceedingly valuable tools in studying the GPIIb-IIIa complex. The first antibody produced was directed against GPIIb.[78] It did not inhibit the binding of ligands to the complex, but it permitted the quantitation of the number of receptors that are present on platelets and reinforced the data on the stability of the complex, because both glycoproteins were immunoprecipitated by the antibody. It also indicated that at least a portion of the GPIIb molecule was accessible to an IgG molecule, even on unactivated platelets.

Subsequently, a substantial number of antibodies directed against the GPIIb-IIIa complex were produced that inhibited the binding of one or more of the ligands to the receptor and also inhibited platelet aggregation, clot retraction, and adhesion to glass in a parallel manner.[20] Because the initial screening for at least one of these antibodies was performed with a functional assay designed to identify clones making antibodies that blocked the interaction of platelets with fibrinogen, the identification of the antibody's epitope as being on GPIIb-IIIa strongly reinforced the emerging consensus that the fibrinogen binding site was on the GPIIb-IIIa complex itself.[24]

These antibodies were also valuable in clarifying the complex interactions between platelets and the fluid-phase adhesive proteins. In particular, they provided convincing evidence that von Willebrand factor can bind to two different platelet receptors, namely GPIb and GPIIb-IIIa, depending on the nature of the stimulus.[51,122] Moreover, asialo-von Willebrand factor was shown to induce platelet aggregation by first binding to GPIb which, in turn, led to the exposure of the GPIIb-IIIa receptor so that the latter could bind fibrinogen or additional asialo-von Willebrand factor.[50] A similar mechanism probably operates when the abnormal von Willebrand factor found in patients with type IIb von Willebrand's disease induces platelet aggregation in vitro (and probably in vivo).[29]

Exogenous fibronectin binding to activated platelets was also inhibited by antibodies to GPIIb-IIIa, indicating that this receptor was at least one of the binding sites for this ligand.[115] Interestingly, such antibodies also blocked the binding of exogenous thrombospondin to platelets, even though studies with thrombasthenic platelets, which lack the GPIIb-IIIa receptor, have reached somewhat differing conclusions about whether or not there is a binding site for thrombospondin on GPIIb-IIIa.[1,56,115] Recently, platelet GPIV was identified as a possible receptor for thrombospondin.[3] This subject thus remains unresolved, and the recent identification of an RGD-containing sequence in thrombospondin heightens the mystery.[74]

The natural extension of the functional studies involving antibody-induced inhibition of ligand binding to platelets was the use of the antibodies themselves as probes of the molecular organization of the receptors. To accomplish this, it was vital to define the epitopes recognized by the antibodies. One striking observation is that several of the antibodies that inhibit fibrinogen binding to activated platelets do not react with either GPIIb or GPIIIa alone when the complex is split by removing calcium with strong chelating agents, at high pH and temperature. From this is was tentatively inferred that these antibodies were "complex-dependent," that is, that they recognized an epitope that existed only when the two proteins were joined together.[9,25,79,110] Identification of the epitope as being complex-specific was crucial to the physiologic interpretation of the binding of the antibodies to unactivated platelets, because if they truly were complex-specific, then the two glycoproteins must exist as a complex even without activation.

A major stumbling block to the unequivocal identification of the epitopes as being complex-dependent was the need to use strong calcium-chelating agents to separate GPIIb from GPIIIa, because it could be argued that the epitope might be present on only one of the two glycoproteins, but in a region where calcium is required to maintain the conformation. Thus, the antibodies might be calcium-dependent rather than complex-dependent, in which case the binding to unactivated platelets would have no bearing on the status of the complex. It has been very difficult to rigorously prove that the antibodies are complex-dependent rather than calcium-dependent, but existing data seem to support this conclusion. In particular, we demonstrated that incubation of the GPIIb–IIIa complex with antibody 10E5 or an alloimmune antibody to GPIIb–IIIa (made by a patient with Glanzmann's thrombasthenia) made the complex resist dissociation by EDTA, and that radiolabeled antibodies 7E3 and 10E5, respectively, would still bind to these antibody-maintained complexes despite the presence of EDTA (Fig. 10-1).[25] Thus, unless 10E5 and the alloimmune antibody prevented EDTA from removing the calcium, an unlikely possibility, these data indicated that both 7E3 and 10E5 could bind to the GPIIb–IIIa complex in the absence of calcium. A recent study from another laboratory showed that after the GPIIb–IIIa complex is dissociated with calcium-chelating agents, it can be reassociated by treating the complex with neuraminidase.[62] The removal of negatively charged sialic acid residues presumably allows the complex to rejoin without the charge-neutralizing effects of the calcium ions. Radiolabeled 10E5 bound to this neuraminidase-reconstituted complex, despite the calcium chelation treatment, reinforcing the conclusion that this antibody is complex-dependent, not calcium-dependent.[62] Finally, it should be emphasized that even if antibody binding is complex-dependent, this need not indicate that the epitope is composed of amino acid segments from both proteins, for it could be argued that an epitope contained solely on one protein might be altered by complex formation, even without the other protein becoming part of the epitope. That is why we chose to designate the epitopes of our antibodies 10E5 and 7E3 as GPIIb and/or GPIIIa.

The calcium sensitivity of different monoclonal antibodies to GPIIb–IIIa has furnished important information about the complex. All of the "complex-dependent" antibodies lose

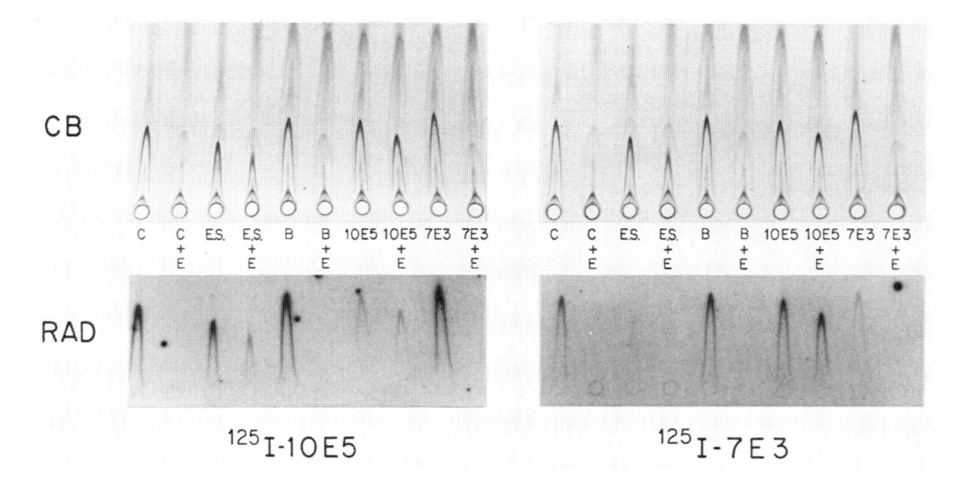

Figure 10-1. Radioimmunoelectroassay of solubilized platelets pretreated with either buffer or antibodies and developed with either radiolabeled 10E5 or 7E3 antibody in conjunction with heterologous antiplatelet IgG. Platelets solubilized in Triton X-100 were incubated with 10-μl control IgG (*C*) (17 mg/ml); IgG from a patient with Glanzmann's thrombasthenia making an antibody that reacts with the GPIIb–IIIa complex (*E.S.*; 15 mg/ml); buffer (*B*) (0.15 M NaCl, 0.01 M TRIS/C1, *p*H 7.4); 10E5 antibody (0.67 mg/ml); or 7E3 antibody (0.6 mg/ml), for 3 h at 22°C. These samples were then run in the assay either without further treatment or after an additional hour of incubation at 37°C with 10 mM EDTA (*E*). *CB* is the Coomassie Blue-stained gel, and *RAD* is the radioautogram. Note that EDTA treatment of the control samples results in the loss of the GPIIb–IIIa complex; preincubation of platelets with E.S. IgG or 10E5 protects the GPIIb–IIIa complex from dissociation by EDTA; radiolabeled 10E5 can bind to the GPIIb–IIa complex held together by the E.S. IgG despite the EDTA-treatment; radiolabeled 7E3 can bind to the GPIIb–IIIa complex held together by antibody 10E5, despite the EDTA-treatment (Coller BS et al: J Lab Clin Med 107:384, 1986,[25] with permission).

their reactivity when the complex is subjected to high concentrations of the chelating agents at high pH and high temperature, because these conditions dissociate the complex.[25,127] The binding of some antibodies (e.g., 10E5) to intact platelets is totally unaffected by calcium chelators at 22 °C and pH 7.4.[25] Other antibodies (e.g.,7E3) are partially inhibited under these conditions, suggesting that calcium plays an additional role for them. Moreover, because the inhibition is consistently incomplete, it suggests that there is heterogeneity of GPIIb–IIIa complexes (or their microenvironments) as they exist in the platelet membrane.[25] Such heterogeneity is also indicated by the existence of other monoclonal antibodies that block the binding of ligands to only a constant fraction of GPIIb–IIIa receptors, even in the presence of calcium.[115] PAC-1 is an IgM murine monoclonal antibody directed at the GPIIb–IIIa receptor that binds poorly to unactivated platelets but much better to platelets activated with ADP, epinephrine, or thrombin (see following discussion).[129,130] Its binding to activated platelets shows a dramatic sensitivity to calcium chelating agents, with the binding decreasing by about 80% when the calcium concentration is below 10^{-7} M, even though the pH and temperature conditions do not favor dissociation of the complex.[129] Finally, PMI-1, an IgG murine monoclonal antibody that inhibits the adhesion of platelets to a collagen-coated surface, has the reverse divalent cation sensitivity—its epitope is cryptic at normal calcium or magnesium concentrations and is increasingly available as the concentrations are reduced, even though there is no dissociation of the GPIIb–IIIa complex.[46] The epitope of this antibody has recently been identified, by using synthetic peptides, as being near the carboxy-terminal region of the GPIIb$_\alpha$ chain.[71]

Monoclonal antibodies 7E3 and PAC-1 have been used to try to better understand the mechanism of GPIIb–IIIa receptor exposure. Kinetic analysis of the binding of 7E3 to platelets demonstrated that the on-rate increased significantly (two- to threefold) when platelets were activated with ADP (Table 10-1).[18]

This was not due to an increase in the total number of GPIIb–IIIa sites, because the total number of 10E5 reactive molecules did not change significantly (Table 10-2). Activation with agents that induce the platelet release reaction (thrombin and ionophore) produced more dramatic increases in the on-rate, but the interpretation of these data was confounded by the increase in the total number of membrane GPIIb–IIIa receptors that occurs under these conditions,[18] presumably by incorporation of intraplatelet stores of GPIIb–IIIa into the plasma membrane (*see* Table 10-2).[92,145] Interestingly, despite the slower on-rate of 7E3 to unactivated platelets, with time, the extent of 7E3 binding to unactivated platelets equaled that to ADP-activated platelets.[18] These data suggested that 7E3 binds, either preferentially

Table 10-1
Binding of ^{125}I-Labeled 7E3 and ^{125}I-Labeled 10E5 to Gel-Filtered Platelets

	7E3		10E5	
Time (min)	*−ADP*	*+ADP*	*−ADP*	*+ADP*
1	250 ± 20*	780 ± 60†	1070 ± 80	1140 ± 70
2	430 ± 30	1100 ± 40†	1380 ± 80	1390 ± 60
3	540 ± 40	1250 ± 50†	1420 ± 70	1420 ± 60
5	860 ± 60	1620 ± 80†	1670 ± 60	1700 ± 60
30	1820 ± 80	1930 ± 100	1790 ± 80	1720 ± 80
60	1950 ± 80	1930 ± 80	1840 ± 80	1750 ± 70

*Molecules per platelet (mean ± SEM).
†$p < 0.001$ comparing values without and with ADP stimulation

Citrated PRP was gel-filtered and adjusted to 2.7–3.2 × 10^{11} platelets per liter. Samples of 1.2 ml were incubated with 133 μl of buffer or ADP (100 μM) for 30 sec and then 4.5 μl of ^{125}I-labeled 7E3 or ^{125}I-labeled 10E5 (both 0.52 μg/ml) was added. Duplicate 0.1-ml aliquots were removed at the indicated times, layered over 0.1 ml of 30% sucrose and centrifuged at 12,000 *g* for 3 min. Results are the mean ± SEM values of four experiments performed with platelets from three separate donors. Note that the initial rate of binding of 7E3 is enhanced approximately three-fold by ADP activation, whereas the rate of 10E5 binding is unaffected. Also note that by 60 min, the total number of 7E3 molecules bound to unactivated platelets is no different from that bound to ADP-activated platelets. (Reproduced with permission from Coller, B.S.: J Clin Invest 76:101, 1985.)

Table 10-2
Effects of Various Agonists on the Rate of ^{125}I-Labeled 7E3 Binding to Platelets and Extent of ^{125}I-Labeled 10E5 Binding to Platelets

	^{125}I-Labeled 7E3 (1.0 μg/ml; 2 min)	^{125}I-Labeled 10E5 (17.9 μg/ml; 30 min)
Buffer	960*	57,030
ADP (10 μM)	3,790	53,570
Epinephrine (10 μM)	2,390	53,570
Thrombin (0.5 U/ml)	5,540	89,860
Ionophore A 23187 (25 μM)	5,080	77,770

*Molecules of antibody bound per platelet (mean of duplicate determinations).

Platelet-rich plasma was prepared from citrated blood (0.01 volume 40% sodium citrate) and gel-filtered. The gel-filtered platelets (3.70×10^{11} platelets per liter) were then incubated for 30 sec at 22°C with buffer (0.15 M NaCl, 0.01 M HEPES, pH 7.4), ADP, epinephrine, thrombin, or ionophore A 23187 at the indicated concentrations. Then 4 μl of ^{125}I-labeled 7E3 (final concentration 1.0 μg/ml) was added at 22°C for 2 min or 20 μl of ^{125}I-labeled 10E5 (final concentration 17.9 μg/ml) was added for 30 min, after which the amount of antibody bound per platelet was determined. Note that ADP and epinephrine increased the initial rate of radiolabeled 7E3 binding without increasing the total number of GPIIb-IIIa receptors, as judged by the binding of a saturating concentration of 10E5 at equilibrium. Thrombin and ionophore A23187 produced a more profound increase in 7E3-binding rate, but the interpretation of these data are confounded by the increased number of GPIIb-IIIa receptors exposed on the platelet surface after activation with these agents. (Reproduced with permission from Collier, B.S.: J Clin Invest 76:101, 1985.)

or exclusively, with an activated state; this could be because 7E3 either recognizes the activated conformation of the complex itself, preferentially or exclusively, or because a change in the microenvironment surrounding the GPIIb–IIIa complex permits 7E3 to gain access to its binding site on the complex. Moreover, the ability of 7E3 to bind to unactivated platelets, albeit slowly, suggests that there may well be a dynamic equilibrium between the different conformations of GPIIb–IIIa itself, or its microenvironment, such that even on unactivated platelets a fraction of the receptors is always in the proper conformation for binding 7E3. Because the off-rate of 7E3, like several other antibodies to the GPIIb–IIIa receptor,[109] is extremely slow,[18] receptors with 7E3 bound would be removed from the equilibrium, and with time, more and more of the receptors would assume the proper conformation for 7E3 binding. This plastic model of the GPIIb–IIIa receptor activation mechanism appears consistent with recent evidence indicating that proteins assume a very large number of different conformations in relatively brief periods.[33] Mathematical models have been constructed to use the immunologic data to derive insight into the percentage of the molecules that are in the different conformations, but we were not able to derive these data because of the unavailability of a receptor that was fully fixed in the activated form.

Whereas the ligands that bind to GPIIb–IIIa are all macromolecular glycoproteins, we wondered if the exposure mechanism might operate by limiting access of large proteins to their binding site(s) on GPIIb–IIIa on unactivated platelets and then making access readily available with platelet activation. In a subsequent study we addressed this possibility by comparing the binding rates to unactivated and activated platelets of intact 7E3, smaller fragments of 7E3 [F(ab′)$_2$ and Fab′], and cross-linked aggregates of 7E3 (dimers, trimers, and tetramers).[15] We found that the smallest fragment bound most rapidly to unactivated platelets, whereas the largest bound least rapidly (Fig. 10-2). Moreover, with activation, the binding rate increased most dramatically for the largest aggregates and only minimally for the Fab′. The rates of binding to activated platelets for all of the antibody species were quite similar, suggesting that they now all had relatively equal access to the binding sites. We recently confirmed the differential binding rates of 7E3 as a function of size by using a rat monoclonal antibody to mouse IgG$_1$ heavy chains prepared by another research group[73] to make a stable tetrameric molecule and then measuring the rates of binding to unactivated and activated platelets.

It is worthwhile to analyze data from other sources to compare with these observations on the possibility that size-selectivity acts as a

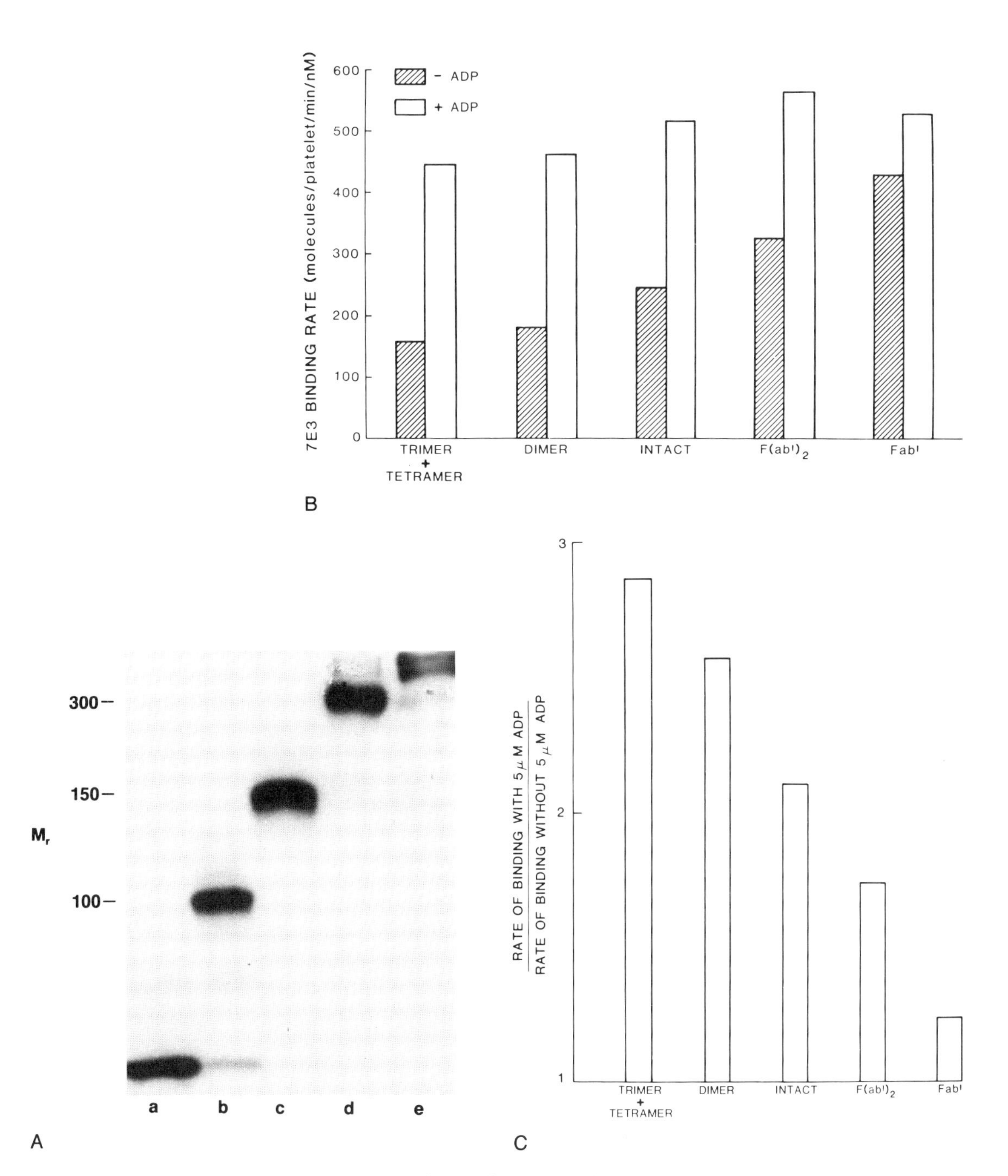

Figure 10-2. (*A*) Radioautographic analysis of cross-linked and digested 7E3 antibody. The radiolabeled antibody species were electrophoresed in a 5.5% SDS–polyacrylamide gel; after drying the gel was subjected to radioautography. *a*, Fab′ 7E3; *b*, $F(ab')_2$ 7E3; *c*, intact 7E3; *d*, 7E3 dimer; *e*, 7E3 trimer plus tetramer. (*B*) Binding of cross-linked, intact, and fragmented 7E3 species to platelets. Data shown are the means of two separate experiments in which duplicate determinations were made. (*C*) Enhancement of binding of cross-linked, intact, and fragmented 7E3 species. Data from the experiment reported in *B* are expressed as the ratio of the binding rate after 5 μM ADP activation to the rate without activation. Similar results were obtained in experiments using 1-, 2-, and 10-μM ADP stimulation. Note that the smaller fragments bound more rapidly to unactivated platelet than did the larger antibody species. After activation with ADP, the binding rates were similar for all of the species, with the largest species, therefore, achieving the greatest increase (Coller BS: J Cell Biol 103:451, 1986,[15] with permission).

mechanism for controlling access to the GPIIb-IIIa receptor-binding sites. It is important to emphasize that even with the largest aggregate of 7E3, which approached fibrinogen in its apparent Stokes radius, the binding to unactivated platelets was considerably greater than that reported for fibrinogen binding to unactivated platelets.[18] This suggests that there may be another mechanism or mechanisms governing exclusion of fibrinogen—perhaps charge or shape. Alternatively, the differences in binding may result from the 7E3 binding site on GPIIb-IIIa differing from that of fibrinogen, with the former somewhat less cryptic on unactivated platelets. In fact, in unpublished studies, we have been unable to inhibit the binding of radiolabeled 7E3 with small RGD-containing peptides, indicating that the sites are not identical. Finally, it is possible that fibrinogen binding requires the exposure of one or more ancillary sites in addition to the RGD-γ-chain site, and that these are maintained in a more cryptic state on unactivated platelets.

In favor of size-exclusion playing some role in the platelets' GPIIb-IIIa exposure mechanism are the preliminary data showing that the γ-chain peptides and small RGD-containing peptides bind equally well to unactivated and activated platelets.[64,70] The M_r 9000 trigramin peptide bound to the same number of sites on unactivated and activated platelets, but activation increased the affinity of binding,[58] much like that 7E3 binding;[18] however, this peptide is much smaller than an Fab′ molecule, and thus, given the 7E3 binding data,[15] one might have thought that it should not have shown so great a difference in binding rate with activation. The observation that purified GPIIb-IIIa can bind fibrinogen, fibronectin, and von Willebrand factor also seems to support the hypothesis that the topographic arrangement of the receptors in the platelet membrane may be responsible for the exclusion of the proteins from receptors that are always competent, even on unactivated platelets. This is also consistent with the ability of proteases to "expose" GPIIb-IIIa receptors, such that they can bind fibrinogen without activators, but as indicated earlier, subtle changes in the GPIIb-IIIa receptor itself may accompany these reactions.[90] Finally, it has recently been shown that neuraminidase more completely desialates the GPIIb-IIIa complex on ADP-treated platelets than on unactivated platelets, suggesting that activation results in greater access of the enzyme to certain regions of the complex.[62]

Several observations, however, are more difficult to reconcile with a size exclusion interpretation and require discussion. (1) When a γ-chain pentapeptide was conjugated to albumin to make it polyvalent, it only supported platelet aggregation when the platelets were activated with ADP, indicating that even though the molecule was much smaller than fibrinogen and somewhere between an Fab′ and $F(ab')_2$ molecule in size, it could not bind to unactivated platelets.[63] One possible explanation for this is the presence of charge exclusion in addition to size exclusion for the highly negatively charged albumin molecule. Alternatively, because platelet aggregation rather than binding of the peptide-albumin was measured, it is possible that the conjugate actually bound to platelets even without activation, but that aggregation required the postbinding modifications induced by ADP. (2) An M_r 12,000 fragment of fibronectin, which is considerably smaller than the Fab fragment of 7E3, did not bind to platelets unless the platelets were activated with thrombin.[38]

When interpreting this study, it is important to recognize the differences between fibronectin and fibrinogen binding. In particular, fibronectin binding requires thrombin activation, with ADP and epinephrine activation being ineffective.[113] In addition, fibronectin cannot inhibit fibrinogen binding to platelets, whereas fibrinogen can inhibit fibronectin binding. Further complicating this matter is the presence of at least one additional fibronectin receptor on platelets composed of the GPIc-IIIa complex, and this receptor can interact with immobilized fibronectin, even without platelet activation.[67] Thus, thrombin must induce alterations in the GPIIb-IIIa receptor (or in its microenvironment) that are fundamentally different from those induced by ADP.

Further support for this notion comes from the finding that the combination of two monoclonal antibodies to GPIIb-IIIa that block ADP-induced platelet aggregation, but not fibrinogen binding, block both fibrinogen binding and platelet aggregation induced by thrombin.[88] In addition, a monoclonal antibody to GPIIb-IIIa has been described (P4) that does not block platelet aggregation or fibrinogen binding induced by ADP or thrombin, but does inhibit thrombin-induced binding of radiolabeled, exogenous fibronectin by about

80%.[81] (3) Radioiodinated photoactivatable derivatives of the γ-chain peptide and RGD-containing peptides labeled GPIIb and GPIIIa to a much greater extent when the platelets were activated with thrombin than when they were unactivated.[126] Similarly, in another study, RGD-containing peptides could be cross-linked to GPIIb–IIIa more readily and with a different pattern when platelets were activated.[32] It is difficult to reconcile these data with the preliminary results indicating that these peptides bind equally well to activated and unactivated platelets. It is possible that the peptides did bind to GPIIb–IIIa, but that thrombin activation enhanced the photoactivated labeling and cross-linking by altering the geometric organization. It would be interesting to know if the enhanced labeling occurred with ADP and epinephrine as well, because these agents can induce fibrinogen receptor exposure without producing the changes peculiar to thrombin activation.

PAC-1 shows a most dramatic increase in binding to GPIIb–IIIa on activated platelets, compared with its binding to platelets treated with prostacyclin (PGI_2) to maintain them in an unactivated state (Fig. 10-3).[129] Epinephrine, ADP, and thrombin are all effective in increasing PAC-1 binding from ~1000 molecules per platelet to ~11,000, 13,500, and 22,000, respectively.[129] Unlike 7E3, PAC-1 does not show a progressive increase in binding with time, indicating that the GPIIb–IIIa complex does not spontaneously assume the PAC-1 epitope or that access is limited so that PAC-1 cannot gain entry to the binding site. Interestingly, PAC-1 is an IgM antibody and thus size-dependent exclusion may operate more effectively on it than on 7E3, which is an IgG. PAC-1 inhibited fibrinogen binding and platelet aggregation, and fibrinogen, in turn, inhibited PAC-1 binding. The RGD-containing peptides can also inhibit PAC-1 binding,[40] indicating that it probably binds to a site different from that of 7E3. As this may be closer to the fibrinogen binding site, it may better reflect the exclusion mechanism(s) that operate on fibrinogen. Most recently, two other antibodies to sites on the GPIIb–IIIa complex have been described that show preference for activated platelets. (1) A human IgM monoclonal autoantibody to GPIIIa bound only to thrombin-activated platelets or platelets that have been stored for some time,[89] and (2) an IgG antibody that does not alter platelet aggregation and thus is not directed at the ligand-binding site of the complex, bound preferentially to thrombin-activated platelets.[82]

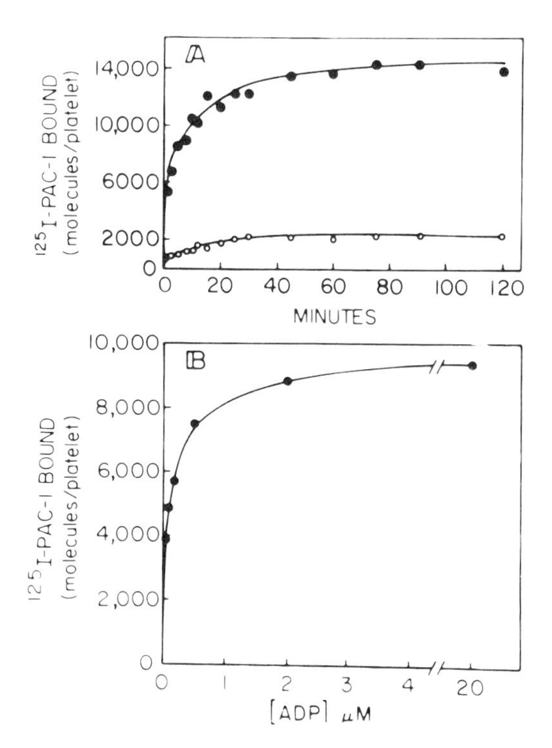

Figure 10-3. Binding of ^{125}I-labeled PAC-1 to platelets. (*A*) Aspirin-treated, gel-filtered platelets were incubated for 5 min at room temperature with 1 μM PGI_2 (open circles) or 10 μM ADP (closed circles). The platelets were then incubated with ^{125}I-labeled PAC-1 (18 μg/ml) at room temperature for various periods, up to 120 min. (*B*) Platelets were incubated for 5 min with concentrations of ADP ranging from 0.05 to 20 μM. Then ^{125}I-labeled PAC-1 (10 μg/ml) was added and the binding of the antibody to the platelets was measured 15-min later. This experiment is representative of three so performed (Shattil SJ et al: J Biol Chem 260:11107, 1985,[129] with permission).

The foregoing analysis highlights the complexity of describing the exposure mechanism of the GPIIb–IIIa receptor, but it may be useful, nonetheless, to offer a working model that incorporates as many of the existing data as possible (Fig. 10-4). The salient features are a single site to which RGD-containing peptides and the γ-chain peptides bind; a region of limited size-dependent access; and ancillary binding sites for fibrinogen, fibronectin, and von Willebrand factor. It is assumed that stable binding of any of the three ligands requires

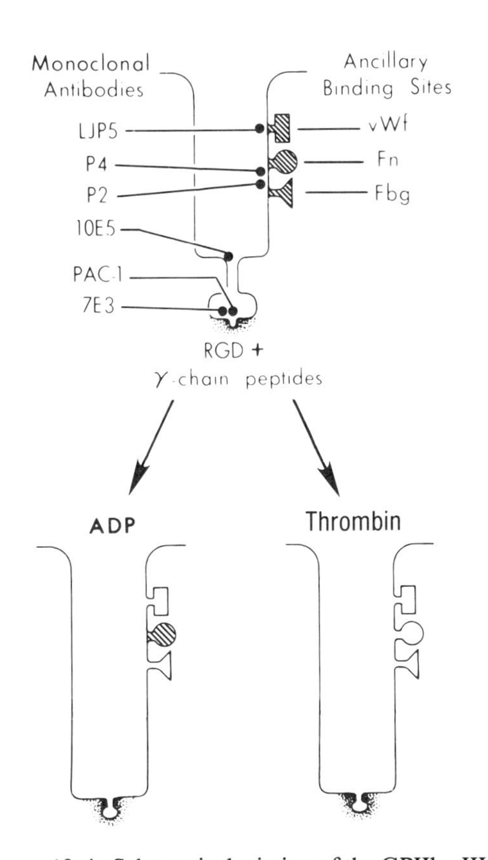

Figure 10-4. Schematic depiction of the GPIIb-IIIa receptor based on data from the binding of the ligands, monoclonal antibodies, and synthetic peptides. RGD and γ-chain peptides bind equally well to unstimulated and stimulated platelets and so their receptor(s) is available on unstimulated platelets; however, because the pattern of photolabeling and cross-linking of such peptides to GPIIb and GPIIIa on activated platelets differs from that on unactivated platelets, this receptor(s) must undergo some alteration with activation. It is assumed that each macromolecular ligand (fibrinogen, fibronectin, and von Willebrand factor) binds to both the RGD-γ-chain-binding site(s) and at least one additional ancillary binding site that is cryptic on unactivated platelets. ADP can expose the ancillary sites for fibrinogen and von Willebrand factor, but not fibronectin, whereas thrombin can expose all of them. Antibody 7E3 is postulated to bind relatively close to the RGD-γ-chain peptide. Its access to its binding site is size-limited in unactivated, but not activated, platelets. Antibody PAC-1 is postulated to bind at, or very near, the RGD-γ-chain peptide-binding site and to overlap the 7E3-binding site. Antibody 10E5 is postulated to be farther away from the RGD-γ-chain peptide-binding site(s), but strategically located. Antibody LJP5, which selectively blocks von Willebrand factor binding is postulated to bind near the von Willebrand factor ancillary-binding site. Antibody P2, which inhibits fibrinogen binding more than fibronectin binding, is postulated to bind between the fibrinogen and fibronectin ancillary-binding site, whereas P4 binds to a separate epitope in the same region but nearer the fibronectin ancillary site.

access to both the RGD-γ-chain site and at least one ancillary site. This seems likely because the intact ligands all have higher affinities for the GPIIb-IIIa receptor than do the RGD and γ-chain peptides. Direct support for this assumption comes primarily from recent studies of fibronectin binding to other cells in which regions distinct from the RGD site play an important role.[95] Further, it is assumed that ADP both increases size-dependent access to the RGD-γ-chain site and exposes the ancillary sites for fibrinogen and von Willebrand factor, whereas thrombin can, in addition, expose the fibronectin ancillary site. Finally, these activators also alter the region surrounding the RGD-γ-chain peptide site. It is interesting to try to propose locations for the epitopes of some of the monoclonal antibodies to GPIIb-IIIa on the basis of this scheme, although this is clearly an exercise in speculation. Antibody LJP5, which selectively blocks von Willebrand factor binding without interfering with fibrinogen or fibronectin binding[137] may be directed at a region near the von Willebrand factor ancillary site. Antibody P4, which blocks fibrinogen binding only minimally, but is a potent inhibitor of fibronectin binding, may be directed at an epitope near the fibronectin ancillary site, with some overlap into the fibrinogen site.[81] Antibody P2, on the other hand, blocks fibrinogen binding more effectively than fibronectin binding, and so its epitope may be in the same region, but closer to the fibrinogen binding site.[81] The P2 and P4 epitopes cannot be very close to each other, however, because P4 binding is not inhibited by excess P2.[81] Antibody 10E5, which blocks the binding of all three ligands, may be situated near the site that limits access to the RGD-γ-chain binding site. 7E3 and PAC-1 are likely to be closer to the RGD-γ-chain site, with the latter perhaps occupying part of the binding region. Their epitopes are shown as overlapping because 7E3 is a potent inhibitor of

PAC-1 binding,* although the reverse is not true. The depicted relationship between the 10E5 and 7E3 epitopes could also explain the paradox of 10E5 partially inhibiting 7E3 binding, with 7E3 causing little or no inhibition of 10E5 binding.[25]

Antibodies 7E3 and PAC-1 have both been applied to analysis of platelets in clinical conditions. We studied the rate of radiolabeled 7E3 binding to unactivated and ADP-activated platelets in patients with renal disease who were receiving long-term hemodialysis, as a way of assessing the activatability of the GPIIb-IIIa receptor.[7] This approach seemed preferable to studying fibrinogen binding, because the latter requires either platelet washing or gel filtration—procedures that can alter platelet function—whereas 7E3 binding can be measured in citrated platelet-rich plasma. We found that before dialysis, 7E3 bound normally to the patients' unactivated platelets, but that the rate failed to increase with ADP activation to the same extent as normal (Table 10-3).[7] This abnormality became more severe during the hemodialysis procedure and partially improved by the end of dialysis. These data suggested that the patients have an intrinsic platelet defect that results in decreased activatability of the GPIIb-IIIa complex and that hemodialysis transiently exacerbates the defect. One hypothesis to explain the deterioration during dialysis is that release of small amounts of ADP from erythrocytes or other cells during dialysis causes the development of a refractory state in which ADP-induced activatability is reduced. In fact, such a condition was simulated in vitro by adding ADP to platelet-rich plasma without stirring and showing a decreased enhancement of the 7E3-binding rate with subsequent ADP activation.[6]

PAC-1 has been used to assess the presence of activated platelets by measuring PAC-1 binding with a fluorescence-activated cell analyzer.[128] PAC-1 binding could be measured in whole blood, offering the advantage of minimal manipulation. Addition of activating agents resulted in an increase in PAC-1 binding, and most impressively, mixing experiments demonstrated that this binding assay could identify as few as 0.8% activated platelets.[128] This technique thus promises to be a very powerful method of assessing platelet activation in vivo (Fig. 10-5).

*Shattil, S.: Personal communication.

Glycoprotein Ib

Although not as extensively studied, GPIb, or its microenvironment, has been reported to undergo changes with platelet activation. In particular, thrombin produced a 60% to 90% reduction in the binding of monoclonal antibodies directed at multiple epitopes on GPIb and decreased platelet agglutination by ristocetin, without producing a decrease in the total amount of platelet GPIb.[43,83] Glycoprotein IX, which has been shown to exist in a noncovalent complex with GPIb,[23] also showed this same phenomenon.[83] Cytochalasin B prevented thrombin from decreasing the reaction of a monoclonal antibody with GPIb, suggesting that a cytoskeletal rearrangement was involved.[43] Proteolysis of GPIb to glycoacalicin was excluded as the cause by showing minimal release of the latter from thrombin-activated platelets.[83] Finally, it is interesting that other alterations in GPIb function in binding von Willebrand factor have been reported in the past with ADP (inhibition) and cytoskeletal-altering agents (enhancement), although GPIb itself was not assessed.[19,21,22,52]

Activation-Dependent Platelet Antigens That Are Recruited from Internal Stores

The Integral α-Granule Membrane Glycoprotein of M_r ~140,000

Two groups initially reported the development of monoclonal antibodies against an integral membrane glycoprotein found in α granules,[57,80] and another group has more recently reported a similar antibody.[28] Although the original reports suggested slightly different biochemical characteristics for the protein, subsequent studies involving direct comparisons clearly indicated that the same protein was being studied.[10,132] Unfortunately, the protein has been given two different designations (GMP-140 and PADGEM).

The protein becomes exposed on activated platelets in concert with α-granule secretion, and maximal secretion results in the presence of ~13,000 molecules on the platelet surface (assuming one antibody molecule binds to one glycoprotein molecule). The binding of antibodies to the protein is not dependent on divalent cations, as chelating agents do not alter the interactions. A small sampling of other cells indicated that the protein is present in endo-

Table 10-3
Binding of ^{125}I-Labeled 7E3 to the Platelets of Normal Subjects and Patients with Chronic Renal Disease Before, During, and at the End of Hemodialysis

	^{125}I-Labeled 7E3 Binding Rate (molecules/platelet/min/nM)		Activation Ratio
	−ADP	*+ADP*	*(+ADP/−ADP)*
Normal Controls ($n = 8$)	210 ± 7*	428 ± 8	2.30
Patients ($n = 11$)			
Before dialysis	214 ± 10	414 ± 23†	1.93
During dialysis	212 ± 11	361 ± 26†	1.71
End of dialysis	232 ± 8	395 ± 12‡	1.70

*Mean ± SEM.
†$p < 0.02$ compared with normal controls.
‡$p < 0.001$ compared with normal controls.

Citrated platelet-rich plasma (0.2 ml; $2-3 \times 10^{11}$ platelets per liter) was incubated with 22 μl of buffer (0.15 M NaCl, 0.01 M HEPES, pH 7.4) or ADP (50 μM in the same buffer; final concentration 5 μM) for 30 sec at 22°C. Radiolabeled 7E3 (1 μl) was then added at a subsaturating concentration (1.48 μg/ml) and, after 2 min, duplicate 0.1-ml samples were layered over 30% sucrose, and platelet-bound antibody was separated from free antibody by centrifugation. The radioactivity of the platelet pellet and the supernatant was then measured. The total number of 7E3-binding sites were determined with the binding assay described above, but with a saturating concentration of ^{125}I-labeled 7E3 (19.0 μg/ml) that was allowed to reach equilibrium (2 hr) at 22°C.

Note that the binding rates of ^{125}I-labeled 7E3 to the unactivated platelets did not differ significantly from those of control platelets, although the rate at the end of dialysis was somewhat greater than the other values. With ADP activation, the normal platelets showed the characteristic increase in binding rate. The rate of binding to ADP-activated platelets from the patients before dialysis, however, was significantly less than control and, thus, the activation ratio was lower. The abnormality appeared to become more severe during dialysis and perhaps to begin to ameliorate by the end of dialysis. [Adapted with permission from Beer, J. et al.: In Marguerie, G. (ed): Platelet Membrane Biochemistry, John Libbey and Co, pp 47–58, 1988.]

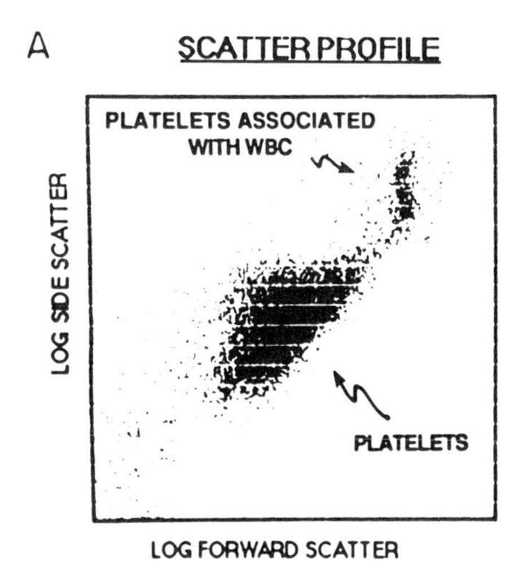

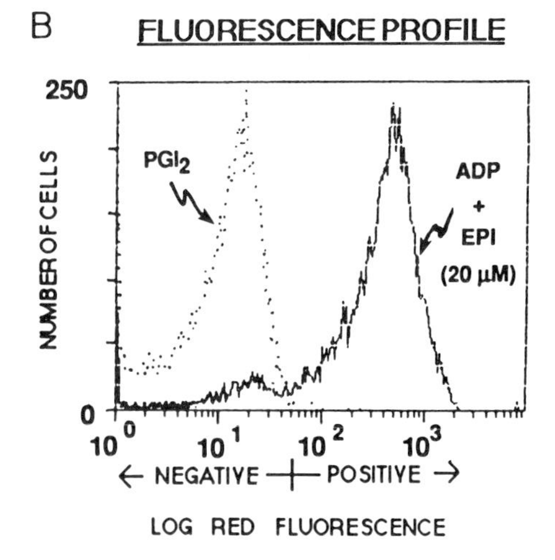

Figure 10-5. Example of the two-color method of flow cytometric analysis of activated platelets with PAC-1. Whole blood was incubated with biotin-PAC-1 and PGI_2 or ADP plus epinephrine. Then phycoerythrin-steptavidin and an FITC-labeled antibody to platelet GPIb (AP1) were added, and the samples were analyzed by flow cytometry. (*A*) Light-scatter profile of AP1-positive cells. These platelets exhibited two separate light-scatter populations. About 95% of the cells appeared to be single platelets, whereas 5% of the platelets exhibited greater light scatter. (*B*) Once the platelets were identified by the AP1 binding, biotin-PAC1 binding was quantitated by analyzing the platelets for phycoerythrin ("red") fluorescence (Shallil SJ et al: Blood 70:307, 1987,[128] with permission).

thelial cells but not other blood cells.[6] No function has yet been ascribed to the protein.

Monoclonal and polyclonal antibodies against this protein have been used in several different studies of platelet physiology and pathology. (1) Serial immunoelectronmicroscopic analyses of platelets after activation with thrombin demonstrated that α granules form large vacuolar structures that are not surface connected before fusion with the plasma membrane.[141] (2) A radiolabeled polyclonal antibody was used to image experimental thrombi formed in an ex vivo Dacron vascular graft in baboons, with good resolution and a high ratio of radioactivity in the graft to radioactivity in the blood pool.[97] The specificity of the antibody for platelets that have undergone the release of α-granule contents should assure its reaction in vivo with platelets in thrombi that have undergone release, but its sensitivity for detecting naturally occurring thrombi remains to be determined. (3) A monoclonal antibody was used to demonstrate that several patients with the gray platelet syndrome, whose platelets lack many of the α-granule proteins, have normal amounts of the M_r 140,000 protein in intracellular vesicles.[121] These structures appear to be aberrant α granules that are essentially devoid of the endogenously synthesized α-granule products (e.g., PF-4, thrombospondin, β-thromboglobulin) but contain some of the proteins that may get incorporated into α granules by megakaryocyte pinocytosis (e.g., albumin, IgG). This study thus suggests that the defect in this disorder is not failure to make α granules but, rather, failure to target the appropriate proteins into the granules. (4) A clinical study in patients who had adult respiratory distress syndrome and in those undergoing cardiopulmonary bypass surgery, indicated that 6/13 patients with the former condition had elevated platelet membrane binding of a monoclonal antibody to the M_r 140,000 protein, whereas only 1/10 patients undergoing cardiopulmonary bypass surgery developed an elevated level of antibody binding.[43] In another study, none of the seven patients undergoing extracorporal circulation showed increased platelet binding of a similar antibody.[28]

Surface Expression of α-Granule Proteins

The induction of the platelet-release reaction results in the expression of some α-granule proteins on the platelet surface; thus, quantitation of this phenomenon can be used as an index of platelet activation, either in vivo or in vitro.[41,42,43] The mechanisms of surface expression have been studied in detail for each of the proteins. Although a comprehensive critical analysis of these data is beyond the scope of this chapter, several general principles seem worthy of emphasis.

The α-granule adhesive glycoproteins fibrinogen, thrombospondin, fibronectin, and von Willebrand factor, all become expressed on the surface of activated platelets.[35,37,41-43,47,86,100,101,108,131,144] Fibrinogen, fibronectin, and von Willebrand factor are present in substantial amounts in plasma, so activation may result in their surface expression by the binding of exogenous protein, by the direct expression of endogenous protein attached to receptors in the α-granule membranes that fuse with the plasma membrane, or by release and subsequent binding of the protein to one or more surface receptors. Because thrombospondin is not present in substantial amounts in normal plasma, only the last two mechanisms pertain to it.

Divalent cations play an important role in the binding of both exogenous and released fibrinogen, von Willebrand factor, fibronectin, and thrombospondin to platelets. Fibrinogen, von Willebrand factor, and fibronectin bind to GPIIb-IIIa; the data are equivocal, however, for thrombospondin because monoclonal antibodies to GPIIb-IIIa can block the binding of exogenous thrombospondin to platelets, but platelets from at least some patients with Glanzmann's thrombasthenia, who express only very low levels of GPIIb-IIIa, bind exogenous thrombospondin in an apparently normal manner, perhaps through GPIV[4] (see foregoing).

Surface expression of von Willebrand factor, fibronectin, and thrombospondin can also occur by divalent cation-independent mechanisms. In each case, however, the number of molecules expressed on the surface of platelets in the presence of chelating agents is only a small fraction of that found in the presence of optimal concentrations of divalent cations. Surface expression of both exogenous and endogenous fibrinogen appears to be divalent cation-dependent.[27]

Platelet factor 4 also becomes expressed on the platelet surface after activation.[13,42] Exogenous PF-4 binds to platelets equally well in the presence or absence of divalent cations, and activation with thrombin does not alter the binding.[13] Approximately 2200 tetrameric molecules of PF-4 bind per platelet.[13] Thus, unlike the mechanism that operates with the adhesive glycoproteins, it appears that thrombin does not induce a receptor with increased affinity for PF-4 but rather it works by simply releasing PF-4 from α granules. The high affinity of PF-4 for sulfated glycosaminoglycans, such as heparin, has led to the suggestion that the sulfated glycosaminoglycans on the surface of platelets and endothelial cells serve as the PF-4 receptors. In contrast to PF-4, the β-thromboglobulin family of molecules (including low-affinity PF-4 and platelet basic protein) does not become expressed on the platelet surface after activation.[13]

The expression of α-granule proteins on the platelet surface has also been exploited for detecting in vivo platelet activation in various disease states. From a practical standpoint, the low plasma concentration of thrombospondin and its high copy number when bound to platelets (25,000–40,000 molecules per platelet) have made it an attractive index of in vivo platelet activation. In the study of patients with acute respiratory distress syndrome and patients undergoing cardiopulmonary bypass surgery alluded to earlier,[43] it was found that 4/13 patients in the former group, but none of the patients in the latter group, showed an increase in platelet-associated thrombospondin.[40] These same characteristics make radiolabeled antibodies to thrombospondin interesting probes for detecting thrombi in vivo because it can be expected that at least some of the platelets involved in thrombus formation have undergone the release reaction and, therefore, ought to have thrombospondin expressed on their surface.

Monoclonal Antibodies That Cause Platelet Activation

Several groups have reported the production of monoclonal antibodies against platelet glycoproteins of low molecular mass that are able to induce platelet activation.[12,30,31,34,49,55,84,136,146] Although there appears to be a major glycoprotein of M_r ~21,000–26,000, additional minor proteins with M_rs extending up to ~28,000 have been reported.[84] Whether these minor protein bands are precursors, products, or identical proteins with different posttranslational modifications remains to be determined, but selective protein- and carbohydrate-labeling studies suggest more extensive glycosylation of the higher M_r bands. It has also been reported that monoclonal antibodies against $GPIIb_\beta$ (M_r 22,000) can induce platelet activation,[60] but a review of the criteria used to establish that these antibodies truly reacted with $GPIIb_\beta$, rather than with a separate glycoprotein of the same M_r, indicates that it is possible that these antibodies were reacting with the glycoprotein(s) indicated above, rather than with $GPIIb_\beta$. The tissue distribution of the antigen recognized by these antibodies has not been reported in detail, but many, if not all, of these antibodies react with acute lymphoblastic leukemia cells.[146] Moreover, at least some of these antibodies react with glomerular and distal tubular cells in the kidney, and with subpopulations of both T cells and B cells; monocytes and granulocytes show only low-level reactivity of questionable specificity.[146]

The platelet activation and aggregation patterns produced by all of these antibodies have been similar, with the antibodies inducing platelet secretion and aggregation in a dose-dependent manner after a variable lag phase. The aggregation is mediated, at least in part, by the GPIIb–IIIa receptor, as indicated by its divalent cation-dependence, inhibition by monoclonal antibodies to the receptor, and failure to occur with Glanzmann's thrombasthenia platelets. Glycoprotein Ib appears to play no role, as judged by the normal aggregation of Bernard Soulier platelets induced by the antibodies and the failure of monoclonal antibodies to the von Willebrand factor-binding site on GPIb to affect aggregation. Although the antibodies to the low-molecular-mass protein(s) can induce thromboxane synthesis, this is not a prerequisite for aggregation, as indomethacin-treated platelets aggregate normally. Release of α granule, dense body, and lysosomal contents can all be induced by these antibodies, and release is not totally aggregation-dependent, for it occurs in unstirred samples. Platelet aggregation and dense body release is totally inhibited by increasing platelet cAMP.

At least one of the antibodies can activate the protein kinase C system, leading to phosphorylation of the M_r 20,000 and 40,000 target proteins.[12] Although the calcium antagonist, TMB-8, blocked phosphorylation, no increase in cytoplasmic free calcium could be demonstrated with quin 2, suggesting that the antibody probably causes release of such small amounts of calcium that they are below the sensitivity limits of quin 2. In fact, calcium mobilization, as judged by quin 2, has been demonstrated with another of the antibodies.[120] Interestingly, platelet activation by this same antibody did not seem to depend on external calcium, which contrasts with thrombin-induced activation.[120] The $F(ab')_2$ fragments of some, but not all, of the antibodies were also able to induce platelet activation; Fab′ and Fab fragments of several antibodies failed to induce aggregation, although at least two augmented the response to ADP and collagen,[49] whereas the Fab′ fragment of the antibody said to be against $GPIIb_\beta$ retained the platelet aggregation activity.[60] Thus, there may, or may not, be a requirement for bifunctional binding to induce aggregation. The Fab fragment of one of the antibodies that did not cause aggregation, also did not inhibit aggregation induced by ADP, epinephrine, collagen, and thrombin, but the Fab fragment of another antibody did inhibit platelet aggregation induced by several agonists, raising the possibility that this low molecular mass protein(s) is involved in aggregation induced by these agonists.[12,84]

Binding studies with one monoclonal antibody indicated that there is an average of about 65,000 molecules of the antigen on platelets.[84] Careful immunoprecipitation and immunoblotting studies indicate that the antigen is distinct from $GPIb_\beta$, $GPII_\beta$, and GPIX, proteins of similar molecular mass.[84] A slight decrease in the relative molecular mass, as determined by SDS-PAGE, accompanies reduction of the protein, raising the possibility that it contains an interchain disulfide bond. An interesting association of this protein with GPIb has been noted; immunoprecipitates produced by one such antibody of solubilized platelets labeled with periodate/[^{3}H]borohydride, but not lactoperoxidase/^{125}I, contained the GPIb-GPIX complex in addition to the M_r 22,000-28,000 bands.[84] Moreover, a radiolabeled band of M_r 210,000 was also immunoprecipitated by this antibody, and it appeared to contain a GPIb-related epitope (or to be noncovalently associated with a protein that did), because "preclearing" the solubilized platelet proteins with an anti-GPIb antibody removed this band. The authors emphasized that only a small fraction of GPIb appears to be associated with the low M_r proteins, and they speculate that there may be heterogeneity of GPIb molecules that are complexed with the lower M_r proteins, with some retaining and others losing the epitope recognized by the monoclonal antibody to GPIb. Interestingly, it was shown that one of these antibodies can inhibit or reverse ristocetin-induced platelet agglutination, suggesting a functional connection to GPIb.[55] However, this phenomenon may operate through a more indirect mechanism because ADP and thrombin have both been implicated in decreasing ristocetin-induced agglutination, as discussed earlier.

A platelet-activating antibody was recently reported in the serum of a patient with autoimmune thrombocytopenia purpura.[133] The IgG and $F(ab')_2$ fragment aggregated normal platelets and induced the release reaction, but the Fab fragment had little or no capacity to aggregate normal platelets. PGI_2 inhibited the aggregation, whereas aspirin did not; EDTA only partially inhibited aggregation. The patient's platelet count rose in response to steroid therapy, thus permitting platelet aggregation studies, which showed a dramatic, but isolated, defect in collagen-induced aggregation. A similar defect could be produced in normal platelets by incubating them with the Fab fragment of the patient's IgG. Immunoprecipitation studies revealed a major band at M_r 57,000 (nonreduced), 62,000 (reduced), but several minor bands were also evident. These data suggest some relationship between this protein and the collagen receptor, but additional confirmatory evidence will be required. Finally, two recent preliminary reports indicate that monoclonal antibodies directed against the GPIIb-IIIa receptor can activate platelets.[85,124] Further analysis of these antibodies' epitopes may furnish important insights into the receptor exposure mechanism.

CONCLUSION

The power of immunologic approaches in investigating the physiologic basis of platelet activation is amply demonstrated in this review. Moreover, there is increasing opportunity for applying these same reagents and techniques to better understanding the functional abnormalities of many different diseases. It is hard to escape the conclusion that this field is still in its infancy and that important new information is certain to be obtained.

This work was supported by the National Heart, Lung, and Blood Institute, grant 19278.

REFERENCES

1. Aiken ML, Ginsberg MH, Plow EF: Identification of a new class of inducible receptors on platelets. Thrombospondin interacts with platelets via a GPIIb-IIIa-independent mechanism. J Clin Invest 78:1713, 1986

2. Aiken ML, Ginsberg MH, Plow EF: Divalent cation-dependent and independent surface expression of thrombospondin on thrombin-stimulated human platelets. Blood 69:1, 1987

3. Amit AG, Mariuzza RA, Phillips SEV, Poljak RJ: Three-dimensional structure of an antigen-antibody complex at 6 A resolution. Nature 313:156, 1985

4. Asch AS, Barnwell J, Silverstein RL, Nachman RL: Isolation of the thrombospondin membrane receptor. J Clin Invest 79:1054, 1987

5. Barlow DJ, Edwards MS, Thornton JM: Continuous and discontinuous protein antigenic determinants. Nature 322:747, 1986

6. Beckstead J, Steinberg PE, McEver RP, Shuman MA, Bainton DF: Immunohistochemical localization of membrane and alpha granule proteins in human megakaryocytes: Application to plastic-embedded bone marrow biopsy specimens. Blood 67:285, 1986

7. Beer J, Kelleher S, Coller BS: Activatability of platelet GPIIb/IIIa receptors by ADP in renal patients on chronic hemodialysis. In Marguerie G (ed): Platelet Membrane Biochemistry, pp 47-58 John Libbey and Co 1988

8. Benjamin DC, Berzofsky JA, East IJ, Gurd FRN, Hannum C, Leach SJ, Margoliash E, Michael JG, Miller A, Prager EM, Reichlin M, Sercanz EE, Smith-Gill SJ, Todd PE, Wilson AC: The antigenic structure of proteins: A reappraisal. Annu Rev Immunol 2:67, 1984

9. Bennett JS: The platelet-fibrinogen interaction. In George JN, Nurden AT, Phillips DR (eds): Platelet Membrane Glycoproteins, p 193, New York, Plenum Press, 1985

10. Berman CL, Yeo EL, Wencel-Drake JD, Furie BC, Ginsberg MH, Furie B: A platelet alpha granule membrane protein that is associated with the plasma membrane after activation: Characterization and subcellular localization of platelet activation-dependent granule-external membrane protein. J Clin Invest 78:130, 1986

11. Berzofsky JA: Intrinsic and extrinsic factors in protein antigenic structure. Science 229:932, 1985

12. Boucher C, Soria C, Mirshahi M, Soria J, Perrot JY, Fournier N, Billard M, Rosenfeld C: Characteristics of platelet aggregation induced by the monoclonal antibody ALB_6 (acute lymphoblastic leukemia antigen p 24). FEBS Lett 161:289, 1983

13. Capitanio AM, Niewiarowski S, Rucinski B, Tuszynski GP, Cierniewski CS, Hershock D, Kornecki E: Interaction of platelet factor 4 with human platelets. Biochim Biophys Acta 839:161, 1985

14. Charo I, Fitzgerald LA, Steiner B, Rall SC, Bekeart LS, Phillips DR: Platelet glycoproteins IIb and IIIa: Evidence for a family of immunologically and structurally related glycoproteins in mammalian cells. Proc Natl Acad Sci USA 83:8351, 1986

15. Coller BS: Activation affects access to the platelet receptor for adhesive glycoproteins. J Cell Biol 103:451, 1986

16. Coller BS: Blood elements at surfaces: Platelets. Ann NY Acad Sci (in press), 1986

17. Coller BS: Mechanism(s) of exposure of the platelet glycoprotein IIb/IIIa complex receptor for adhesive glycoproteins. In McGregor JL, (ed): Monoclonal Antibodies and Human Blood Platelets, Amsterdam. Elsevier, 1986

18. Coller BS: A new murine monoclonal antibody reports on activation-dependent change in the conformation and/or microenvironment of the platelet GPIIb/IIIa complex. J Clin Invest 76:101, 1985

19. Coller BS: Platelet-von Willebrand factor interactions. In George JN, Nurden AT, Phillips DR, (eds): Platelet Membrane Glycoproteins, p 215, New York, Plenum Press, 1985

20. Coller BS: Report of the working party on hybridoma-derived monoclonal antibodies to platelet. Thromb Haemostasis 51:169, 1984

21. Coller BS: Effects of tertiary amine local anesthetics on von Willebrand factor-dependent platelet function: Alteration of membrane reactivity and degradation of GPIb by a calcium-dependent protease(s). Blood 60:731, 1982

22. Coller BS: Inhibition of von Willebrand factor-dependent platelet function by increased platelet cyclic AMP and its prevention by cytoskeleton-disrupting agents. Blood 57:846, 1981

23. Coller BS, Peerschke EI, Scudder LE, Sullivan CA: Studies with a murine monoclonal antibody that abolishes ristocetin-induced binding of von Willebrand factor to platelets: Additional evidence in support of GPIb as a platelet receptor for von Willebrand factor. Blood 61:99, 1983

24. Coller BS, Peerschke EI, Scudder LE, Sullivan CA: A murine monoclonal antibody that completely blocks the binding of fibrinogen to platelets produces a thrombasthenic-like state in normal platelets and binds to glycoproteins IIb and/or IIIa. J Clin Invest 72:325, 1983

25. Coller BS, Peerschke EI, Seligsohn U, Scudder LE, Nurden AT, Rosa J-P: Studies on the binding of an alloimmune and two murine monoclonal antibodies to the platelet glycoprotein IIb-IIIa complex receptor. J Lab Clin Med 107:384, 1986

25a. Coller BS, Steinberg M, Beer JH, Scudder LE: A murine monoclonal antibody to platelet GPIa/IIa inhibits platelet-collagen interactions. Clin Res 36:563a, 1988 (abst)

26. Colman PM, Laver WG, Varghese JN, Baker AT, Tulloch PA, Air GM, Webster RG: Three-dimensional structure of a complex of antibody with influenza virus neuramindase. Nature 326:358, 1987

27. Courtois G, Ryckewaert J-J, Woods VL, Ginsberg MH, Plow EF, Marguerie GA: Expression of intracellular fibrinogen on the surface of stimulated platelets. Eur J Biochem 159:61, 1986

28. Dechavanne U, Ffrench M, Page J, Ffrench P, Boukerche H, Bryon PA, McGregor JL: Significant reduction in the binding of a monoclonal antibody (LYP18) directed against the IIb/IIIa glycoprotein complex to platelets of patients having undergone extracorporal circulation. Thromb Haemostasis 57:106, 1987

29. DeMarco L, Del Ben MG, Budde U, Federici AB, Girolami A, Zimmerman TS, Ruggeri ZM: The platelet aggregating properties of type IIb von Willebrand factor: The role of sialic acid and two distinct membrane receptors. Circulation (Suppl. II):II-96, 1987

30. Deng C-T, Terasaki PI, Iwaki Y, Hofman FM, Koeffler P, Cahan L, Awar NE, Billing R: A monoclonal antibody cross-reactive with human platelets, megakaryocytes, and common acute lymphocytic leukemia cells. Blood 61:759, 1983

32. Dowel BL, Tuck FL, Borowitz MJ, LeBien TW, Metzger RS: Phylogenetic distribution of a 24,000 dalton human leukemia-associated antigen on platelets and kidney cells. Develop Compar Immunol 8:187, 1984

32. D'Souza SE, Ginsberg MH, Lam S, Plow EF: Activation dependent alterations in the chemical crosslinking of arginyl-glycyl-aspartic acid (RGD) peptides with platelet glycoprotein (GP) GPIIb–IIIa. Thromb Haemostasis 58:243, 1987

33. Elber R, Karplus M: Multiple conformational states of proteins: A molecular dynamics analysis of myoglobin. Science 235, 1987

34. Enouf J, Bredou R, Boucheix C, Mirshahi M, Soria C, Levy-Toledano S: Possible involvement of two proteins [phosphoprotein and CD9 (p24)] in regulation of platelet calcium fluxes. FEBS Lett 183:398, 1985

35. Fernandez MFL, Ginsberg MH, Ruggeri ZM, Batelle FJ, Zimmerman TS: Multimeric structure of platelet factor VIII/von Willebrand factor: The presence of larger multimers and their reassociation with thrombin-stimulated platelets. Blood 60:1132, 1982

36. Frelinger AL III, Lam S C-T, Smith MA, Plow EF, Ginsberg MH: Arg-Gly-Asp peptides induce changes in platelet membrane glycoprotein IIB–IIIA associated with loss of adhesive protein binding function (abstr). Clin Res 35:598A, 1987

37. Furby FH, Berndt MC, Castaldi PA, Koutts J: Characterization of calcium-dependent binding of endogenous factor VIII/von Willebrand factor to surface activated platelets. Thromb Res 35:501, 1984

38. Gardner JM, Hynes RO: Interaction of fibronectin with its receptor on platelets. Cell 42:439, 1985

39. Gartner TK, Bennett JS: The tetrapeptide analogue of the cell attachment site of fibronectin inhibits platelet aggregation and fibrinogen binding to activated platelets. J Biol Chem 260:11891, 1985

40. Gartner TK, Power JW, Beachey EH, Bennett JS, Shattil J: The tetrapeptide analogue of the alpha chain and decapeptide analogue of the gamma chain of fibrinogen bind to different sites on the platelet receptor (abstr). Blood 66:305a, 1985

41. George JN, Lyons RM, Morgan RK: Membrane changes associated with platelet activation. J Clin Invest 66:1, 1980

42. George JN, Onofre AR: Human platelet surface binding of endogenous secreted factor VIII–von Willebrand factor and platelet factor 4. Blood 59:194, 1982

43. George JN, Pickett EB, Soucerman S, McEver RP, Kunicki TJ, Kieffer N, Newman PJ: Platelet surface glycoproteins: Studies on resting and activated platelets and platelet membrane microparticles in normal subjects, and observations in patients during adult respiratory distress syndrome and cardiac surgery. J Clin Invest 78:340, 1986

44. Geysen HM, Tainer JA, Rodda SJ, Mason TJ, Alexander H, Getzoff ED, Lerner RA: Chemistry of antibody binding to a protein. Science 235:1184, 1987

45. Giancotti FG, Languino LR, Zanetti A, Peri G, Tarone G, Dejana E: Platelets express a membrane protein complex immunologically related to the fibroblast fibronectin receptor and distinct from GPIIb/IIIa. Blood 69:1535, 1987

46. Ginsberg MH, Lightsey A, Kunicki TJ, Kaufman A, Marguerie G, Plow EF: Divalent cation regulation of the surface orientation of platelet membrane glycoprotein IIb: Correlation with fibrinogen binding function and definition of a novel variant of Glanzmann's thrombasthenia. J Clin Invest 78:1103, 1986

47. Ginsberg MH, Painter RG, Forsyth J, Birdwell C, Plow EF: Thrombin increases expression of fibronectin antigen on the human platelet surface. Proc Natl Acad Sci USA 77:1049, 1980

48. Girma JP, Kalafatis M, Pietu G, Lavergne JM, Chopek MW, Edington TS, Meyer D: Mapping of distinct von Willebrand factor domains interacting with platelet GPIb and GPIIb/IIIa and with col-

lagen using monoclonal antibodies. Blood 67:1356, 1986

49. Gorman DJ, Castaldi PA, Zola H, Berndt MC: Preliminary functional characterization of a 24,000 dalton platelet surface protein involved in platelet activation. Nouv Rev Fr Hematol 27:155, 1985

50. Gralnick HR, Williams SB, Coller BS: Asialo von Willebrand factor interactions with platelets. Interdependence of glycoproteins Ib and IIb/IIIa for binding and aggregation. J Clin Invest 75:19, 1985

51. Gralnick HR, Williams SB, Coller BS: Fibrinogen competes with von Willebrand factor for binding to the glycoprotein IIb/IIIa complex when platelets are stimulated with thrombin. Blood 64:797, 1984

52. Grant RA, Zucker MD, McPherson J: ADP-induced inhibition of von Willebrand factor-mediated platelet agglutination. Am J Physiol 230:1406, 1976

53. Hagen I, Solum NO: Structure and function of platelet membrane glycoproteins as studied by crossed immunoelectrophoresis. In George JN, Nurden AT, Phillips DR (eds): Platelet Membrane Glycoproteins. p 105. New York, Plenum Press, 1985

54. Haverstick DM, Cowan JF, Yamada KM, Santoro SA: Inhibition of platelet adhesion to fibronectin, fibrinogen and von Willebrand factor substrates by a synthetic tetrapeptide derived from the cell-binding domain of fibronectin. Blood 66:946, 1985

55. Higashihara M, Maeda H, Shibata Y, Kume S, Ohashi T: A monoclonal antihuman platelet antibody: A new platelet aggregating substance. Blood 65:382, 1985

56. Hourdille P, Hasitz M, Belloc F, Nurden AT: Immunocytochemical study of the binding of fibrinogen and thrombospondin to ADP- and thrombin-stimulated human platelets. Blood 65:912, 1985

57. Hsu-Liu S-C, Berman CL, Furie BC, August D, Furie B: A platelet membrane protein expressed during platelet activation and secretion: Studies using a monoclonal antibody specific for thrombin-activated platelets. J Biol Chem 259:9121, 1984

58. Huang T-F, Lukasiewicz H, Holt, JC, Niewiarowski S: Trigramin. A low molecular weight peptide inhibiting fibrinogen interaction with platelet receptors expressed on glycoprotein IIb/IIIa complex. J Biol Chem 262:16157, 1987

59. Isenberg WM, McEver RP, Phillips DR, Shuman MA, Bamton DF: The platelet fibrinogen receptor: An immunogold-surface replica study of agonist-induced ligand binding and receptor clustering. J Cell Biol 104:1655, 1987

60. Jennings LK, Phillips DR, Walker WS: Monoclonal antibodies to human platelet glycoprotein IIb_{β} that initiate distinct platelet responses. Blood 65:1112, 1985

61. Jolles P, Levy-Toledano S, Fiat A-M, Soria C, Gillessen D, Thomaidis A, Dunn FW, Caen JP: Analogy between fibrinogen and casein: Effect of an undecapeptide isolated from kappa-casein on platelet function. Eur J Biochem 158:279, 1986

62. Karpatkin S, Ferziger R, Dorfman D: Crossed immunoelectrophoresis of human platelet membranes. Effect of charge on association and dissociation of the glycoprotein GPIIb–GPIIIa membrane complex. J Biol Chem 261:14266, 1986

63. Kloczewiak MA, Timmons DS, Lukas TJ, Hawiger J: Platelet receptor recognition site on human fibrinogen: Synthesis and structure-function relationship of peptides corresponding to the carboxy-terminal segment of the gamma chain. Biochemistry 23:1767, 1984

64. Kloczewiak MA, Timmons SD, Lukas TJ, Hawiger JJ: Structural attributes of synthetic peptides inhibiting and promoting aggregation of human platelets. Circulation 70(Suppl. II):II-358, 1984

65. Kornecki E, Lukaslewicz H, Eckardt A, Egbring R, Ehrlich YH, Niewiarowski S: Enzymatic proteolysis of the platelet membrane glycoprotein IIb/IIIa complex and exposure of fibrinogen receptors. Blood 68(Suppl.1):320a, 1986

66. Kornecki E, Tuszynski GP, Niewiarowski S: Inhibition of fibrinogen receptor mediated platelet aggregation by heterologous anti-human platelet membrane antibody: Significance of a 66,000 M_r protein derived from glycoprotein IIIa. J Biol Chem 258:9349, 1983

67. Kunicki TJ, Nugent DJ, Staats SJ, Orchekowski RP, Wayner EA, Carter WG: The human fibroblast Class II extracellular matrix receptor mediates platelet adhesion to collagen and is identical to the platelet glycoprotein Ia-IIa complex. J Biol Chem 263:4516, 1988

68. Kunicki TJ: Organization of glycoproteins within the platelet plasma membrane. In George JN, Nurden AT, Phillips DR (eds): Platelet Membrane Glycoproteins, p 87. New York, Plenum Press, 1985

69. Kunicki TJ, Newman PJ: Synthesis of analogs of human platelet membrane glycoprotein IIb–IIIa complex by chicken peripheral blood thrombocytes. Proc Natl Acad Sci USA 82:7319, 1985

70. Lam SC-T, Forsyth J, Pierschbacher MD, Ruoslahti E, Plow EF, Ginsberg MH: A synthetic peptide containing a fibronectin cell attachment sequence inhibits platelet aggregation and binds specifically and saturably to platelets. Fed Proc 44:1994, 1985

71. Lam S, Plow EF, Frelinger AL, Smith MA, Loftus JC, Ginsberg MH: Arg-Gly-Asp (RGD) pep-

tides increase the exposure of the carboxyl terminal region of the heavy chain of GPIIb on the platelet surface. Thromb Haemostasis 58:243, 1987

72. Lam SC-T, Plow EF, Smith MA, Andrieux A, Ryckwaert J-J, Marguerie G, Ginsberg MH: Evidence that arginyl-glycyl-aspartate peptides and fibrinogen γ-chain peptides share a common binding site on platelets. J Biol Chem 262:947, 1987

73. Lansdorp PM, Aalberse RC, Bos R, Schutter WG, van Bruggen EFJ: Cyclic tetramolecular complexes of monoclonal antibodies: A new type of cross-linking reagent. Eur J Immunol 16:679, 1986

74. Lawler J, Hynes RO: The structure of human thrombospondin, an adhesive glycoprotein with multiple calcium-binding sites and homologies with several different proteins. J Cell Biol 103:1636, 1986

75. Lerner RA: Tapping the immunological repertoire to produce antibodies of predetermined specificity. Nature 299:592, 1982

76. Leung LLK, Kinoshita T, Nachman RL: Isolation, purification and partial characterization of platelet membrane glycoprotein IIb and IIIa. J Biol Chem 256:1994, 1981

77. Loftus J, Plow EF, Pytela R, Pierschbaker M, Ryckewaert JJ, Ruoslahti E, Ginsberg M: Immunochemical and structural comparison of GPIIb-IIIa and the vitronectin receptor. Circulation (Suppl. II):II-63, 1986

78. McEver RP, Baenziger NL, Majerus PW: Isolation and quantitation of the platelet membrane glycoprotein deficient in the thrombasthenia using a monoclonal hybridoma antibody. J Clin Invest 66:1311, 1980

79. McEver RP, Bennett EM, Martin MN: Identification of two structurally and functionally distinct sites on human platelet membrane glycoprotein IIb-IIIa using monoclonal antibodies. J Biol Chem 258:5269, 1983

80. McEver RP, Martin MN: A monoclonal antibody to a membrane glycoprotein binds only to activated platelets. J Biol Chem 259:9799, 1984

81. McGregor JL, McGregor L, Bauer A-S, Catimel B, Brochier J, Dechavanne M, Clemetson KJ: Identification of two distinct regions within the binding sites for fibrinogen and fibronectin on the IIb-IIIa human platelet membrane glycoprotein complex by monoclonal antibodies P2 and P4. Eur J Biochem 159:443, 1986

82. Metzelaar MJ, Nieuwenhuis HK, Sixma JJ: Detection of activated platelets with monoclonal antibodies. Thromb Haemostasis 58:281, 1987

83. Michelson AD, Barnard MR: Thrombin-induced changes in platelet membrane glycoproteins Ib, IX, and IIb-IIIa complex. Blood 70:1673, 1987

84. Miller JL, Kupinski JM, Hustad KO: Characterization of a platelet membrane protein of low molecular weight associated with platelet activation following binding by monoclonal antibody AG-1. Blood 68:743, 1986

85. Modderman PW, Huisman JG, van Mourik JA, von dem Bourne AEG Kr: Platelet activation induced by a monoclonal antibody against the platelet GPIIb/IIIa complex. Thromb Diath 58:193, 1987

86. Mosher DF, Pesciotta DM, Loftus JC, Albrecht RM: Secreted alpha granule proteins. The race for receptors. In George JN, Nurden AT, Phillips DR (eds): Platelet Membrane Glycoproteins, p 171. New York, Plenum Press, 1985

87. Nardet C, Semeriva M, Yamada KM, Thiery JP: Peptides containing the cell-attachment recognition signal Arg-Gly-Asp prevent gastrulation in *Drosophila* embryos. Nature 325:348, 1987

88. Newman PJ, McEver RP, Doers MP, Kunicki TJ: Synergistic action of two murine monoclonal antibodies that inhibit ADP-induced platelet aggregation without blocking fibrinogen binding. Blood 69:668, 1987

89. Nieuwenhuis HK, Akkerman JWN, Hondijk WPM, Sixma JJ: Human blood platelets with a defect of response to collagen fail to express surface glycoprotein Ia. Nature 318:470, 1985

90. Niewiarowski S, Budynski AZ, Morinelli TA, Budzynski TM, Stewart GJ: Exposure of fibrinogen receptor on human platelets by proteolytic enzymes. J Biol Chem 256:917, 1981

91. Niewiarowski S, Eckard TA, Lukasiewicz H, Norton K, Huang T-F, Kornecki E: Products of limited proteolysis of glycoprotein IIIa on the platelet membranes. Thromb Haemostasis 58:197, 1987

92. Niiya K, Hodson E, Bader R, Byers-Ward, Koziol JA, Plow EF, Ruggeri ZM: Increased surface expression of the membrane glycoprotein IIb/IIIa complex induced by platelet activation. Relationship to the binding of fibrinogen and platelet activation. Blood 70:475, 1987

93. Niman HL, Houghten RA, Walker LE, Reisfeld RA, Wilson IA, Hogle JM, Lerner RA: Generation of protein-reactive antibodies by short peptides is an event of high frequency: Implications for the structural basis of immune recognition. Proc Natl Acad Sci USA 80:4949, 1983

94. Nugent DJ, Kunicki TJ, Berglund C, Bernstein ID: A human monoclonal autoantibody recognizes a neoantigen on glycoprotein IIIa expressed on stored and activated platelets. Blood 70:16, 1987

95. Obara M, Kang MS, Rocher-Dufour S, Kornbliht A, Thiery JP, Yamada KM: Expression of the cell-binding domain of human fibronectin in *E. coli.* FEBS Lett 213:261, 1987

96. Oi VT, Vuong TM, Hardy R, Reidler J, Dangl J, Herzenberg LA, Stryer L: Correlation be-

tween segmental flexibility and effector function of antibodies. Nature 307:136, 1984

97. Palabrica T, Furie BC, Konstam MA, Connolly R, Ramberg K, Brockway B, Aronovitz M, Furie B: Imaging of thrombi using anti-PADGEM antibodies specific for activated platelets. Circulation 74(suppl. II):II-237, 1986

98. Parise LV, Phillips DR: Fibronectin-binding properties of the purified glycoprotein IIb–IIIa complex. J Biol Chem 261:14011, 1986

99. Parise LV, Steiner L, Nannizzi L, Phillips DR: Peptides from fibrinogen and fibronectin change the conformation of purified platelet glycoprotein IIb–IIIa. Thromb Haemostasis 58:243, 1987

100. Parker RI, Gralnick HR: Identification of platelet glycoprotein IIb/IIIa as the major binding site for released platelet von Willebrand factor. Blood 68:732, 1986

101. Parker RI, Rick ME, Gralnick HR: The effect of calcium on the availability of platelet von Willebrand factor. J Lab Clin Med 106:336, 1985

102. Peerschke EIB: The platelet fibrinogen receptor. Semin Hematol 22:241, 1985

103. Peerschke EI, Coller BS: A murine monoclonal antibody that blocks fibrinogen binding to normal platelets also inhibits interactions with chymotrypsin-treated platelets. Blood 64:59, 1984

104. Peerschke EIB, Francis CW, Marder VJ: Fibrinogen binding to human blood platelets: Effect of γ chain carboxyterminal structure and length. Blood 67:385, 1986

105. Peerschke EIB, Galanakis DK: The synthetic RGDS peptide inhibits the binding of fibrinogen lacking intact α chain carboxyterminal sequences to human blood platelets. Blood 69:950, 1987

106. Peerschke EIB, Galanakis DK: Binding of fibrinogen to ADP-treated platelets: Importance of the A-alpha chain. In Henschen A, Hessel B, McDonagh J, Saldeen T (eds): Fibrinogen-Structural Variants and Interactions, p 369. Berlin, Walter de Gruyter & Co., 1985

107. Peerschke EI, Zucker MB: Fibrinogen receptor exposure and aggregation of human platelets produced by ADP and chilling. Blood 57:663, 1981

108. Phillips DR, Jennings LK, Prasanna HR: Ca^{2+}-mediated association of glycoprotein G (thrombin-sensitive protein, thrombospondin) with human platelets. J Biol Chem 255:11629, 1980

109. Pidard D, Bouillot C, Didry D, Nurden AT: Differential effects of α-chymotrypsin on the GPIIb–IIIa complex of intact platelets at 22°C and at 37°C: Relation to platelet aggregability. Blood 68(Suppl. 1):323a, 1987

110. Pidard P, Montgomery RR, Bennett JS, Kunicki TJ: Interaction of AP-2, a monoclonal antibody specific for the human platelet glycoprotein IIb–IIIa complex with intact platelets. J Biol Chem 258:12482, 1983

111. Piereschbacher MD, Ruoslahti E: Variants of the cell recognition site of fibronectin that retain attachment-promoting activity. Proc Natl Acad Sci USA 81:5985, 1984

112. Pischel KD, Hemler ME, Huang C, Bluestein HG, Woods VL: Use of the monoclonal antibody 12F1 to characterize the differentiation antigen VLA-2. J Immunol 138:226, 1987

113. Plow EF, Ginsberg MH: Specific saturable binding of plasma fibronectin to thrombin-stimulated platelets. J Biol Chem 256:9477, 1981

114. Plow EF, Loftus JC, Levin EG, Fair DS, Dixon D, Forsyth J, Ginsberg MH: Immunologic relationship between platelet membrane glycoprotein GPIIb/IIIa and cell surface molecules expressed by a variety of cells. Proc Natl Acad Sci USA 83:6002, 1986

115. Plow EF, McEver RP, Coller BS, Woods VL, Marguerie GA, Ginsburg MH: Related binding mechanisms for fibrinogen, fibronectin, von Willebrand factor and thrombospondin on thrombin-stimulated human platelets. Blood 66:724, 1985

116. Plow EF, Pierschbacher M, Ruoslahti E, Marguerie GA, Ginsberg MH: The effect of Arg-Gly-Asp containing peptides on fibrinogen and von Willebrand factor binding to platelets. Proc Natl Acad Sci USA 82:8057, 1985

117. Plow EF, Srouji AH, Meyer D, Marguerie G, Ginsberg MH: Evidence that three adhesive proteins interact with a common recognition site on activated platelets. J Biol Chem 259:5388, 1984

118. Pytela R, Pierschbacher MD, Ginsberg MH, Plow EF, Ruoslahti E: Platelet membrane glycoprotein IIb/IIIa: Member of a family of Arg-Gly-Asp-specific adhesion receptors. Science 231:1559, 1986

119. Pytela R, Pierschbacher MD, Ruoslahti E: A 125/115 kDa cell surface receptor specific for vitronectin interacts with the arginine-glycine-aspartic acid adhesion sequence derived from fibronectin. Proc Natl Acad Sci USA 82:5766, 1985

120. Rendu F, Boucheix C, Lebret M, Soria C, Levy-Toledano S: Comparison of the platelet membrane signal transmission induced by thrombin or the mAb ALB6 (CD9). Thromb Haemostasis 58:454, 1987

121. Rosa J-P, George JN, Bainston DF, Nurden AT, Caen JP, McEver RP: Gray platelet syndrome. Demonstration of alpha granule membranes that can fuse with the cell surface. J Clin Invest 80:1834, 1987

122. Ruggeri ZM, DeMarco L, Gatti L, Bader R, Montgomery RR: Platelets have more than one binding site for von Willebrand factor. J Clin Invest 72:1, 1983

123. Ruggeri ZM, Houghten R, Russel S, Zimmerman TS: Inhibition of platelet function with synthetic peptides designed to be high affinity antagonists of fibrinogen binding to platelets. Proc Natl Acad Sci USA 83:5708, 1986

124. Ryckewaert JJ, Valiron O, Newton IA, Concord E, Prenant M, Berthier R: Studies on the involvement of GPIIb/IIIa complex in platelet aggregation with two monoclonal antibodies. Thromb Haemostasis 58:245, 1987

125. Sanchez-Madrid T, Nagy JA, Robbins E, Simon P, Springer TA: A human leukocyte differentiation antigen family with distinct α subunits and a common β-subunit: The lymphocyte function-associated antigen, the C3bi complement receptor, and the p150,95 molecule. J Exp Med 158:1785, 1983

126. Santoro SA, Lawing WJ Jr: Competition for related but nonidentical binding sites on the glycoprotein IIb–IIIa complex by peptides derived from platelet adhesive proteins. Cell 48:867, 1987

127. Shattil SJ, Brass LF, Bennett JS, Pandhi P: Biochemical and functional consequences of dissociation of the platelet membrane glycoprotein IIb–IIIa complex. Blood 66:92, 1985

128. Shattil SJ, Cunningham N, Hoxie JA: Detection of activated human platelets in whole blood using activation-dependent monoclonal antibodies and flow cytometry. Blood 70:307, 1987

129. Shattil SJ, Hoxie J, Cunningham M, Brass LF: Changes in the platelet membrane glycoprotein IIb–IIIa complex during platelet activation. J Biol Chem 260:11107, 1985

130. Shattil SJ, Motulsky HJ, Insel PA, Flaherty L, Brass LF: Expression of fibrinogen receptors during activation and subsequent desensitization of human platelets by epinephrine. Blood 68:1224, 1986

131. Silverstein RL, Leung LLK, Nachman RL: Thrombospondin: A versatile multifunctional glycoprotein. Arteriosclerosis 6:245, 1986

132. Steinberg PE, McEver RP, Shuman MA, Jacques VV, Bainton DF: A platelet alpha-granule membrane protein (GMP-140) is exposed on the plasma membrane after activation. J Cell Biol 101:880, 1985

133. Sugiyama T, Okuma M, Ushikubi F, Sensaki S, Kanaji K, Uchino H: A novel platelet aggregating factor found in a patient with defective collagen-induced platelet aggregation and autoimmune thrombocytopenia. Blood 69:1712, 1987

134. Takada Y, Huang C, Hemler ME: Fibronectin receptor structures in the VLA family of heterodimers. Nature 326:607, 1987

135. Tamkun JW, DeSimone DW, Fonda D, Patel RS, Buck G, Horwitz AF, Hynes RO: Structure of integrin, a glycoprotein involved in the transmembrane linkage between fibronectin and actin. Cell 46:271, 1986

136. Thiagarajan P, Perussia B, DeMarco L, Wells K, Trinchieri G: Membrane proteins on human megakaryocytes and platelets identified by monoclonal antibodies. Am J Hematol 14:255, 1983

137. Trapani Lombardo V, Hodson E, Roberts JR, Kunicki TJ, Zimmerman TS, Ruggeri ZM: Independent modulation of von Willebrand factor and fibrinogen binding to the platelet membrane glycoprotein IIb/IIIa complex as demonstrated by monoclonal antibodies. J Clin Invest 76:1950, 1985

138. Urushihara H, Yamadu KM: Evidence for involvement of more than one class of glycoprotein in cell interactions with fibronectin. J Cell Physiol 126:323, 1986

139. van Regenmortel MH: Antigenic cross-reactivity between proteins and peptides: New insights and applications. Trends Biol Sci 12:237, 1987

140. Watt KWK, Cottrell BA, Strong DD, Doolittle RF: Amino acid sequence studies on the α-chain of human fibrinogen. Overlapping sequences providing the complete sequence. Biochemistry 18:5410, 1979

141. Wencel-Drake JD, Wilhite MR, Kunicki TJ, Furie BC, Furie B, Ginsberg MH:Direct evidence of compound granule formation during secretion of platelet alpha granule constituents. Circulation 74 (Suppl. II):II-422, 1986

142. Westhof E, Altschuh D, Moras D, Bloomer AC, Mondragon A, Klug A, van Regenmortel MHV: Correlation between segmental mobility and the location of antigenic determinants in proteins. Nature 311:123, 1984

143. Williams S, Gralnick H: Inhibition of von Willebrand factor binding to platelets by two recognition site peptides: The pentadecapeptide of the carboxy terminus of the fibrinogen gamma chain and the tetrapeptide Arg-Gly-Asp-Ser. Thromb Res 46:457, 1987

144. Wolff R, Plow EF, Ginsberg MH: Interaction of thrombospondin with resting and stimulated human platelets. J Biol Chem 261:6840, 1986

145. Woods V, Wolff LE, Keller DM: Resting platelets contain a substantial centrally located pool of glycoprotein IIb–IIIa complex which may be accessible to some but not other extracellular proteins. J Biol Chem 261:15242, 1986

146. Zola H, Moore HA, McNamara PJ, Hunter IK, Bradley J, Brooks DA, Gorman DJ, Berndt MC: A membrane protein antigen of platelets and non-T All Dis Markers 2:399, 1984

Part Four Application of Antibody Probes to the Study of Platelet Biochemistry and Molecular Biology

11

The Application of Crossed-Immunoelectrophoresis and Related Immunoassays to the Characterization of Glycoprotein Structure and Function

DOMINIQUE PIDARD

The two-dimensional, crossed-immunoelectrophoresis (CIE) technique was introduced to protein chemistry more than 20 years ago by Laurell and by Clarke and Freeman, as both a qualitative and a quantitative analytical procedure.[28,100,101] Since then, CIE and related techniques have been widely applied to the characterization and quantitation of water-soluble proteins present in various biologic fluids. A comprehensive review of the principles, the practice, and some exemplary applications of these techniques to clinical chemistry can be found in Axelsen, et al.[3]

It is only more recently that CIE has been applied to the study of cell membrane glycoproteins.[8-12,14,27,44,46,63,64,71,73,78,135,140,150,179] One major limitation for the use of CIE in the analysis of amphiphilic molecules, such as membrane glycoproteins, lies in the difficulty in recovering amphiphilic molecules in a soluble form without the loss of their antigenicity and other biologic properties. Such is the case when using powerful but denaturing ionic detergents such as sodium dodecyl sulfate (SDS) for the solubilization of lipid membranes.[74] The solution to this problem has been realized in the use of mild, nonionic detergents of the polyethylene oxide adduct series (known by trade names such as Triton, Berol, Nonidet, Lubrol, Brij, and Tween) which will disperse the lipid bilayer and bind to the hydrophobic domain(s) of intrinsic membrane glycoproteins, generally without major modification of overall protein conformation and biologic activities.[8,10,74,108]

Agarose gel immunoprecipitation techniques thus permit the separate identification of membrane protein components in a complex protein mixture; the characterization of membrane glycoproteins for structure, organization, and function, without the necessity of prior purification; and the quantitation and the comparative analysis of a single membrane component and its analogues in different cell types or various biologic fluids.[8,10] Crossed-immunoelectrophoresis has proved to be highly effective for these purposes, and this technique has been applied to the analysis of plasma membrane and cell wall antigens from various microorganisms and to the characterization of the polypeptide composition of subcellular organelles isolated from eukaryotic cells.[12,27,46,63,73,78,135,140,150] Isolated human vascular endothelial cells and human blood cells of various types, including erythrocytes, platelets, and lymphocytes, have been used to produce polyclonal polyspecific antibodies in rabbits.[9,11,15,44,64,71,179] With use of these antibodies the plasma membranes of these cells have been extensively investigated and characterized by CIE and related techniques.

The aim of this chapter is to review the contributions derived from this particular immunochemical approach that have contributed to our current knowledge of the organization and physiologic functions of platelet plasma membrane glycoproteins.

REFERENCE PATTERN AND IDENTIFICATION OF THE MAJOR ANTIGENIC COMPONENTS OF HUMAN PLATELETS AS SEEN BY CROSSED-IMMUNOELECTROPHORESIS

The establishment of a reproducible reference pattern requires that the different components of the analytical system (i.e., the antibody preparation, the cell extracts, and the agarose gel support) are prepared according to rigorous protocols.[8,10] The salient features of the protocols that we have found to be successful are outlined in the following:

1. *Antibodies:* In all instances, polyclonal, polyspecific antihuman platelet antibodies have been raised in rabbits using either washed intact platelets or isolated plasma membranes.[66,97,155] In the latter, membranes ought to be isolated in the presence of broad-spectrum protease inhibitors to minimize the potential for degradation of the membrane glycoproteins and consequent loss of immunogenic determinants.[10,155] Sera should be harvested over a period of several months from a number of identically immunized rabbits and pooled to minimize the individual variations between rabbits and between bleeds from an individual rabbit that are normally encountered during the immune response to a mixture of antigens.[8,66,97] Furthermore, we have found it useful to regularly replace a number of older animals in the immunization protocol (e.g., those immunized for the longest period) with newly sensitized ones to keep the overall immunization status of the lot as constant as possible and to minimize temporal variations observed in CIE patterns obtained with successive batches of antisera.[10] For optimum results, a purified immunoglobulin G (IgG) fraction of these antisera is almost requisite.[10,66,97] Contaminating plasmin in the IgG preparation must be inhibited by the addition of an inhibitor such as aprotinin, again, to avoid proteolysis of antigens during the second-dimension immunoelectrophoresis.[10,66,97]
2. *Antigens:* Among all of the nonionic detergents mentioned earlier, the one most widely used for the solubilization of proteolipidic cell membranes has been octoxynol (octylphenoxypolyethoxyethanol), commonly known as Triton X-100.[8,10,74] Solutions of 1% v/v Triton X-100 (equivalent to 10.6 g/liter, or 16.7 mmol/liter) in TRIS-glycine or TRIS-barbital buffers, *p*H 8.6, have been used to achieve near complete solubilization of intact platelets or subcellular membrane fractions.[66,97,155] The high efficiency of solubilization is reflected in the recovery of more than 90% of the total platelet protein in the soluble phase as nonsedimentable material.[66,97] The Triton X-100-insoluble fraction consists mainly of cytoskeletal and contractile proteins, such as actin and myosin, and must be eliminated by ultracentrifugation.[129] Because Triton X-100, and nonionic detergents in general, do not inactivate the endogenous cell proteases released at the time of solubilization, the entire solubilization procedure has to be performed rapidly at 4°C, and the solubilized material has to be stored in aliquots at −80°C until use.[10] Depending upon the type of experiment and its purpose(s), protease inhibitors can be added to the solubilization medium. Considerations of the effect(s) of endogenous proteases upon the CIE profile of platelet membrane glycoproteins will be presented in the following sections. Samples should also be analyzed shortly after preparation, to circumvent the formation of nonspecific protein aggregates caused by prolonged storage.[99] For this, high-speed centrifugation of the platelet lysates before frozen storage, and after thawing, will eliminate the nidus for further precipitation by removing insoluble cytoskeletal proteins and protein aggregates.
3. *Agarose gels:* Electrophoresis and immunoprecipitation are performed in gels made of 1% w/v agarose in TRIS-glycine or TRIS-barbital buffers, *p*H 8.6, in the presence of 0.5% to 1.0% v/v Triton X-100.[8,10,66,97,155] The types of agarose that have generally been chosen are those with a moderate electroendosmosis coefficient.[66,97] These allow a moderate passive counter-migration of IgG molecules toward the cathode during the second-dimension electrophoresis. An intermediate gel is usually intercalated between the first-dimension gel strip and the

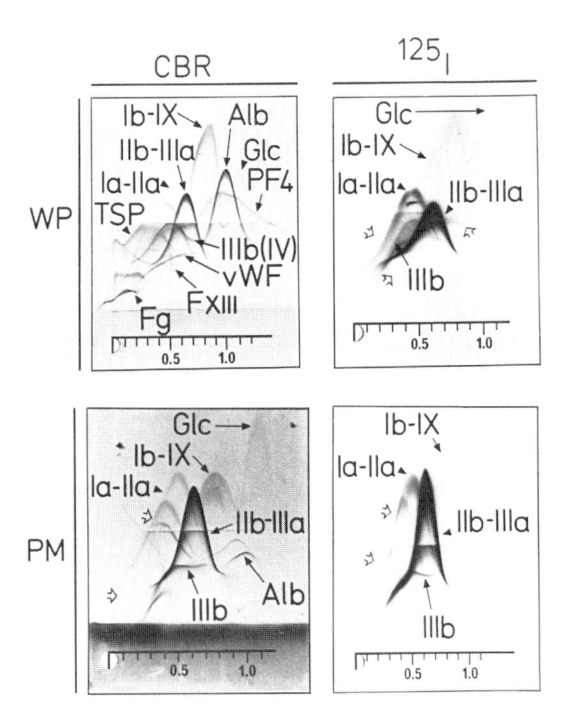

Figure 11-1. Reference patterns of CIE of Triton X-100-soluble proteins from ^{125}I-labeled normal whole platelets (WP, *upper panels*) and isolated plasma membranes (PM, *lower panels*): Coomassie Blue R-stained gels (CBR, *left-hand panels*) and autoradiographs (^{125}I, *right-hand panels*). Platelets were labeled with ^{125}I by the lactoperoxidase-catalyzed method, washed, then solubilized in 0.038 mol/liter TRIS, 0.1 mol/liter glycine (T/G), pH 8.6, by addition of 1% Triton X-100. Plasma membranes were isolated from ^{125}I-labeled platelets by the technique of Barber and Jamieson,[5] then similarly solubilized. Soluble platelet proteins (100 μg) or membrane proteins (20 μg) were separated by first-dimension electrophoresis in the lower gel sections (left to right) at 10 V/cm for 1 h, then electrophoresed at 2 V/cm for 18 h (bottom to top) through a blank intermediate gel into the upper gel sections containing purified rabbit IgG antibodies (1.0–1.3 mg/cm^2) with multispecific antihuman platelet activity. Gels were made of 1% agarose prepared in the T/G buffer containing 0.5% Triton X-100, and T/G also served as the electrode solution. After electrophoresis, gels were washed, dried, stained, and exposed to Kodak X-Omat MA films for 5–10 days. The scale at the bottom of each gel and autoradiograph represents the relative mobility index (RMI) values (one division corresponds to 0.1 unit): The position (in cm) of each given protein or protein complex relative to the center of the sample application well was deduced from the apex of the corresponding immunoprecipitate, and the RMI was calculated by dividing this value by that measured on each plate for albumin (Alb), taken this latter protein as an internal standard (RMI = 1.0). Identified here are α-granule proteins: von Willebrand factor (VWF), thrombospondin (TSP), fibrinogen (Fg), platelet factor 4 (PF4), albumin (Alb); cytosolic proteins: factor XIIIa, α chain (FXIII); plasma membrane glycoproteins (GP) and glycoprotein complexes (*see also* Table 11-1): the GPIb–IX, GPIIb–IIIa, and GPIa–IIa complexes, GPIIIb (GPIV). Open arrowheads point to unidentified, ^{125}I-labeled membrane (glyco)proteins.

second-dimension, antibody-containing upper gel to increase the resolution of the immunoprecipitation pattern in that region of the gel and to provide a convenient mode for inclusion of a specific ligand or a purified antigen between the separated antigenic proteins and the precipitating, polyspecific antibodies (see later discussion).[66,97,155] The CIE is performed at *p*H 8.6, which corresponds to the mean isoelectric point (*p*I) of IgG molecules. At this *p*H, most of the platelet (glyco)proteins, except those with a very basic *p*I, are negatively charged and will migrate toward the anode, according to their net, intrinsic charge.[3,72,116] Concentrations of antibodies in the range of 500–800 μg IgG/cm^2 in the upper gel are usually optimum for the analysis of total platelet proteins (50–100 μg) or plasma membrane proteins (20–50 μg).[66,97,155]

By using these guidelines, a CIE reference pattern has been established for Triton X-100-soluble proteins obtained from whole platelets (Fig. 11-1). This pattern is typical of those obtained with the platelets from more than 200 different healthy individuals. For a given batch of antiplatelet antibodies, excellent reproducibility of the CIE profile for a single platelet sample, analyzed on different occasions, can be obtained.[98] When samples from different subjects are simultaneously analyzed, only minor variations are observed in the relative areas beneath individual immunoprecipitates. These probably reflect individual differences in the content of given platelet constituents. Such differences do not impair straightforward qualitative comparisons of different CIE profiles. However, if one changes from one batch of antisera to another, more appreciable modifications will occur in the reference pattern, affecting the number of immunoprecipitates observed on Coomassie Blue R250(CBR)-stained gels, the relative area that they encompass, and the sharpness of certain precipitin arcs.[10,64,97] Although such modifications are not an obstacle to the identification of the more prominent and best-characterized immunoprecipitates, they may render difficult the comparison of reference patterns established in different laboratories, especially when considering minor or poorly characterized immunoprecipitates.[66,97,99,155]

A CBR-stained immunoplate, similar to that presented in Figure 11-1, would contain at least 20 immunoprecipitates.[66,97,98] As a first approach, most of these immunoprecipitates can be accurately identified from one gel to the next on the basis of the position in the first-dimension gel, drawn from the apex of the precipitin line, relative to that of a chosen internal standard such as albumin (*see* Fig. 11-1 and refer to Table 11-1); the staining intensity and sharpness of the precipitin line; the shape; and the area encompassed on the gel.[8,10] Under standard conditions, all of these characteristics are fairly consistent for a given immunoprecipitate.

Most of the immunoprecipitates seen in whole-platelet extracts are symmetric, but a few are constantly asymmetric, appearing with a trailing edge, "spur," or "shoulder" on the cathodal side, such as the GPIIb–IIIa precipitate, or as a bimodal precipitate, such as those given by thrombospondin or the GPIb–IX complex and glycocalicin (*see* Fig. 11-1). Such asymmetric shapes for membrane or soluble proteins, when analyzed by CIE, have been consistently noted in various cell systems and are commonly regarded as an indication of charge heterogeneity within a single antigenic species, immune cross-reactivity between different but related antigens, or a combination of both.[8,9,10,46,61,63,135] This would be the case for a proteolytic product and its precursor form(s) or for a multiprotein complex and its subunits.[8,10] It should be noted that heterogeneity in the relative molecular mass (M_r) within a single molecular species should have only a slight effect upon the appearance of immunoprecipitates because the agarose gels used for CIE have no sieving properties (unless the molecular mass of a protein complex is higher than 10^8).[8] On the other hand, the area encompassed by a given precipitate is directly proportional, for a given antibody preparation, to the amount of antigen initially present in the protein extract applied to the gel, and this property can be used to make CIE a very quantitative procedure.[28]

Identification and characterization of platelet antigens originating from various subcellular compartments, as described in the following sections, have been carried out using several modifications and adaptations of the basic CIE technique, the details of which have been published in excellent reviews.[8,10]

α-Granule Proteins

Use of Monospecific Antibodies and Purified Antigens

Several of the platelet proteins stored in α granules are strong immunogens and give rise to prominent immunoprecipitates on a typical CIE profile. The location of the precipitation lines formed by proteins, such as fibrinogen, fibronectin, albumin, von Willebrand factor (VWF), or platelet factor 4 (PF4), has been revealed by incorporating into the intermediate gel either a polyclonal, monospecific antibody raised against the purified protein to competitively immunoprecipitate the corresponding antigen present in the platelet extract (Fig. 11-2), or the purified antigen itself.[54,66,68,131,155] In both cases, this results in the displacement of the corresponding immunoprecipitate present within the CIE profile.

In an alternative approach, the addition of trace amounts of ^{125}I-labeled β-thromboglobulin (β-TG) to the platelet extract revealed, upon autoradiographic analysis of the immunoplate, the location of the precipitate given by this protein.[131]

Analysis of Congenitally Deficient Platelets

Platelets of patients with the gray platelet syndrome (GPS) have been shown to be profoundly deficient in most of the secretable proteins normally stored in the platelet α granules (*see also* Chap. 5).[131] The CIE analysis of whole-platelet extracts obtained from two GPS patients with less than 10% of the normal amounts of fibrinogen, VWF, and fibronectin, not only confirmed, by the absence of the corresponding precipitates, the location of these three adhesive proteins and that of PF4 on a normal profile, but also showed the disappearance of a previously unidentified cathodal precipitate with a characteristic bimodal shape.[131] The sodium dodecyl sulfate–polyacrylamide

Table 11-1
Major Properties of the Platelet Membrane Glycoproteins Identified in the CIE Gel System

Glycoprotein	Relative Mobility Index*	Molecular Mass †	Isoelectric Point‡	Specific Interactions Observed in CIE with	Involvement(s) in Platelet Functions§
Plasma Membrane					
IIb–IIIa complex	0.632 ± 0.022			Fibrinogen; Ca^{2+}	Binding site for fibrinogen, fibronectin, von Willebrand factor, and vitronectin (platelet adhesion and aggregation)
IIb	0.623 ± 0.038	142,000	4.6–5.2	Ca^{2+}	
IIIa(III)	0.410 ± 0.026	99,000	4.8–6.0	Ca^{2+}	
Ib–IX complex	0.821 ± 0.025	170,000 (Ib) 17,000 (IX)‖	5.0–6.0 (Ib) 5.8–6.5 (IX)‖	Thrombin; heparin	Receptor for thrombin (Ib); binding site for von Willebrand factor (Ib) (platelet activation and adhesion)
Glycocalicin#	1.114 ± 0.031	140,000‖	4.0–5.0‖	Thrombin	
Ia-IIa complex	0.512 ± 0.031	153,000 (Ia) 138,000 (IIa)	4.8–5.4 (Ia)	Ca^{2+}; heparin	Binding site for collagen (platelet adhesion?)
IIIb (IV)	0.518 ± 0.035	97,000	3.4–5.0		Binding site for thrombospondin (platelet adhesion and aggregation?)
α-Granule Membrane **					
G4 (GMP140/PADGEM?)		146,000		Fibrinogen; heparin	?
G8					?
G18		130,000		Ca^{2+}	?

*Calculated upon CIE analysis of Triton X-100-soluble platelet or plasma membrane proteins as indicated in the legend to Figure 11-1. Each value represents the mean + one standard deviation of at least ten measurements made on different CIE plates.

†Listed are the apparent molecular masses (M_r) estimated for each glycoprotein upon SDS–PAGE analysis performed without disulfide bonds reduction. (Data from Phillips DR, Agin PP: J Biol Chem 252:2121 1977).

‡(Data from McGregor JL, Clemetson KJ, James E, Luscher EF, Dechavanne M: Biochim Biophys Acta 599:473, 1980).

§(Data from Nurden AT: In Vertraete M, Vermylen J, Lijnen R, Arnout J (eds): Thrombosis and Haemostasis 1987. Leuven, Leuven University Press, 1987).

‖(Data from Clemetson KJ: In George JN, Nurden AT, Phillips DR (eds): Platelet Membrane Glycoproteins. New York, Plenum Press, 1985).

#Glycocalicin represents the larger proteolytic product of the outer GPIb α chain. It carries the thrombin- and von Willebrand factor-binding sites associated with GPIb.

**All the data in this section are from Gogstad GO, et al; refer to the text and see Refs. 53, 54, 58, and 59. The GPIIb–IIIa complex has not been taken into account in this section.

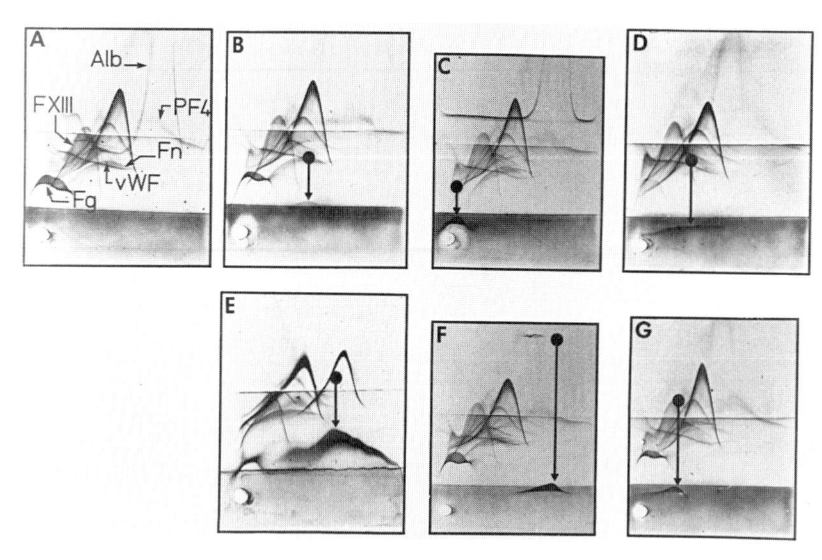

Figure 11-2. Identification of platelet protein antigens in CIE by competitive immunoprecipitation. Triton X-100-soluble platelet proteins (100 μg) were submitted to CIE as described in the legend to Figure 11-1, while the second-dimension intermediate gel contained 50–100 μl of a monospecific goat or rabbit antiserum raised against one of the following purified plasma proteins: fibronectin, Fn (*B*); fibrinogen, Fg (*C*); von Willebrand factor (factor VIII-related antigen), VWF (*D*); platelet factor 4, PF4 (*E*); albumin, Alb (*F*); and factor XIII α chain, FXIII (*G*). In each instance, the black dot and arrow indicate the displacement of the corresponding immunoprecipitate relative to its normal location seen on a CIE profile for which the intermediate gel contains no or a nonimmune rabbit serum (*A*). Shown here are CBR-stained gels.

gel electrophoresis (SDS–PAGE) analysis of this precipitate after its excision from immunoplates obtained using Triton X-100-soluble extracts of normal platelet, demonstrated that thrombospondin (TSP) was the antigen contained within this precipitation line.[131] This particular procedure for polypeptide analysis has been commonly used to identify antigens present in CIE immunoprecipitates, as well as to establish the multipolypeptide nature of certain apparently homogeneous antigenic components.[8,10,125,134]

Analysis of Subcellular Fractions

Crossed-immunoelectrophoresis has also been used to characterize homogeneous fractions of isolated platelet α granules.[51,54] The CIE profile obtained for Triton X-100-soluble extracts of α granules electrophoresed against polyspecific antiplatelet antibodies showed the presence of at least 20 immunoprecipitates, among which those given by fibrinogen, TSP, and PF4 were predominant.[54] Comparison of the CIE profiles obtained for the nonsedimentable fraction of sonicated α granules with those obtained using the soluble proteins secreted from intact platelets upon stimulation by thrombin led Gogstad et al. to conclude that most of those proteins found in purified α granules that can be revealed by CIE are secretable proteins, only a few of which have now been identified.[55]

Cytosolic Antigens

Platelets contain appreciable amounts of the α subunit of the coagulation factor XIII (FXIII), which is found in the platelet cytosol and is recovered as the enzymatically active factor XIII (FXIIIa) in the nonsedimentable fraction of platelets disrupted by sonication.[21,31] The platelet FXIII α chain generates a major cathodal precipitate upon CIE of whole-platelet protein extracts (*see* Fig. 11-1). This precipitate has been identified by using monospecific anti-FXIII antibodies in competitive immunoprecipitation experiments (*see* Fig. 11-2) and by SDS–PAGE polypeptide analysis of this particular precipitate.[68,131] Gogstad et al.[52] have demonstrated that platelet FXIIIa, similar to many other soluble or membrane-associated enzymes, remains an active transglutaminase even after its immunoprecipitation in the presence of a nonionic detergent.[8,12,52,135] This observation further substantiates the contention that CIE is a nondestructive analytical procedure that may thus allow functional investigations of biologically active enzymes or receptors (see later discussion).

It is remarkable that, except for FXIII, no other cytosolic platelet proteins have yet been identified by CIE when using an anti-whole-platelet antibody preparation. Of interest is the observation of Gogstad et al. that addition of semipurified actomyosin to a whole platelet extract did not result in any modification of the CIE profile, suggesting an absence of specific antibodies against contractile proteins in their rabbit antiserum.[54] The inability to visualize functionally and structurally important platelet cytoskeletal or contractile proteins thus appears to be one limitation of the CIE technique.

Plasma Membrane Glycoproteins

Identification and characterization of platelet plasma membrane glycoprotein antigens that give rise to immunoprecipitates in CIE have been based on a comparison of CIE profiles obtained with extracts of isolated plasma membrane versus intact platelets and on various modifications of the CIE technique. These modifications take advantage of particular properties of membrane proteins, such as their availability on the cell surface, the presence of oligosaccharide side chains in their structure, and their status as amphiphilic proteins whose sequence contains hydrophobic, membrane-spanning domain(s).[8,10]

Crossed-Immunoelectrophoresis Pattern of Isolated Plasma Membranes

More than 10 immunoprecipitates can be routinely observed on CBR-stained immunoplates obtained with Triton X-100-soluble extracts of isolated plasma membranes, when electrophoresed against rabbit antiplatelet antibodies (*see* Fig. 11-1).[66] When the CIE analysis is performed using polyspecific antibodies raised against isolated plasma membranes, up to 20 immunoprecipitates can be detected after CBR-staining.[155] Except for traces of fibrinogen, VWF, or albumin, none of the previously mentioned α-granule or cytosolic antigens are detected in the CIE profile of isolated membranes (*see* Fig. 11-1).[58,66,97] On the basis of simply shape and position, only a few of the immunoprecipitates seen with isolated membranes can be related directly to the immunoprecipitates observed in the more complex pattern given by whole platelets.[58,66] These include the major, well-stained immunoprecipitate containing the GPIIb-IIIa complex and that given by the GPIb-IX complex; the latter, because of its typical anodal location.

Surface Modifications of Membrane Proteins

Chemical or biochemical modifications of membrane components using membrane-impermeable reagents, including radioisotope-labeling procedures, are widely used to assess the structure, organization, and functions of membrane proteins. Among various radiolabeling procedures, the lactoperoxidase-catalyzed iodination technique has the advantage that it has little or no effect on intrinsic properties of platelet membrane proteins, including molecular mass, isoelectric point, subunit organization, and biologic activities, features that can all be analyzed when using a nondenaturing, analytical procedure such as CIE.[30,116,141,143,146]

Crossed-immunoelectrophoresis of ^{125}I-labeled platelets or isolated membranes followed by autoradiography allows the identification of five to six immunoprecipitates containing ^{125}I-labeled, surface-oriented membrane proteins (*see* Fig. 11-1).[58,64,66,97,99] Excision and SDS-PAGE analysis of the labeled antigens has made possible the identification of GPIa, GPIb, GPIIa, GPIIb, GPIIIa, and GPIIIb as those membrane glycoproteins detectable in CIE (*see* Fig. 11-1 and Table 11-1), as shown by Kunicki et al. and Gogstad et al.[58,97,125,134] Later investigations by Berndt et al. have also revealed the presence of GPIX on the CIE profile (discussed later).[7] No major qualitative differences were noted between the autoradiographic profiles observed with ^{125}I-labeled extracts of whole platelets and isolated plasma membranes, indicating that isolation of plasma membranes under rigorous conditions does not result in extensive modifications of the membrane protein composition and organization, and that isolated membranes should accurately reflect the physicochemical and biochemical properties of native plasma membranes.[58,99]

Treatment of intact platelets by α-chrymotrypsin resulted in the nearly complete disappearance of those immunoprecipitates corresponding to membrane glycoproteins, such as the GPIIb-IIIa and the GPIb-IX complexes, whereas the immunoadsorption of the polyspecific antiserum with increasing concentrations of intact, washed platelets led to the progressive elimination of all precipitates seen on the CIE profile of isolated membranes, confirming that most of the platelet membrane proteins immunoprecipitated during CIE are restricted to the outer surface of the membrane.[66,155]

Interactions Specific for Membrane Glycoproteins in Nondenaturing Agarose Gels

Because of their stereospecificity toward particular oligosaccharide sequences, lectins are potent tools in procedures designed for identification, characterization, and purification of glycosylated membrane proteins.[30,115,119] A special procedure, called crossed-immunoaffinoelectrophoresis, has been designed to use lectins during the CIE analysis of a complex mixture of glycoproteins.[13] According to this technique, a purified lectin can be either directly added to the protein extract, incorporated into the first-dimension gel, or incorporated into the intermediate gel before the onset of the second-dimension electrophoresis. Depending on the chosen approach and whether or not the lectin chosen can itself precipitate the ligand, its addition to the CIE system will result in modifications in the appearance of one, or of several, immunoprecipitates, allowing the identification of glycoprotein antigens and the partial characterization of their usually complex carbohydrate moieties (Fig. 11-3).[8,10,13,66]

With this procedure, most of the membrane proteins identified in CIE profiles have been found to be substantially glycosylated.[66] Furthermore, the differential specificity seen in CIE toward certain major membrane glycoproteins by several common lectins, including wheat germ agglutinin, *Ricinus communis* agglutinin, *Lens culinaris* agglutinin, and concanavalin A (*see* Fig. 11-3), agreed well with data previously reported concerning the relative specificity of these lectins for the same platelet membrane glycoproteins, as well as with the more recently characterized structure of the major oligosaccharide side chains that are found in GPIb, GPIIb, and GPIIIa.[66,115,119,155,171,172]

Treatment of intact platelets with neuraminidase before the solubilization with Triton X-100 resulted in a cathodic shift in the position of immunoprecipitates containing platelet surface sialoglycoproteins.[66] This effect was the consequence of a reduced negative charge resulting from the removal of terminal sialic acid residues. Three membrane antigens present in the CIE pattern were thus affected by desialation, including the GPIIb-IIIa complex and β_2-microglobulin.[66,155] Although there is still some uncertainty about whether platelet-associated HLA antigens should be considered as integral membrane components or as adsorbed antigens, β_2-microglobulin has been shown to be present on the platelet surface and to be immunoprecipitated during CIE, giving rise to a very cathodal precipitate that has been identified by incubating pre-formed immunoplates with ^{125}I-labeled antibodies to this protein.[58,64,65,83]

The potential amphiphilic nature of the platelet membrane glycoproteins, detected by CIE, was first investigated by use of charge-shift electrophoresis.[66] This method is based on the fact that only proteins containing a hydrophobic (membrane) domain can bind appreciable amounts of nonionic detergent.[29,74,108] If small amounts of a charged detergent, such as the cationic detergent cetyltrimethylammonium bromide (CTAB) or the anionic detergent deoxycholate (DOC), are added to the neutral detergent Triton X-100, this will result in the formation of mixed, charged detergent micelles that will bind to any amphiphilic protein and, thereby, significantly contribute to its apparent net charge, resulting in a slower or a faster mobility of this protein during the first-dimension of electrophoresis.[8,10,75] Alternatively, protein hydrophobicity has been evaluated by incorporating a hydrophobic, phenyl-Sepharose matrix into the intermediate gel (crossed-hydrophobic interaction-immunoelectrophoresis), in which event only amphiphilic proteins will be retained or retarded during the second-dimension electrophoresis because of hydrophobic interactions with the matrix.[8,10] These two approaches have both indicated that all major platelet membrane glycoproteins identified in the CIE pattern are amphiphilic molecules and can be thus regarded as integral membrane glycoproteins.[66]

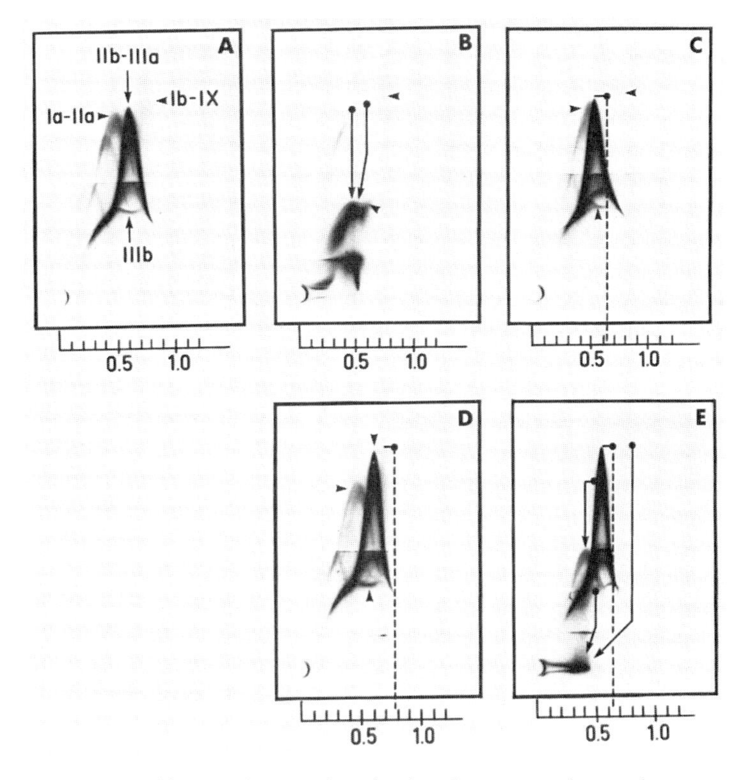

Figure 11-3. Use of lectins to identify and characterize platelet plasma membrane glycoproteins in CIE (crossed-immunoaffinoelectrophoresis). Triton X-100-soluble membrane proteins (20 μg) obtained from ^{125}I-labeled platelets were submitted to CIE essentially as described in the legend to Figure 11-1, except that the first-dimension agarose gels contained various lectins and, when necessary for lectin activity, divalent cations (Ca^{2+}, Mg^{2+}, Mn^{2+}). The autoradiographs were obtained for CIE plates exposed for 5 days on Kodak X-Omat MA films and show the pattern of precipitation seen with: (*A*) no lectins in the first-dimension gel; (*B*) concanavalin A (ConA), 100 μg/ml; (*C*) *Lens culinaris* agglutinin (LcA), 100 μg/ml; and (*D*) wheat germ agglutinin (WGA), 10 μg/ml and (*E*) 100 μg/ml. The black dots and arrows indicate the displacement of immunoprecipitates, the dashed lines indicate the retardation of glycoproteins during first-dimension electrophoresis. Note that the GPIIb–IIIa complex strongly interacts with ConA (monosaccharide specificity: αMan, αGlc) (*B*) and is retarded through interactions with LcA (monosaccharide specificity: αMan, αGlc) (*C*) and WGA (monosaccharide specificity: βNeuAc, GlcNAc) (*E*), whereas the highly sialylated GPIb–IX complex is a major ligand for WGA (*D*) and can even be directly precipitated by the multimeric lectin, together with GPIIIb (*E*). The GPIa–IIa complex appears to interact with both ConA (*B*) and WGA (*E*).

Inherited Molecular Abnormalities of the Platelet Plasma Membrane

Analysis of Triton X-100-soluble extracts of platelets obtained from patients affected with specific and well-characterized membrane molecular defects affecting glycoprotein composition has helped to identify certain antigens detected by CIE.[44,70,97,98]

Thus, analysis of platelets from patients with type I Glanzmann's thrombasthenia, which are almost devoid of both GPIIb and GPIIIa, demonstrated a complete disappearance of the major, central immunoprecipitate seen on both CBR-stained gels and autoradiographs (*see* Fig. 11-1), suggesting that one or both of the missing glycoprotein(s) is (are) the major antigen(s) found in this immunoprecipitate (see next section).[70,97,98] Similarly, analysis of platelets obtained from patients with the Bernard-Soulier syndrome, lacking the GPIb–

IX complex, showed the disappearance of an anodal precipitate, later confirmed to contain GPIb–IX by SDS–PAGE polypeptide analysis and use of monoclonal antibodies.[7,70,97] A detailed discussion of these and other inherited abnormalities of platelet membrane glycoproteins is found in Chapter 5 of this book.

ORGANIZATION AND DISTRIBUTION OF PLATELET MEMBRANE GLYCOPROTEINS AS DETERMINED BY CROSSED-IMMUNOELECTROPHORESIS

As will be evident in the following sections, the recent availability of monospecific antibodies, either polyclonal or monoclonal, has made an immunochemical procedure such as CIE a major approach to investigating the supramolecular organization and distribution of membrane glycoproteins.

The Glycoprotein IIb–IIIa Complex

Immunochemical Evidence that Glycoproteins IIb and IIIa Exist as Complexes in Solution

That GPIIb and GPIIIa do indeed exist as a complex (designated GPIIb–IIIa) in Triton X-100-soluble extracts of whole platelets or isolated plasma membranes was suggested by a series of observations made in early CIE studies: (1) a single, major ^{125}I-labeled immunoprecipitate is absent from the CIE pattern of thrombasthenic platelets, which lack both GPIIb and GPIIIa; (2) this immunoprecipitate contains both glycoproteins, as revealed by SDS–PAGE polypeptide analysis; and (3) this immunoprecipitate sometimes appears with a pattern of partial dissociation into multiple components.[66,70,155] One initial hypothesis was that dissociation arose from the proteolytic processing of a single antigen, but this explanation was later dismissed, and it is likely that what is now recognized as a partial dissociation of the GPIIb–IIIa complex resulted, during these early experiments, from the addition of ethylenediaminetetraacetic acid (EDTA) to the medium used to isolate the platelet plasma membranes.[65,66,99,155,156]

Because no clear-cut conclusions could be drawn from the SDS–PAGE polypeptide analysis of major immunoprecipitates when using the polyspecific antiplatelet rabbit antibodies, owing to the considerable overlap of multiple immunoprecipitates with the one of interest, an alternative approach was designed by Kunicki et al., who used, as precipitating antibody, a monospecific human alloantibody, IgG-L.[66,99] This IgG alloantibody, which had been generated by a polytransfused thrombasthenic patient, was reactive with all normal platelets, nonreactive with the patient's own platelets, and induced a thrombasthenialike state when added to normal platelets.[36,104] The IgG-L antibody was shown to specifically react with, and precipitate during CIE, a major membrane antigen, giving rise to a single precipitin arc that is identical with the major arc seen in a normal CIE profile.[70,99,152] As determined by SDS–PAGE analysis, this precipitate contained both GPIIb and GPIIIa.[99]

Findings similar to that reported by Kunicki et al. have also been obtained by Jenkins et al., who used polyclonal rabbit antibodies raised against copurified GPIIb and GPIIIa. These antibodies specifically immunoprecipitated both glycoproteins within a single arc during CIE analysis of Triton X-100-soluble extracts of whole platelets or isolated plasma membranes.[81]

A trailing, and even a partial splitting, of the cathodal arm of the GPIIb–IIIa arc is frequently observed, indicating antigenic heterogeneity of the GPIIb–IIIa complex.[61,66,70,99,155,156] Polypeptide analysis of that part of the precipitate does not reveal the presence of any ^{125}I-labeled membrane proteins other than GPIIb and GPIIIa nor is there any difference in the relative amounts of the two glycoproteins or in their relative molecular masses, thus this immunochemical heterogeneity does not result from partial dissociation or limited proteolysis of the complex.[99] Such heterogeneity could arise from the existence of soluble polymers containing, in addition to the GPIIb–IIIa complex itself, cytoskeletal and contractile proteins such as actin.[42,110,136]

Solubilization of platelets or isolated plasma membranes with Triton X-100 in the presence of EDTA, or addition of EDTA to the extracts before CIE analysis, results in the progressive disappearance of the major precipitate, accompanied by the concomitant appearance of two new immunoprecipitates at separate locations.[65,79,89,99,152] A large body of evidence now exists that supports the contention that, upon dissociation of the GPIIb–IIIa complex, each of the immunoprecipitated glycoprotein subunits is restricted to one of these new precipitates. The GPIIb precipitate has an electrophoretic mobility similar to that of the complex during the first-dimension separation, whereas GPIIIa is found within a more cathodal precipitate (*see* Table 11-1 and Fig. 11-4).[99] Such evidence includes SDS-PAGE analysis of antigens in each of these new precipitates, showing the presence of ^{125}I-labeled polypeptide antigens with the characteristics of GPIIb and GPIIIa, respectively; the relative intensity of ^{125}I-surface-labeled antigens in each precipitate, consistent with the known capacity of each glycoprotein to incorporate iodine; the marked interaction of the more cathodal antigen with concanavalin A in crossed-affinoimmunoelectrophoresis studies, consistent with the known specificity of this lectin for GPIIIa; and the specific competitive precipitation of either of these two precipitates when monospecific rabbit antibodies to GPIIb or GPIIIa are incorporated in the intermediate gel.[65,71,79,99,115,143]

As noted by Hagen et al., only free GPIIIa shows a line of partial immunochemical identity with the GPIIb-IIIa complex (*see*, for instance, Fig. 11-4), whereas free GPIIb appears to express, following dissociation from GPIIIa, otherwise cryptic antigenic determinants.[65,79,99] On the other hand, as previously mentioned, free GPIIb has a mobility during the first-dimension electrophoresis that is very similar to that of the GPIIb-IIIa complex, whereas free GPIIIa, with a lower mobility, appears to be slightly less negatively charged. Taken together, these observations would suggest that, under the conditions used for CIE analysis, GPIIb contributes a major part to the net electric charge of the complex, whereas GPIIIa contributes significantly to its antigenicity.

It is often noted that each free glycoprotein does not form a single immunoprecipitate but, rather, generates a series of closely superimposed precipitation lines.[65,79,99] Although this has not been investigated further in detail, such immunochemical heterogeneity of each free subunit may result from various causes, such as (1) limited proteolytic degradation of one or both glycoproteins, either "in vivo," "in vitro" during isolation and solubilization of the platelets, or subsequent to the dissociation of the complex, as GPIIb has been shown to be more susceptible to the attack by proteolytic enzymes when dissociated from GPIIIa; (2) the formation of homopolymers, particularly GPIIIa which contains several intrachain disulfide bonds and can form aggregates through disulfide exchange; and (3) the existence of true polymorphisms of these two glycoproteins, for example, reflecting the existence of several platelet-specific, multiallelic alloantigens associated with either GPIIIa or GPIIb (*see* Chap. 6).[24,43,82,93,143,156] Any of these factors may thus result in modifications of the antigenic structure of the molecule.

Unless the GPIIb-IIIa complex is exposed to well-defined physicochemical conditions (*see* later discussion), it reproducibly appears in CIE gels as the single major immunoprecipitate described previously. In particular, there is no evidence for appreciable amounts of "spontaneously" dissociated or preexisting free GPIIb and free GPIIIa within the membrane of resting platelets, given the limits of sensitivity of the CIE technique.[56,65,99] Furthermore, GPIIb and GPIIIa are restricted to those precipitates just described, which contain no other proteins.[97] Finally, replacement of Triton X-100 with other nonionic detergents, or a decrease in the concentration of Triton X-100 in the solubilizing medium to 0.05% (0.53 g/liter) does not result in the separation of GPIIb from GPIIIa during first-dimension electrophoresis.[97,152] Decreasing the amounts of nonionic detergent that are bound to amphiphilic proteins has been shown to result in an increased mobility of such proteins in gels, which then facilitates the separation of two closely migrating, but still noncomplexed, proteins.[14] It is, thus, most likely that the GPIIb-IIIa complex, as detected by CIE, reflects a true membrane association of the two glycoproteins rather than a nonspecific association of these proteins in solution.

The precise physicochemical characterization of the GPIIb-IIIa complex and its subunits has been accomplished through the use of various chromatographic procedures and by sucrose density gradient ultracentrifugation of Triton X-100-soluble extracts of isolated, ^{125}I-labeled plasma membranes.[82,144] This information is presented in detail in Chapter 2 and can also be found in a recent review by Nurden et al.[130]

Factors Regulating Complex Formation Between Glycoprotein IIb and Glycoprotein IIIa

Effect of Divalent Cations, *p*H, and Temperature. In their initial studies, both Kunicki et al.[99] and Gogstad et al.[56] noted that the minimal concentration of EDTA required to obtain partial dissociation of the GPIIb-IIIa complex slightly exceeds the total concentration of calcium (Ca^{2+}) and magnesium (Mg^{2+}) normally present in extracts of either whole platelets or isolated plasma membranes. Furthermore, dissociation was found to proceed to completion as a function of both time and EDTA concentration.[99] Divalent cation chelators other than EDTA, such as ethylene glycol-bis(β-aminoethyl ether)-*N*, *N'*-tetraacetic acid (EGTA) and sodium citrate, also have similar deleterious effects on the GPIIb-IIIa complex.[56,79,99]

The chelator does not interfere directly with one or both glycoproteins but, rather, acts on the availability of divalent cations as shown by: (1) dissociation of GPIIb-IIIa can be induced by dialyzing Triton X-100-soluble extracts against a Ca^{2+}-free, chelator-free buffer; (2) [^{14}C]EDTA does not label any of the immunoprecipitates containing GPIIb, GPIIIa, or the GPIIb-IIIa complex, when added to the protein sample before CIE;* (3) dissociation can be prevented by the simultaneous addition of equimolar amounts of EDTA and $CaCl_2$ to the sample; and (4) dissociation can be reversed by the addition of a molar excess of $CaCl_2$ to the sample after incubation with EDTA.[56,79,88,99] This latter observation is important because it clearly indicates that dissociation of the GPIIb-IIIa complex in solution is a fully reversible process, one not involving proteolysis or denaturation.

Similar observations have been made with isolated plasma membranes that were incubated for short periods with EDTA or EGTA before washing and solubilization in the absence of chelators.[56,99] Here, appearance of free GPIIb and free GPIIIa in the CIE pattern clearly indicated that the state of association of the two glycoproteins truly depends upon the availability of membrane-bound calcium.[99] Again, as observed by Gogstad et al., reassociation of GPIIb and GPIIIa, which had been first separated within intact, isolated membranes by exposure to EDTA, could be obtained by readdition of $CaCl_2$ to the membrane preparation.[56] As judged by CIE, the time course of reassociation is slower at *p*H 8.6 than that of dissociation (a phenomenon also noted to be more pronounced for Triton X-100-solubilized glycoproteins).[56,99] This suggests that (re)association of GPIIb and GPIIIa in the plane of the lipid bilayer might be facilitated, compared with that observed with glycoproteins in solution, by a favorable orientation and a restricted mobility of the two molecules, together with the presence of potentially high local concentrations of Ca^{2+}, a result of loose interactions of this cation with membrane lipids. These findings favor the hypothesis that GPIIb and GPIIIa are already present as complexes within isolated plasma membranes.[43,56,79,99]

There is some inconsistency in reports on use of the CIE approach about the relative ability of different divalent cations to support complex formation. Although there is a general agreement concerning the central role played by calcium in this phenomenon, there is some disagreement concerning the replacement of Ca^{2+} by other divalent cations for the maintenance of the GPIIb-IIIa complex.[56,79,99] Actually, two different experimental situations have to be considered: that in which a given divalent cation is added simultaneously with the chelator, to test its protective effect on the dissociation of the complex, in which case Mg^{2+} (but not Mn^{2+}, Cu^{2+}, Sr^{2+}, or Zn^{2+}) was occasionally found to behave similarly to Ca^{2+} when added in molar amounts similar to that of the chelator; and second; that in which a divalent cation is added in molar excess to the chelator to investigate its ability to support reassociation of already separated glycoproteins, in which case only Ca^{2+} has been reported to support the re-formation of the GPIIb-IIIa complex.[56,79,99] Magnesium and other divalent cations have generally been found ineffective in the latter, with the exception of data reported by Howard et al.,[79] who noted a complete reassociation upon addition of Ca^{2+}, Mg^{2+}, Mn^{2+}, or Zn^{2+}.[56,79,99] Although a rather complex situation may arise from rapid exchanges or displacements of one given cation for another that affects the chelator, the GPIIb-IIIa complex, and its separated subunits, it would seem that the GPIIb-IIIa complex still shows a rather restricted specificity toward calcium ions for its formation and stability.

Similar findings have been reported, in parallel to the forementioned CIE studies, by Jennings and Phillips and by Fujimura and Phillips, who used different biochemical approaches, about the stability of the GPIIb-IIIa complex in solution and within isolated plasma membranes (*see also* Chap. 2).[43,82,130]

Physicochemical variables other than divalent cation availability can also affect the stability of the GPIIb-IIIa complex, i.e., *p*H and

*Kunicki, T.J.: Personal communication, 1981.

temperature. On the basis of CIE analysis, Rosa et al. have noted that dissociation of Triton X-100-solubilized GPIIb–IIIa complexes in the presence of EDTA is much faster at 22°C than at 4°C, an effect that can be ascribed, in part, to the influence of temperature upon the rate of chemical reactions.[152] However, information gained through an examination of the effects of EDTA on the GPIIb–IIIa complex in intact platelets have raised the possibility that temperature may also influence the conformation of the complex and, thus, the accessibility of complex-bound Ca^{2+} to chelators.

On the other hand, *p*H appears to also affect the stability of GPIIb–IIIa, as shown by Gogstad et al. and Rosa et al., who found that at *p*H 7.4, both Triton X-100-solubilized and membrane-borne GPIIb–IIIa complexes are only minimally dissociated in the presence of EDTA or EGTA at either 4°C or 22°C.[56,152] Dissociation progressively increases, as judged by CIE analysis, when the medium is alkalinized, up to a *p*H 8.7 to 9.0.[56,152] The stabilizing effect of neutral *p*H or, inversely, the deleterious effect of alkaline *p*H toward the GPIIb–IIIa complex is also evident from reassociation experiments. Reassociation takes place more rapidly, and with a lower requirement for Ca^{2+}, at *p*H 7.5 than at *p*H 9.0.[56] Although the apparent association constant of EDTA for Ca^{2+} is lowered at neutral *p*H, increasing the concentration of the chelator at *p*H 7.4 to compensate for this effect did not facilitate the dissociation of the complex.[56] A direct influence of *p*H upon the stability of the GPIIb–IIIa complex is also evident from the observation that elution of purified GPIIb–IIIa from immunoaffinity columns by alkalinization of the medium to *p*H 11.5 ultimately results in the dissociation of the two subunits, even in the continuous presence of 0.5 mmol/liter $CaCl_2$, unless the *p*H of the effluent is rapidly neutralized.*

Glycoprotein IIb and Glycoprotein IIIa as Calcium-Binding Proteins. Because the purified or specifically immunoprecipitated GPIIb–IIIa complex appears to consist solely of GPIIb and GPIIIa in a 1 : 1 molar ratio, with no evidence that additional polypeptides are part of this complex (including the ubiquitous, regulatory calcium-binding protein calmodulin), and in view of the findings presented earlier, an obvious question is whether either GPIIb, GPIIIa, or both, can directly interact with divalent cations.[82] The CIE procedure again has been of major use in solving this particular question.

Incubating preformed CIE immunoplates with $^{45}Ca^{2+}$, followed by the autoradiographic analysis of the washed and dried gels, has enabled Gogstad et al. to demonstrate a marked labeling of the GPIIb–IIIa complex by $^{45}Ca^{2+}$, together with few other platelet membrane (glyco)proteins.[59] Incorporation of $^{45}Ca^{2+}$ increased after the unlabeled, complex-bound Ca^{2+} had been depleted with an EDTA-containing medium.[59] As noted by the authors, the binding of $^{45}Ca^{2+}$ to the immunoprecipitated GPIIb–IIIa occurs at *p*H 7.4, even in the presence of a twofold molar excess of EDTA, whereas binding at *p*H 9.0 is abolished in the presence of chelators, suggesting that the binding is specific and involves site(s) of high affinity at neutral *p*H.[59] Desialation of membrane glycoproteins on intact platelets, after incubation with neuraminidase, partly decreased the capacity of the GPIIb–IIIa immunoprecipitate to bind $^{45}Ca^{2+}$, suggesting that some of the labeling may have proceeded through the loose interaction of Ca^{2+} with negatively charged sialic acid residues, whereas the labeling of the highly sialylated GPIb was found to be totally abolished by a prior treatment with neuraminidase.[59]

With intact platelets that have been incubated with $^{45}CaCl_2$ before sedimentation, solubilization, and CIE analysis, it was observed that only preincubation of platelets with EDTA permitted the incorporation of $^{45}Ca^{2+}$ into the GPIIb–IIIa complex, providing further support for the hypothesis that there exists a tightly bound, GPIIb–IIIa-associated Ca^{2+} pool and indicating that at least some of this Ca^{2+} is present on the extracellular portion of the complex.[59] Addition of ADP and fibrinogen to $^{45}Ca^{2+}$-labeled platelets and their subsequent aggregation did not result in a further incorporation of $^{45}Ca^{2+}$ into the GPIIb–IIIa complex.[59]

These data appear to agree well with those reported by Peerschke et al. and by Brass and Shattil, who both investigated, in detail, the capacity of intact platelets to take up and bind $^{45}Ca^{2+}$.[16,138,139] Their findings led to the conclusion that each GPIIb–IIIa complex should contain at least two high-affinity ($K_d = 1 \times$

*Pidard, D.: Unpublished observation, 1982.

10^{-9} mol/liter) and six low-affinity ($K_d = 4 \times 10^{-7}$ mol/liter) Ca^{2+}-binding sites, whose occupancy appears to be essential for both the stability and the functional properties of the complex.[16,138,139] It appears that the high-affinity sites show an absolute specificity for Ca^{2+}, whereas, at the low-affinity sites, Ca^{2+} might be partly replaceable by Mg^{2+} (*see* following section).[16,139]

A crucial observation made by Gogstad et al. was that free (EDTA-dissociated) GPIIb and GPIIIa are both able to bind some $^{45}Ca^{2+}$ when pre-formed CIE immunoplates are incubated with $^{45}Ca^{2+}$ at *p*H 7.4, even in the presence of a twofold molar excess of EDTA.[59] This would thus establish both glycoproteins as calcium-binding proteins (CaBPs), rather than as proteins susceptible to association through "Ca^{2+} bridges." That binding of calcium ions to free GPIIb may affect its conformation was later demonstrated by Charo et al., who showed that GPIIb has a different mobility during SDS-PAGE depending on whether the electrophoresis is performed in the presence of $CaCl_2$ or in the presence of EDTA.[25] This entails a change in the relative molecular mass from 130,000 (in the presence of EDTA) to 118,000 (in the presence of $CaCl_2$).[25] Although data on the primary amino acid sequence of GPIIb indicates the presence of four "calcium-binding loops" within the GPIIb α subunit, no similar domains have been found in the amino acid sequence of GPIIIa, thus raising some questions concerning the mechanism(s) by which this glycoprotein may bind divalent cations (*see also* Chap. 2).[40,148]

Effects of Chelators on the Glycoprotein IIb-IIIa Complex in Intact Platelets. Early CIE experiments have shown that no dissociation of the GPIIb-IIIa complex occurs in the plasma membrane of intact platelets that have been isolated from plasma and washed in the presence of EDTA at *p*H 7.4 and 20°C.[66,97,155] This finding suggests that on intact platelets not all complex-bound Ca^{2+} is displaceable under these conditions. Subsequently, evidence has been presented that, in platelets exposed for short periods (less than 15 min) to millimolar concentrations of EDTA at 37°C, the GPIIb-IIIa complex may undergo structural changes "in situ," as revealed by CIE analysis.[144] These include a marked decrease of the major immunoprecipitate, the appearance of precipitates given by free GPIIb and free GPIIIa and, most notably, the appearance of a new cathodal immunoprecipitate in a position identical with that of free GPIIIa. This new antigenic species is immunologically related to the GPIIb-IIIa complex and has been found to contain both GPIIb and GPIIIa.[144] However, it loses antigenic and biologic properties specific to the functional GPIIb-IIIa complex, i.e., the capacity to bind "complex-specific" monoclonal antibodies and fibrinogen.[144]

By using a similar CIE approach, Zucker et al. have noted an absence of modifications to the GPIIb-IIIa complex in platelets exposed to EDTA at 37°C.[183] Nonetheless, these findings corroborate previous observations made by Shattil et al. and by Fitzgerald and Phillips, who used a nondenaturing polyacrylamide gel electrophoresis system, and sucrose density gradient ultracentrifugation, respectively, to investigate the state of association of GPIIb and GPIIIa in platelets exposed to EDTA at 37°C.[39,154] Both studies demonstrated that formation of homo- or heteropolymers of GPIIb, GPIIIa and, potentially, other proteins, may follow an initial dissociation of the GPIIb-IIIa complex in the membrane of intact platelets exposed to chelators at 37°C.[39,154] This polymerization step is an irreversible process that cannot be reversed by a subsequent readdition of Ca^{2+}.[39,130,146,154] Thus, this phenomenon could explain both the irreversible loss of aggregability and the reduced capacity to bind $^{45}Ca^{2+}$ that are observed with platelets treated at 37°C with EDTA (*see also* Chap. 2).[139,144,154,182]

Other Factors. Inclusion of protease inhibitors in the solubilizing medium has not been found to have any significant effect upon the structure or the stability of the GPIIb-IIIa complex, as estimated by CIE.[56,65,99]

Similarly, neither the addition of ADP and fibrinogen to Triton X-100-soluble extracts of isolated plasma membranes prepared in the presence of EDTA, nor the prior activation of intact platelets by ADP or thrombin, appears to modify the reassociation/dissociation or the Ca^{2+}-binding capacities of the GPIIb-IIIa complex.[56,59] These findings suggest that the activation of platelets does not result in gross modifications in the conformation of the GPIIb-IIIa complex.

A charge effect has been suggested, by Karpatkin et al., to play a role in the formation of the GPIIb-IIIa complex.[85] They noted, using

CIE, that for Triton X-100-solubilized membrane glycoproteins that have been treated by neuraminidase a "spontaneous" reassociation of GPIIb and GPIIIa, which had been first dissociated with EDTA, could be obtained in the absence of calcium. That negatively charged sialic acid residues may affect the association of GPIIb and GPIIIa into heterodimers was further suggested in this study by the observation that addition of the cationic peptide tetralysine permitted the reassociation of separated and fully sialated GPIIb and GPIIIa in the absence of free Ca^{2+}, most likely through the neutralization of negative charges.[85] Further investigations are clearly required to confirm and elucidate this potential influence of glycoprotein charge upon the stability of the GPIIb-IIIa complex.

In conclusion to this section, it might be said that given the data accumulated by CIE and other analytical techniques, briefly summarized here, the GPIIb-IIIa complex is most likely to be found as such in the membrane of intact, resting platelets that are immersed in a plasma milieu containing millimolar concentrations of divalent cations. This view is entirely supported by the positive reactivity of intact platelets with well-characterized, complex-specific monoclonal antibodies (*see* the following section and Chap. 12).

Several physicochemical variables, including *p*H and temperature, however, may exert some influence on the stability of the complex or on the conformation of its subunits, thus modifying its propensity to dissociate in the presence of chelators. This latter point should be remembered when manipulating platelets for experimental purposes under drastic conditions of low calcium concentrations, *p*H, and temperature, because such manipulations may lead to the irreversible denaturation of the GPIIb-IIIa complex.

Interaction of the Glycoprotein IIb-IIIa Complex with Monospecific Antibodies: Crossed-Immunoelectrophoresis as an Approach to the Analysis of Epitope Specificity

Possibly, one of the most important applications of CIE has been its use in defining the antigenic specificity of various monospecific, polyclonal or monoclonal antibodies, particularly those directed against the GPIIb-IIIa complex. So far, only the CIE permits the unambiguous, reliable, rapid separation and visualization simultaneously on the same agarose gel of the three molecular species of interest, namely, GPIIb, GPIIIa, and GPIIb-IIIa complex. This can be accomplished through partial dissociation of this complex in the presence of EDTA under controlled conditions of *p*H and temperature. Furthermore, membrane glycoproteins retain much of their antigenic properties under the conditions used for the CIE and are thus amenable to immunochemical characterization.

Other techniques designed for the determination of antigen specificity, such as immunoaffinity chromatography or indirect immunoprecipitation in aqueous phase, require an independent analytical procedure, routinely SDS-PAGE, for analysis and identification of the reactive antigens. At the same time, immunoblotting techniques coupled to high-resolution SDS-PAGE separation of antigenic proteins are limited in their application by the denaturing effects of SDS on noncovalent protein complexes and by the incomplete renaturation of proteins during electrotransfer onto blotting membranes.

Monoclonal Antibodies. An increasing number of murine monoclonal antibodies are now being produced that show reactivity with the GPIIb-IIIa complex on intact platelets. However, only a few have been precisely characterized for epitope specificity. When this has been done, CIE has proved to be the technique of choice. The experimental procedure is simple, in that it merely involves addition of trace amounts of a purified, ^{125}I-labeled monoclonal immunoglobulin in the intermediate gel before second-dimension electrophoresis. The antibody can thus bind to its antigenic determinant(s) when the platelet antigens move through the intermediate gel before being immunoprecipitated by the polyspecific rabbit antibodies present in the upper gel. Assuming that the membrane glycoprotein(s) of interest is (are) precipitated by the polyspecific antibodies and that the binding of the monoclonal immunoglobulin does not modify the pattern of precipitation (which is usually the case when only trace amounts of a heavily ^{125}I-labeled antibody are added into the gel), the protein(s) bearing the epitope specific for this antibody will be identified in the autoradiographic analysis of the dried, CBR-stained immunoplate. Such an analysis is illustrated in Figure 11-4 for three different monoclonal antibodies known to interact with the intact GPIIb-IIIa complex and shown here to bind to their respective epitopes on GPIIb (Tab), GPIIIa (AP3), or the GPIIb-IIIa complex (AP2).[111,121,145] The point should be stressed here that, as exemplified by AP-2, this is the only direct way to demonstrate a "complex-specific" antibody while showing its lack of reactivity with free GPIIb or free GPIIIa.

Over 17 murine monoclonal anti-GPIIb-IIIa antibodies reported thus far have been tested in CIE for epitope identification. Only 2 have been found to react with an epitope on

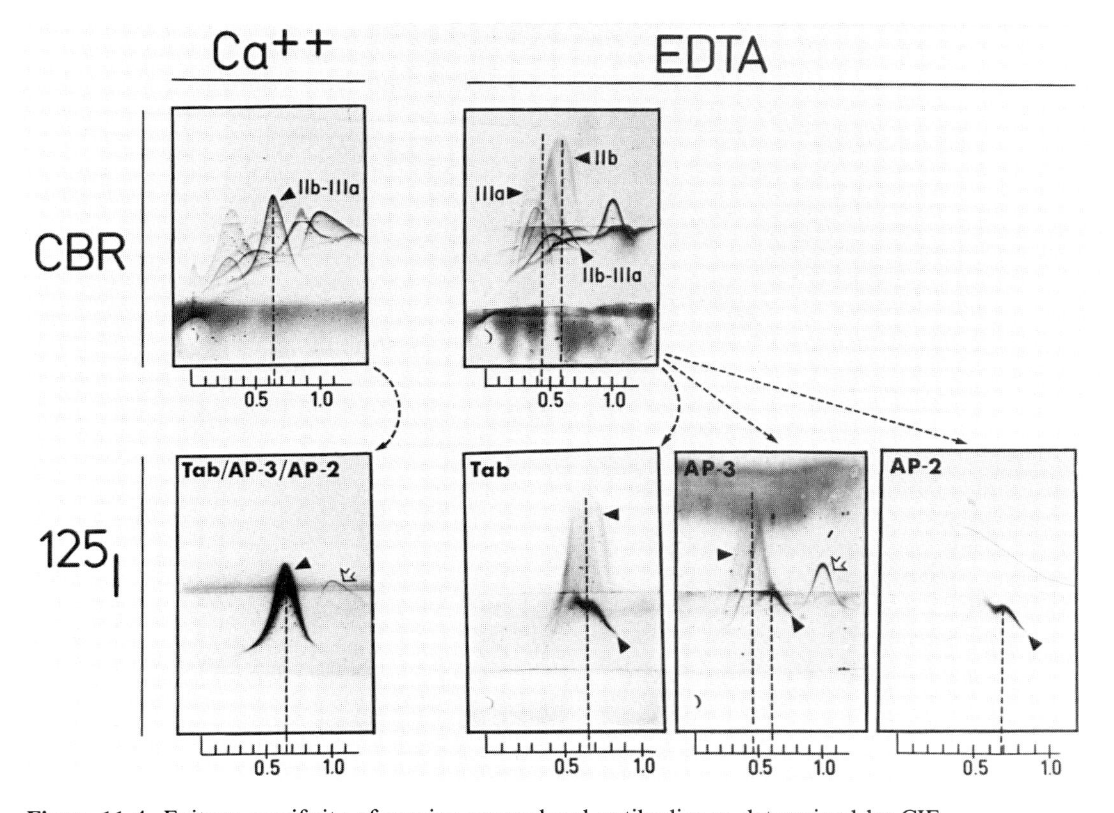

Figure 11-4. Epitope specificity of murine monoclonal antibodies as determined by CIE. Triton X-100-soluble platelet proteins were first incubated for 30 min at 22°C with 2 mmol/liter $CaCl_2$ (Ca^{2+}, *left-hand panels*) or 2 mmol/liter EDTA-Na_2 (EDTA, *right-hand panels*) before being submitted to CIE as indicated in the legend to Figure 11-1. Here, three different murine monoclonal antibodies that are reactive with the GPIIb-IIIa complex were labeled with ^{125}I and incorporated into the second-dimension intermediate gels (5×10^5 cpm/plate, 0.5-2 μg of IgG) and were free to react with the platelet antigens before immunoprecipitation by the polyspecific antiplatelet rabbit antibodies took place. Representative CBR-stained gels showing the intact and partially dissociated GPIIb-IIIa complex (CBR, *upper panels*) and autoradiographs obtained after exposure of the plates for 1 week on Kodak X-Omat AR films (^{125}I, *lower panels*) are shown for the antibodies Tab (a gift of Dr. R. P. McEver, Oklahoma City, Oklahoma), AP3* and AP2.† Note that AP2 reacts solely with the GPIIb-IIIa complex but neither with free GPIIb nor with free GPIIIa, whereas Tab reacts with both complexed and free GPIIb, and AP3 with both complexed and free GPIIIa. For an easier comparison, dashed lines have been drawn to indicate the RMI value of each molecular species (*see also* Table 11-1). Traces of ^{125}I-labeled albumin contaminated the ^{125}I-AP3 IgG and were precipitated with the platelet albumin during CIE (indicated by an open arrow).
*A gift of Dr. P.J. Newman, Milwaukee, Wisconsin.
†A gift of Dr. T.J. Kunicki, Milwaukee, Wisconsin.

GPIIIa (AP3, SZ-21*), 4 recognize an epitope on GPIIb (Tab, 3B2, PMI-1, ITI-P11), whereas 11 have been categorized as "complexspecific" (AP-2, T10, A2A9, 10E5, 7E3, EDU-3,* 4F10, P2, P4, LJP5, and LJP9).[17,49,105,111,117,121,145,153,169,174,175,180] Two of the latter (7E3 and 10E5) have been characterized by single-dimension radioimmunoelectroassay instead of CIE.[33]

The technique, as it is currently used, however, has its own inherent limitations. First, what is termed "free" GPIIb or GPIIIa actually represents the dissociated glycoproteins seen in CIE. They would be better defined as "Ca^{2+}-free" glycoproteins, as CIE of EDTA-treated extracts is routinely performed in the absence of re-added Ca^{2+}. Thus, any monoclonal antibody reacting with a Ca^{2+}-dependent epitope on either glycoprotein, independently of complex integrity, would not interact with the Ca^{2+}-free form and could be inaccurately classified as "complex-specific." However, "Ca^{2+}-dependent epitopes" can be distinguished from "complex-dependent epitopes" in CIE by adding back calcium to the CIE plate on which GPIIb, GPIIIa, and the GPIIb-IIIa complex have been resolved (in so doing, AP2 still did not react with "free" GPIIb or "free" GPIIIa).* Second, the CIE approach does not permit a distinction between epitopes restricted to one or the other subunits but expressed only after complex formation owing to conformational changes of the protein (complexation-dependent epitopes) and those truly made of sequences arising from both glycoproteins (mixed, or combinatorial epitopes); nor does any other method now permit this distinction. The expression "complex-specific monoclonal antibody" should be regarded in consequence (with some caution) as describing antibodies that do not recognize the Ca^{2+}-free, dissociated forms of GPIIb or GPIIIa.

Of interest is the recent description of an immunoblotting procedure, applied to CIE gels for the characterization of monoclonal antibodies to platelet antigens, that may add further versatility to the technique and help define more precisely the expression of conformational epitopes on some antigenic proteins.[169] Examples of this particular technical adaptation of CIE are illustrated in Figure 11-5.

*Pidard, D.: unpublished results, 1983 and 1987.
*Kunicki, T.J.: personal communication, 1987.

A detailed description of the applications of such well-characterized murine monoclonal antibodies to the study of the structural and functional properties of GPIIb-IIIa is largely beyond the scope of this chapter.[17,33,49,111,117,121,144,145,154,175,180] These have been recently reviewed and are presented again in Chapter 12 in this book.[113]

The same approach has been used to partially characterize a human monoclonal antibody (5E5) that appears to recognize a neoantigen on GPIIIa that is expressed on intact platelets only after stimulation or prolonged storage.[127] Upon CIE analysis, ^{125}I-labeled 5E5 reacts with the GPIIb-IIIa complex of fresh platelet extracts while it labels, in addition, a neoprecipitate seen only with stored platelet extracts.[126] This neoantigen may represent an as yet unidentified, modified form of platelet GPIIIa or the GPIIb-IIIa complex (*see also* Chap. 14).

Heterologous Polyclonal Antibodies. Leung et al. have used a particular adaptation of the two-dimensional immunoelectrophoresis technique to demonstrate the absence of immunologic identity between GPIIb and GPIIIa.[103] Here, proteins to be analyzed are first separated by SDS-PAGE, according to their relative molecular mass after denaturation by SDS, before being electrophoresed perpendicularly: first, through an agarose gel layer containing a large excess of a nonionic detergent that will displace the SDS bound to the proteins and will permit the renaturation of amphiphilic membrane proteins in solution and, second, through an agarose gel containing a precipitating antibody.[27,35] When using polyclonal rabbit antisera raised against either purified GPIIb or GPIIIa in the second-dimension agarose gels, Leung et al. have noted that only a single immunoprecipitate formed, in each case, in a position corresponding to the well-separated GPIIb or GPIIIa, respectively.[103] This was an indication for an absence of immunologic cross-reactivity between the two molecules, as it established the monospecificity for each antibody preparation.

That GPIIb and GPIIIa are immunologically different molecular entities is further confirmed by the absence of cross-reactivity of all monoclonal antibodies whose specificity is restricted to either one of the molecules and by the absence of any partial antigenic identity between the precipitation arcs

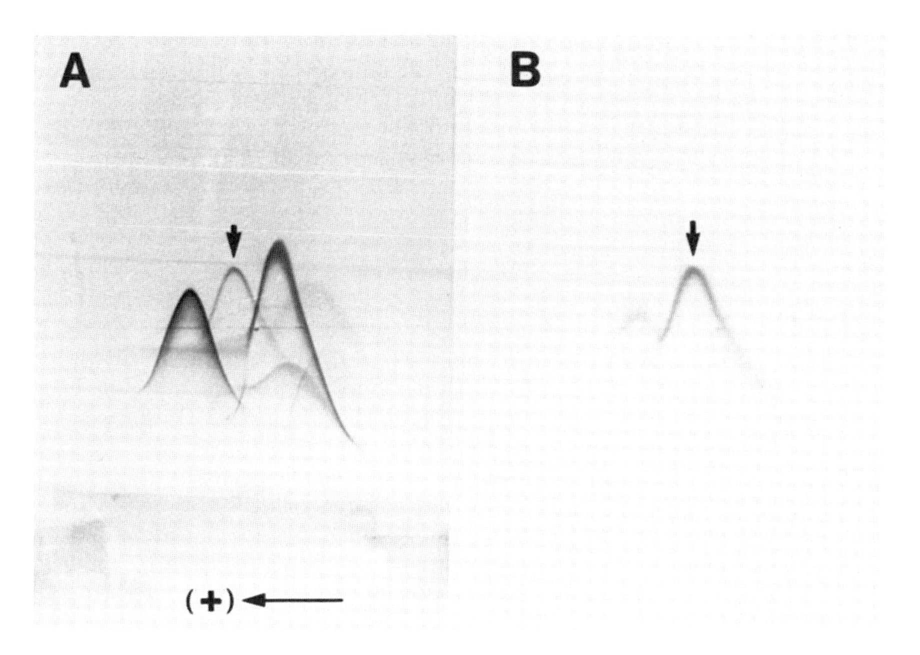

Figure 11-5. Immunoblot of the GPIb-IX complex separated by CIE. Total platelet antigens were separated by CIE. Ten micrograms of nonradiolabeled monoclonal antibody, API, specific for GPIb was incorporated into the intermediate gel of the second dimension. After electrophoresis, the gel was washed three times as described in the text and pressed overnight at ambient temperature in a humidified container against a nitrocellulose sheet that had been presoaked in T/G. After transfer, the sheet was trimmed to the dimensions of the CIE plate, carefully removed from the gel and incubated in a blocking solution (1.5% gelatin in T/G) for 1 h. The sheet was then washed for 10 min twice in T/G plus 0.5% gelatin. Visualization of the precipitin arc that had bound AP1 was then achieved by incubation of the sheet for 3 hr in T/G containing horse radish peroxidase (HRP)-conjugated goat antimouse IgG, followed by a fivefold wash in T/G, followed by incubation in the HRP color reagent. Note that the nitrocellulose sheet provides a reverse image of the CIE gel. Therefore, the CIE gel depicted in this figure has been photographed in a reverse direction compared with the others depicted in this chapter; the anode to the left, the sample well to the right. (*A*) The CIE gel following the immunoblot procedure that has been stained with CBR; (*B*) the corresponding immunoblot. The arrow indicates the precipitin arc given by GPIb-IX and bound by AP1. The fainter and smaller peak in (*B*) to the left (anodic side) of the GPIb-IX arc represents glycocalicin, a proteolytic derivative of GPIb that also reacts with AP1.

formed by the free glycoproteins in CIE.[49,56,65,79,99,111,113,121,169,174,180] All biochemical, physicochemical, and biosynthetic characteristics also point toward GPIIb and GPIIIa being unrelated molecules (*see also* Chaps. 2, 6, and 15.)[18,77,82,131,143]

Human Isoantibodies, Alloantibodies, and Autoantibodies. Few investigations with CIE have been performed, so far, to characterize the antigenic specificity of human iso-, allo- or autoantibodies that can arise in various immunopathologic situations, such as posttransfusion purpura, fetomaternal alloimmunization, or autoimmune thrombocytopenic purpura (*see also* Chaps. 6, 7, and 19).

The best-characterized human isoantibody, so far, remains IgG-L, which served to demonstrate the existence of GPIIb and GPIIIa as noncovalent complexes in solution and which has a marked inhibitory effect upon platelet aggregation and binding of fibrinogen to activated platelets.[99,104,152] Further studies with this antibody demonstrated that, in CIE, it reacts mainly with the GPIIb-IIIa complex immunoprecipitate, although it also shows some reactivity with free GPIIb.[89,152] Immunoblotting experiments confirmed this latter finding, and indicated that the reactivity of IgG-L toward GPIIb was not dependent upon the presence of calcium ions.[152]

These observations further confirm that GPIIb-IIIa is a major immunogenic component of the membrane of normal, nonstimulated platelets. The specificity of these isoantibodies, as well as platelet-specific alloantibodies, is described in greater detail in Chapter 6 of this book.

Subcellular, Tissue, and Species Distribution of the Glycoprotein IIb-IIIa Complex

This particular aspect of platelet membrane glycoprotein antigens is detailed in Chapter 9 and will be mentioned only briefly here, for the CIE technique has been of special interest in this case.

Subcellular Distribution of the Platelet Glycoprotein IIb-IIIa Complex. Crossed-immunoelectrophoretic examination of isolated, human platelet α granules solubilized with Triton X-100 has led Gogstad et al. to conclude that a fraction of the total platelet GPIIb-IIIa complex is present intracellularly as a granular pool.[54] This fraction of GPIIb-IIIa appears to be, in all respects, immunochemically and biochemically identical with its plasma membrane counterpart, except that it is not normally available for chemical or enzymatic surface modifications, including radioisotopic labeling.[54]

This granular pool of GPIIb-IIIa complexes is retained within the isolated α-granule membrane fraction, from which it is solubilized only in the presence of nonionic detergents.[55,58] It is not released in the extracellular medium upon the activation-dependent secretion of α granules, indicating that GPIIb-IIIa is an intrinsic component of the granular membrane.[55,58] Because secretion of granular contents probably occurs through an exocytotic mechanism by which granular membranes fuse with the plasma membrane, it appears that an extra pool of membrane glycoproteins implicated in platelet adhesiveness is made available on the cell surface after platelet activation.[55,58] As judged by CIE, GPIIb-IIIa appears to be the only well-characterized plasma membrane glycoprotein also present in the α-granule membrane, of which it appears as a major antigenic component.[54,55,58]

Although the possibility for a contamination of isolated α granules by plasma membrane fragments or vesicles, of which the GPIIb-IIIa complex is a major immunogenic and antigenic component, cannot be totally ruled out, these findings appear to be supported by light and electron microscopic examination of intact platelets and platelet frozen sections using a panel of monoclonal and polyclonal anti-GPIIb-IIIa antibodies and immunogold labeling of subcellular compartments.[176] It has been observed, using these techniques, that only polyclonal, but not monoclonal, antibodies to the GPIIb-IIIa complex labeled the α-granule membrane, whereas both types of antibody heavily labeled the plasma membrane and the luminal surface of vacuolar structures believed to represent the open, surface-connected canalicular system.[176] This striking differential reactivity of the α-granule GPIIb-IIIa complex might be explained, in part, by the possibility that the platelet fibrinogen stored in the granules is already bound to the complex and, thus, sterically blocks the access of various monoclonal, complex-specific antibodies to their respective epitopes on GPIIb-IIIa. This hypothesis would be supported by the observations of Gogstad et al. that a fraction of several adhesive proteins present in α granules, such as VWF and fibrinogen, tend to remain associated with the granular membrane after disruption of isolated α granules by ultrasonication.[55,58] This would further suggest that, upon exocytosis of α granules, pre-formed GPIIb-IIIa-fibrinogen complexes are expressed on the cell surface that can directly participate in the adhesive properties of stimulated platelets.[55,176]

Cellular and Species Distribution of the Platelet Glycoprotein IIb-IIIa Complex. An exhaustive discussion of this point is beyond the scope of this chapter as it is still the subject of intensive investigations. The reader is referred to a recent review by Kunicki et al. and to Chapter 9 of this book.[98]

Human Megakaryocytes and Promegakaryocytic Cell Lines. Although it has long been known that both GPIIb and GPIIIa are expressed as noncovalent complexes on the surface of human bone marrow megakaryocytes, as early as the promegakaryoblast stage, no further attempt has been made to characterize these complexes using the CIE technique.[20] There is, however, no evidence that the megakaryocyte GPIIb-IIIa complex should be immunologically different from its platelet counterpart, considering its similar reactivity toward a panel of monoclonal and polyclonal antibodies.[20]

Of considerable interest is the observation that several immortalized leukemic cell lines can synthesize and express on their surface what appears to be a close analogue of the GPIIb-IIIa complex. The HEL cell line is primarily an erythroleukemic cell line that expresses megakaryocytic antigenic markers, including GPIIb and GPIIIa.[165] Crossed-immunoelectrophoresis examination of Triton X-100-soluble extracts of HEL cell membranes, using antiplatelet antibodies, has revealed the presence of a major immunoprecipitate that reacts with ^{125}I-labeled monoclonal antibodies specific for GPIIb (Tab) or for the GPIIb-IIIa complex (T10).[165] Further CIE investigations have indicated that the HEL GPIIb-IIIa complex dissociates upon chelation of divalent cations to give rise to immunoprecipitates, corresponding to free GPIIb and free GPIIIa, that are similar to those observed with the platelet glycoproteins.[167] The HEL GPIIb-IIIa has also been shown to bind ^{125}I-labeled fibrinogen.[167] These data, combined with other biochemical and immunochemical evidence, clearly indicate the HEL cells can synthesize and express a membrane glycoprotein complex structurally and functionally similar to the platelet GPIIb-IIIa complex. Accordingly, HEL cells have been a major source of mRNAs in studies aimed at an elucidation of the molecular genetics and the cellular biosynthesis of these two glycoproteins.[18]

Leukemic and sarcoma cell lines other than HEL have been shown to synthesize and express GPIIb, GPIIIa, or the GPIIb-IIIa complex, but none have yet been characterized by the CIE approach.[95,165,167]

Human Endothelial Cells and Leukocytes. Biochemical and immunochemical approaches, such as metabolic radioisotopic labeling and indirect immunoprecipitation, have been used to establish that human endothelial cells (HEC) synthesize two glycoproteins, analogous to GPIIb and GPIIIa, that are expressed on the surface of HEC as noncovalent complexes (*see also* Chaps. 2 and 9).[38,95,102,122]

A CIE analysis of Triton X-100-soluble extracts of HEC has revealed that this complex is immunoprecipitated by polyspecific rabbit antiplatelet antibodies and that it forms a precipitate similar to, but not identical with, that given by the platelet GPIIb-IIIa complex.[15,102,122] Differences in the CIE pattern of these two glycoprotein complexes include a slower mobility of the HEC complex during the first-dimension electrophoresis, and the lack of susceptibility of the HEC complex to chelator-induced dissociation.[102] This latter finding confirms previous observations based on sucrose density gradient ultracentrifugation of Triton X-100-soluble extracts of HEC prepared in the presence of either EDTA or divalent cations.[38]

Although there is no doubt that human endothelial cells contain closely related analogue, or analogues, of the platelet GPIIb-IIIa complex, the differences noted by CIE analysis, the differential immunologic reactivities observed with a panel of monoclonal antibodies specific for the two complexes, and a comparison of their relative molecular masses, all point to the existence of marked structural (and functional) differences between the platelet GPIIb and GPIIIa and their HEC counterparts (*see also* Chaps. 2 and 9).[15,38,50,95,102,122] That the expression of the two classes of membrane complexes is under separate genomic regulation is further emphasized by the observation that thrombasthenic patients express normal levels of the HEC GPIIb-IIIa analogue, as judged by CIE analysis, although they totally lack the platelet GPIIb-IIIa complex.[48]

That strong analogies may also exist between GPIIb-IIIa and the leukocyte-adhesion molecules, LFA-1, Mac-1, and p150,95, appears less certain. All of these proteins belong to the same superfamily of membrane proteins (the so-called cytoadhesins, or integrins) implicated in the adhesive properties of various cell types.[25]

By CIE analysis of Triton X-100-soluble extracts of intact monocytes or isolated monocyte plasma membranes and by using polyspecific rabbit antiplatelet or anti-GPIIb-IIIa antibodies, Gostad et al. have demonstrated the presence of noncovalent, Ca^{2+}-dependent complexes of GPIIb and GPIIIa in the membrane of monocytes.[57] Monocyte GPIIb-IIIa appeared in all respects identical with its platelet counterpart and was missing from the monocytes of a type I thrombasthenic patient.[57] However, later investigations, which were based on metabolic radioisotopic labeling, on immunoprecipitation experiments, and on electron microscopy examination of immunolabeled monocytes, failed to confirm these early observations.[95] As noted by Kunicki et al., artifacts may well have arisen in the former CIE study because of the tight adherence of platelets or platelet fragments to monocytes, a phenomenon known as *satellism*.[19,98] Alternatively, it cannot be excluded that some polyclonal anti-GPIIb-IIIa antibodies may cross-react with some of the leukocyte-adhesion molecules, because these cytoadhesins all share structural and, potentially, functional homologies.[25] Very rarely, however, has a common antigenic reactivity been described between the platelet GPIIb-IIIa complex and the leukocyte-adhesion molecule family, when one considers the large panel of monoclonal antibodies directed at either type of molecular complex.[2,22] It is doubtful, therefore, that the platelet GPIIb-IIIa complex is expressed as such in the leukocyte plasma membrane, and no close immunochemical similarities between the platelet and leukocyte cytoadhesins appear to exist.

Species Distribution of Glycoprotein IIb, Glycoprotein IIIa, and Glycoprotein IIb-IIIa-Like Antigens. On the basis of immunochemical and biochemical approaches, more or less closely related analogues of GPIIb, GPIIIa, or the GPIIb-IIIa complex have been described in various animal cell types, including bovine endothelial cells, mouse leukocytes, mammalian platelets and megakaryocytes, and avian thrombocytes (*see* Chap. 9).[38,92,95,109,162] As none of these cell types have yet been investigated with the CIE technique, the existence of the GPIIb and GPIIIa analogues as complexes in these cells usually remains to be established. The observation of Kunicki et al. that avian thrombocytes can bind a number of the well-characterized, GPIIb-IIIa complex-specific monoclonal antibodies (including AP-2) would indicate that complex formation between these two glycoproteins is a common ancestral feature that is of primary importance for both the expression and the function(s) of these molecules.[92,95]

The Glycoprotein Ib-IX Complex

Glycoprotein Ib Is a Major Substrate for Proteolysis on the Platelet Surface

Glycoprotein Ib has been identified on CIE gels as giving rise to a major anodal immunoprecipitate (*see* Fig. 11-1), although this had not been fully appreciated as such in early CIE studies because of an extreme anodic location in the CIE profile and because of its poor staining with CBR and ofttimes diffuse outline.[66,70,97,99,155]

A peculiar feature of this immunoprecipitate is that it consistently appears as a bimodal, but continuous, line of precipitation when whole-platelet extracts are used (*see* Fig. 11-1); the slow-moving, cathodic component is always predominant. This pattern of antigenic heterogeneity has been examined by Solum et al., who used a monospecific rabbit antibody against purified glycocalicin, a major glycopeptide easily released into the aqueous environment from the platelet glycocalyx. It was found that this antiglycocalicin antibody produced, from whole-platelet extracts, the same double-peaked immunoprecipitate and that the fast-moving, anodic component comigrates with purified glycocalicin.[71,157,158] Charge-shift CIE and crossed-hydrophobic interaction-immunoelectrophoresis (*see* earlier discussion) showed that the slow-moving component was an amphiphilic membrane protein, and SDS-PAGE polypeptide analysis of the excised immunoprecipitates and two-dimensional, SDS-PAGE-immunoelectrophoresis analysis enabled the definitive identification of the slow- and fast-moving components as the membrane GPIb and the soluble glycoprotein, glycocalicin, respectively.[71,157,158]

That glycocalicin is derived from GPIb through enzymatic proteolysis of the latter was further confirmed by the observation that the glycocalicin antigen is absent from the soluble fraction obtained from platelets disrupted in the presence of inhibitors of the cytosolic, Ca^{2+}-activated neutral protease(s) (CANPs, or calpains), whereas the particulate fraction showed a major, single-peaked immunoprecipitate in the position of that given by GPIb when analyzed with the antiglycocalicin antibody.[158] Both molecular species can be found when endogenous platelet calpains are not inhibited.[158] Similar findings, also based on CIE, have been subsequently reported by Ali-Briggs et al.[1]

The detailed biochemical analysis of both molecules has later proved that glycocalicin represents a major, highly glycosylated polypeptide of the externally oriented portion of the GPIb α subunit, from which it is released as a proteolytic product by calpains.[30,130,177] Neuraminidase-treated, desialated GPIb exhibits a much lower mobility during first-dimension electrophoresis, resulting in a marked shift of the GPIb precipitate toward the cathode, which suggests that sialic acid residues normally account for most of its negative charge.[157] Interestingly, in detergent-aqueous phase partitioning experiments that used Triton X-114 (a nonionic detergent with a low "cloud point" near 20°C), GPIb was found to partition into the aqueous phase, rather than into the detergent phase, as would be expected from an amphiphilic protein.[123,178] Such a behavior has been thought to result from the extreme hydrophilicity of the extracellular portion of this glycoprotein, which can be attributed to its high content in carbohydrates.[71,123]

Because of the marked susceptibility of GPIb to proteolysis, an "in vivo" degradation of this membrane glycoprotein is an expected phenomenon, possibly as the consequence of aging for circulating platelets, or in pathophysiologic situations in which increased levels of active plasma proteases are to be found. Indeed, by using an electrophoretic immunodiffusion technique that employed a polyclonal antiglycocalicin antibody and an immunoradiometric assay with ^{125}I-labeled, monoclonal antiglycocalicin antibody, Coller et al. were able to detect a soluble antigen, indistinguishable from glycocalicin, in the plasma of healthy individuals, in amounts ranging from 1.5 to 3.0 mg/liter.[32]

As with the GPIIb–IIIa complex and its subunits, advantage has been taken of the coprecipitation of glycocalicin and intact GPIb into distinct, but related, precipitates, to test for the specificity of monoclonal anti-GPIb antibodies (*see* Fig. 11-6).[89] In so doing, Nugent et al. showed that the monoclonal antibody, AP-1, reacts with an epitope located on the glycocalicin portion of GPIb, whereas the C7E10 antibody labels only intact GPIb, suggesting that it probably recognizes either the GPIb β subunit or that part of the α chain close to the plasma membrane that is not released after cleavage.[127] As illustrated in Figure 11-6, the monoclonal antibodies AN 51 and WM 23 recognize, similarly to AP-1, epitopes located on glycocalicin.

Glycoprotein Ib Is Linked to the Cytoskeleton of Resting Platelets Through Direct Interactions with Actin-Binding Protein

The observation that GPIb is partially proteolyzed after the release of endogeneous, active calpains during solubilization of intact platelets by nonionic detergent has prompted several investigators to consider the effects of inhibition of this proteolytic activity upon the appearance in CIE of GPIb-related immunoprecipitates. By use of a polyclonal and an ^{125}I-labeled monoclonal antibody directed against glycocalicin, to selectively visualize the GPIb-related precipitates, Solum et al. and Okita et al. have noted that inclusion of EDTA or leupeptin (both inhibitors of calpains) in the solubilizing medium results in a major decrease of the bimodal GPIb–glycocalicin precipitate as well as in the appearance of a new precipitation line that contains glycocalicin-related material and is formed in a more cathodic region of the CIE gel.[71,133,161] This new arc showed antigenic cross-reactivity with both the residual GPIb precipitate and a rocket-shaped precipitate located directly above the antigen well (*see* Fig. 11-6).[133,161] There was, however, no indication of antigenic heterogeneity (such as the presence of spurs) along the entire precipitation line (*see* Fig. 11-6).[71] This is consistent with the absence of degradation or covalent cross-linking of GPIb in these extracts, as indicated by SDS–PAGE analysis of the total GPIb-related material purified from the Triton X-100/leupeptin extract by affinity chromatography.[161] Solum et al. have further noted that for platelet extracts that have been prepared in the presence of EDTA, increased amounts of GPIb are sedimented with the Triton X-100-insoluble cytoskeletal fraction, which is essentially composed of actin-binding protein (ABP, M_r 250,000), α-actinin (M_r 105,000), and actin (M_r 43,000).[159] The GPIb-glycocalicin antigens can be released from this fraction upon readdition of calcium, as judged by CIE, whereas ABP in the Triton X-100-insoluble fraction is selectively degraded by a leupeptin-sensitive protease activity.[159]

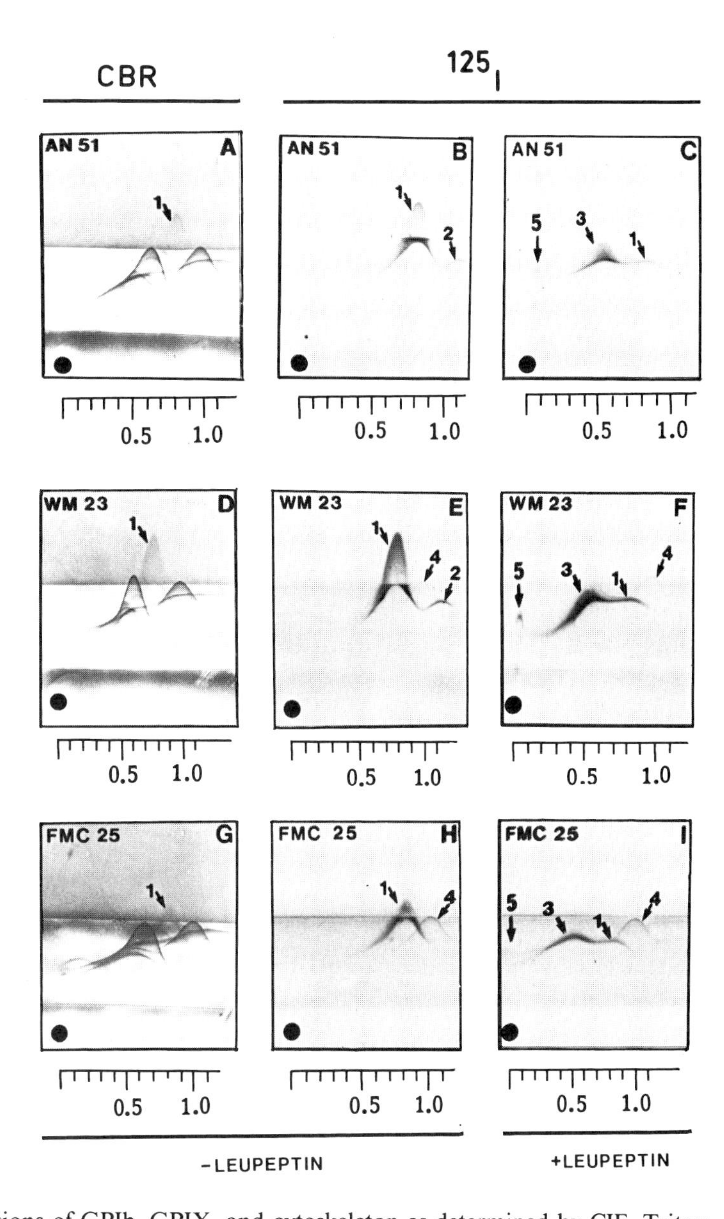

Figure 11-6. Interactions of GPIb, GPIX, and cytoskeleton as determined by CIE. Triton X-100-soluble platelet proteins (100 μg) were submitted to CIE as indicated in the legend to Figure 11-1. Platelet lysates were prepared in the absence *(A, B, D, E, G, H)* or in the presence *(C, F, I)* of 0.5 mg/ml of leupeptin, to maintain active or to inhibit platelet endogenous calpains, respectively. As indicated, ^{125}I-labeled murine monoclonal antibodies with epitopes on the α chain of GPIb (AN 51 and WM 23) or reactive with GPIX (FMC 25) were incorporated into the intermediate gel (5×10^5 cpm/plate, 0.5–2 μg of IgG) before the second-dimension electrophoresis. Autoradiographs of dried CIE plates were developed for 5 days on Kodak X-Omat MA films. Shown here are the CBR-stained gels (CBR: *A, D, G*) and corresponding autoradiographs (^{125}I; *B, E, H*) obtained for the protein lysates prepared in the absence of leupeptin (−leupeptin), and the autoradiographs *(C, F, I)* obtained with the same platelet sample solubilized in the presence of leupeptin (+leupeptin). Black dots locate the sample application wells. Immunoprecipitate identification is based on studies described in the text (*see* Ref. 71) and on the specificity of the monoclonal antibodies: *1*, the GPIb–IX complex; *2*, glycocalicin; *3*, the GPIb–IX complex linked to cytoskeletal component(s), most likely ABP; *4*, albumin (due to contamination of the original monoclonal IgG preparations); *5*, high-molecular-mass complexes (actin filaments?) containing GPIb–IX-related material. Note that FMC 25 (anti-GPIX) reacts only with those immunoprecipitates containing intact GPIb and no longer reacts with that corresponding to the major proteolytic product of the GPIb α chain, glycocalicin (adapted from Berndt MC, Gregory C, Kabral A, et al: Eur J Biochem 151:637, 1985).

That the cathodal shift noted on CIE for the GPIb-related immunoprecipitate most likely reflects the direct interaction of this membrane glycoprotein with ABP is supported by the finding that GPIb and ABP copurify upon immunoaffinity chromatography of Triton X-100-soluble extracts of whole platelets prepared in the presence of leupeptin, when the monoclonal antiglycocalicin antibody, AP-1, is used.[133] On the other hand, the rocketlike precipitate is regarded as given by slow-moving, high-molecular-mass complexes, possibly containing G-actin or small filaments of F-actin, in addition to ABP and GPIb.[159]

Of particular interest are the observations of Solum et al., showing that (1) intact platelets incubated with the local anesthetic, dibucaine, show a progressive intracellular degradation of ABP, whereas the CIE analysis of Triton X-100–leupeptin extracts of these same platelets shows a shift of the GPIb-related precipitate from the cathodal form (GPIb–ABP) to the anodal form (free GPIb–glycocalicin); and (2) incubation of intact platelets with diamide results in an intracellular cross-linking of cytoskeletal proteins, that is accompanied by an increased incorporation of GPIb into the Triton X-100-insoluble cytoskeleton, whereas GPIB–ABP complexes, giving rise to the cathodal precipitate during CIE, are found in the Triton X-100-soluble extracts.[160] These findings have been interpreted as evidence that calpains are intracellularly activated after incubation with dibucaine, resulting in the proteolysis of ABP and in the release of "free" GPIb, whereas diamide can intracellularly inactivate the same proteases, thus resulting in the appearance of stable GPIb–ABP complexes upon solubilization with Triton X-100.[160] Interestingly, prior treatment of platelets with dibucaine or diamide was found to potentiate and to reduce, respectively, the GPIb-mediated platelet agglutination induced by bovine VWF.[160] These observations have been ascribed to the differential mobility of GPIb within the plane of the membrane, depending upon its linkage to the cytoskeleton of the resting platelet through interactions with ABP.[160] Moreover, this suggests that the interaction between GPIb and ABP, as it is observed in solution using CIE, most likely reflects a true, native membrane glycoprotein–cytoskeleton interaction of potential physiologic significance.[133] Similar conclusions have been reached in parallel by Fox et al., with use of different biochemical and immunochemical approaches.[41,42]

Interactions of Glycoprotein Ib with Other Glycoproteins of the Plasma Membrane: The Glycoprotein Ib–IX Complex

Early attempts to purify GPIb to homogeneity by immunoaffinity chromatography, using monoclonal antibodies specific for this glycoprotein, have shown that another membrane glycoprotein, GPIX, is consistently copurified with GPIb.[7,89,130] Glycoprotein IX, also designated GP17, is an integral membrane glycoprotein with an M_r in the range of 17,000 to 22,000, which is best identified after tritium labeling of the glycoprotein carbohydrate moieties on intact platelets and then protein separation by SDS–PAGE followed by fluorographic analysis of the polyacrylamide gels.[30] This is why GPIX has escaped detection when conventional CBR- or PAS-staining procedures or ^{125}I-labeling techniques have been used to identify the molecular species present in the immunopurified GPIb–ABP complex or in the GPIb-related immunoprecipitate(s).[89,97,133]

Berndt et al. have further shown that GPIb and GPIX are coadsorbed on affinity columns made of monoclonal antibodies to either glycoprotein, whereas the direct binding of the same ^{125} I-labeled antibodies to intact platelets reveals that an equal number of copies of both glycoproteins are present on the platelet surface.[7] The same investigators have used the CIE technique to establish that both ^{125}I-labeled, monoclonal anti-GPIX and anti-GPIb antibodies react with the "GPIb" immunoprecipitate, whereas only anti-GPIb antibodies react with the precipitate given by glycocalicin; and that the anti-GPIX antibody also labels the GPIb–ABP complex immunoprecipitate seen when calpains have been inhibited in the Triton X-100-soluble extracts (*see* Fig. 11-6).[7] Taken together, these data indicate that GPIb and GPIX are tightly associated in nonionic detergent solutions as noncovalent, 1:1 heterodimers.[7] Accordingly, the GPIb immunoprecipitate identified on conventional CIE patterns should be designated as the GPIb–IX precipitate (*see* Fig. 11-1).

That this association in solution actually reflects a true protein–protein interaction in the platelet membrane has been subsequently demonstrated through the characterization of GPIb–IX complex-specific monoclonal antibodies that bind to intact platelets to the same extent that anti-GPIb or anti-GPIX antibodies do (*see also* Chap. 12).[37] Although it has been shown that acidifying the medium to *p*H 3.0 results in the reversible dissociation of the GPIb–IX complex, the physicochemical or biochemical factors regulating its formation under physiologic conditions have not been yet characterized.[7] There is no doubt that the existence of such a complex is of a great functional significance, considering the role of GPIb as a membrane-binding site for von Willebrand factor and for α-thrombin (see later discussion). The implication of the complex in the binding of drug-dependent antibodies, most likely through the GPIX component (*see also* Chap. 8), as well as its absence or reduction in the platelets of patients with the Bernard-Soulier syndrome (*see* Chap. 5) remain areas of intense investigation.[7,130]

Wicki and Clemetson have shown that a "GPIb complex," isolated from plasma membranes by aqueous-detergent phase partitioning, using the nonionic detergent Trixon X-114, contains GPIX in addition to other, as yet, unidentified membrane or peripheral proteins of M_r 27,000, 35,000, 43,000, and 120,000, suggesting that the GPIb, GPIX, and ABP might be part of a larger macromolecular membrane structure(s).[178] It should be noted that these studies present no direct biochemical or immunochemical evidence that glycoprotein V is part of the GPIb complex.[30,130,177]

Other features of the GPIb–IX complex that have been revealed by the CIE approach include its absence from the membrane of purified α granules; its inability to bind $^{45}Ca^{2+}$, except through relatively weak interactions with the negatively charged sialic acid residues; and its capacity to be intracellularly phosphorylated (a phosphorylation site has been identified on the GPIbβ subunit).[54,58,59,161,181]

The presence of a differently glycosylated form of the platelet GPIb α subunit in subclones of the erythroleukemic, promegakaryocytic HEL cell line has been recently reported, but it has not yet been characterized by CIE.[86]

Glycoproteins Ia and IIa

Very little is known about these two major platelet membrane glycoproteins (GPIa: M_r 153,000/167,000, and GPIIa: M_r 138,000/157,000, nonreduced/reduced), although new information concerning both their membrane organization and potential involvement in platelet physiology is now emerging.

Early CIE investigations aimed at identifying the ^{125}I-labeled plasma membrane glycoprotein antigens present in major immunoprecipitates assigned GPIa and GPIIa to a single precipitation line in a position slightly more cathodal than that of the GPIIb–IIIa complex precipitate (*see* Fig. 11-1).[97] Although some antigenic heterogeneity can be noted, such as a splitting of the precipitation line along its cathodal side, no dissociation was noted upon chelation of divalent cations, by inclusion of various lectins in the gel, or by substitution of Triton X-100 for other nonionic detergents, suggesting that a tight association may exist between these two glycoproteins.[97,99,130] Gogstad et al. have later reported that GPIa is present within a major immunoprecipitate similar to that identified by Kunicki et al., although in their studies, GPIIa appeared to be located in a distinct precipitate.[58,64]

More recently, Van Mourik et al. have characterized a monoclonal antibody, CLB-HEC 75, that recognizes a membrane antigen present on both human endothelial cells and platelets.[173] By means of indirect immunoprecipitation coupled to SDS–PAGE analysis and by CIE analysis, this antigen was found to be strictly identical on both cells, and similar in all respects to GPIIa. Again, CIE analysis with the ^{125}I-labeled CLB-HEC 75 antibody showed the platelet GPIIa to be located in a precipitate slightly more cathodal than that formed by GPIIb–IIIa.[173] Later studies by Borsum et al. have shown that human endothelial cells and platelet plasma membranes share three common glycoprotein antigens in this system, one of which may represent GPIIa.[15]

In their studies, Gogstad et al. have shown that the GPIa-related precipitate is absent from the membrane of purified α granules and that this antigen may also represent a minor Ca^{2+}-binding protein of the platelet plasma membrane.[58,59] Alternatively, that GPIIa could well be engaged, at least in solution, in glycoprotein complexes in which divalent cations may play some role is suggested by the observations of Pidard et al. and Fitzgerald et al. that two ^{125}I-labeled plasma membrane proteins with M_r similar to the those of GPIa and GPIIa cosediment during sucrose density gradient ultracentrifugation, when it is performed in the presence of Ca^{2+}, with a velocity similar to that of the GPIIb–IIIa complex, whereas inclusion of EDTA results in a much lower mobility for GPIIa, similar to that of free GPIIb.[39,146]

Complex interactions between GPIb, GPIa, and ABP have also been postulated to exist, based on the observations that GPIb and GPIa are coprecipitated by a number of antiplatelet membrane monoclonal antibodies and that fractions of both GPIb and GPIa cosediment with a membrane-associated network of actin filaments, which appear to represent the cytoskeleton of resting platelets, most likely through their common attachment to ABP.[41,114] Because the CIE analysis of platelet lysates does not indicate even a partial antigenic relationship between the precipitates given by GPIa and GPIb, it would seem likely that these glycoproteins do not interact directly within the membrane, and that their coprecipitation or copurification, rather, would be the result of conditions of membrane solubilization that ensure the integrity of ABP.[41,64,97,114]

Data recently have been reported that point toward the involvement of GPIa and GPIIa in platelet function. These are the examination of pathologic platelets that lack the membrane GPIa and are unable to spread normally on collagen-coated surfaces; the potency of a murine monoclonal antibody, PlH5, originally raised against the human fibroblast class II extracellular matrix receptor, but that also binds to GPIa and precipitates GPIa–IIa complexes, to specifically inhibit adhesion of platelets to collagen; and the observation of biochemical and immunochemical similarities between the multipolypeptide membrane receptors for fibronectin found on mouse or chicken fibroblasts and human platelet membrane complexes involving glycoproteins similar to GPIIa and GPIc (*see also* Chap. 2).[47,96,124,147]

Although the availability of monospecific immunochemical probes will help to identify the exact location of GPIa, GPIIa and, possibly, GPIc within CIE patterns and to elucidate their potential interactions with each other and with other proteins, a still speculative view would be that GPIa and GPIIa on one side, GPIc and GPIIa on the other side, can form complexes within the plasma membrane of unstimulated platelets, which may participate in the interaction of platelets with adhesive proteins present in the subendothelium, such as collagen and fibronectin, whereas GPIa might also have a pivotal role because of its transmembrane linkage, through ABP, with the submembranous cytoskeleton.

Glycoproteins Specific for the Membrane of α Granules

The CIE examination of purified α granules has led Gogstad et al. to identify several immunoprecipitates that appear to contain granule-specific antigens: the G18 protein has a very anodal location, similar to that of albumin, whereas the G4 and G8 antigens have similar mobilities during the first-dimension electrophoresis and give superimposed immunoprecipitates, slightly more cathodal than that given by the GPIIb–IIIa complex.[58] All antigens have a mobility that is modified after neuraminidase treatment, and they are retained with the isolated α-granule membrane and not released in the external medium upon activation of intact platelets by thrombin, suggesting that they represent intrinsic α-granule membrane sialoglycoproteins.[55,58] However, both the G4 and G18 antigens can incorporate some iodine during the lactoperoxidase-catalyzed, ^{125}I-labeling of the platelet surface, and the G4 glycoprotein also appears to coisolate with plasma membranes, although in low amounts, suggesting that both antigens may also be expressed on the platelet surface, possibly owing to a basal activation of isolated and surface-labeled platelets.[45,58]

An SDS–PAGE polypeptide analysis of excised precipitates has shown the G4 antigen to be a polypeptide of M_r 146,000/132,000 (nonreduced/reduced), whereas G18 corresponds to a polypeptide of M_r 130,000–135,000 under both conditions.[58] The G18 antigen has also been shown to be a major Ca^{2+}-binding protein in Triton X-100 extracts of whole platelets.[59]

These findings have to be corroborated with those reported by McEver and Martin, and by Hsu-Lin et al., who separately described an integral α-granule membrane sialoglycoprotein of M_r 140,000 under both nonreduced and reduced conditions, using two monoclonal antibodies, S12 and KC4, that recognized different epitopes on the same molecule.[80,112] This glycoprotein, designated granule membrane protein (GMP)-140 or PADGEM (for platelet activation-dependent granule-external membrane), appears to be essentially absent from the plasma membrane of resting platelets (or present in small amounts owing to background activation) and to be restricted to the α-granule membrane, whereas it is fully translocated to the surface of thrombin-activated platelets after exocytosis of the α granules.[6,45,80,112,163] McEver and Martin, using the CIE technique with the ^{125}I-labeled S12 antibody, have shown that S12 labels an immunoprecipitate very similar in its location and shape to that described by Gogstad et al. as G4, although the subcellular distribution of the S12-reactive antigen in resting and stimulated platelets has not yet been investigated with the CIE approach.[58,112]

Of note is the observation that the GMP-140/PADGEM protein is also present in endothelial cells.[45] Besides its potential use as a marker for in vivo or in vitro platelet activation, it has yet no known physiologic function.[45]

EVALUATION OF THE INTERACTION BETWEEN PLATELET MEMBRANE GLYCOPROTEINS AND THEIR NATURAL LIGANDS WITH CROSSED-IMMUNOELECTROPHORESIS: THE SEARCH FOR "RECEPTORS"

The technical modifications of the basic CIE technique that have been developed through studies described in the preceding sections of this chapter have received further application in the tentative characterization of receptor function(s) for several platelet membrane glycoproteins.[71]

One can distinguish between primary and secondary platelet membrane receptors. *Primary receptors* are those involved in the initial interaction of the plasma membrane with soluble agonists or antagonists of platelet activation pathways that can be generated or secreted within its environment or with some of the adhesive proteins present in the vascular subendothelium that mediate the initial attachment of platelets to this surface. *Secondary receptors* are those whose expression depends upon the prior activation of the intracellular machinery as part of the cellular response to a stimulus and that are involved in the transformation of the platelet plasma membrane into a procoagulant and adhesive surface following cell activation.[142] This process often involves the binding of various coagulation factors, some of which, such as fibrinogen, also have properties of adhesive proteins.

It should be made clear, however, that by using the CIE technique, one can only define "ligand-binding proteins" rather than "receptors," because the existence of a functional response, which would truly define a receptor, cannot be considered in this system.

Investigating Primary Receptors in Crossed-Immunoelectrophoresis: The Thrombin-Binding Proteins

Numerous investigations have been conducted on intact platelets or subcellular fractions to identify potential thrombin receptor(s) on the platelet surface and to elucidate the mechanism of action of one of the most potent platelet agonists. Both the experimental procedures used and the major conclusions drawn from these studies have been recently reviewed by Phillips,[142] and all point to a major involvement of GPIb, and possibly GPV, in the initial interaction between thrombin and the platelet surface.[142,177,178] However, other proteins contained in the platelets, such as TSP, fibrinogen, and FXIII, can also interact with thrombin.[142]

Because most of these (glyco)proteins can be identified on the CIE profile of whole-platelet extracts, the CIE approach described here could be of interest in further defining the platelet thrombin-binding proteins. Two different approaches have been used by Hagen et al.[68,69] First, purified bovine thrombin that had been coupled to Sepharose beads was incorporated into the intermediate gel, assuming that the immobilized ligand should retain or retard any thrombin-binding protein antigen during second-dimension electrophoresis. Indeed, immunoprecipitates corresponding to PF4, to FXIIIa, to GPIb and glycocalicin, and to an unidentified and very anodal antigen, were retained in the intermediate gel.[64,67,68] Surprisingly, no retardation of any of these proteins was noted when thrombin had been inhibited at its serine-active site.[64,68] Among these particular molecules, evidence for a proteolytic, substrate–enzyme-type of interaction has been obtained only for FXIII. The interaction between thrombin and PF4 has been thought to occur through the proteoglycan carrier of PF4.[67,68] In the second approach, ^{125}I-labeled bovine thrombin was first allowed to interact with intact platelets, then platelet extracts were prepared in Triton X-100 and analyzed by

CIE.[69] Autoradiographic analysis of the gels revealed that three immunoprecipitates contained ^{125}I-thrombin, namely, those given by the GPIb-IX and by the GPIIb-IIIa complexes, and an additional, strongly labeled immunoprecipitate, which could not be seen on CBR-stained gels, with a position intermediate between those of GPIIb-IIIa and GPIb-IX.[69] Again, the use of inactivated, ^{125}I-labeled thrombin resulted in a complete inhibition of its interaction with membrane glycoproteins, as judged by the CIE procedure.[69] The same approach was applied to soluble, α-granule-secreted proteins and revealed a marked labeling of the precipitation lines formed by albumin and TSP and only a partial labeling of the precipitate given by secreted PF4.[69] Because of technical problems, an interaction of platelet fibrinogen with thrombin could not be observed.

These findings thus confirmed previous observations that on the surface of unstimulated platelets thrombin binds to the glycocalicin portion of GPIb, without noticeable proteolysis of the glycoprotein receptor, whereas it can also interact with various α-granule (TSP, PF4) or cytosolic (FXIIIa) proteins once they are released from their intracellular compartments.[142,177,178] A marked discrepancy exists, however, between the CIE observations and studies performed on intact platelets, in that the binding of inactivated thrombin to intact cells has been found to be identical with that of the active enzyme.[69,142] No satisfactory explanations have been given for this discrepancy. Also surprising is the observation that GPIIb-IIIa can bind ^{125}I-labeled thrombin. A similar observation, based on CIE, has been made using purified, ^{125}I-labeled human α-thrombin chemically cross-linked to the surface of intact platelets (conditions under which GPIb remains a major thrombin-binding protein). This has been proposed to result from the presence of an Arg-Gly-Asp sequence at position 197-199 of the β chain of thrombin.*

The description by Hagen et al. of a heavily and previously unidentified ^{125}I-labeled thrombin precipitate remains a puzzling observation. Hagen's study suggests that the antigen, or antigens, contained in this precipitate appears to represent a loosely attached, nonglycosylated membrane component(s) that does not show the properties that would be expected of the heavily glycosylated GPV or its thrombin proteolytic fragment.[69,142,177] Membrane proteins other than GPIb and GPV have been identified that show specific interactions with thrombin. These include a noncovalent complex of two membrane-associated polypeptides of M_r 74,000 and 55,000 and, more recently, a membrane-bound, platelet antithrombin inhibitor of the serpin family, similar to the fibroblast protease nexin I.[26,62] The potential relationship of one of these components to the major thrombin-binding protein identified in CIE remains to be established.

*Jandrot-Perrus, M.: Personal communication, 1986.

Investigating Secondary Receptors in Crossed-Immunoelectrophoresis: The Fibrinogen-Binding Proteins

The binding of fibrinogen molecules to the surface of activated platelets is certainly a major and, possibly, obligatory event in the physiologic process of platelet thrombus formation, a key step in primary hemostasis. Upon stimulation of resting platelets by any physiologic agonist, a specific binding site for fibrinogen is expressed on the platelet surface, whose occupancy is a prerequisite for platelet aggregation to occur.[137] Over the past 10 years, extensive investigations have been devoted to the characterization of this platelet fibrinogen-binding site and to the elucidation of its biochemical identity (*see also* Chap. 2).[137] Investigations conducted with intact platelets have concluded that the GPIIb-IIIa complex contains such an inducible binding site for fibrinogen, based on the absence of binding of fibrinogen to type I thrombasthenic platelets, which otherwise totally lack the GPIIb-IIIa complex; the inhibitory effect of GPIIb-IIIa complex-specific monoclonal antibodies on the binding of fibrinogen to normal stimulated platelets; and the covalent cross-linking of platelet-bound, chemically derivatized fibrinogen to the GPIIb-IIIa complex.[130,137]

Only a few analytic procedures, however, have permitted the visualization and quantitative or qualitative evaluation of a direct interaction between fibrinogen molecules and GPIIb-IIIa complexes. This has been realized through reconstitution experiments that use artificial proteoliposomes or through the use of a solid-phase enzymoimmunoassay.[4,120,137] Although informative, these approaches require the prior purification of functionally active

GPIIb-IIIa complexes and, in the latter, the preparation of monospecific polyclonal antibodies. Again, the CIE technique has offered an accurate and simple alternative.

With use of the same methodology as that implemented in the investigation of platelet calcium-binding proteins (*see* section on GPIIb and GPIIIa as calcium-binding proteins), Gogstad et al. have characterized the interaction of ^{125}I-labeled, soluble fibrinogen with pre-formed immunoprecipitates in CIE gels.[53] Four immunoprecipitates were found to be specifically labeled upon incubation of immunoplates with a solution containing ^{125}I-labeled fibrinogen, namely, those given by platelet fibrinogen, cytosolic FXIIIa, α-granule membrane glycoprotein G4, and the plasma membrane GPIIb-IIIa complex.[53] No binding occurred to dissociated, free GPIIb or free GPIIIa and, except for platelet fibrinogen, addition of EDTA prevented the binding of soluble fibrinogen to all immunoprecipitated, fibrinogen-binding proteins at *p*H 8.7 but had no effect at *p*H 7.4.[53] THe GPIIb-IIIa complex showed no preference toward Ca^{2+} or Mg^{2+} ions to bind fibrinogen, whereas FXIIIa and the G4 protein exhibited a marked specificity for Ca^{2+} and Mg^{2+}, respectively.[53]

Later CIE studies by Thorsen et al. revealed that fragments X, Y, and D, generated from intact fibrinogen by plasminolysis, all bound to the GPIIb-IIIa complex, whereas fragments E and fragments D that lacked a large amino acid sequence at the COOH-terminus of the γ chain, did not.[168] These results are similar to those previously reported by Nachman et al., who employed an unidimensional immunoelectrophoresis technique in which purified GPIIb-IIIa had to pass through an intermediate gel containing either fragments D or fragments E before being precipitated in an upper gel by monospecific anti-GPIIb-IIIa antibodies.[120] The bound fragments were then revealed by immunoblotting of the gel, with ^{125}I-labeled antifibrinogen antibodies.[120] The observations of Thorsen et al. that immunoprecipitated GPIIb-IIIa also interacts with the E_1 domain of the D dimer-E fragments of polymerized fibrin, and with the NH_2-terminal disulfide knot of intact fibrinogen, remain to be evaluated by alternative biochemical methods, although they may provide some evidence for a new class of adhesive sites (or adhesiotopes) within the fibrinogen molecule.[168,170]

Thus, except for the absence of an inhibitory effect of EDTA on the interaction between GPIIb-IIIa and fibrinogen at *p*H 7.4, all the data obtained by CIE studies appear to fit with the characteristics previously ascribed to the fibrinogen-binding site on intact platelets, including the existence of a single class of sites associated with GPIIb-IIIa, the requirement for intact GPIIb-IIIa complexes, a similar requirement for the presence of Ca^{2+} or Mg^{2+}, and a marked specificity toward the D domain of fibrinogen.[17,137,144,154]

On the other hand, the observation that the α-granule membrane glycoprotein G4 (possibly identical with the GMP140/PADGEM protein, discussed earlier) can interact with fibrinogen might be of physiologic significance because fibrinogen is a major component among the secretable proteins stored in α granules.

A striking feature of the interaction between fibrinogen and immunoprecipitated GPIIb-IIIa is that it does not require, nor is it potentiated by, the presence of an agonist, such as ADP.[53] This is a consistent finding, i.e., purified GPIIb-IIIa complexes appear to exist in an "activated" state.[4,120] This might indicate that the dispersion of plasma membrane lipids by a nonionic detergent results in the relaxation of the GPIIb-IIIa complex from a constrained, "nonactive" conformation, a phenomenon that may also occur upon physiologic stimulation of the intact platelet (*see* Shattil et al. and Coller in Ref. 113). Alternatively, this may result from an irreversible modification of the GPIIb-IIIa complex, such as the proteolytic processing of one or both of its subunits or from the association of GPIIb-IIIa with an, as yet, unidentified polypeptide or lipid component(s). A third possibility is that only a fraction of the total immunoprecipitated GPIIb-IIIa complex (for instance, that present in the membrane of α granules) takes part in this interaction, possibly owing to its native, "preactivated" state.* Clearly, further investigations are required to distinguish between these possibilities and to elucidate this crucial aspect of GPIIb-IIIa complex function.

Because platelet fibrinogen appears to be immunochemically and functionally identical with its plasma counterpart, one would expect to observe some degree of interaction between

*Legrand, C.: Personal communication, 1986.

this molecule and the GPIIb–IIIa complex in a CIE pattern, appearing as a coprecipitation of the two antigens or as a line of partial antigenic identity between the two immunoprecipitates.[84,94] This is clearly not so (*see* Fig. 11-2), although some evidence for confluence between the two precipitates has been occasionally observed.[53] One possibility is that preformed GPIIb–IIIa–fibrinogen complexes are unstable and rapidly dissociate because of the combination of an alkaline milieu, the presence of detergent, and the application of an electric field during electrophoresis. However, inclusion of leupeptin in the solubilizing medium results in marked modifications in the appearance of the precipitate given by fibrinogen, which here appears with a trailing line of precipitation extending from its anodal part toward the cathodal edge of the GPIIb–IIIa complex precipitate.† As fibrinogen is susceptible to degradation by endogenous platelet calpains, proteolytic degradation of this molecule at the time of solubilization when leupeptin is omitted, may well destroy or impair any possible interaction with its receptor.[91] The same situation may apply to platelet VWF, another ligand for the GPIIb–IIIa complex and a substrate for platelet calpains[90] (*see also* Ruggeri in Ref. 113). In any event, these observations emphasize the necessity to control potential proteolytic events when investigating molecular interactions in such analytic systems.

Of interest is the observation of Gogstad et al. that ^{125}I-labeled fibronectin incubated with pre-formed CIE immunoplates, under these conditions, does not bind to the GPIIb–IIIa complex, yet GPIIb–IIIa has been identified as a specific receptor for fibronectin on activated, intact platelets.[53,149]

Heparin-Binding Proteins

The binding of heparin to the platelet surface has been postulated to play a major role in the pathogenesis of heparin-associated thrombocytopenia (HAT).[106] Heparin-associated thrombocytopenia is a severe abnormal condition that occurs in a significant percentage of patients receiving antithrombotic heparin therapy and that sometimes associates thrombocytopenia with arterial thrombosis.[118] Development of antiplatelet, heparin-dependent antibodies in some of patients with HAT has been described, and Western blot analysis of HAT sera has shown that at least three platelet polypeptides, of M_r 180,000, 124,000, and 82,000 (nonreduced), are reactive with HAT antibodies.[106,118] The M_r 82,000 component was further shown to be accessible to iodogen-catalyzed iodination on the platelet surface.[106] However, all three polypeptides also directly interacted with ^{125}I-labeled heparin.[106] These findings support the contention that, in addition to potentially functioning as a hapten, heparin could also bind to some platelet membrane (glyco)protein(s) and, through conformational changes of its receptor(s), could reveal otherwise cryptic antigenic determinants (*see also* Chap. 8 and 19).[106]

Interesting observations have been reported by Gogstad et al., who used the CIE technique to characterize platelet heparin-binding proteins.[60] Immobilized heparin covalently coupled to a Sepharose matrix was incorporated into the intermediate gel and was found, in this system, to specifically retain TSP and PF4, all secretable heparin-binding proteins present in the platelet α granules.[60] On the other hand, the α-granule membrane G4 glycoprotein was also retained, whereas the plasma membrane GPIb–IX complex (but not glycocalicin) and the GPIa-related antigen, as well as an unidentified antigen (precipitate 25), were specifically retarded, suggesting that several major plasma membrane glycoproteins may directly interact with heparin.[60] Although obtained under nonphysiologic conditions, these results confirm other findings obtained with intact platelets, indicating that the observations made with CIE might be physiologically relevant.[107]

†Pidard, D.: Unpublished observations, 1984.

THE USE OF CROSSED-IMMUNOELECTROPHORESIS AND OTHER IMMUNOELECTROPHORETIC TECHNIQUES IN THE DELINEATION OF MOLECULAR ABNORMALITIES IN PLATELET MEMBRANE DISORDERS

The use of the CIE technique has allowed a refined characterization of some of the (glyco)protein deficiencies encountered in various inherited platelet disorders, including the gray platelet syndrome, the Bernard-Soulier syndrome, and Glanzmann's thrombasthenia. In turn, analyses of such abnormalities that are restricted to a few membrane or granular (glyco)proteins have helped to identify some of the major immunoprecipitates present in the CIE pattern of normal platelets.[44,64,70,79,97,130,131,156]

Our current knowledge of the phenotypic expression and pathogenesis of platelet membrane glycoprotein disorders is discussed in detail in Chapter 5 of this book. This section will be limited to the description of some of the applications that CIE and related immunoelectrophoretic techniques have received in the evaluation of quantitative defects affecting membrane antigens and in the biochemical and immunochemical characterization of qualitative platelet abnormalities.

Quantitative Assessments of Membrane Antigens in Abnormal Conditions

The CIE technique has been found to be sensitive enough to permit the detection of less than 5% of the normal content of the GPIIb-IIIa complex in Triton X-100-soluble extracts of whole platelets. Although type I thrombasthenic platelets show a complete absence of the GPIIb-IIIa complex immunoprecipitate, type II platelets contain, as judged by CIE, from less than 5% to up to 20% of the normal levels of GPIIb-IIIa.[70,76,98,130,164]

Single-dimension, rocket immunoelectrophoresis provides a simpler and more efficient alternative to CIE for measuring residual amounts of antigens because it relies uniquely on the height of the precipitate arcs, rather than on the area covered by the bell-shaped immunoprecipitate arcs seen on CIE profiles.[87,164] When coupled with the use of ^{125}I-labeled monoclonal antibodies incorporated into the agarose gel to specifically label the antigen of interest, it can provide a very sensitive radioelectroimmunoassay (REIA).[34,87] This technique has been applied to the study of both type I and type II Glanzmann's thrombasthenia and to Bernard-Soulier syndrome platelets.[34,87]

The status of individuals heterozygous for the Glanzmann's thrombasthenia trait, relative to the content of the GPIIb-IIIa complex in their platelets, is far from clear. Both CIE and REIA techniques have indicated values ranging from 35% to 70% of the normal content, in both type I and type II kindreds of various ethnic origins, with sometimes marked differences between obligate carriers within the same family.[34,76,98,130,164] In all instances, however, heterozygotes could be clearly distinguished from normal individuals.[34,98,164] Such heterogeneity in the quantitative abnormalities affecting the GPIIb-IIIa complex, in both homozygous and heterozygous individuals, is strongly indicative of a complex genetic regulation of the disease (*see also* Chap. 5).

Residual levels of total GPIIb-IIIa complexes in type II or heterozygous thrombasthenic platelets, as measured by CIE or REIA, are very similar to those quantitated on the platelet surface through the direct binding of ^{125}I-labeled monoclonal antibodies, suggesting a surface orientation for most of these residual complexes.*[34]

A puzzling situation is offered by the fibrinogen content in type I, type II, and heterozygous thrombasthenic platelets. Fibrinogen is found to be variably decreased, as judged by CIE, although there is no evidence for a direct correlation between the level of residual GPIIb-IIIa complexes and that of platelet fibrinogen.[70,84,98,130,164]

Investigating Qualitative Defects of Membrane Glycoproteins

Inherited Disorders: The Case of Variants of Glanzmann's Thrombasthenia

Variants of Glanzmann's thrombasthenia constitute a heterogeneous category of patients whose platelets unambiguously exhibit a functional disorder typical of that encountered in thrombasthenia type I (i.e., a total absence of platelet aggregation resulting from the deficient expression of binding sites for adhesive proteins upon stimulation), whereas normal or subnormal amounts of plasma membrane GPIIb and GPIIIa are detected, as judged by radioisotopic surface labeling and SDS-PAGE analysis.[23,49,130,132] These findings are usually considered to reflect a deficient transmembrane or intracellular stimulus-response coupling or a qualitative abnormality intrinsic to the GPIIb-IIIa complex. The CIE analysis of some of these platelets has proved to be of great interest in defining the molecular abnormality(ies) responsible for the functional defect.

*Pidard, D. et al.: Unpublished data, 1987.

Thus, Nurden et al. have reported a patient (C.M.) whose platelets exhibit normal amounts of surface-exposed GPIIb and GPIIIa.[132] When kept in the continuous presence of physiologic concentrations of divalent cations, the patient's platelets showed evidence, upon CIE analysis, of apparently normal GPIIb-IIIa complexes. However, exposure of these platelets to EDTA before solubilization with Triton X-100, under conditions of *p*H and temperature that do not affect the stability of the complex in normal platelets, resulted in nearly complete dissociation of the complex.[132] An increased susceptibility of GPIIb-IIIa to displacement of the complex-bound calcium by chelators was ascertained, here, by the rate of dissociation of the complex upon addition of EDTA to Triton X-100-soluble extracts, that was much faster than that observed with normal platelets.[132] That an apparently abnormal organization of the two glycoproteins resulted in a functionally defective complex was further assessed by the inability of the intact patient's complex to bind ^{125}I-labeled fibrinogen in CIE, using an assay adapted from that of Gogstad et al. in which the labeled ligand is incorporated into the intermediate gel, rather than used to label pre-formed immunoprecipitates (*see also* Chap. 5).[53,132] In contrast, the residual GPIIb-IIIa complexes present in type II thrombasthenic platelets appear to be functional, as they do bind fibrinogen in this same assay.*

Patients who may express a similar abnormal organization of the GPIIb-IIIa complex have been described by Ginsberg et al.[49] As with the patient C.M., these individuals, who belong to the same family, appear indistinguishable from classic type I thrombasthenic patients, given their platelet function test results, but their platelets contain near normal levels of surface-exposed GPIIb and GPIIIa.[49] Their platelets differ from normals in that, in the presence of physiologic concentrations of Ca^{2+}, they do bind significant amounts of a monoclonal antibody, PMI-1, whose epitope is located on the GPIIb α chain and is expressed on the surface of normal platelets only when external divalent cations are lowered to the micromolar range.[49] This is indicative of an abnormal divalent cation-dependent regulation of the conformation of GPIIb, possibly linked to the inability of these platelets to bind fibrinogen.[49] The CIE analysis of these particular platelets has shown the presence of an intact GPIIb-IIIa complex, although some subtle modifications of its shape and appearance have been noted.[49] No attempts have been made, however, to further characterize its capacity to dissociate nor its ability to interact with fibrinogen in this system.

Another patient (R.P., Paris-Lariboisière I), whose platelets express reduced amounts of membrane GPIIb-IIIa complexes (30% to 40% of the normal value) but functionally behave like those of a typical type I thrombasthenic patient, has been described by Caen.[23] Preliminary studies indicate that the residual complexes of this patient do not show an increased susceptibility to chelating agents and that they can directly interact with ^{125}I-labeled fibrinogen, as judged by the CIE approach described earlier.* In this particular case, a defect involving a stimulus-response-coupling mechanism of intact platelets can be hypothesized.

Yet, another patient has been described by Tanoue et al., who appears to have a mild form of the disease because her washed platelets aggregate nearly normally in response to thrombin, although they do not respond to ADP, collagen, or epinephrine in plasma.[166] In this patient, CIE analysis has revealed the presence of normal amounts of the GPIIb-IIIa complex, which dissociates normally in the presence of EDTA.[166] By crossed-affinoimmunoelectrophoresis, a reduced interaction of GPIIb-IIIa with the lectin concanavalin A (Con A) was observed.[166] An abnormal glycosylation pattern restricted to GPIIb and GPIIIa was confirmed by a reduced PAS-staining of these two glycoproteins upon separation by SDS-PAGE.[166]

Acquired Disorders: The Tn Syndrome

The Tn syndrome is clinically characterized by polyagglutinability of red blood cells accompanied, more or less, by severe thrombocytopenia and leukopenia.[128,130] It is an acquired disorder, with a clonal expression, that affects a percentage of the circulating erythrocytes, platelets, and granulocytes, variably from case to case, suggesting that the pathogenesis of the disease may lie in the somatic mutation of a pluripotent stem cell.[128,130] The basic biochemical defect resides in an absent or abnormal

*Fournier, D. et al.: Unpublished data, 1985.

β-galactosyl transferase (T-transferase) resulting in an incomplete synthesis of oligosaccharide side chains that leaves *N*-acetyl-D-galactosamine (GalNAc) residues unsubstituted by sialic acid or by sialic acid–galactose disaccharides.[130] Unsubstituted GalNAc residues linked to serine or threonine thus represent or participate in the expression of the Tn antigen, for which natural antibodies are present in the plasma of most individuals.[130] The presence of incomplete oligosaccharide side chains is the particular feature of several major blood cell membrane sialoglycoproteins, including red cell glycophorins A and B, leukocyte sialophorin(s), and platelet GPIb.[128,130,151]

Extensive investigations have been performed by Nurden et al. on a patient presenting with more than 80% of Tn-positive circulating platelets.[128] Analysis of the patient's platelets by CIE revealed an abnormal immunochemical behavior of the incompletely glycosylated GPIb, reflected by a markedly decreased area of the GPIb immunoprecipitate (Fig. 11-7) in contrast to the presence, in these

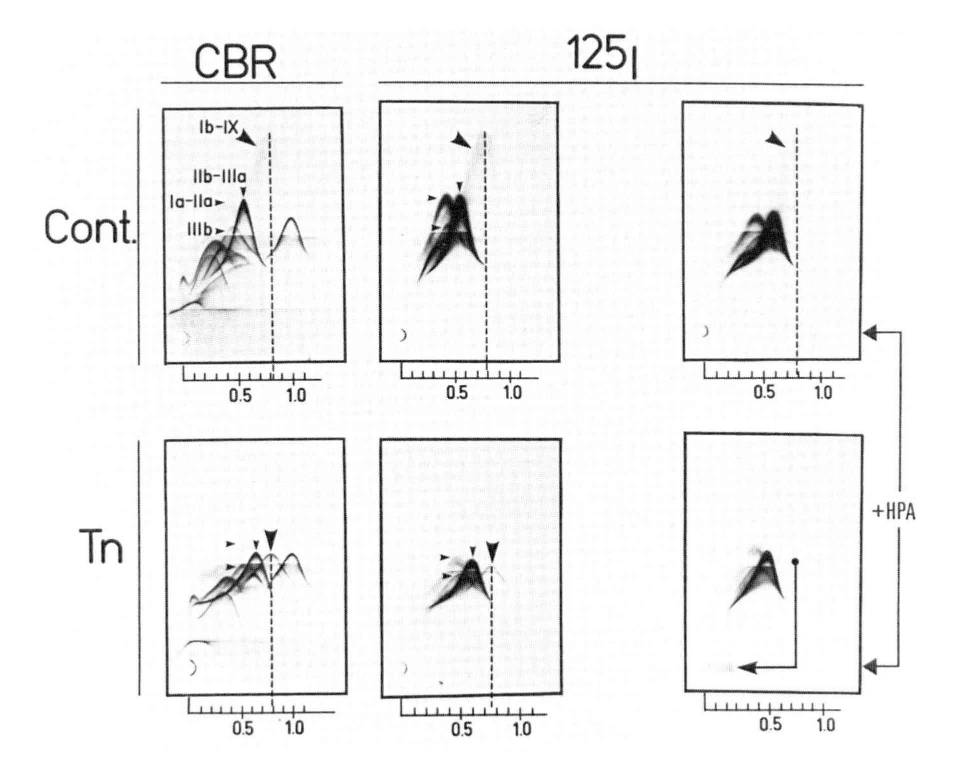

Figure 11-7. CIE and crossed-affinoimmunoelectrophoresis analysis of Tn platelets. Triton X-100-soluble proteins (100 μg) prepared from ^{125}I-labeled platelets obtained from an healthy control donor (Cont.) and from a patient affected with the Tn syndrome (Tn) were submitted to CIE essentially as described in the legend to Figure 11-1. The CBR-stained gels (CBR) and the corresponding autoradiographs (^{125}I) obtained after 2 days of exposure on Kodak X-Omat MA films (*left-hand panels*) are shown, together with the autoradiographic profiles observed when *Helix pomatia* agglutinin (HPA; monosaccharide specificity: GalNAc) was present at 50 μg/ml during the first-dimension electrophoresis (*right-hand panels*). The dashed lines refer to the location of the GPIb–IX complex. Note that the abnormally glycosylated GPIb–IX complex has a normal location but gives rise to an immunoprecipitate of decreased area, whereas it is directly precipitated by the lectin into the first-dimension gel. In contrast, fully glycosylated GPIb–IX complexes are unaffected by the lectin. Other major membrane glycoproteins appear unmodified in the Tn platelets (adapted from Nurden AT, Dupuis D, Pidard D et al; reproduced from the Journal of Clinical Investigation, 1982, 70:1281, by copyright permission of the American Society for Clinical Investigation.)

platelets, of near normal amounts of the GPIb polypeptide core.[128] This would suggest that the pattern of glycosylation of GPIb can strongly influence its antigenicity. The abnormal glycosylation of GPIb could be demonstrated, here, through crossed-affinoimmunoelectrophoresis experiments, because the abnormal GPIb was directly precipitated by *Helix pomatia* agglutinin (HPA), which has a specificity for GalNAc residues, when this was incorporated into the first-dimension agarose gel, whereas this lectin had no effect on the mobility of normally glycosylated GPIb (*see* Fig. 11-7).[128]

Rather surprisingly, the absence of negatively charged sialic acid residues on this abnormal GPIb did not result in a slower mobility during the first-dimension electrophoresis. This may indicate that factors other than its own intrinsic negative charge are involved in the mobility of GPIb during agarose gel electrophoresis, such as its association with GPIX or the presence of acidic glycolipids in the complex. Alternatively, the terminal GalNac residues may compensate for the negative charge normally provided by sialic acid.

That GPIb and GPIX exist as complexes was not suspected or known at the time of that study. Differential effects upon GPIb, GPIX, or the GPIb-IX complex have not been investigated further in patients with the Tn syndrome.

CONCLUSIONS

Investigations of the platelet plasma membrane glycoproteins as diverse as those described throughout this chapter clearly establish crossed-immunoelectrophoresis and related immunochemical techniques as simple, fast, reproducible, and versatile approaches to the functional and structural analyses of complex mixtures of soluble and membrane (glyco)proteins (*see* Table 11-1).

The resolution of numerous molecular species into separate entities, appearing here as immunoprecipitates, may seem relatively poor when compared with the SDS-PAGE system (for comparison, *see* Clemetson[30]). However, the point has to be stressed that, because of the use of nonionic detergents, several major antigenic components of human platelets appear in CIE as multipolypeptide complex structures. This has been observed also for other cell systems or subcellular fractions and is generally not the result of artifactual interactions or aggregations of proteins in solution but, rather, of an accurate reflection of native membrane or cellular (glyco)protein organization.[8,10,12,97,99,150] Thus, every macromolecular structure that has been described through CIE of platelet or plasma membrane extracts (i.e., GPIIb-IIIa, GPIb-IX, GPIb-ABP, and GPIa-IIa; *see* Table 11-1) has subsequently been shown to exist in the intact platelet by other methods. Moreover, the resolution and sensitivity of the technique can be increased by varying the antigen/antibody ratio, by using subcellular fractions (such as plasma membranes or isolated granules) instead of whole cell extracts, and by utilizing antibodies of a more restricted specificity.[8,10,54,58,155] In whole-platelet extracts, the sensitivity of CIE can best be appreciated by considering that 100 ng of total platelet protein should not contain more than 250 ng of fibronectin, an amount that is, nonetheless, sufficient to produce a detectable immunoprecipitate (*see* Fig. 11-1). For strongly immunogenic proteins, as little as 10 to 100 ng of antigen can generate precipitation lines.[8,10]

Because it is a nondenaturing approach, much information can be gained, through the use of CIE, about certain biologic activities of the platelet plasma membrane glycoproteins, such as their metal-binding properties and receptorlike activities (*see* Table 11-1).

A major application of the CIE technique is also found in the characterization of monospecific antibodies, particularly those generated through hybridoma technology. This technique remains, thus far, the easiest and least ambiguous approach to defining epitope specificity for a large number of monoclonal antibodies. The application of protein transfer and immunoblotting procedures to CIE gels should assist in this purpose by increasing the sensitivity and by extending the applicability of the technique.[169] Except for IgG-L, no attempts have been reported to characterize the antigenic specificity of human iso-, allo-, or autoantibodies using CIE.[152] This is clearly an underutilization of the potential of this technique, and new investigations in this area should be prompted in the near future.

Finally, CIE and related unidimensional immunoelectrophoretic techniques have proved to be most useful for the quantitative or qualitative characterization of platelet membrane glycoproteins, as well as their metabolic products, or structural analogues, in various biologic fluids, cells types, animal species, and disease states.

I believe that, when used to complement other, well-established analytic procedures, and with the availability of new immunochemical reagents, CIE will contribute to a better understanding of the structure and function of the platelet plasma membrane glycoproteins, both in physiology and pathology.

REFERENCES

1. Ali-Briggs EF, Clemetson KJ, Jenkins CSP: Antibodies against platelet membrane glycoproteins. I. Crossed immunoelectrophoresis studies with antibodies that inhibit ristocetin-induced platelet aggregation. Br J Haematol 48:305, 1981

2. Altieri DC, Mannucci PM, Capitanio AM: Binding of fibrinogen to human monocytes. J Clin Invest 78:968, 1986

3. Axelsen NH, Kroll J, Weeke B: A manual of quantitative immunoelectrophoresis. Methods and applications. Scan J Immunol 2 (Suppl 1), 1973

4. Baldassare JJ, Kahn RA, Knipp MA, Newman PJ: Reconstitution of platelet proteins into phospholipid vesicles. Functional proteoliposomes. J Clin Invest 75:35, 1985

5. Barber JA, Jamieson GA: Isolation and characterization of plasma membranes from human blood platelets. J Biol Chem 245:6357, 1970

6. Berman CL, Yeo EL, Wencel-Drake JD, Furie BC, Ginsberg MH, Furie B: A platelet alpha-granule membrane protein that is associated with the plasma membrane after activation. Characterization and subcellular localization of platelet activation-dependent granule-external membrane protein. J Clin Invest 78:130, 1986

7. Berndt MC, Gregory C, Kabral A, Zola E, Fournier D, Castaldi PA: Purification and preliminary characterization of the glycoprotein Ib complex in the human platelet membrane. Eur J Biochem 151:637, 1985

8. Bjerrum OJ: Immunochemical investigation of membrane proteins. A methodological survey with emphasis placed on immunoprecipitation in gels. Biochim Biophys Acta 472:135, 1977

9. Bjerrum OJ, Bog-Hansen TC: The immunochemical approach to the characterization of membrane proteins. Human erythrocyte membrane proteins analyzed as a model system. Biochim Biophys Acta 455:66, 1976

10. Bjerrum OJ, Bog-Hansen TC: Immunochemical gel precipitation techniques for analysis of membrane proteins. In Maddy AH (ed): Contribution to Biochemical Analysis of Membrane. London, Chapman & Hall, 1976

11. Bjerrum OJ, Lundahl P: Crossed immunoelectrophoresis of human erythrocyte membrane proteins. Immunoprecipitation patterns for fresh and stored samples of membranes extensively solubilized with nonionic detergents. Biochim Biophys Acta 342:69, 1974

12. Blomberg F, Raftell M: Enzyme polymorphism in rat-liver microsomes and plasma membranes. 1. An immunochemical study of multienzyme complexes and other enzyme-active antigens. Eur J Biochem 49:21, 1979

13. Bog-Hansen TC: Crossed immuno-affinoelectrophoresis. An analytical method to predict the result of affinity chromatography. Anal Biochem 56:480, 1973

14. Borsum T, Bjerrum OJ: Electrophoretic migration velocity of amphiphilic proteins increases with decreasing Triton X-100 concentration: A new characteristic of their identification. Electrophoresis 7:197, 1986

15. Borsum T, Hagen I, Bjerrum OJ: Electroimmunochemical characterization of endothelial cell proteins: Antigenic relationship with platelet and erythrocyte membrane proteins. Thromb Haemostasis 58:686, 1987

16. Brass LF, Shattil SJ: Identification and function of the high affinity binding sites for Ca^{2+} on the surface of platelets. J Clin Invest 73:626, 1984

17. Brass LF, Shattil SJ, Kunicki TJ, Bennett JS: Effect of calcium on the stability of the platelet membrane glycoprotein IIb–IIIa complex. J Biol Chem 260:7875, 1985

18. Bray PF, Rosa J-R, Lingappa VR, Kan YW, McEver RP, Shuman MA: Biogenesis of the platelet receptor for fibrinogen: Evidence for separate precursors for glycoproteins IIb and IIIa. Proc Natl Acad Sci USA 83:1480, 1986

19. Breton-Gorius J, Lewis JC, Guichard J, Kieffer N, Vainchenker W: Monoclonal antibodies specific for human platelet membrane glycoproteins bind to monocytes by focal absorption of platelet membrane fragments: An ultrastructural immunogold study. Leukemia 1:131, 1987

20. Breton-Gorius J, Vainchenker W: Expression of platelet proteins during the in vitro and in vivo differentiation of megakaryocytes and morphological aspects of their maturation. Semin Hematol 23:43, 1986

21. Broekman MJ, Handin RI, Cohen P: Distribution of fibrinogen, and platelet factors 4 and XIII in subcellular fractions of human platelets. Br J Haematol 31:51, 1975

22. Burns GF, Cosgrove L, Triglia T, Beall JA, Lopez AF, Werkmeister JA, Begley CG, Haddad AP, d'Apice AJF, Vaclas MA, Cawley JC: The IIb-IIIa glycoprotein complex that mediates platelet aggregation is directly implicated in leukocyte adhesion. Cell 45:269, 1986

23. Caen JP: Variant thrombasthénie Paris-I-Lariboisière. Trouble fonctionnel de l'agrégation des plaquettes humaines indépendant des glycoprotéines. CR Seances Acad Sci Sér. III 300:417, 1985

24. Calvete JJ, McGregor JL, Rivas G, Gonzalez-Rodriguez J: Identification of a glycoprotein IIIa dimer in polyacrylamide gel separation of human platelet membranes. Thromb Haemostasis 58:694, 1987

25. Charo IF, Fitzgerald LA, Steiner B, Rall SC, Bekeart LS, Phillips DR: Platelet glycoproteins IIb and IIIa: Evidence for a family of immunologically and structurally related glycoproteins in mammalian cells. Proc Natl Acad Sci USA 83:8351, 1986

26. Chelladurai M, Fossett NG, Ganguly P: A novel thrombin-reactive protein complex in human platelets. J Biol Chem 258:1407, 1983

27. Chua N-H, Blomberg F: Immunochemical studies of thylakoid membrane polypeptides from spinach and *Chlamydomonas reinhardtii.* J Biol Chem 254:215, 1979

28. Clarke HGM, Freeman T: Quantitative immunoelectrophoresis of human serum proteins. Clin Sci 35:403, 1968

29. Clarke S: The size and detergent binding of membrane proteins. J Biol Chem 250:5459, 1975

30. Clemetson KJ: Glycoproteins of the platelet plasma membrane. In George JN, Nurden AT, Phillips DR (eds): Platelet Membrane Glycoproteins. New York, Plenum Press, 1985

31. Cohen I, Glaser T, Veis A, Bruner-Lorand J: Ca^{2+}-dependent cross-linking processes in human platelets. Biochim Biophys Acta 676:137, 1981

32. Coller BS, Kalomiris E, Steinberg M, Scudder LE: Evidence that glycocalicin circulates in normal plasma. J Clin Invest 73:794, 1984

33. Coller BS, Peerschke EI, Seligsohn U, Scudder LE, Nurden AT, Rosa J-P: Studies on the binding of an alloimmune and two murine monoclonal antibodies to the platelet glycoprotein IIb-IIIa complex receptor. J Lab Clin Med 107:384, 1986

34. Coller BS, Seligsohn U, Zivelin A, Zwang E, Lusky A, Modan M: Immunologic and biochemical characterization of homozygous and heterozygous Glanzmann thrombasthenia in the Iraqi-Jewish and Arab populations of Israel: Comparison of techniques for carrier detection. Br J Haematol 62:723, 1986

35. Converse CA, Papermaster DS: Membrane protein analysis by two-dimensional immunoelectrophoresis. Science 189:469, 1975

36. Degos L, Dautigny A, Brouet JC, Colombani M, Ardaillou N, Caen JP, Colombani J: A molecular defect in thrombasthenic platelets. J Clin Invest 56:236, 1975

37. Du X, Beutler L, Ruan C, Castaldi PA, Berndt MC: Glycoprotein Ib and glycoprotein IX are fully complexed in the intact platelet membrane. Blood 69:1524, 1987

38. Fitzgerald LA, Charo IF, Phillips DR: Human and bovine endothelial cells synthesize membrane proteins similar to human platelet glycoproteins IIb and IIIa. J Biol Chem 260:10893, 1985

39. Fitzgerald LA, Phillips DR: Calcium regulation of the platelet membrane glycoprotein IIb-IIIa complex. J Biol Chem 260:11366, 1985

40. Fitzgerald LA, Steiner B, Rall SC, Lo S, Phillips DR: Protein sequence of endothelial glycoprotein IIIa derived from a cDNA clone. J Biol Chem 262:3936, 1987

41. Fox JEB: Identification of actin-binding protein as the protein linking the membrane skeleton to glycoproteins in platelet plasma membranes. J Biol Chem 260:11970, 1985

42. Fox JEB, Phillips DR: Actin-membrane interactions in platelets. In Bennett V, Cohen CM, Lux SE, Palek J (eds): Membrane Skeletons and Cytoskeletal-Membrane Associations. New York, Alan R Liss, 1986

43. Fujimura K, Phillips DR: Calcium cation regulation of glycoprotein IIb-IIIa complex formation in platelet plasma membranes. J Biol Chem 258:10247, 1983

44. George JN, Nurden AT, Phillips DR: Molecular defects in interactions of platelets with the vessel wall. N Engl J Med 311:1084, 1984

45. George JN, Pickett EB, Saucerman S, McEver RP, Kunicki TJ, Kieffer N, Newman PJ: Studies on resting and activated platelets and platelet membrane microparticles in normal subjects, and observations in patients during adult respiratory distress syndrome and cardiac surgery. J Clin Invest 78:340, 1986

46. Gerlach JH, Bjerrum OJ, Rank GH: Electroimmunochemical analysis of plasma vesicles from *Saccharomyces cerevisiae.* Can J Biochem 60:659, 1982

47. Giancotti FG, Languino LR, Zanetti A, Peri G, Tarone G, Dejana E: Platelets express a membrane protein complex immunologically related to the fibroblast fibronectin receptor and distinct from GP IIb-IIIa. Blood 69:1535, 1987

48. Giltay JC, Leeksma OC, Breederveld C, Van Mourik JA: Normal synthesis and expression of endothelial IIb/IIIa in Glanzmann's thrombasthenia. Blood 69:809, 1987

49. Ginsberg MH, Lightsey A, Kunicki TK, Kaufman A, Marguerie GA, Plow EF: Divalent cat-

ion regulation of the surface orientation of platelet membrane glycoprotein IIb. Correlation with fibrinogen binding function and definition of a novel variant of Glanzmann's thrombasthenia. J Clin Invest 78:1103, 1986

50. Ginsberg MH, Loftus J, Ryckwaert J-J, Pierschbacher M, Pytela R, Ruoslahti E, Plow EF: Immunochemical and amino-terminal sequence comparison of two cytoadhesins indicates they contain similar or identical β subunits and distinct α subunits. J Biol Chem 262:5437, 1987

51. Gogstad GO: A method for the isolation of α-granules from human platelets. Thromb Res 20:669, 1980

52. Gogstad GO, Brosstad F: Platelet factor XIII is an active enzyme after solubilization and crossed immunoelectrophoresis. Thromb Res 29:237, 1983

53. Gogstad GO, Brosstad F, Krutnes M-B, Hagen I, Solum NO: Fibrinogen-binding properties of the human platelet glycoprotein IIb–IIIa complex: A study using crossed-immunoelectrophoresis. Blood 60:663, 1982

54. Gogstad GO, Hagen I, Korsmo R, Solum NO: Characterization of the proteins of isolated human platelet α-granules. Evidence for a separate α-granule-pool of the glycoproteins IIb and IIIa. Biochim Biophys Acta 670:150, 1981

55. Gogstad GO, Hagen I, Korsmo R, Solum NO: Evidence for release of soluble, but not of membrane-integrated, proteins from human platelet α-granules. Biochim Biophys Acta 702:81, 1982

56. Gogstad GO, Hagen I, Krutnes M-B, Solum NO: Dissociation of the glycoprotein IIb–IIIa complex in isolated human platelet membranes. Dependence of *p*H and divalent cations. Biochim Biophys Acta 689:21, 1982

57. Gogstad GO, Hetland O, Solum NO, Prydz H: Monocytes and platelets share the glycoproteins IIb and IIIa that are absent from both cells in Glanzmann's thrombasthenia type I. Biochem J 214:331, 1983

58. Gogstad GO, Krutnes M-B, Hetland O, Solum NO: Comparison of protein and lipid composition of the human platelet α-granule membranes and glycerol lysis membranes. Biochim Biophys Acta 732:519, 1983

59. Gogstad GO, Krutnes M-B, Solum NO: Calcium-binding proteins from human platelets. A study using crossed immunoelectrophoresis and $^{45}Ca^{2+}$. Eur J Biochem 133:193, 1983

60. Gogstad GO, Solum NO, Krutnes M-B: Heparin-binding platelet proteins demonstrated by crossed affinity immunoelectrophoresis. Br J Haematol 53:563, 1983

61. Golovtchenko-Matsumoto AM, Osawa T: Heterogeneity of band 3, the major intrinsic protein of human erythrocyte membranes. Studies by crossed immunoelectrophoresis and crossed immuno-affinoelectrophoresis. J Biochem 87:847, 1980

62. Gronke RS, Bergman BL, Baker JB: Thrombin interaction with platelets. Influence of a platelet protease nexin. J Biol Chem 262:3030, 1987

63. Guerillon J, Barray S, Devauchelle G: Crossed immunoelectrophoresis of Chilo iridescent virus surface antigens. Arch Virol 73:161, 1982

64. Hagen I: Electroimmunochemical characterization of platelet proteins: Their subcellular location and involvement in platelet adhesion, aggregation and secretion. In Bjerrum OJ (ed): Electroimmunochemical Analysis of Membrane Proteins. Amsterdam, Elsevier Science Publishers, 1983

65. Hagen I, Bjerrum OJ, Gogstad GO, Korsmo R, Solum NO: Involvement of divalent cations in the complex between the platelet glycoproteins IIb and IIIa. Biochim Biophys Acta 701:1, 1982

66. Hagen I, Bjerrum OJ, Solum NO: Characterization of human platelet proteins solubilized with Triton X-100 and examined by crossed immunoelectrophoresis. Reference patterns of extracts from whole platelets and isolated membranes. Eur J Biochem 99:9, 1979

67. Hagen I, Brosstad F, Gogstad GO, Solum NO, Korsmo R: Demonstration of variable forms of the platelet factor 4 immunoprecipitate using crossed immunoelectrophoresis. Thromb Res 27:77, 1982

68. Hagen I, Brosstad F, Solum NO, Korsmo R: Crossed immunoelectrophoresis using immobilized thrombin in intermediate gel. A method for demonstration of thrombin-binding proteins. J Lab Clin Med 97:213, 1981

69. Hagen I, Gogstad GO, Brosstad F, Solum NO: Demonstration of ^{125}I-labelled thrombin binding platelet proteins by use of crossed immunoelectrophoresis and autoradiography. Biochim Biophys Acta 732:600, 1983

70. Hagen I, Nurden AT, Bjerrum OJ, Solum NO, Caen J: Immunochemical evidence for protein abnormalities in platelets from patients with Glanzmann's thrombasthenia and Bernard-Soulier syndrome. J Clin Invest 65:722, 1980

71. Hagen I, Solum NO: Structure and function of platelet membrane glycoproteins as studied by crossed immunoelectrophoresis. In George JN, Nurden AT, Phillips DR (eds): Platelet Membrane Glycoproteins. New York, Plenum Press, 1985

72. Hanash SM, Neel JV, Baier LJ, Rosenblum BB, Niezgoda W, Markel D: Genetic analysis of thirty-three platelet polypeptides detected in two-dimensional polyacrylamide gels. Am J Hum Genet 38:352, 1986

73. Hearn VM, MacKenzie DWR: Analysis of wall antigens of *Aspergillus fumigatus* by two-di-

mensional immunoelectrophoresis. J Med Microbiol 14:119, 1981

74. Helenius A, Simons K: Solubilization of membranes by detergents. Biochim Biophys Acta 415:29, 1975

75. Helenius A, Simons K: Charge-shift electrophoresis: Simple method for distinguishing between amphilic and hydrophilic proteins in detergent solution. Proc Natl Acad Sci USA 74:529, 1977

76. Herrmann FH, Meyer M, Gogstad GO, Solum NO: Glycoprotein IIb-IIIa complex in platelets of patients and heterozygotes of Glanzmann's thrombasthenia. Thromb Res 32:615, 1983

77. Hiraiwa A, Matsukage A, Shiku H, Takahashi T, Naito K, Yamada K: Purification and partial amino acid sequence of human platelet membrane glycoproteins IIb and IIIa. Blood 69:560, 1987

78. Hofstra H, Van Tool MJD, Dankert J: Cross-reactivity of major outer membrane proteins of *Enterobacteriaceae,* studied by crossed immunoelectrophoresis. J Bacteriol 143:328, 1980

79. Howard L, Shulman S, Sadamandan S, Karpatkin S: Crossed immunoelectrophoresis of human platelet membranes. The major antigen consists of a complex of glycoproteins IIb and IIIa, held together by Ca^{2+} and missing in Glanzmann's thrombasthenia. J Biol Chem 257:8331, 1982

80. Hsu-Lin S-C, Berman CL, Furie BC, August D, Furie B: A platelet membrane protein expressed during platelet activation and secretion. Studies using a monoclonal antibody specific for thrombin-activated platelets. J Biol Chem 259:9121, 1984

81. Jenkins CSP, Ali-Briggs EF, Clemetson KJ: Antibodies against platelet membrane glycoproteins. II. Influence on ADP- and collagen-induced platelet aggregation, crossed immunoelectrophoresis and relevance to Glanzmann's thrombasthenia. Br J Haematol 49:439, 1981

82. Jennings LK, Phillips DR: Purification of glycoproteins IIb and IIIa from human platelet plasma membranes and characterization of a calcium-dependent glycoprotein IIb-IIIa complex. J Biol Chem 257:10458, 1982

83. Kao KJ, Cook DJ, Scornik JC: Quantitative analysis of platelet surface HLA by W6/32 anti-HLA monoclonal antibody. Blood 68:627, 1986

84. Karpatkin M, Howard L, Karpatkin S: Studies on the origin of platelet-associated fibrinogen. J Lab Clin Med 104:223, 1984

85. Karpatkin S, Ferziger R, Dorfman D: Crossed immunoelectrophoresis of human platelet membranes. Effect of charge on association and dissociation of the glycoprotein GP IIb-IIIa membrane complex. J Biol Chem 261:14266, 1986

86. Kieffer N, Debili N, Wicki A, Titeux M, Henri A, Mishal Z, Breton-Gorius J, Vainchenker W, Clemetson KJ: Expression of platelet glycoprotein Ibα in HEL cells. J Biol Chem 261:15854, 1986

87. Kristopeit SM, Kunicki TJ: Quantitation of platelet membrane glycoproteins in Glanzmann's thrombasthenia and the Bernard-Soulier syndrome by electroimmunoassay. Thromb Res 36:133, 1984

88. Kronman MJ, Bratcher SC: An experimental artifact in the use of chelating metal ion buffers. Binding of chelators to bovine α-lactalbumin. J Biol Chem 258:5707, 1983

89. Kunicki TJ: Organization of glycoproteins within the platelet plasma membrane. In George JN, Nurden AT, Phillips DR (eds): Platelet Membrane Glycoproteins. New York, Plenum Press, 1985

90. Kunicki TJ, Montgomery RR, Schullek J: Cleavage of human von Willebrand factor by platelet calcium-activated protease. Blood 65:352, 1985

91. Kunicki TJ, Mosesson MW, Pidard D: Cleavage of fibrinogen by human platelet calcium-activated protease. Thromb Res 35:169, 1984

92. Kunicki TJ, Newman PJ: Synthesis of analogs of human platelet membrane glycoprotein IIb-IIIa complex by chicken peripheral blood thrombocytes. Proc Natl Acad Sci USA 82:7319, 1985

93. Kunicki TJ, Newman PJ: The biochemistry of platelet-specific alloantigens. Curr Stud Hematol Blood Transf 52:18, 1986

94. Kunicki TJ, Newman PJ, Amrani DL, Mosesson MW: Human platelet fibrinogen: Purification and hemostatic properties. Blood 66:808, 1985

95. Kunicki TJ, Newman PJ, Montgomery RR, Kawai Y, Furihata K: The human platelet membrane glycoprotein IIb-IIIa complex: A prototype for cytoadhesins. In Jolles G, Legrand YJ, Nurden AT (eds): Biology and Pathology of Platelet-Vessel Wall Interactions. London, Academic Press Inc, 1986

96. Kunicki TJ, Nugent DJ, Staats S, Orchekowski RP, Wayner EA, Carter WG: The human fibroblast class II extracellular matrix receptor (ECMR II) mediates platelet adhesion to collagen and is identical to the platelet glycoprotein Ia-IIa complex. J Biol Chem 263:4516, 1988

97. Kunicki TJ, Nurden AT, Pidard D, Russell NR, Caen JP: Characterization of human platelet glycoprotein antigens giving rise to individual immunoprecipitates in crossed immunoelectrophoresis. Blood 58:1190, 1981

98. Kunicki TJ, Pidard D, Cazenave J-P, Nurden AT, Caen JP: Inheritance of the human platelet alloantigen, Pl^{A1}, in type I Glanzmann's thrombasthenia. J Clin Invest 67:717, 1981

99. Kunicki TJ, Pidard D, Rosa J-P, Nurden AT: The formation of Ca^{2+}-dependent complexes of platelet membrane glycoproteins IIb and IIIa in so-

lution as determined by crossed immunoelectrophoresis. Blood 58:268, 1981

100. Laurell C-B: Antigen-antibody crossed electrophoresis. Anal Biochem 10:358, 1965

101. Laurell C-B: Quantitative estimation of proteins by electrophoresis in agarose gel containing antibodies. Anal Biochem 15:45, 1966

102. Leeksma OC, Zandbergen-Spaargaren J, Giltay JC, Van Mourik JA: Cultured human endothelial cells synthesize a plasma membrane protein complex immunologically related to the platelet glycoprotein IIb/IIIa complex. Blood 67:1176, 1986

103. Leung LLK, Kinoshita T, Nachman RL: Isolation, purification and partial characterization of platelet membrane glycoproteins IIb and IIIa. J Biol Chem 256:1994, 1981

104. Levy-Toledano S, Tobelem G, Legrand C, Bredoux R, Degos L, Nurden AT, Caen JP: Acquired IgG antibody occurring in a thrombasthenic patient: Its effect on human platelet function. Blood 51:1065, 1978

105. Lombardo VT, Hodson E, Roberts JR, Kunicki TJ, Zimmerman TS, Ruggeri ZM: Independant modulation of von Willebrand factor and fibrinogen binding to the platelet membrane glycoprotein IIb/IIIa complex as demonstrated by monoclonal antibody. J Clin Invest 76:1950, 1985

106. Lynch DM, Howe SE: Heparin-associated thrombocytopenia: Antibody binding specificity to platelet antigens. Blood 66:1176, 1985

107. Makhoul RG, Devine DV, Breuckman WD, McCann RL, Greenberg CS: Evidence for the involvement of platelet glycoproteins other than GP Ib in heparin-associated thrombocytopenia and thrombosis. Thromb Res 45:421, 1987

108. Makino S, Reynolds JA, Tanford C: The binding of deoxycholate and Triton X-100 to proteins. J Biol Chem 248:4926, 1973

109. McCaffery PJ, Berridge MV: Expression of the leukocyte functional molecule (LFA-1) on mouse platelets. Blood 67:1757, 1986

110. McEver RP, Baenziger NL, Majerus PW: Isolation and quantitation of the platelet membrane glycoprotein deficient in thrombasthenia using a monoclonal hybridoma antibody. J Clin Invest 66:1311, 1980

111. McEver RP, Bennett EM, Martin MN: Identification of two structurally and functionally distinct sites on human platelet membrane glycoprotein IIb–IIIa using monoclonal antibodies. J Biol Chem 258:5269, 1983

112. McEver RP, Martin MN: A monoclonal antibody to a membrane glycoprotein binds only to activated platelets. J Biol Chem 259:9799, 1984

113. McGregor JL: Monoclonal Antibodies and Human Blood Platelets. Amsterdam, Elsevier Science Publishers, 1986

114. McGregor JL, Brochier J, Wild F, Follea G, Trzeciak M-C, James E, Dechavanne M, McGregor L, Clemetson KJ: Monoclonal antibodies against platelet membrane glycoproteins. Characterization and effect on platelet function. Eur J Biochem 131:427, 1983

115. McGregor JL, Clemetson KJ, James E, Greenland T, Dechavanne M: Identification of human platelet glycoproteins in SDS-polyacrylamide gels using ^{125}I-labelled lectins. Thromb Res 16:825, 1979

116. McGregor JL, Clemetson KJ, James E, Luscher EF, Dechavanne M: Characterization of human platelet membrane proteins and glycoproteins by their isoelectric point (*p*I) and apparent molecular weight using two-dimensional electrophoresis and surface-labelling techniques. Biochim Biophys Acta 599:473, 1980

117. McGregor JL, McGregor L, Bauer A-S, Catimel B, Brochier J, Dechavanne M, Clemetson KJ: Identification of two distinct regions within the binding sites for fibrinogen and fibronectin on the IIb–IIIa human platelet membrane glycoprotein complex by monoclonal antibodies P2 and P4. Eur J Biochem 159:443, 1986

118. McMillan R: Immune thrombocytopenia. Clin Haematol 12:69, 1983

119. Moroi M, Jung SM: Selective staining of human platelet glycoproteins using nitrocellulose transfer of electrophoresed proteins and lactoperoxidase-conjugated lectins. Biochim Biophys Acta 798:295, 1984

120. Nachman RL, Leung LLK, Kloczewiak M, Hawiger J: Complex formation of platelet membrane glycoprotein IIb and IIIa with the fibrinogen D domain. J Biol Chem 259:8584, 1984

121. Newman PJ, Allen RW, Kahn RA, Kunicki TJ: Quantitation of membrane glycoprotein IIIa on intact human platelets using the monoclonal antibody AP-3. Blood 65:227, 1985

122. Newman PJ, Kawai Y, Montgomery RR, Kunicki TJ: Synthesis by cultured human umbilical vein endothelial cells of two proteins structurally and immunologically related to platelet membrane glycoproteins IIb and IIIa. J Cell Biol 103:81, 1986

123. Newman PJ, Knipp MA, Kahn RA: Extraction and identification of human platelet integral membrane proteins using Triton X-114. Thromb Res 27:221, 1982

124. Nieuwenhuis HK, Akkerman JWN, Houdijk WPH, Sixma JJ: Human blood platelets showing no response to collagen fail to express surface glycoprotein Ia. Nature 318:470, 1985

125. Norrild B, Bjerrum OJ, Vestergaard BF:

Polypeptide analysis of individual immunoprecipitates from crossed immunoelectrophoresis. Anal Biochem 81:432, 1977

126. Nugent D, Kunicki TJ, Berglund C, Bernstein VD: A human monoclonal autoantibody recognizes a neoantigen on glycoprotein IIIa expressed on stored and activated platelets. Blood 70:16, 1987

127. Nugent D, Kunicki TJ, Montgomery RR, Bernstein I: A monoclonal antibody to platelet glycoprotein Ib (GPIb) blocks ristocetin-induced agglutination but does not bind to glycocalicin (abstr). Circulation 70(Suppl.II):356, 1984

128. Nurden AT, Dupuis D, Pidard D, Kieffer N, Kunicki TJ, Cartron J-P: Surface modifications in the platelets of a patient with α-*N*-acetyl-D-galactosamine residues, the Tn-syndrome. J Clin Invest 70:1281, 1982

129. Nurden AT, Dupuis D, Pidard D, Kunicki TJ, Caen JP: Biochemistry and immunology of platelet membranes with reference to glycoprotein composition. Ann NY Acad Sci 370:72, 1981

130. Nurden AT, George JN, Phillips DR: Platelet membrane glycoproteins: Their structure, function, and modifications in disease. In Phillips DR, Shuman MA (eds): Biochemistry of Platelets. New York, Academic Press, 1986

131. Nurden AT, Kunicki TJ, Dupuis D, Soria C, Caen JP: Specific protein and glycoprotein deficiencies in platelets isolated from two patients with the gray platelet syndrome. Blood 59:709, 1982

132. Nurden AT, Rosa J-P, Fournier D, Legrand C, Didry D, Parquet A, Pidard D: A variant of Glanzmann's thrombasthenia with abnormal glycoprotein IIb-IIIa complexes in the platelet membrane. J Clin Invest 79:962, 1987

133. Okita JR, Pidard D, Newman PJ, Montgomery RR, Kunicki TJ: On the association of glycoprotein Ib and actin-binding protein in human platelets. J Cell Biol 100:317, 1985

134. Owen P: An improved procedure for polypeptide analysis of radiolabeled antigens resolved by crossed immunoelectrophoresis and its application to the study of inner and outer membranes of *Escherichia coli*. Electrophoresis 7:19, 1986

135. Owen P, Kaback HR: Immunochemical analysis of membrane vesicles from *Escherichia coli*. Biochemistry 18:1413, 1979

136. Painter RG, Prodouz KN, Gaarde W: Isolation of a subpopulation of glycoprotein IIb-IIIa from platelet membranes that is bound to membrane actin. J Cell Biol 100:652, 1985

137. Peerschke EIB: The platelet fibrinogen receptor. Semin Hematol 22:241, 1985

138. Peerschke EIB: *p*H and magnesium alter ^{45}calcium binding at sites other than glycoproteins I or IIb/IIIa. Proc Soc Exp Biol Med 179:232, 1985

139. Peerschke EI, Grant RA, Zucker MB: Decreased association of ^{45}calcium with platelets unable to aggregate due to thrombasthenia or prolonged calcium deprivation. Br J Haematol 46:247, 1980

140. Perille-Collins ML, Salton MRJ: Preparation and crossed immunoelectrophoretic analysis of cytoplasmic and outer membrane fractions from *Neisseria gonorrhoeae*. Infect Immun 30:281, 1980

141. Phillips DR: Surface labeling as a tool to determine structure-function relationships of platelet plasma membrane glycoproteins. Thromb Haemostasis 42:1638, 1979

142. Phillips DR: Receptors for platelet agonists. In George JN, Nurden AT, Phillips DR (eds): Platelet Membrane Glycoproteins. New York, Plenum Press, 1985

143. Phillips DR, Agin PP: Platelet plasma membrane glycoproteins. Evidence for the presence of nonequivalent disulfide bonds using nonreduced-reduced two-dimensional gel electrophoresis. J Biol Chem 252:2121, 1977

144. Pidard D, Didry D, Kunicki TJ, Nurden AT: Temperature-dependent effects of EDTA on the membrane glycoprotein IIb-IIIa complex and platelet aggregability. Blood 67:604, 1986

145. Pidard D, Montgomery RR, Bennett JS, Kunicki TJ: Interaction of AP-2, a monoclonal antibody specific for the human platelet glycoprotein IIb-IIIa complex, with intact platelets. J Biol Chem 258:12582, 1983

146. Pidard D, Rosa J-P, Kunicki TJ, Nurden AT: Further studies on the interaction between human platelet membrane glycoproteins IIb and IIIa in Triton X-100. Blood 60:894, 1982

147. Piotrowicz RS, Orchekowski RP, Nugent DJ, Yamada KM, Kunicki TJ: Glycoprotein Ic-IIa functions as an activation-independent fibronectin receptor on human platelets. J Cell Biol 106:1359, 1988

148. Poncz M, Eisman R, Heidenrich R, Silver SM, Vilaire G, Surrey S, Schwartz E, Bennett JS: Structure of the platelet membrane glycoprotein IIb. Homology to the α subunits of the vitronectin and fibronectin receptors. J Biol Chem 262:8476, 1987

149. Pytela R, Pierschbacher MD, Ginsberg MH, Plow EF, Ruoslahti E: Platelet membrane glycoprotein IIb/IIIa: Member of a family of Arg-Gly-Asp-specific adhesion receptors. Science 231:1559, 1986

150. Raftell M, Blomberg F: Enzyme polymorphism in rat-liver microsomes and plasma membranes. 2. An immunochemical comparison of enzyme-active antigens solubilized by detergents, papain or phospholipases. Eur J Biochem 49:31, 1974

151. Remold-O'Donnell E, Zimmerman C, Kenney D, Rosen FS: Expression on blood cells of sialo-

phorin, the surface glycoprotein that is defective in Wiskott-Aldrich syndrome. Blood 70:104, 1987

152. Rosa J-P, Kieffer N, Didry D, Pidard D, Kunicki TJ, Nurden AT: The human platelet membrane glycoprotein complex GP IIb–IIIa expresses antigenic sites not exposed on the dissociated glycoproteins. Blood 64:1246, 1984

153. Ruan C, Du X, Wan H, Hu X, Xi X, Li P: Characterization of the fibrinogen binding sites using monoclonal antibodies to human platelet membrane glycoproteins IIb/IIIa (abstr). Thromb Haemostasis 58:243, 1987

154. Shattil SJ, Brass LF, Bennett JS, Pandhi P: Biochemical and functional consequences of dissociation of the platelet membrane glycoprotein IIb–IIIa complex. Blood 66:92, 1985

155. Shulman S, Karpatkin S: Crossed immunoelectrophoresis of human platelet membranes. Diminished major antigen in Glanzmann's thrombasthenia and Bernard-Soulier syndrome. J Biol Chem 255:4320, 1980

156. Shulman S, Wiesner R, Troll W, Karpatkin S: Reevaluation of the presence of the major antigen–Ca^{2+} complex in Bernard-Soulier syndrome platelets. Elastase degradation of the complex in Bernard-Soulier syndrome platelet preparations. Thromb Res 30:61, 1983

157. Solum NO, Hagen I, Filion-Myklebust C, Stabaeck T: Platelet glycocalicin. Its membrane association and solubilization in aqueous media. Biochim Biophys Acta 597:235, 1980

158. Solum NO, Hagen I, Slettbakk T: Further evidence for glycocalicin being derived from a larger amphiphilic platelet membrane glycoprotein. Thromb Res 18:773, 1980

159. Solum NO, Olsen TM: Glycoprotein Ib in the Triton-insoluble (cytoskeletal) fraction of blood platelets. Biochim Biophys Acta 799:209, 1984

160. Solum NO, Olsen TM: Effects of diamide and dibucaine on platelet glycoprotein Ib, actin-binding protein and cytoskeleton. Biochim Biophys Acta 817:249, 1985

161. Solum NO, Olsen TM, Gogstad GO, Hagen I, Brosstad F: Demonstration of a new glycoprotein Ib-related component in platelet extracts prepared in the presence of leupeptin. Biochim Biophys Acta 729:53, 1983

162. Stenberg PE, Beckstead JH, McEver RP, Levin J: Immunohistochemical localization of membrane and α-granule proteins in plastic-embedded mouse bone marrow megakaryocytes and murine megakaryocyte colonies. Blood 68:696, 1986

163. Stenberg PE, McEver RP, Shuman MA, Jacques YV, Bainton DF: A platelet alpha-granule membrane protein (GMP-140) is expressed on the plasma membrane after activation. J Cell Biol 101:880, 1985

164. Stormorken H, Gogstad GO, Solum NO, Pande H: Diagnosis of heterozygotes in Glanzmann's thrombasthenia. Thromb Haemostasis 48:217, 1982

165. Tabilio A, Rosa J-P, Testa U, Kieffer N, Nurden AT, Del Canizio MC, Breton-Gorius J, Vainchenker W: Expression of platelet membrane glycoproteins and α-granule proteins by human erythroleukemia cell line (HEL). EMBO J 3:453, 1984

166. Tanoue K, Hasegawa S, Yamaguchi A, Yamamoto N, Yamasaki H: A new variant of thrombasthenia with abnormally glycosylated GP IIb/IIIa. Thromb Res 47:323, 1987

167. Thiagarajan P, Shapiro SS, Sweterlitsch L, McCord S: A human erythroleukemia cell line synthesizes a functionally active glycoprotein IIb–IIIa complex capable of binding fibrinogen. Biochim Biophys Acta 924:127, 1987

168. Thorsen LI, Brosstad F, Gogstad GO, Sletten K, Solum NO: Binding of ^{125}I-labelled fibrin(ogen) fragments to platelets and to immunoprecipitated glycoprotein IIb–IIIa complex. Thromb Res 42:645, 1986

169. Thorsen LI, Gaudernack G, Brosstad F, Pedersen TM, Solum NO: Identification of platelet antigens by monoclonal antibodies using crossed immunoelectrophoresis with immunoblotting of the monoclonal antibody. Thromb Haemostasis 57:212, 1987

170. Thorsen LI, Hessel B, Brosstad F, Gogstad GO, Solum NO: The N-DSK γ-chain binds to immunoprecipitated GP IIb–IIIa. Thromb Res 47:315, 1987

171. Tsuji T, Osawa T: Structures of the carbohydrate chains of membrane glycoproteins IIb and IIIa of human platelets. J Biochem 100:1387, 1986

172. Tsuji T, Tsunehisa S, Watanabe Y, Yamamoto K, Tohyama H, Osawa T: The carbohydrate moiety of human platelet glycocalicin. The structure of the major Ser/Thr-linked sugar chain. J Biol Chem 258:6335, 1983

173. Van Mourik JA, Leeksma OC, Reinders JH, de Groot PG, Zandbergen-Spaargaren J: Vascular endothelial cells synthesize a plasma membrane protein indistinguishable from the platelet membrane glycoprotein IIa. J Biol Chem 260:11300, 1985

174. Varon D, Karpatkin S: A monoclonal antiplatelet antibody with decreased reactivity for autoimmune thrombocytopenic platelets. Proc Natl Acad Sci USA 80:6992, 1983

175. Villela R, Lozano T, Mila J, Bordie L, Ercilla G, Ordinas T, Vives J: An antiplatelet monoclonal antibody that inhibits ADP- and epinephrine-induced aggregation. Thromb Haemostasis 51:93, 1984

176. Wencel-Drake JD, Plow EF, Kunicki TJ, Woods VL, Keller DM, Ginsberg MH: Localization of internal pools of membrane glycoproteins involved in platelet adhesive responses. Am J Pathol 124:324, 1986

177. Wicki AN, Clemetson KJ: Structure and function of platelet membrane glycoproteins Ib and V. Effects of leukocyte elastase and other proteases on platelets response to von Willebrand factor and thrombin. Eur J Biochem 153:1, 1985

178. Wicki AN, Clemetson KJ: The glycoprotein Ib complex of human blood platelet. Eur J Biochem 163:43, 1987

179. Wilk AS, Bankhurst AD, Williams RC: Crossed radioimmunoelectrophoresis for the analysis of lymphocyte surface antigens. J Immunol Methods 30:309, 1979

180. Woods VL, Wolff LE, Keller DM: Resting platelets contain a substantial centrally located pool of glycoprotein IIb–IIIa complex which may be accessible to some but not other extracellular proteins. J Biol Chem 261:15242, 1986

181. Wyler B, Bienz D, Clemetson KJ, Luscher EF: Glycoprotein Ibβ is the only phosphorylated major membrane glycoprotein in human platelets. Biochem J 234:373, 1986

182. Zucker MA, Grant RA: Nonreversible loss of platelet aggregability induced by calcium deprivation. Blood 52:505, 1978

183. Zucker MA, Varon D, Masiello NC, Karpatkin S: The combining ability of glycoproteins IIb, IIIa and Ca^{2+} in EDTA-treated nonaggregable platelets. Thromb Haemostas is 50:848, 1983

12

Use of Murine Monoclonal Antibodies to Determine Platelet Membrane Glycoprotein Structure and Function

ZAVERIO M. RUGGERI · ELISABETH M. HODSON

Monoclonal antibodies are a powerful tool for the study of protein structure and function. They are specific reagents capable of high-affinity interaction with identifiable domains of molecules and, therefore, offer unique opportunities for exploring structure–function relationships. In this chapter, we shall review some of their applications relating to platelet biology, with particular emphasis on two membrane glycoproteins (GP), GPIb and the GPIIb–IIIa complex.

As in all review articles, the balance of the topics treated is influenced by the primary research interests of the authors. Much of what will appear in the next pages has to do with the interaction between platelets and von Willebrand factor. It is hoped that the reader will be able to identify a message of more general relevance in these specific topics of discussion.

THE GLYCOPROTEIN Ib COMPLEX

Structure and Function of the Glycoprotein Ib Complex

Glycoprotein Ib and GPIX are two distinct integral membrane proteins that form a noncovalent equimolar complex.[8,21,95,96] Glycoprotein Ib has a relative molecular mass (M_r) of approximately 170 kDa and represents the predominant component of the complex; GPIX has a molecular mass of approximately 20 kDa. Glycoprotein Ib is a disulfide-linked two-chain molecule that comprises a heavy (α) chain of approximately 140 kDa and a light (β) chain of 24 kDa; GPIX is a single-chain polypeptide. Glycoprotein Ib participates in hemostasis by acting as one of the two presently known platelet receptors for von Willebrand factor.[76] Its function is to mediate the anchoring of platelets at sites of vascular injury.[91] In addition to its function as a von Willebrand factor receptor, GPIb has been identified as one of the platelet-binding sites for thrombin,[23,35,100,101] although at least one published report questions this identification.[85] The binding of both von Willebrand factor and thrombin appears to be mediated by the glycocalicin portion of GPIb.[60,62]

Glycocalicin is a soluble proteolytic fragment of the heavy (α) chain of GPIb that is generated by a cleavage in a position close to the transmembrane domain of the molecule.[61, 63, 82, 96, 99] Thus, glycocalicin constitutes most of the extracellular domains of the heavy chain of GPIb.[33] Free glycocalicin can be detected in normal plasma,[15] a finding that reflects ongoing catabolism of platelet GPIb and whose potential clinical relevance has not yet been explored.

Glycoprotein IX has no known function of its own. It also is not now known if it plays any role in modulating the receptor function of GPIb. Glycoprotein IX has been shown to be important for the recognition of platelets by quinine/quinidine drug-dependent antibodies (*see* Chap. 8 in this volume). Glycoprotein Ib and GPIX are concurrently decreased in the congenital disease known as the Bernard-Soulier syndrome.[7,9,11]

Monoclonal Antibodies in the Study of Glycoprotein Ib

Much of our current knowledge about the GPIb molecule and its functional properties is derived from studies of patients with the Bernard-Soulier syndrome[52,91] and from the use of monoclonal antibodies. In either type study, the lack of GPIb on platelets or the functional blockage of relevant epitopes of the GPIb molecule result in decreased binding of von Willebrand factor and impaired platelet adhesion to exposed subendothelial surfaces.

The effects of an anti-GPIb monoclonal antibody on platelet function were initially described by Ruan and coworkers[75] and Michael and coworkers.[50] The antibody developed and used by these authors (AN 51) had a pronounced inhibitory effect on platelet aggregation induced by ristocetin, but it only partially inhibited the ristocetin-mediated von Willebrand factor binding to platelets. Subsequently, other monoclonal anti-GPIb antibodies were selected for their ability to inhibit ristocetin-induced platelet agglutination and were used to obtain additional evidence that GPIb is a binding site for von Willebrand factor. Two such antibodies, AP1[53,76] and 6D1[16] were shown to completely block von Willebrand factor binding to platelets in the presence of ristocetin. Antibodies with these properties also proved instrumental in demonstrating that platelets have more than one binding site for von Willebrand factor. This became apparent when it was possible to show that the binding of von Willebrand factor to thrombin-stimulated platelets was not blocked by AP1.[76]

When the binding of monoclonal anti-GPIb antibodies to normal platelets is quantitated, approximately 15,000 to 30,000 molecules are bound per cell, and this is considered to reflect the number of GPIb molecules present on the membrane of normal platelets. In patients with the Bernard-Soulier syndrome (homozygotes), the binding is markedly reduced or undetectable, whereas the binding is reduced by approximately 50% in heterozygote individuals.[18,53] The measurement of anti-GPIb monoclonal antibody binding to platelets, therefore, provides a rapid and sensitive method for the detection of carriers of the Bernard-Soulier syndrome.

The function of von Willebrand factor and GPIb in promoting platelet adhesion to exposed subendothelium can be studied in perfusion systems, thus allowing one to monitor simultaneously several important rheological parameters and to recreate the flow conditions found in different segments of the vasculature. The use of antibodies directed against GPIb has been useful to confirm and extend the findings obtained with platelets congenitally deficient in this surface receptor.[78,92] When platelets lack GPIb, or its function is blocked by specific antibodies, platelet adhesion, i.e., the initial attachment of platelets to an exposed subendothelium followed by spreading, is markedly impaired. Thus, a simple schematic representation of the initial events in hemostasis has evolved that considers the function of GPIb and von Willebrand factor essential for the initial adhesion of platelets to thrombogenic surfaces, whereas the GPIIb-IIIa receptor and other adhesive proteins, among them fibronectin and fibrinogen, are considered important for the subsequent additional recruitment of platelets into the growing thrombus (platelet-platelet interaction, or aggregation). The reality of biologic events, however, often proves more complicated than our schematic representations. In fact, it is now clear that optimal platelet adhesion, i.e., the initial attachment to and spreading onto thrombogenic surfaces, requires the functional integrity of GPIIb-IIIa in addition to that of GPIb,[45] particularly under conditions of high-shear stress.

Other possible functions of GPIb have been explored with monoclonal antibodies. Thrombin-induced aggregation of platelets, as well as thrombin binding to the platelet membrane, have been shown to be inhibited by antibodies, directed against GPIb.[100,101] Moreover, at least two anti-GPIb antibodies, SZ 2 and AP1,[74] have been shown to inhibit the collagen-induced aggregation of platelets. SZ 2, but not AP1, also inhibits platelet aggregation induced by platelet aggregating factor (PAF). Here, the effects of the anti-GPIb monoclonal antibodies are thought to be the consequence of steric hindrance, as both GPIb and the putative collagen receptor (perhaps the GPIa-IIa complex or other membrane glycoproteins) may lie in close proximity in the platelet membrane. A similar explanation has been proposed for the inhibitory effect of SZ 2 on aggregation induced by platelet aggregating factor. Here, either an unknown membrane receptor for platelet aggregating factor, or a membrane glycoprotein involved in aggregation induced by platelet-aggregating factor, may lie in proximity of GPIb. Platelets from patients with the Bernard-Soulier syndrome, lacking GPIb, exhibit normal aggregatory response when stimulated with both collagen and platelet-aggregating factor, a finding that excludes any direct role of GPIb in the responses mediated by these two agonists. Accordingly, SZ 2, which does not bind to Bernard-Soulier platelets, does not inhibit their aggregation induced by collagen or platelet-aggregating factor.[74]

The von Willebrand Factor-Binding Domain of Glycoprotein Ib

We have used three murine monoclonal antibodies to define the von Willebrand factor-binding domain of GPIb.[33] One of these antibodies was prepared using washed platelets as immunogen, and positive clones were selected for their reactivity with human platelets. All of the positive clones were then tested for their capacity to inhibit ristocetin-induced platelet agglutination. Ten antiplatelet antibodies were identified in the first screening, one of which inhibited agglutination in the second screening. This antibody was designated LJ-P3.

The specificity of the inhibitory monoclonal antibody was confirmed in two ways: the antibody bound to normal platelets but not to platelets from a patient with the Bernard-Soulier syndrome; and when the antibody was incubated with ^{125}I-labeled or ^{3}H-labeled solubilized platelet membrane proteins, it reacted with a single glycoprotein having the electrophoretic characteristics of GPIb. This antibody inhibited the binding of von Willebrand factor to GPIb but only to about 50% of the control values.

The anti-GPIb antibody, LJ-P3, was used as an immunoadsorbent in one of the purification steps for the preparation of glycocalicin and GPIb. Purified glycocalicin was then used as immunogen in the preparation of a second series of monoclonal antibodies. Twelve positive clones were identified in this manner, all reacting with the glycocalicin portion of the α chain of GPIb. One of the monoclonal antibodies, designated LJ-Ib1, completely inhibited von Willebrand factor-mediated platelet agglutination and von Willebrand factor binding to GPIb, whereas all of the others were without effect in this regard. One other antibody, designated LJ-Ib10, reacted with denatured, reduced and *S*-carboxymethylated glycocalicin and could be used to detect the protein after Western blotting.

Purified IgG was prepared from each of the three antibodies, LJ-P3, LJ-Ib1 and LJ-Ib10, and used to determine the number of corresponding binding sites on the platelet membrane. These were found to range from 2.1 to 2.7×10^4 per platelet (Table 12-1), values in good agreement with previously reported estimates.[16,50,53] Antibody LJ-P3, prepared using whole platelets as immunogen, had an affinity 10 to 20 times greater than that of the two antibodies prepared against purified GPIb (*see* Table 12-1). The effect of the three antibodies on the von Willebrand factor-platelet interaction is shown in Figure 12-1.

Table 12-1
Properties of the Monoclonal Antibodies Directed Against GPIb

Antibody	Subtype	K_d (nM)	Molecules Bound per Platelet ($\times 10^{-4}$)	Inhibition of VWF Binding to Platelets
LJ-P3	IgG_1	4.7	2.12	Incomplete
LJ-Ib1	IgG_1	97.0	2.67	Complete
LJ-Ib10	IgG_{2a}	31.2	2.43	Absent

(Subtype of IgG was determined by immunodiffusion using monospecific rabbit antisera. Dissociation constant (K_d) and number of binding sites were determined from computerized Scatchard-type analysis, using the program Ligand, described by Munson in Methods in Enzymology, 92:542–576, 1983. Handa M, Titani K, Holland LZ, Roberts JR, Ruggeri ZM: The von Willebrand factor-binding domain of platelet membrane glycoprotein Ib. Characterization by monoclonal antibodies and partial amino acid sequence analysis of proteolytic fragments. J Biol Chem 261:12579, 1986; reprinted with permission from Handa et al.)

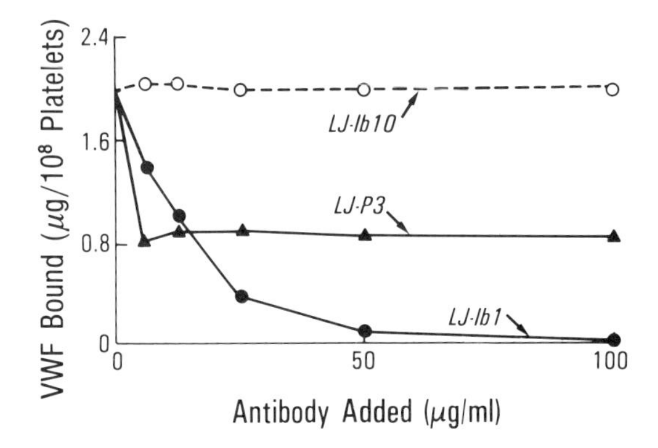

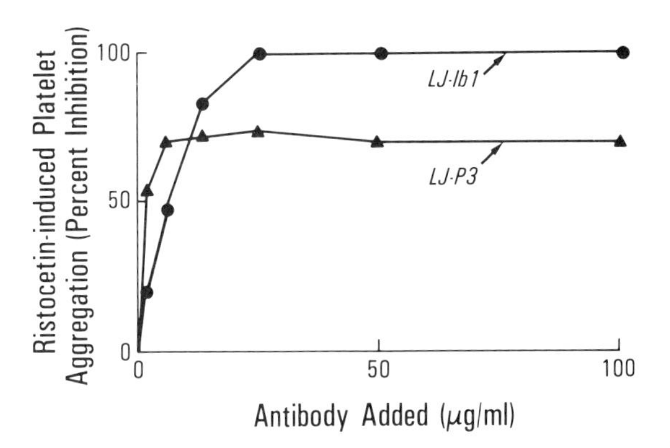

Figure 12-1. Effect of antibodies on von Willebrand factor–platelet interaction. *Upper panel.* Washed platelets (1×10^8/ml) were mixed with monoclonal IgG (at the concentrations indicated) and ristocetin (1 mg/ml) for 5 min at 22–25°C. ^{125}I-labeled VWF (7 μg/ml) was then added to the mixture and incubated for 30 min. *Lower panel*: Platelet-rich plasma (2.8×10^8/ml) was stirred at 1100 rpm in the aggregometer cuvette, 37°C, and preincubated for 1 min with varying concentrations of monoclonal IgG before addition of ristocetin (1.2 mg/ml). The effect of the antibodies was expressed as percent inhibition of maximal aggregation observed in the control curve containing control monoclonal IgG. LJ-Ib10 (not shown) had no effect on platelet aggregation induced by ristocetin (Handa M; Titani K; Hollan LZ, Roberts JR, Ruggeri ZM: The von Willebrand factor-binding domain of platelet membrane glycoprotein Ib. Characterization by monoclonal antibodies and partial amino acid sequence analysis of proteolytic fragments. J Biol Chem 261:12579–12585, 1986; reprinted with permission)

Our efforts to localize the von Willebrand factor-binding domain within the glycocalicin portion of GPIb were based on the previous demonstration that glycocalicin in solution can inhibit the ristocetin-dependent binding of von Willebrand factor to GPIb. This finding suggested that a region of the α chain of GPIb, separated from the β chain, retains structural features that are essential for expressing the binding function. We used three different proteases, namely, trypsin, *Staphylococcus aureus* V8 protease, and *Serratia marcescens* protease, to generate proteolytic fragments of ^{125}I-labeled GPIb or glycocalicin. A tryptic fragment of 45 kDa, with a relatively low content of carbohydrate, reacted with the three monoclonal antibodies used, including the two that inhibited von Willebrand factor binding to GPIb (Fig. 12-2). Upon prolonged exposure to trypsin, an additional cleavage occurred within the 45-kDa fragment. The two resulting polypeptides (35 kDa and 7 kDa) remained linked by disulfide bonds[88] (*see* Fig. 12-2). The 45-kDa fragment was isolated and its amino-terminal sequence was determined. It was found to be the same as the amino-terminal sequence of GPIb

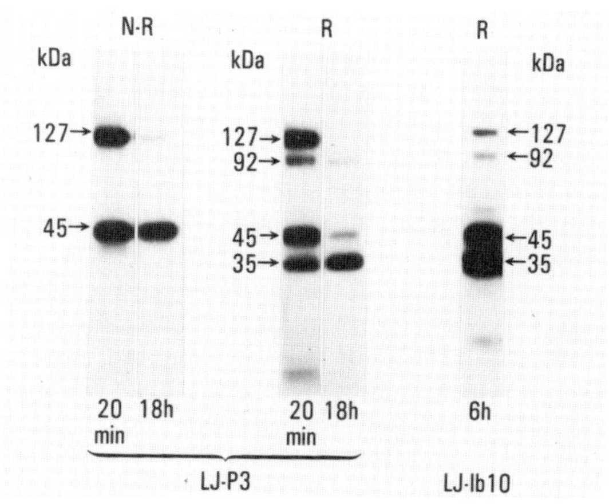

Figure 12-2. Analysis of immunoisolated tryptic fragment of GPIb. The fragments generated by L-1-tosylamido-2-phenylethylchloromethyl ketone–trypsin digestion of ^{125}I-labeled GPIb at 37°C (incubation times are indicated) were subjected to solid-phase immunoisolation using the monoclonal antibodies LJ-P3 and LJ-Ib10. The immunoisolated fragments were then analyzed by 5–15% gradient SDS–PAGE under nonreducing (N-R) or reducing (R) conditions, followed by autoradiography. The relative molecular mass of the polypeptides is indicated (Handa M, Titani K, Holland LZ, Roberts JR, Ruggeri ZM: The von Willebrand factor-binding domain of platelet membrane glycoprotein Ib. Characterization by monoclonal antibodies and partial amino acid sequence analysis of proteolytic fragments. J Biol Chem 261:12579–12585, 1986; reprinted with permission)

α chain and glycocalicin. Another major tryptic fragment of apparently 84 kDa, very rich in carbohydrate, had a distinct amino-terminus and did not react with any of the monoclonal antibodies tested. A fragment of apparently 38 kDa, generated by digestion with *S. marcescens* protease, had the same amino-terminus as the tryptic fragment of 45 kDa and reacted with the same monoclonal antibodies (Fig. 12-3).

The 45-kDa tryptic fragment was subsequently purified in sufficient amounts to assess its inhibition of von Willebrand factor binding. Indeed, this fragment in solution could inhibit the ristocetin-dependent binding of von Willebrand factor to platelets. The conclusions reached were the following:

- Glycocalicin, a large water-soluble fragment of the GPIb α chain, has the same amino-terminus as the intact α chain; as glycocalicin is detached from the platelet surface by proteolysis, this proves that the amino-terminus of the α chain is oriented away from the platelet membrane and toward the surrounding environment.
- The von Willebrand factor-binding domain of GPIb resides in proximity to the amino terminus of the α chain, in a region of the molecule that is relatively poor in carbohydrate.
- Monoclonal antibodies that inhibit von Willebrand factor binding to GPIb react with this region of the molecule.

A schematic representation of the structural organization of the GPIb α chain, based on the results of these studies, is presented in Figure 12-4.

More recently, we have obtained the complete amino acid sequence of the 45-kDa tryptic fragment of glycocalicin,[88] and Lopez et al. have successfully cloned the α chain of GPIb.[46] The sequence deduced from the cDNA clones and that derived from the purified platelet protein are in complete agreement. Considering the scheme shown in Figure 12-4, it is obviously erroneous to designate the von Wille-

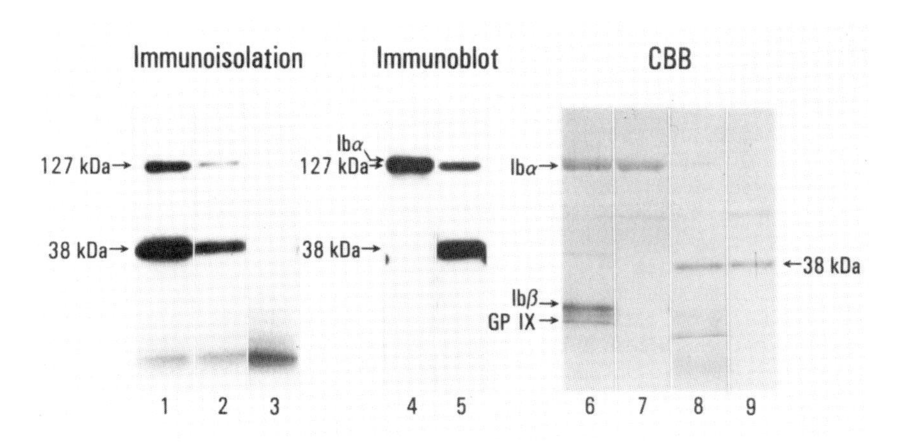

Figure 12-3. Immunoisolation, immunoblotting, and electroelution of GPIb fragments generated by *S. marcescans* protease digestion. A 6-hr digest of ^{125}I-labeled GPIb was subjected to solid-phase immunoisolation using monoclonal antibodies LJ-P3 (lane 1) and LJ-Ib1 (lane 2) and the control anti-GPIIb–IIIa antibody LJ-P5 (lane 3). The autoradiography of a reduced 5–15% gradient gel is shown. Purified intact GPIb (lane 4) and a 6-hr digest (lane 5) were also analyzed by immunoblot analysis using the monoclonal antibody LJ-Ib10. Electroeluted GPIb α chain (lane 7) derived from purified GPIb (lane 6) and the electroeluted 38-kDa fragment (lane 9) obtained from the whole digest of purified GPIb (lane 8) are also shown after analysis by 5–15% gradient SDS–PAGE and staining with Coomassie Brilliant Blue R (CBB). The relative molecular mass of the polypeptides is indicated (Handa M, Titani K, Holland LZ, Roberts JR, Ruggeri ZM: The von Willebrand factor-binding domain of platelet membrane glycoprotein Ib. Characterization by monoclonal antibodies and partial amino acid sequence analysis of proteolytic fragments. J Biol Chem 261:12579–12585, 1986; reprinted with permission)

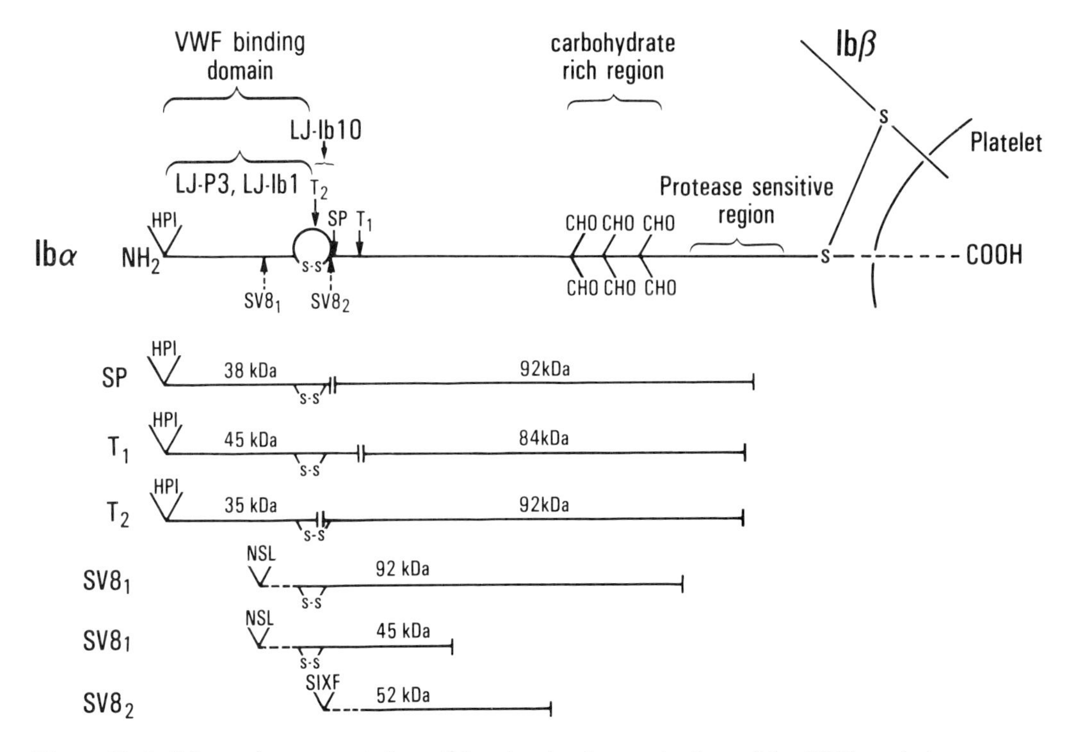

Figure 12-4. Schematic representation of the structural organization of the GPIb α chain. The orientation of the major proteolytic fragments generated by digestion of the GPIb α chain with *S. marcescans* protease (SP), trypsin (T), and *S. aureus* V8 protease (SV8) is indicated by the corresponding NH_2-terminal sequence and reactivity with three distinct monoclonal antibodies. Localization of the epitopes corresponding to these antibodies (LJ-P3, LJIb-1, LJ-Ib10) is tentative, but within regions of the GPIb α chain that can be defined with certainty. The localization of the NH_2-terminus of the fragments generated by *S. aureus* V8 protease digestion is indicated with broken lines because it cannot be established on the basis of these results (*see* Ref. 88). Because all these fragments react with LJ-Ib10, however, their NH_2-termini must be distal to the LJ-Ib10 epitope. The relative molecular masses of the fragments are indicated. The von Willebrand factor (VWF)-binding domain lies within the NH_2-terminal region of the α chain. The COOH-terminus of the GPIb α chain is indicated with a broken line because it was not known at the time of this work, as it is now,[46] that it has a transmembrane portion. One-letter abbreviation for amino acids indicates the NH_2-terminal sequence of fragments (Handa M, Titani K, Holland LZ, Roberts JR, Ruggeri ZM: The von Willebrand factor-binding domain of platelet membrane glycoprotein Ib. Characterization by monoclonal antibodies and partial amino acid sequence analysis of proteolytic fragments. J Biol Chem 261:12579–12585, 1986; reprinted with permission)

brand factor-binding domain of GPIb α chain as the "peptide tail" of the molecule. This name finds its origin in the concept that the "macroglycopeptide" (carbohydrate-rich region) was oriented toward the exterior of the platelet surface and the "peptide" (carbohydrate-poor) region was close to the surface. The designation of "peptide head" seems more appropriate, because this domain of the α chain of GPIb has a globular shape and contains the amino-terminus.

THE GLYCOPROTEIN IIb–IIIa COMPLEX

Structure and Function of the Glycoprotein IIb–IIIa Complex

Glycoprotein IIb and GPIIIa are two major integral membrane glycoproteins that are markedly decreased or absent in platelets from patients with the congenital disease, Glanzmann's thrombasthenia (structure and function of platelet membrane glycoproteins, and their congenital abnormalities, are reviewed in other chapters of this book). Glycoprotein IIb is a disulfide-linked, two-chain molecule composed of a heavy (α) chain of approximately 135 kDa and a light (β) chain of 22 kDa. Glycoprotein IIIa is a single-chain molecule with internal disulfide bonds and apparent molecular mass of 95 kDa under nonreducing conditions that increases to 105 kDa after reduction. Glycoprotein IIb and GP IIIa form a calcium-dependent heterodimer complex that is present as such in the membrane of resting platelets.

Monoclonal Antibodies in the Study of the Glycoprotein IIb–IIIa Complex

Monoclonal antibodies have proved very useful for the definition of several aspects of the structure and function of the GPIIb–IIIa complex. They were used initially to purify and quantitate GPIIb and GPIIIa and, then, to assess their structural and functional organization in the membrane of resting and activated platelets.[17,47,48,55,67,86]

The GPIIb–IIIa complex functions as a receptor for adhesive molecules like fibrinogen, fibronectin, and von Willebrand factor.[4,6,17,20,30,48,54,64,67,68,71,76,89] Its role in primary hemostasis is important for platelet adhesion and thrombus formation upon exposed thrombogenic surfaces.[45,78,92]

Although GPIIb–IIIa is present on the surface of unstimulated platelets, its binding function becomes apparent only after stimulation of the cells with agonists, such a ADP, thrombin, and epinephrine. Little is known about the mechanisms that impart this receptor activity. The two prevailing hypotheses suggest that agonists either induce a conformational transition, possibly calcium-dependent, directly within GPIIb–IIIa to render it a competent receptor, or they cause changes in the microenvironment such that a hidden receptor becomes accessible to macromolecular ligands. It has proved difficult to discriminate between these two possibilities, but this is not surprising when one considers the complexity of the structural organization of the platelet membrane. Moreover, the two possibilities are not mutually exclusive. A detailed description of these topics is found in Chapter 10 in this volume.

Ginsberg and coworkers have provided evidence for a divalent cation-dependent regulation of the surface orientation of GPIIb.[27] These authors have described a monoclonal antibody, identified as PMI-1, that binds to isolated GPIIb as well as to the GPIIb–IIIa complex, and whose binding is inhibited by the presence of magnesium or calcium, in a manner that inversely correlates with the divalent cation dependency of fibrinogen binding to stimulated platelets. Interestingly, in patients with a variant form of Glanzmann's thrombasthenia the binding of PMI-1 to platelets was not affected by the presence of divalent cations, a finding that correlated with the inability of the patients' GPIIb–IIIa to express fibrinogen-binding capacity. Thus, these elegant studies performed with a unique monoclonal antibody have provided evidence that the surface orientation of GPIIb can be modulated by physiologic concentrations of calcium and magnesium ions, resulting in functionally significant changes that correlate with the capacity of platelets to bind fibrinogen.

Nugent and coworkers have reported that a neoantigen appears on GPIIIa in connection with thrombin-induced platelet activation or under suboptimal conditions of platelet storage.[59] Their findings are relevant in several respects. They provide evidence for an activation-dependent conformational change of GPIIIa, in addition to that involving GPIIb discussed previously, thus adding further support to the concept that physical rearrangements within the GPIIb–IIIa complex are likely to be part of the mechanisms that lead to expression of receptor function. Moreover, they provide insights into the processes that may be involved in removal of aging platelets from the circulation and, possibly, in the generation of autoimmune responses through the exposure of neoantigens. It is relevant that the antibody described by Nugent and coworkers was a human monoclonal IgM derived from Epstein-Barr virus-transformed lymphocytes fused to a mouse–human heterohybrid line.

In addition to its role as a binding site for adhesive proteins, the GPIIb–IIIa complex may participate in events that occur after protein binding and may be important in the process of platelet–platelet interaction. For example, Newman and coworkers have shown that two monoclonal antibodies, one specific for GPIIb and the other for GPIIIa, could inhibit ADP-induced aggregation without blocking ADP-induced fibrinogen binding.[56] This was seen only when the two antibodies were used together; neither antibody, when used by itself, had any effect on platelet aggregation. It is relevant that the inhibitory effect on aggregation was observed with ADP but not with other agonists, such as thrombin. The nature of the events that follow fibrinogen binding and are important for aggregation remains to be defined. The findings of Newman and coworkers suggest that these events may differ depending upon the agonist involved. Moreover, it has been shown that, after the binding of monoclonal antibodies, GPIIb-IIIa molecules cluster and tend to localize to limited areas of the platelet surface (capping).[80] In contrast, GPIb remains scattered over the entire platelet surface, even after monoclonal antibody binding. Thus, membrane reorganization of GPIIb-IIIa may follow an interaction with multivalent ligands and may be involved in the processes of cell-to-cell and cell-to-surface contact (particularly spreading) mediated by GPIIb-IIIa.

Quantitation of the Glycoprotein IIb-IIIa Complex on Resting and Stimulated Platelets

It is generally accepted that the transitional events that render GPIIb-IIIa a functional receptor are efficient, because all the GPIIb-IIIa molecules present on the surface of the platelet membrane may become a binding site for adhesive molecules. This conclusion is based on the similarity between the estimated number of fibrinogen-binding sites on stimulated platelets [5,37,66,69,70] and that of GPIIb-IIIa molecules on the platelet surface, as determined by binding of several monoclonal antibodies.[17,47,48,55,67,76] In addition to that exposed on the cell surface, other pool(s) of GPIIb-IIIa have been detected. For example, GPIIb-IIIa molecules have been identified on the intraluminal surface of vacuolar structures[93] that may correspond to the canalicular system of platelets.[3,94] In intact platelets, the accessibility of this pool to antibody probes is uncertain.[102] In addition, by subcellular fractionation[31,32,90] and electron microscopy,[93] GPIIb-IIIa has been identified as a constituent of platelet α granule membranes. When platelets are stimulated to undergo a secretory reaction, α-granule constituents, including their membrane components, as well as other intracellular species, become expressed upon the cell surface.[40,84,93] Therefore, the number of GPIIb-IIIa molecules available on the surface of unstimulated and stimulated platelets may differ with the extent of platelet activation.[25] This, in turn, may affect the number of functional receptors for extracellular fibrinogen or other adhesive proteins.

We have used three monoclonal antibodies to characterize GPIIb-IIIa on unstimulated and stimulated platelets.[58] Each of these antibodies bound to platelets only when the integrity of the GPIIb-IIIa complex was maintained. This was shown for LJ-P9 in a previous publication,[89] and similar properties were also observed for LJ-CP3 and LJ-CP8. The binding of these three antibodies to unstimulated and thrombin-stimulated platelets was examined using Fab′ fragments and measured as a function of antibody concentration. All three antibodies showed clear evidence of saturable binding to both thrombin-stimulated and unstimulated platelets (Fig. 12-5). With all three antibodies, the maximum number of binding sites observed with thrombin-stimulated platelets was significantly greater ($p < 0.001$) than that observed with unstimulated cells. This was most evident with LJ-CP3 (220% increase), followed by LJ-P9 (212% increase) and LJ-CP8 (200% increase). The K_d of LJ-CP3 tended to be lower after thrombin-stimulation, although this difference was not statistically significant. In contrast, the K_ds of LJ-CP8 and LJ-P9 were significantly higher ($p < 0.01$) with thrombin-stimulated than with unstimulated platelets. These findings may explain the observation that, when single concentrations of the antibodies were tested at or below their K_d for unstimulated platelets, increased binding to thrombin-stimulated platelets was readily demonstrated with LJ-CP3, but it was less apparent with the other two antibodies.

A certain degree of variability was found in the extent of antibody binding to platelets from different individuals, with a broader range (molecules/platelet) observed for LJ-CP3 (resting: 33,500-81,100; thrombin-stimulated: 88,600-196,000) and LJ-CP8 (resting: 27,500-67,100; thrombin-stimulated: 45,200-131,900) than for LJ-P9 (resting: 42,400-55,200; thrombin-stimulated: 102,400-113,900). It is important that the increase in antibody binding was specific for GPIIb-IIIa because binding of a monoclonal antibody to another major membrane glycoprotein, GPIb, was not increased but, rather, it was decreased, after thrombin stimulation. This effect of thrombin on the binding of a

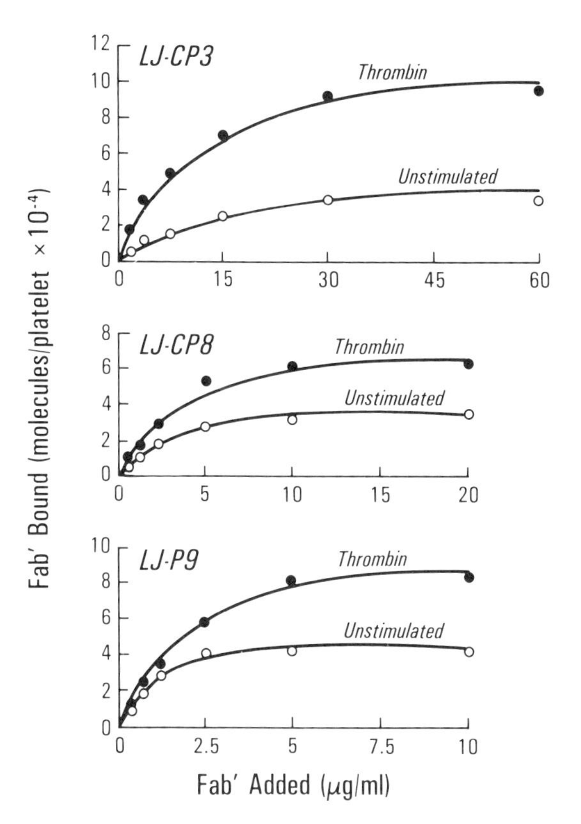

Figure 12-5. Binding of anti-GPIIb–IIIa monoclonal Fab′ fragments to unstimulated and stimulated platelets. These binding isotherms demonstrate the dose-dependent saturable interaction of three different monoclonal antibodies (as indicated) to either unstimulated or thrombin-stimulated platelets. Increasing amounts of antibody (monovalent Fab′ fragment) were added in the presence of 2 mmol/liter of Ca^{2+} and 2 mmol/liter of Mg^{2+}. It is apparent that platelets exposed to thrombin bind more anti-GPIIb–IIIa antibody than do the unstimulated ones (Niiya K, Hodson E, Bader R, Byers-Ward V, Koziol JA, Plow EF, Ruggeri ZM: Increased surface expression of the membrane glycoprotein IIb/IIIa complex induced by platelet activation. Relationship to the binding of fibrinogen and platelet aggregation. Blood 70:475–483, 1987; reprinted with permission)

monoclonal antibody to GPIb had previously been described by George and coworkers.[25] Stimulation of platelets with phorbol myristate acetate (PMA) gave results similar to those observed with thrombin. In contrast, stimulation of platelets with ADP, at concentrations that caused maximal fibrinogen binding with this agonist, yielded no statistically significant changes in the binding of LJ-CP3, compared with unstimulated platelets.

Our findings are in agreement with those reported by other investigators, who found no effect of ADP on the surface expression of GPIIb–IIIa measured with a number of different monoclonal antibodies.[12,13,20,48,81] Again, in analogy with our results, others have found that platelets stimulated with thrombin bind more anti-GPIIb–IIIa antibodies than do resting platelets.[25] The studies performed by Shattil and coworkers also demonstrated that more PAC-1 (an anti-GPIIb–IIIa monoclonal antibody whose binding is dependent upon platelet activation) bound to thrombin-stimulated than to ADP-stimulated platelets.[81] The reasons for the different effect of ADP, when compared with stronger agonists, on the surface expression of GPIIb–IIIa remain unclear at present.

To prove that the increased surface expression of GPIIb–IIIa-related epitopes was due to the binding of antibody to sites unavailable on resting platelets, we performed experiments with antibody labeled with two different isotopes. In this manner, the GPIIb–IIIa molecules exposed on the surface of unstimulated platelets were saturated with ^{131}I-labeled LJ-CP3 F(ab′)$_2$ and then reacted, before or after stimulation, with ^{125}I-labeled antibody. The results shown in Figure 12-6 demonstrate that thrombin-stimulated platelets, unlike resting platelets, bound a significant amount of ^{125}I-labeled antibody at a time when the pool of GPIIb–IIIa molecules exposed on unstimulated platelets was still blocked by the ^{131}I-labeled antibody. The minimal binding of ^{125}I-labeled antibody to the resting platelets coated with ^{131}I-labeled antibody can be explained by occupation of sites from which ^{131}I-labeled antibody had dissociated. The modest increase in binding of the ^{125}I-labeled antibody to ADP-stimulated platelets is consistent with the increase observed in all experiments with antibody LJ-CP3. The increased binding of monoclonal anti-GPIIb–IIIa antibodies to platelets stimulated with strong agonists has at least two possible explanations: (1) The number of GPIIb–IIIa molecules on the platelet surface, or in a position accessible to antibody molecules, increases; or (2) the number of GPIIb–IIIa molecules remains unchanged, but the number of accessible epitopes per molecule increases. The latter possibility seems unlikely, however, because different monoclonal antibodies that recognize unrelated epitopes exhibit a similar increase in binding, and it is difficult to imagine conformational changes of

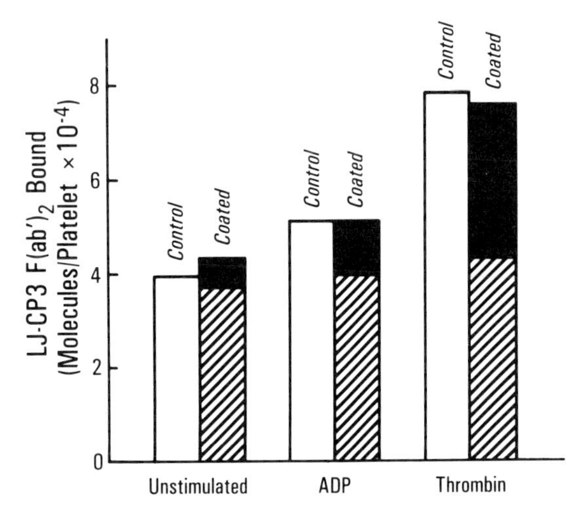

Figure 12-6. Binding of ^{125}I-labeled antibody to resting or stimulated platelets coated with ^{131}I-labeled antibody. The purpose of this experiment was to saturate with monoclonal antibody the GPIIb–IIIa molecules accessible to $F(ab')_2$ fragment on unstimulated platelets. To monitor occupancy of the corresponding epitopes, the antibody was labeled with ^{131}I. Unbound antibody was removed by gel filtration and the precoated platelets were either left unstimulated or exposed to activating agonists. Saturating amounts of antibody, this time labeled with ^{125}I, were then added to monitor the appearance of new binding sites (most likely GPIIb–IIIa molecules not accessible to antibody on unstimulated platelets) while, at the same time, monitoring the continued occupancy of the previously exposed epitopes. Open columns indicate the binding of ^{125}I-labeled LJ-CP3 $F(ab')_2$ (added at a concentration of 50 μg/ml) to control platelets, either unstimulated or stimulated with ADP (10 μmol/liter) or α-thrombin (0.1 NIH U/ml), as indicated. Shaded columns indicate the amount of antibody remaining bound to platelets precoated with ^{131}I-labeled LJ-CP3 $F(ab')_2$. Solid columns indicate the additional amount of ^{125}I-labeled antibody bound to these precoated platelets, either resting or stimulated (Niiya K, Hodson E, Bader R, Byers-Ward V, Koziol JA, Plow EF, Ruggeri ZM: Increased surface expression of the membrane glycoprotein IIb/IIIa complex induced by platelet activation. Relationship to the binding of fibrinogen and platelet aggregation. Blood 70:475–483, 1987; reprinted with permission)

a molecule resulting in the concurrent duplication of several distinct epitopes.

The increased surface expression of GPIIb–IIIa-related epitopes observed upon stimulation with certain agonists correlates with increased fibrinogen binding. In fact, α-thrombin and PMA induced greater fibrinogen binding than either ADP or epinephrine. At saturation, the binding of fibrinogen (mean ± standard deviation) to platelets stimulated with PMA (10 nM) was 76,100 ± 13,200 molecules per platelet (range: 58,500–87,900) and was significantly greater ($p < 0.001$) than its binding to platelets stimulated with ADP (10 μM), 17,600 ± 9100 molecules per platelet (range: 9800–30,600). On the other hand, dissociation constants, $K_d = 4.78 \pm 3.9 \times 10^{-7}$ M for PMA and $K_d = 5.78 \pm 2.6 \times 10^{-7}$ M for ADP, were not significantly different.

Thus, we have obtained evidence for the existence of at least two compartments of GPIIb–IIIa molecules. One is exposed on the surface of resting platelets and exhibits receptor function for adhesive molecules upon stimulation with appropriate agonists. The other is not accessible to antibody molecules on the membrane of unstimulated platelets but becomes exposed upon activation with "strong" stimuli. The GPIIb–IIIa molecules in both compartments exhibit the ability to bind fibrinogen. The functional activity of the newly expressed GPIIb–IIIa molecules appears to contribute to the enhanced fibrinogen-binding capacity and aggregation of platelets seen in response to certain physiologic agonists, such as thrombin.

Woods and coworkers have also obtained evidence for the existence of what they call a "centrally located pool" of GPIIb–IIIa that becomes expressed on the surface of platelets stimulated with thrombin.[98] They also found, in agreement with our results discussed earlier, that translocation of this pool of GPIIb–IIIa to the platelet surface correlates with an increase in fibrinogen and fibronectin binding.

Independent Modulation of von Willebrand Factor and Fibrinogen Binding to Platelets

One of the functional attributes of the GPIIb–IIIa receptor on platelets is its broad specificity, in that it can bind at least three major adhesive proteins, namely fibrinogen,[4,6,17,20,30,48,54,64,67,89] fibronectin,[65,71] and von Willebrand factor.[76] There are two lines of evidence suggesting that the binding of different adhesive proteins to GPIIb–IIIa may be mediated by common mechanisms. First, monoclonal anti-GPIIb–IIIa antibodies have been described that block equally well the binding of the three different ligands;[71] second, synthetic peptides with the sequence of the carboxyl-terminus of the fibrinogen γ chain (His-His-Leu-Gly-Gly-Ala-Lys-Gln-Ala-Gly-Asp-Val) or with the sequence Arg-Gly-Asp, found at least once in each of the three ligands considered (fibrinogen, fibronectin, and von Willebrand factor), block effectively the binding of all three adhesive proteins to GPIIb-IIIa.[24,36,44,72,73,77,87,97] Even though these results do not prove that the foregoing sequences represent the functional domain(s) responsible for receptor recognition in the proteins in which they are present, they certainly suggest that a common binding site on GPIIb-IIIa may mediate the interaction of a family of adhesive glycoproteins with stimulated platelets.

In contrast to this hypothesis, however, we have obtained results that suggest that the binding of von Willebrand factor and fibrinogen to GPIIb-IIIa may be independently modulated at the receptor level.[89] We have characterized a monoclonal anti-GPIIb-IIIa antibody, LJ-P5, and used this antibody together with others to obtain evidence that the blocking of distinct epitopes on the GPIIb-IIIa complex has distinct effects upon the binding of von Willebrand factor and fibrinogen to stimulated platelets. By using a similar approach, others have demonstrated that monoclonal anti-GPIIb-IIIa antibodies may selectively block fibronectin binding without affecting fibrinogen binding, and vice versa.[49]

In our studies, the binding of von Willebrand factor to ADP-stimulated platelets was completely blocked by two different anti-GPIIb-IIIa monoclonal antibodies, LJ-P5 and LJ-P9 (Fig. 12-7, upper panel). The latter antibody also blocked the binding of fibrinogen, whereas LJ-P5 had no effect on this binding (Fig. 12-7, lower panel). Similar results were obtained with thrombin-stimulated platelets. The amount of each antibody necessary to achieve maximum inhibition agreed with the amount that gave saturation of binding to platelets. Nevertheless, LJ-P5 Fab had no effect on fibrinogen binding, even when added in a tenfold excess over saturating amounts. In evaluating the meaning of these observations, one has to consider the possibility of allosteric effects resulting from the much larger molecular mass of von Willebrand factor (up to several million daltons) as compared with fibrinogen (360,000 Dal). To address this question we have used a proteolytic fragment of von Willebrand factor (fragment II) obtained by digestion with *S. aureus* V8 protease.[28] Fragment II is a homodimer with a molecular mass of 220,000 Dal and is composed of two identical fragments of von Willebrand factor subunit linked by disulfide bonds; it retains the ability to bind to thrombin-stimulated platelets.[29] The binding of this fragment of von Willebrand factor, smaller than fibrinogen, was completely blocked by LJ-P5,* thus suggesting that the differential effect of LJ-P5 on von Willebrand factor and fibrinogen binding is not simply related to the different mass of the two ligands.

The concentration of von Willebrand factor or fibrinogen added to the platelets had no effect on the extent of inhibition obtained with the antibodies, and results were compatible with a noncompetitive inhibitory mechanism (*see* Fig. 12-7). The binding of von Willebrand factor added at concentrations between 0.5 μg/ml and 30 μg/ml could be completely inhibited by LJ-P5 and LJ-P9. LJ-P9 also markedly inhibited the binding of fibrinogen when the latter was added at concentrations between 5 μg/ml and 600 μg/ml, whereas LJ-P5 was consistently without effect at all concentrations of fibrinogen tested. Experiments measuring the inhibition of von Willebrand factor and fibrinogen binding were performed several times (only three are reported in Fig. 12-7) using platelets from several different donors and different Fab preparations. The results were always in close agreement.

Antibody LJ-P5 Fab had no effect on ADP-induced platelet aggregation, whereas LJ-P9 Fab completely inhibited it (Fig. 12-8), a result in agreement with the concept that fibrinogen binding to GPIIb-IIIa is important for platelet aggregation, as measured in the aggregometer. Identical results were observed when α-thrombin or collagen were used as agonists instead of ADP. In accordance with the fact that LJ-P5 and LJ-P9 competed for binding to platelets, excess LJ-P5 Fab could prevent the inhibitory effect of LJ-P9 on aggregation (*see* Fig. 12-8), thus demonstrating that the inhibitory effect was indeed related to LJ-P9 binding to GPIIb-IIIa. The results of aggregation studies were identical for either citrated platelet-rich plasma or washed platelet suspensions containing purified fibrinogen and 2 mM Ca^{2+}. Neither LJ-P5 nor LJ-P9 affected von Willebrand factor binding to platelets in the presence of ristocetin nor ristocetin-induced aggregation of platelet-rich plasma, in agreement with the concept that these events are mediated by the binding of von Willebrand factor to GPIb and not the GPIIb-IIIa complex.

Antibody LJ-P5 was also used to demon-

*Ruggeri, Z. M.: Unpublished observations

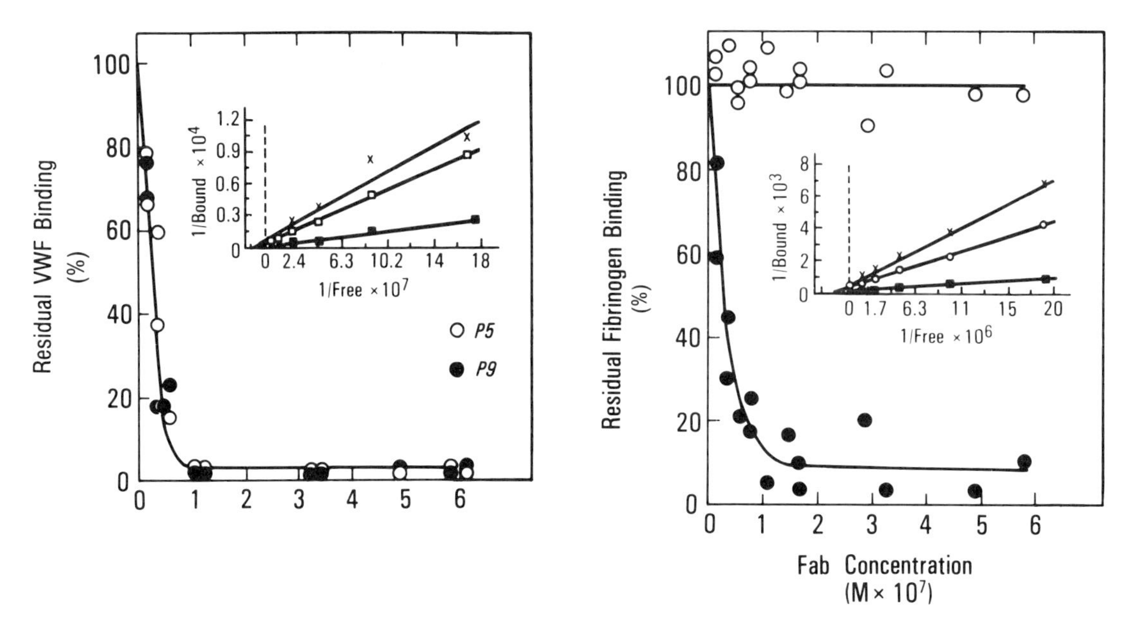

Figure 12-7. Effect of LJ-P5 and LJ-P9 fibrinogen and VWF binding to platelets. Washed platelet suspensions (1×10^8/ml) were mixed with 100 μg/ml of ^{125}I-fibrinogen (2.9×10^{-7} M) (*right panel*), or 5 μg/ml of ^{125}I-VWF (*left panel*). This was followed by 2 mmol/liter $CaCl_2$, the indicated concentration of Fab from LJ-P5 (P5) or LJ-P9 (P9), or an equal volume of Tyrode buffer, and 20 μM ADP. All indicated concentrations were final. The mixture, also containing 2% bovine serum albumin, was incubated for 30 min at room temperature, after which the platelets were separated from free ligand by centrifugation through 20% sucrose. The radioactivity in the platelet pellets was then counted. Nonspecific binding was measured in the presence of a 100-fold excess of unlabeled ligand. Specific binding was calculated by subtracting nonspecific from total binding and expressed as percentage of the binding measured in the absence of Fab (as shown). The latter values corresponded to 38,600 molecules/platelet for fibrinogen and 0.6 μg/10^8 platelets for VWF. These results are the aggregate of three separate experiments performed with different platelet preparations. The inset in the upper panel shows the results of a competition binding study in which increasing amounts of ^{125}I-VWF (between 1.3 and 37 μg/ml) were added to platelets either in the absence (solid squares) or in the presence of LJ-P5 (x, 1.5 μg/ml; open square, 0.8 μg/ml). The reciprocal of specific binding was plotted against the reciprocal of the free VWF concentration added. Even at the highest concentrations of VWF tested, the inhibitory effect of LJ-P5 could not be overcome. A change in position of the intersect on the y-axis, but not on the x-axis, was observed in the presence of the antibody, a finding compatible with a noncompetitive mechanism of inhibition. The inset in the right panel shows the results of a similar experiment performed with ^{125}I-labeled fibrinogen (concentrations between 15 and 366 μg/ml) either in the absence (solid squares) or in the presence of LJ-P9 (x, 15 μg/ml; 0, 3 μg/ml). Results could be interpreted in a similar way as those obtained in the experiment with VWF. In both instances, platelets were stimulated with 0.1 NIH U/ml of α-thrombin (Trapani Lombardo V, Hodson E, Roberts JR, Kunicki TJ, Zimmerman TS; Ruggeri ZM: Independent modulation of von Willebrand factor and fibrinogen binding to the platelet membrane glycoprotein IIb/IIIa complex as demonstrated by monoclonal antibody. J Clin Invest 76:1950–1958, 1985; reprinted with permission)

strate that the binding of von Willebrand factor to GPIIb–IIIa can mediate platelet aggregation under certain conditions. This was shown in the platelet-rich plasma of individuals affected by afibrinogenemia, in whom substantial aggregation can be elicited by "strong" stimuli, such as α-thrombin, despite the complete absence of fibrinogen in plasma or platelets.[19] Here, contrary to what is observed with normal platelet-rich plasma, antibody LJ-P5 inhibits platelet aggregation (Fig. 12-9). This finding demonstrates that platelet aggregation occurring in the absence of fibrinogen is mediated by von Willebrand factor, for it can be blocked by

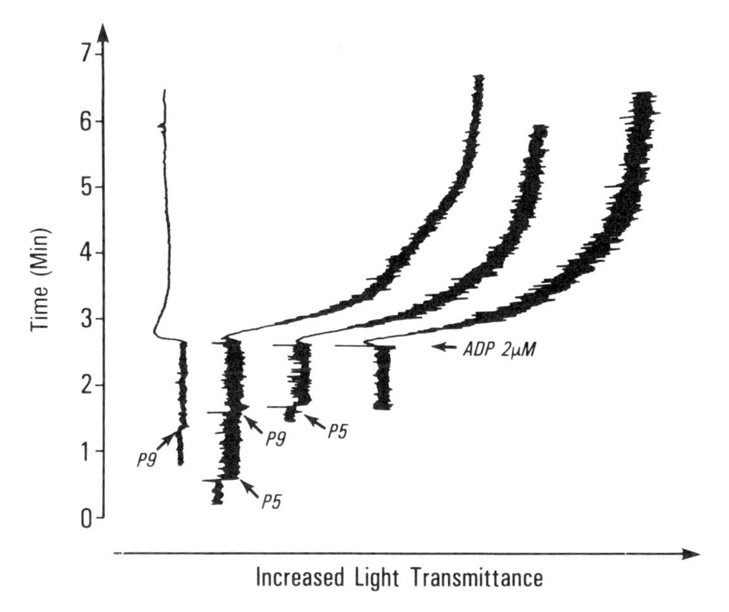

Figure 12-8. Effect of LJ-P5 and LJ-P9 on platelet aggregation. Washed platelet suspensions (2×10^8/ml) were added to an aggregometer cuvette, under stirring conditions, and mixed with 2 mmol/liter $CaCl_2$ and 300 μg/ml of fibrinogen (8.8×10^{-7} M). Then either LJ-P5 (P5) or LJ-P9 (P9) Fab was separately added to the mixture (20 μg/ml each, $\sim 4.2 \times 10^{-7}$ M), or LJ-P5 (200 μg/ml), followed by LJ-P9 (20 μg/ml). A control mixture containing Tyrode's buffer instead of Fab (curve on the right). All indicated concentrations were final. After equilibration and establishment of a straight baseline, ADP (2 μM, final concentration) was added to the mixtures (at arrow) and platelet aggregation recorded as increased light transmittance through the cuvette. The decrease in light transmittance immediately after addition of ADP represents the platelet shape change. Note the inhibitory effect of LJ-P9 on platelet aggregation, but its lack of inhibition of the platelet shape change. Note also the lack of inhibition in the presence of LJ-P5 and the blocking effect of the latter on the inhibition exerted by LJ-P9. Results similar to those seen with ADP could be observed when platelets were stimulated with thrombin or collagen (Trapani Lombardo V, Hodson E, Roberts JR, Kunicki TJ, Zimmerman TS, Ruggeri ZM: Independent modulation of von Willebrand factor and fibrinogen binding to the platelet membrane glycoprotein IIb/IIIa complex as demonstrated by monoclonal antibody. J Clin Invest 76:1950–1958, 1985; reprinted with permission)

an antibody that selectively blocks the binding of von Willebrand factor, but not of fibrinogen or of fibronectin, to GPIIb–IIIa. This inhibition can be overcome by the addition of purified fibrinogen to the system, restoring fibrinogen-dependent platelet aggregation that is not blocked by LJ-P5 (Fig. 12-10).

Other Studies on Glycoprotein IIb–IIIa Structure and Function Using Monoclonal Antibodies

Jennings and coworkers have described monoclonal antibodies directed against the light chain (β chain) of GPIIb that induce platelet activation, as measured by the release reaction, followed by aggregation.[41] These responses could be elicited not only by the intact IgG molecule but also by the monovalent Fab fragment, suggesting that antibody interaction with its specific epitope, independent of receptor clustering (which requires divalent antibody) or Fc-mediated responses because the Fab fragment of the antibody was also effective), was responsible for the observed effects. The physiologic significance of these findings remains obscure. It is possible that occupancy of specific epitopes on the GPIIb–IIIa complex result in a transmembrane signal, mediated through linkage to the membrane skeleton, triggering responses similar to those seen with traditional platelet stimuli. Monoclonal antibodies thus may be helpful in identifying cru-

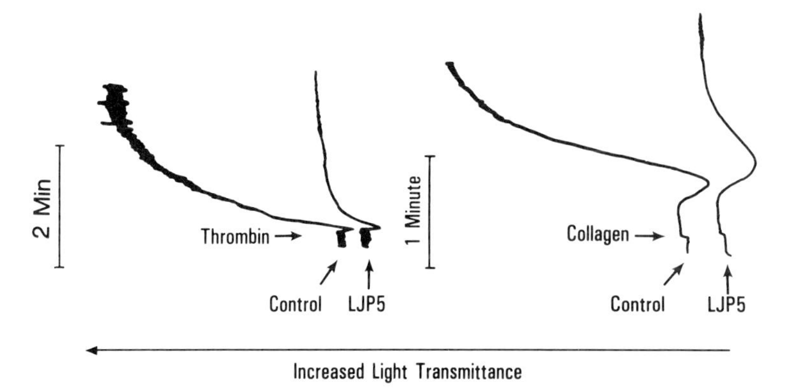

Figure 12-9. Aggregation of afibrinogenemic platelet-rich plasma. The two curves on the right (patient B.P.) demonstrate the aggregating effect of collagen (1 μg/ml) in the absence (control) or in the presence of antibody LJ-P5 (50 μg/ml). The two curves on the left (patient V.M.) demonstrate the aggregating effect of human α-thrombin (2 NIH U/ml) in the absence (control) or in the presence of antibody LJ-P5 (200 μg/ml). The platelet count was 3×10^8/ml in both studies. It is clear that, unlike in normal platelet-rich plasma (*see* Fig. 12-8), the aggregation seen in afibrinogenemic platelet-rich plasma is blocked by LJ-P5. Thus, these results show that, in the absence of fibrinogen, VWF supports platelet aggregation (DeMarco L, Girolami A, Zimmerman TS, Ruggeri ZM: Von Willebrand factor interaction with the glycoprotein IIb/IIIa complex. Its role in platelet function as demonstrated in patients with congenital afibrinogenemia. J Clin Invest 77:1272–1277, 1986; reprinted with permission)

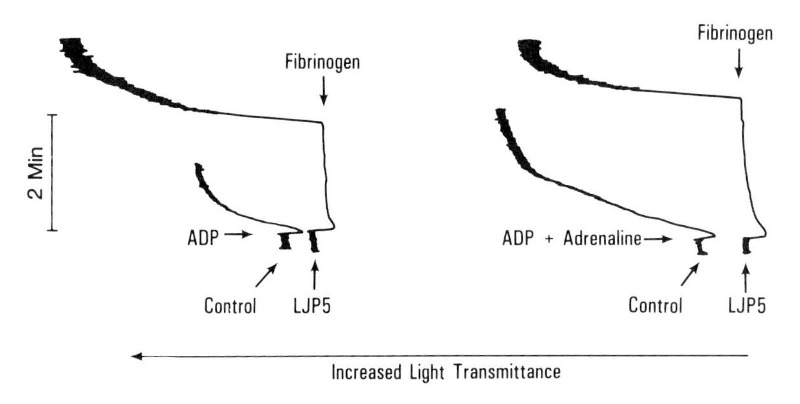

Figure 12-10. Aggregation of afibrinogenemic platelet-rich plasma. The two curves on the right show the aggregation induced by the combination of ADP and epinephrine (control curve, 6.25 μM each) and the blocking effect exerted by antibody LJ-P5 (140 μg/ml) in the presence of the same agonists. Addition of purified fibrinogen (800 μg/ml) to the mixture containing LJ-P5 resulted in prompt platelet aggregation. The two curves on the left show a similar experiment performed using ADP alone, 6.25 μM, as platelet agonist. LJ-P5 concentration was 70 μg/ml. Platelet-rich plasma (platelet count, 3×10^8/ml) was from patient V.M. in both studies. These experiments demonstrate that the inhibitory effect of LJ-P5 is specific for the aggregation mediated by VWF (DeMarco L, Girolami A, Zimmerman TS, Ruggeri ZM: Von Willebrand factor interaction with the glycoprotein IIb/IIIa complex. Its role in platelet function as demonstrated in patients with congenital afibrinogenemia. J Clin Invest 77:1272–1277, 1986; reprinted with permission)

cial domains of GPIIb–IIIa involved in initiating proaggregatory responses.

Monoclonal antibodies against GPIIb–IIIa are being considered as potential antithrombotic agents because of their ability to block the receptor function that mediates binding of adhesive proteins and is crucial for thrombus formation. Experimental animal models in dogs[14] and baboons[34] have shown that injection of monoclonal anti-GPIIb–IIIa monoclonal antibodies in quantities sufficient to saturate the corresponding epitopes on platelets leads to impairment of platelet function, as demonstrated by prolongation of the bleeding time. Moreover, the deposition of platelets onto thrombogenic surfaces or the vascular occlusion caused by platelet thrombi can be markedly inhibited in parallel with an inhibition of GPIIb–IIIa function. These concepts are developed more extensively in another chapter of this book.

MONOCLONAL ANTIBODIES AND THE STUDY OF THE STRUCTURE AND FUNCTION OF OTHER PLATELET MEMBRANE GLYCOPROTEINS

Glycoprotein Ib and GPIIb–IIIa are the best-known and better-characterized platelet membrane glycoproteins, but several others exist whose functions are largely unknown. In recent years, several investigators have started to approach the problem of unveiling the structure and function of these components of the platelet membrane.[22,38] Monoclonal antibodies are proving essential to the success of these efforts.

Thrombospondin is an adhesive molecule that, similar to von Willebrand factor, fibrinogen, and fibronectin, plays an important role in platelet function. Thrombospondin binds to stimulated platelets but, unlike the other three adhesive molecules, it binds equally well to platelets from normal individuals or patients with Glanzmann's thrombasthenia. Thus, another class of inducible receptors (i.e., that function only upon platelet stimulation but distinct from GPIIb–IIIa) must exist on platelets to bind thrombospondin.[1] Asch and coworkers have identified a platelet membrane protein of 88 kDa that appears to be the thrombospondin receptor.[2] This protein, also present on endothelial cells, monocytes, and a variety of human tumor cell lines, reacts with a monoclonal antibody, OKM5, which can block the binding of thrombospondin to platelets and other cells. Moreover, thrombospondin binding to platelets was shown to be blocked by a polyclonal antibody against GPIV, suggesting that this glycoprotein may be the thrombospondin receptor.

The interaction of platelets with collagen in the subendothelial matrix is likely to represent an important step in the initial events of hemostasis, participating as one of the mechanisms that lead to platelet adhesion at the site of endothelial cell damage. Several membrane proteins are being investigated as possible collagen receptors on the platelet membrane. A protein reported as 65-kDa molecular mass has been shown by Chiang and coworkers to react with a monoclonal antibody that inhibits collagen-induced platelet aggregation.[10] The isolated glycoprotein binds to collagen directly. Kotite and Cunningham have identified a platelet membrane glycoprotein of 61 kDa, which also binds specifically to insolubilized collagen.[42] The two proteins, in spite of the similar molecular mass, appear to be different. If this proves to be true, the isolation of two different receptors may have resulted from the use of different collagens by the two groups of investigators. There is certainly the possibility that platelets possess more than one collagen-binding site. For example, another membrane glycoprotein, GPIa, has been implicated in the divalent cation-dependent adhesion of platelets to collagen. Santoro has reported that a protein of 160-kDa molecular mass, possibly GPIa, interacts with collagen in a reaction supported by Mg^{2+} but not by Ca^{2+}.[79] This divalent cation specificity is identical with that observed for the adhesion of intact platelets to collagen. Additional evidence for the possible role of GPIa as collagen receptor comes from the description of a patient with a bleeding diathesis who was shown to be deficient in GPIa and to have a selective defect of collagen-induced aggregation.[57] It is now becoming clear that GPIa forms a noncovalent heterodimeric complex with GPIIa in the platelet membrane (*see* the following).

Platelets possess a number of membrane glycoproteins that appear to be closely related to, if not identical with, the very late activation antigens (VLA) expressed by T-lymphocytes. Five separate VLA structures are presently known, each composed of a distinct α subunit, noncovalently associated with a common β

subunit.[39] Glycoprotein IIa (M_r 145 kDa) reacts with antibodies directed against the β subunit of VLA; GPIa (M_r 160 kDa) and GPIc (M_r 140 kDa) react with antibodies against the α subunit of VLA-2 and VLA-3, respectively (*see* Chap. 2 in this book). A heterodimer complex between GPIc and GPIIa has, in fact, been identified with a rat monoclonal antibody.[83] It is important to note that VLA structures appear to be related to molecules that exhibit receptor function for fibronectin and laminin. In fact, they share common structural features with components of a superfamily of adhesion receptors, still expanding at the present time, that react with Arg-Gly-Asp sequences and are expressed on a variety of cells. It has been reported that platelets have a fibronectin receptor composed of a heterodimer complex (150/135 kDa) distinct from GPIIb–IIIa and immunologically related to the fibroblast fibronectin receptor.[26] This may very well be related to the VLA structures. Glycoprotein IIb and GPIIIa, in fact, are also part of this superfamily and exhibit structural similarities with heterodimer complexes expressed on a variety of cells. The terms *integrins* and *cytoadhesins* have been used by different groups to identify these structures (*see* Chap. 2 in this book).

We have mentioned earlier that monoclonal antibodies to the β chain of GPIIb appear to be involved in the initiation of proaggregatory responses. Other monoclonal antibodies against membrane glycoproteins have been shown to induce platelet activation and aggregation. One such antibody, AG-1, has been characterized in detail by Miller and coworkers.[51] This antibody recognizes a glycoprotein of approximate M_r 21 kDa, apparently complexed with GPIb (or a subset of GPIb molecules) but distinct from GPIX; the glycoprotein also appears to be different from the β (light) chains of GPIb and GPIIb. Thiagarajan and coworkers have described an antibody, B1-12, with similar properties that may, in fact, recognize the same glycoprotein.[86] The physiologic significance of these observations remains obscure.

CONCLUSIONS

The use of monoclonal antibodies has been of the utmost importance in promoting the explosive growth in our knowledge of the platelet membrane within the last decade. Still, we know only a fraction of what we would like to understand. Undoubtedly, our need for reagents of defined specificity will continue to grow as we proceed in the structural and functional mapping of platelet membrane molecules.[43] The ever-expanding use of newer technologies, including molecular biology and peptide chemistry, promises to be rewarding both for the tailoring of antibody molecules to fit specific needs and in better defining the specificity of those already available. This will prove essential for unraveling important pathophysiologic mechanisms related to platelet function.

This work was supported in part by National Institutes of Health grants HL 31950 and HL 37522.

This is publication number 5101 BCR from the Research Institute of Scripps Clinic, La Jolla, California.

REFERENCES

1. Aiken ML, Ginsberg MH, Plow EF: Identification of a new class of inducible receptors on platelets. Thrombospondin interacts with platelets via a GPIIb–IIIa-independent mechanism. J Clin Invest 78:1713, 1986

2. Asch AS, Barnwell J, Silverstein RL, Nachman RL: Isolation of the thrombospondin membrane receptor. J Clin Invest 79:1054, 1987

3. Behnke O: Electron microscopic observations on the membrane systems of the rat blood platelet. Anat Rec 158:121, 1967

4. Bennet JS, Hoxie JA, Leitman SF, Vilaire G, Cines DB: Inhibition of fibrinogen binding to stimulated human platelets by a monoclonal antibody. Proc Natl Acad Sci USA 80:2417, 1983

5. Bennett JS, Vilaire G: Exposure of platelet fibrinogen receptors by ADP and epinephrine. J Clin Invest 64:1393, 1979

6. Bennett JS, Vilaire G, Cines DB: Identification of the fibrinogen receptor on human platelets by photoaffinity labeling. J Biol Chem 257:8049, 1982

7. Berndt MC, Gregory C, Chong BH, Zola H, Castaldi PA: Additional glycoprotein defects in Bernard-Soulier's syndrome: Confirmation of genetic basis by parental analysis. Blood 62:800, 1983

8. Berndt MC, Gregory C, Kabral A, Zola H, Fournier D, Castaldi PA: Purification and preliminary characterization of glycoprotein Ib complex in the human platelet membrane, Eur J Biochem 151:637, 1985

9. Caen JP, Nurden AT, Jeanneau C, Michel H, Tobelem G, Levy-Toledano S, Sultan Y, Valensi F,

Bernard J: Bernard-Soulier syndrome: A new platelet glycoprotein abnormality. Its relationship with platelet adhesion to subendothelium and with the factor VIII von Willebrand protein. J Lab Clin Med 4:586, 1976

10. Chiang TM, Jin A, Kang AH: Platelet-collagen interaction. Inhibition by a monoclonal antibody raised against collagen receptor. J Immunol 139:887, 1987

11. Clemetson KJ, McGregor JL, James E, Dechavanne M, Luscher EF: Characterization of the platelet membrane glycoprotein abnormalities in Bernard-Soulier syndrome and comparison with normal big surface-labelling techniques and high-resolution two-dimensional gel electrophoresis. J Clin Invest 70:304, 1982

12. Coller BS: A new murine monoclonal antibody reports an activation-dependent change in the conformation and/or microenvironment of the platelet glycoprotein IIb/IIIa complex. J Clin Invest 76:101, 1985

13. Coller BS: Activation affects access to the platelet receptor for adhesive glycoproteins. J Cell Biol 103:451, 1986

14. Coller BS, Folts JD, Scudder LE, Smith SR: Antithrombotic effect of a monoclonal antibody to the platelet glycoprotein IIb/IIIa receptor in an experimental animal model. Blood 68:783, 1986

15. Coller BS, Kalomiris E, Steinberg M, Scudder LE: Evidence that glycocalicin circulates in normal plasma. J. Clin Invest 73:794, 1984

16. Coller BS, Peerschke EI, Scudder LE, Sullivan CA: Studies with a murine monoclonal antibody that abolishes ristocetin-induced binding of von Willebrand factor to platelets: Additional evidence in support of GPIb as a platelet receptor for von Willebrand factor. Blood 61:99, 1983

17. Coller BS, Peerschke EI, Scudder LE, Sullivan CA: A murine monoclonal antibody that completely blocks the binding of fibrinogen to platelets produces a thrombasthenic-like state in normal platelets and binds to glycoproteins IIb and/or IIIa. J Clin Invest 72:325, 1983

18. De Marco L, Fabris F, Casonato A, Fabris P, Del Ben MG, Barbato A, Girolami A: Bernard-Soulier syndrome: Diagnosis by an ELISA method using monoclonal antibodies in 2 new unrelated patients. Acta Haematol 75:203, 1986

19. De Marco L, Girolami A, Zimmerman TS, Ruggeri ZM: von Willebrand factor interaction with the glycoprotein IIb/IIIa complex. Its role in platelet function as demonstrated in patients with congenital afibrinogenemia. J Clin Invest 77:1272, 1986

20. Di Minno G, Thiagarajan P, Perussia B, Martinez J, Shapiro SS, Trinchieri G, Murphy S: Exposure of platelet fibrinogen-binding sites by collagen, arachidonic acid, and ADP: Inhibition by a monoclonal antibody to the glycoprotein IIb–IIIa complex. Blood 61:140, 1983

21. Du X, Beutler L, Ruan C, Castaldi PA, Berndt MC: Glycoprotein Ib and glycoprotein IX are fully complexed in the intact platelet membrane. Blood 69:1524, 1987

22. Furukawa K, Hayashi K, Shiku H, Yamada K: Analysis of cell surface molecules on human platelets with monoclonal antibodies. II. Diversity of antibody-binding sites on molecules and its relation to platelet function. Acta Haematol 75:147, 1986

23. Ganguly P: Binding of thrombin to functionally defective platelets: A hypothesis on the nature of the thrombin receptor. Br J Haematol 37:47, 1977

24. Gartner TK, Bennett JS: The tetrapeptide analogue of the cell attachment site of fibronectin inhibits platelet aggregation and fibrinogen binding to activated platelets. J Biol Chem 260:11891, 1985

25. George JN, Pickett EB, Saucerman S, McEver RP, Kunicki TJ, Kieffer N, Newman PJ: Platelet surface glycoprotein. Studies on resting and activated platelets and platelet membrane microparticles in normal subjects, and observations in patients during adult respiratory distress syndrome and cardiac surgery. J Clin Invest 78:340, 1986

26. Giancotti FG, Languino LR, Zanetti A, Peri G, Tarone G, Dejana E: Platelets express a membrane protein complex immunologically related to the fibroblast fibronectin receptor and distinct from GPIIb/IIIa. Blood 69:1535, 1987

27. Ginsberg MH, Lightsey A, Kunicki TJ, Kaufmann A, Marguerie G, Plow EF: Divalent cation regulation of the surface orientation of platelet membrane glycoprotein IIb. Correlation with fibrinogen binding function and definition of a novel variant of Glanzmann's thrombasthenia. J Clin Invest 78:1103, 1986

28. Girma J-P, Chopek MW, Titani K, Davie EW: Limited proteolysis of human vWF by *Staphylococcus aureau* V-8 protease: Isolation and partial characterization of a platelet-binding domain. Biochemistry 25:3156, 1986

29. Girma J-P, Kalafatis M, Pietu G, Lavergne J-M, Chopek MW, Edgington TS, Meyer D: Mapping of distinct von Willebrand factor domains interacting with platelet GPIb and GPIIb/IIIa and with collagen using monoclonal antibodies. Blood 67:1356, 1986

30. Gogstad GO, Brosstad F, Krutnes M-B, Hagen I, Solum NO: Fibrinogen-binding properties of the human platelet glycoprotein IIb–IIIa complex: A study using crossed-radioimmunoelectrophoresis. Blood 60:663, 1982

31. Gogstad GO, Hagen I, Korsmo R, Solum NO: Characterization of the proteins of isolated human platelet alpha-granules: Evidence for a sepa-

rate alpha-granule pool of the glycoproteins IIb and IIIa. Biochim Biophys Acta 670:150, 1981

32. Gogstad GO, Hagen I, Korsmo R, Solum NO: Evidence for release of soluble but not of membrane-integrated proteins from human platelet alpha granules. Biochim Biophys Acta 702:81, 1982

33. Handa M, Titani K, Holland LZ, Roberts JR, Ruggeri ZM: The von Willebrand factor-binding domain of platelet membrane glycoprotein Ib. Characterization by monoclonal antibodies and partial amino acid sequence analysis of proteolytic fragments. J Biol Chem 261:12579, 1986

34. Hanson SR, Pareti FI, Ruggeri ZM, Marzec UM, Kunicki TJ, Montgomery RR, Zimmerman TS, Harker LA: Effects of monoclonal antibodies against the platelet glycoprotein IIb/IIIa complex on thrombosis and hemostasis in the baboon. J Clin Invest 81:149, 1988

35. Harmon JT, Jamieson GA: The glycocalicin portion of platelet glycoprotein Ib expresses both high and moderate affinity receptor sites for thrombin. J Biol Chem 28:13224, 1986

36. Haverstick DM, Cowan JF, Yamada KM, Santoro SA: Inhibition of platelet adhesion to fibronectin, fibrinogen, and von Willebrand factor substrates by a synthetic tetrapeptide derived from the cell-binding domain of fibronectin. Blood 66:946, 1985

37. Hawiger J, Parkinson S, Timmons S: Prostacyclin inhibits mobilisation of fibrinogen-binding sites on human ADP- and thrombin-treated platelets. Nature 283:195, 1980

38. Hayashi K, Furukawa K, Takamoto S, Shiku H, Yamada K: Analysis of cell surface molecules on human platelets with monoclonal antibodies. I. Identification of four platelet-specific surface molecules. Acta Haematol 75:141, 1986

39. Hemler ME, Huang C, Schwarz L: The VLA protein family. Characterization of five distinct cell surface heterodimers each with a common 130,000 molecular weight beta subunit. J Biol Chem 262:3300, 1987

40. Hsu-Lin S-C, Berman CL, Furie BC, August D, Furie B: A platelet membrane protein expressed during platelet activation and secretion. Studies using a monoclonal antibody specific for thrombin-activated platelets. J Biol Chem 259:9121, 1984

41. Jennings LK, Phillips DR, Walker WS: Monoclonal antibodies to human platelet glycoprotein IIb beta that initiate distinct platelet responses. Blood 65:1112, 1985

42. Kotite NJ, Cunningham LW: Specific adsorption of a platelet membrane glycoprotein by human insoluble collagen. J Biol Chem 261:8342, 1986

43. Kunicki TJ, Nugent DJ, Piotrowicz RS, Lai C-S: Covalent attachment of sulfhydryl-specific, electron spin resonance spin-labels to Fab′ fragments of murine monoclonal antibodies that recognize human platelet membrane glycoproteins. Development of membrane protein specific spin probes. Biochemistry 25:4979, 1986

44. Lam SC-T, Plow EF, Smith MA, Andrieux A, Ryckwaert J-J, Marguerie G, Ginsberg MH: Evidence that arginyl-glycyl-aspartate peptides and fibrinogen gamma chain peptides share a common binding site on platelets. J. Biol Chem 262:947, 1987

45. Lawrence JB, Gralnick HR: Monoclonal antibodies to the glycoprotein IIb–IIIa epitopes involved in adhesive protein binding: Effects on platelet spreading and ultrastructure on human arterial subendothelium. J Lab Clin Med 109:495, 1987

46. Lopez JA, Chung DW, Fujikawa K, Hagen FS, Papayannopoulou T, Roth GJ: Cloning of the alpha chain of human platelet glycoprotein Ib: A transmembrane protein with homology to leucine-rich alpha^2-glycoprotein. Proc Natl Acad Sci USA 84:5615, 1987

47. McEver RP, Baenziger NL, Majerus PW: Isolation and quantitation of the platelet membrane glycoprotein deficient in thrombasthenia using a monoclonal hybridoma antibody. J Clin Invest 66:1311, 1980

48. McEver RP, Bennett EM, Martin MN: Identification of two structurally and functionally distinct sites on human platelet membrane glycoprotein IIb–IIIa using monoclonal antibodies. J Biol Chem 258:5269, 1983

49. McGregor JL, McGregor L, Bauer A-S, Catimel B, Brochier J, Dechavanne M, Clemetson KJ: Identification of two distinct regions within the binding sites for fibrinogen and fibronectin on the IIb–IIIa human platelet membrane glycoprotein complex by monoclonal antibodies P2 and P4 Eur J Biochem 159:443, 1986

50. McMichael AJ, Rust NA, Pilch JR, Sochynsky R, Morton J, Mason DY, Ruan C, Tobelem G, Caen J: Monoclonal antibody to human platelet glycoprotein I. I. Immunological studies. Br J Haematol 49:501, 1981

51. Miller JL, Kupinski JM, Hustad KO: Characterization of a platelet membrane protein of low molecular weight associated with platelet activation following binding by monoclonal antibody AG-1. Blood 68:743, 1986

52. Moake JL, Olson JD, Troll JH, Tang SS, Funicella T, Peterson DM: Binding of radioiodinated human von Willebrand factor to Bernard-Soulier, thrombasthenic and von Willebrand's disease platelets. Thromb Res 19:21, 1980

53. Montgomery RR, Kunicki TJ, Taves C, Pidard D, Corcoran M: Diagnosis of Bernard-Soulier syndrome and Glanzmann's thrombasthenia with a

monoclonal assay on whole blood. J Clin Invest 71:385, 1983

54. Nachman RL, Leung LLK: Complex formation of platelet membrane glycoproteins IIb and IIIa with fibrinogen. J Clin Invest 69:263, 1982

55. Newman PJ, Allen RW, Kahn RA, Kunicki TJ: Quantitation of membrane glycoprotein IIIa on intact human platelets using the monoclonal antibody, AP-3. Blood 65:227, 1985

56. Newman PJ, McEver RP, Doers MP, Kunicki TJ: Synergistic action of two murine monoclonal antibodies that inhibit ADP-induced platelet aggregation without blocking fibrinogen binding. Blood 69:668, 1987

57. Nieuwenhuis HK, Akkerman JWN, Houdijk WPM, Sixma JJ: Human blood platelets showing no response to collagen fail to express surface glycoprotein Ia. Nature 318:470, 1985

58. Niiya K, Hodson E, Bader R, Byers-Ward V, Koziol JA, Plow EF, Ruggeri ZM: Increased surface expression of the membrane glycoprotein IIb/IIIa complex induced by platelet activation. Relationship to the binding of fibrinogen and platelet aggregation. Blood 70:475, 1987

59. Nugent DJ, Kunicki TJ, Berglund C, Bernstein ID: A human monoclonal autoantibody recognizes a neoantigen on glycoprotein IIIA expressed on stored and activated platelets. Blood 70:16, 1987

60. Okumura T, Hasitz M, Jamieson GA: Platelet glycocalicin. Interaction with thrombin and role as thrombin receptor of the platelet surface. J Biol Chem 253:3435, 1978

61. Okumura T, Jamieson GA: Platelet glycocalicin. I. Orientation of glycoproteins of the human platelet surface. J Biol Chem 251:5944, 1976

62. Okumura T, Jamieson GA: Platelet glycocalicin: A single receptor for platelet aggregation induced by thrombin or ristocetin. Thromb Res 8:701, 1976

63. Okumura T, Lombart C, Jamieson GA: Platelet glycocalicin. II. Purification and characterization. J Biol Chem 251:5950, 1976

64. Parise LV, Phillips DR: Reconstitution of the purified platelet fibrinogen receptor. J Biol Chem 260:10698, 1985

65. Parise LV, Phillips DR: Fibronectin-binding properties of the purified platelet glycoprotein IIb/IIIa complex. J Biol Chem 261:14011, 1986

66. Peerschke EI, Zucker MB, Grant RA, Egan JJ, Johnson MM: Correlation between fibrinogen binding to human platelets and platelet aggregability. Blood 55:841, 1980

67. Pidard D, Montgomery RR, Bennett JS, Kunicki TJ: Interaction of AP-2, a monoclonal antibody specific for the human platelet glycoprotein IIb-IIIa complex, with intact platelets. J Biol Chem 258:12582, 1983

68. Plow EF, Ginsberg MH: Specific and saturable binding of plasma fibronectin to thrombin-stimulated human platelets. J Biol Chem 256:9477, 1981

69. Plow EF, Marguerie GA: Induction of the fibrinogen receptor on human platelets by epinephrine and the combination of epinephrine and ADP. J Biol Chem 255:10971, 1980

70. Plow EF, Marguerie GA: Participation of ADP in the binding of fibrinogen to thrombin-stimulated platelets. Blood 56:553, 1980

71. Plow EF, McEver RP, Coller BS, Woods VL Jr, Marguerie GA, Ginsberg MH: Related binding mechanisms for fibrinogen, fibronectin, von Willebrand factor, and thrombospondin on thrombin-stimulated human platelets. Blood 66:724, 1985

72. Plow EF, Pierschbacher MD, Ruoslahti E, Marguerie GA, Ginsberg MH: The effect of Arg-Gly-Asp-containing peptides on fibrinogen and von Willebrand factor binding to platelets. Proc Natl Acad Sci USA 82:8057, 1985

73. Plow EF, Srouji AH, Meyer D, Marguerie G, Ginsberg MH: Evidence that three adhesive proteins interact with a common recognition site on activated platelets. J Biol Chem 259:5385, 1984

74. Ruan C, Du X, Xi X, Castaldi PA, Berndt MC: A murine antiglycoprotein Ib complex monoclonal antibody, SZ 2, inhibits platelet aggregation induced by both ristocetin and collagen. Blood 69:570, 1987

75. Ruan G, Tobelem G, McMichael J, Drouet L, Legrand Y, Degos L, Kieffer N, Lee H, Caen JP: Monoclonal antibody to human platelet glycoprotein I. II. Effects on human platelet function. Br J Haematol 49:511, 1981

76. Ruggeri ZM, De Marco L, Gatti L, Bader R, Montgomery RR: Platelets have more than one binding site for von Willebrand factor. J Clin Invest 72:1, 1983

77. Ruggeri ZM, Houghten RA, Russell SR, Zimmerman TS: Inhibition of platelet function with synthetic peptides designed to be high-affinity antagonists of fibrinogen binding to platelets. Proc Natl Acad Sci USA 83:5708, 1986

78. Sakariassen KS, Nievelstein PF, Coller BS, Sixma JJ: The role of platelet membrane glycoproteins Ib and IIb-IIIa in platelet adherence to human artery subendothelium. Br J Haematol 63:681, 1986

79. Santoro SA: Identification of a 160,000 dalton platelet membrane protein that mediates the initial divalent cation-dependent adhesion of platelets to collagen. Cell 46:913, 1986

80. Santoso S, Zimmerman U, Neppert J, Mueller-Eckhardt C: Receptor patching and capping of platelet membranes induced by monoclonal antibodies. Blood 67:343, 1986

81. Shattil SJ, Hoxie JA, Cunningham M, Brass

LF: Changes in the platelet membrane glycoprotein II/IIIa complex during platelet activation. J Biol Chem 20:11107, 1985

82. Solum NO, Hagen I, Filion-Myklebust C, Stabaek T: Platelet glycocalicin: Its membrane association and solubilization in aqueous media. Biochim Biophys Acta 597:235, 1980

83. Sonnenberg A, Janssen H, Hogervorst F, Calafat J, Hilgers J: A complex of platelet glycoproteins Ic and IIa identified by a rat monoclonal antibody. J Biol Chem 262:10376, 1987

84. Stenberg PE, Shuman MA, Levine SP, Bainton DF: Redistribution of alpha-granules and their contents in thrombin-stimulated platelets. J Cell Biol 98:748, 1984

85. Tam SW, Fenton JW, Detwiler TC: Platelet thrombin receptors. Binding of alpha-thrombin is coupled to signal generation by a chymotrypsin-sensitive mechanism. J Biol Chem 255:6626, 1980

86. Thiagarajan P, Perussia B, De Marco L, Wells K, Trinchieri G: Membrane proteins on human megakaryocytes and platelets identified by monoclonal antibodies. Am J Hematol 14:255, 1983

87. Timmons S, Kloczewiak M, Hawiger J: ADP-dependent common receptor mechanism for binding of von Willebrand factor and fibrinogen to human platelets. Proc Natl Acad Sci USA 81:4935, 1984

88. Titani K, Takio K, Handa M, Ruggeri ZM: Amino acid sequence of the von Willebrand factor-binding domain of platelet membrane glycoprotein Ib. Proc Natl Acad Sci USA 84:5610, 1987

89. Trapani-Lombard V, Hodson E, Roberts J, Kunicki TJ, Zimmerman TS, Ruggeri ZM: Independent modulation of von Willebrand factor and fibrinogen binding to the platelet membrane glycoprotein IIb/IIIa complex as demonstrated by monoclonal antibody. J Clin Invest 76:1950, 1985

90. Van der Meulen J, Furuya W, Grinstein S: Isolation and partial characterization of platelet alpha-granule membranes. J Membr Biol 71:47, 1983

91. Weiss HJ, Tschopp TB, Baumgartner HR, Sussman II, Johnson MM, Egan JJ: Decreased adhesion of giant (Bernard-Soulier) platelets to subendothelium. Further implications on the role of the von Willebrand factor in hemostasis. Am J Med 57:920, 1974

92. Weiss HJ, Turitto VT, Baumgartner HR: Platelet adhesion and thrombus formation on subendothelium in platelets deficient in glycoproteins IIb–IIIa, Ib, and storage granules. Blood 67:322, 1986

93. Wencel-Drake JD, Plow EF, Kunicki TJ, Woods VL, Keller DM, Ginsberg MH: Localization of internal pools of membrane glycoproteins involved in platelet adhesive responses. Am J Pathol 124:324, 1986

94. White JG: Interaction of membrane systems in blood platelets. Am J Pathol 66:295, 1972

95. Wicki AN, Clemetson KJ: Structure and function of platelet membrane glycoproteins Ib and V. Effects of leukocyte elastase and other proteases on platelets response to von Willebrand factor and thrombin. Eur J Biochem 153:1, 1985

96. Wicki AN, Clemetson KJ: The glycoprotein Ib complex of human blood platelets. Eur J Biochem 163:43, 1987

97. Williams S, Gralnick H: Inhibition of von Willebrand factor binding to platelets by two recognition site peptides: The pentadecapeptide of the carboxy terminus of the fibrinogen gamma chain and the tetrapeptide Arg-Gly-Asp-Ser. Thromb Res 46:457, 1987

98. Woods VL Jr, Wolff LE, Keller DM: Resting platelets contain a substantial centrally located pool of glycoprotein IIb/IIIa complex which may be accessible to some but not other extracellular proteins. J Biol Chem 261:15242, 1986

99. Yamamoto K, Kosaki G, Suzuki K, Tanoue K, Yamazaki H: Cleavage site of calcium-dependent protease in human platelet membrane glycoprotein Ib. Thromb Res 43:41, 1986

100. Yamamoto K, Yamamoto N, Kitagawa H, Tanoue K, Kosaki G, Yamazaki H: Localization of a thrombin-binding site on human platelet membrane glycoprotein Ib determined by a monoclonal antibody. Thromb Haemostasis 55:162, 1986

101. Yamamoto N, Kitagawa H, Tanoue K, Yamazaki H: Monoclonal antibody to glycoprotein Ib inhibits both thrombin-and ristocetin-induced platelet aggregations. Thromb Res 39:751, 1985

102. Zucker-Franklin D: Endocytosis by human platelets: Metabolic and freeze fracture studies. J Cell Biol 91:706, 1981

13

Homologous Functions and Interactions of Platelets and Endothelial Cells

ROBERT R. MONTGOMERY · YOHKO KAWAI · J. PAUL SCOTT

The glycoprotein surfaces of cells contain membrane receptors that are important to cell–surface and cell–cell interaction. Communication between cells also occurs by means of soluble molecular and macromolecular ligands that interact with these receptors to control cellular response and function. The surface structure of normal human platelets has been studied in great detail and is extensively reviewed in other chapters of this book. Because of the circulating nature of platelets, they are in a unique position to modulate hemostasis and thrombosis and to transport functional messages to distal organs or tissues. They are carried through the body within an endothelial cell network. This network is stationary and can modulate the local hemostatic milieu. Thus, activated platelets and activated clotting factors are carried from one area of the body to another, where they can turn on the stationary (endothelial) system that can then augment or diminish the biologic response and regulate the continuation of this biologic response. Unlike the platelet, the endothelial cell is a "true" cell that cannot only have a preexisting response to this communication but can also alter its synthetic machinery to create new responses. Many structural and functional similarities are being discovered between platelets and endothelial cells. The endothelial cell's function as an "organ" is only beginning to be elucidated. Until recently, little has been known about the surface structure and function of the endothelial cell. Although the immunology of platelet surface antigens has been reasonably well-characterized, the structural basis for endothelial cell antigens is just emerging. This chapter will summarize some of the current knowledge concerning endothelial cells, with particular emphasis on the structural, antigenic, and functional similarities between endothelial cells and platelets.

Endothelium has traditionally been regarded as a tubular conduit for transporting the cellular elements of blood and the circulating proteins of plasma.[28,45] It was thought to be little more than a passive participant in the functional interactions between blood and the tissues that the blood nurtures. However, even in 1856, Virchow included endothelium in his triad of the etiology of vascular thrombosis,[111] and Brucke observed that the integrity of endothelium must be maintained to prevent thrombosis.[7] Little progress was made over the next 100 years in the understanding of its active role in thrombosis and organ biology. The endothelial cell was thought to provide the blood vessel with a smooth, nonthrombogenic surface, with its only participation in vascular events occurring after it was denuded. With this resultant exposure of the subendothelium, platelet adhesion was initiated, followed by platelet aggregation, and blood clotting. As our understanding of the variety of its functions has evolved, the endothelium has come to be considered an active, not a passive, participant in hemostasis.

Today, the endothelium is generally recognized as a multifunctional "organ" that is positioned at the intravascular/extravascular interface. This interface is one cell thick and occupies a surface estimated to be in excess of 1000 to 6300 m^2.[43,53] The quantitative distribution of endothelial cells in the vascular tree is > 95% in capillaries. This distribution of cells has made the study of functional diversity of various endothelial beds very difficult. The cells that are usually cultured are large-vessel endothelium, yet many functions of the endothelium may occur at or near the capillary level. This large, unique interface is the focus of much current research on endothelial cell biology and its relation to hemostasis, thrombosis, fibrinolysis, cellular communication, and cellular transport.

The study of endothelial cell structure and function has been made possible by the introduction in the late 1960s and early 1970s of techniques to culture endothelial cells.[29,31,44] Even today most studies are performed on cells derived from large vessels, such as umbilical vein endothelium (Fig. 13-1). The techniques for microvascular endothelial cell culture are just beginning to emerge,[18,51,69] and there remain the problems in sorting out specialized endothelial functions using cultured cells that may be modified under culture conditions. The impact of vessel source, cell species, growth factors, and other culture conditions on the cell biology of the endothelial cell remain as important variables, requiring further investigation.

THE STRUCTURE OF ENDOTHELIAL CELLS

General

Endothelium exists as a monolayer—both in vivo and in culture. These cells have a characteristic cobblestone appearance and are approximately 50 μm in diameter and 3 μm in thickness. Each endothelial cell has three distinct surfaces: the luminal surface is the nonthrombogenic surface; the abluminal surface is an adhesive surface bound to the subendothelial matrix; and the junctional surface abuts two endothelial surfaces and is described as being cohesive. The manner by which endothelial surfaces join to one another varies from one vascular bed to another. The endothelium in the central nervous system has fused junctions, whereas those in the liver, spleen, and kidneys are looser and permit the regulation of permeability and the exchange of nutrients and plasma constituents. Characterization of surface proteins may prove to be more difficult because, in culture, surface-labeling techniques may only label the luminal side.

Like the platelet, the endothelial cell possesses a glycocalyx, but its constituents are not as well characterized as those of the platelet. The endothelial cell surface may present neoantigens or modified surface antigen after perturbation by various cytokines which, like the platelet, permit it to be the target of autoimmune antibodies. Once the endothelial cell surface is fully characterized, it can be expected to possess a wide diversity of surface antigens, which may account for its susceptibility to immune injury.[10,35]

Weibel-Palade Bodies and Other Subcellular Structures

Within the endothelial cell are unique subcellular organelles that are oblong, rod-shaped structures (0.1 × 3 μm) termed "Weibel-Palade bodies" (Fig. 13-2). The interior is composed of cylindrical tubes (diameter, 20 nm) that have also been recently identified in the α granule of platelets.[16] These rod-shaped bodies are present in cultured umbilical vein endothelial cells and are rarely seen in capillary endothelium, although they are present in CNS endothelium[104] and may represent von Willebrand factor itself. These organelles are probably involved in the regulated secretion of von Willebrand factor and von Willebrand antigen II and will be described in greater detail later in this chapter.

Endothelial cells contain large numbers of pinocytotic vesicles[70] that are involved in transcellular transport. Cells in culture may possess more pinocytotic vesicles during rapid proliferation, and these vesicles may be particularly important in CNS endothelium, where transport must be through the cell, not around the cell, because of tight endothelial cell junctions.[104]

Endothelial Cell Surface Proteins

The endothelial cell possesses three surfaces with discrete functions, which have been reviewed by Stemerman and coworkers.[104] The

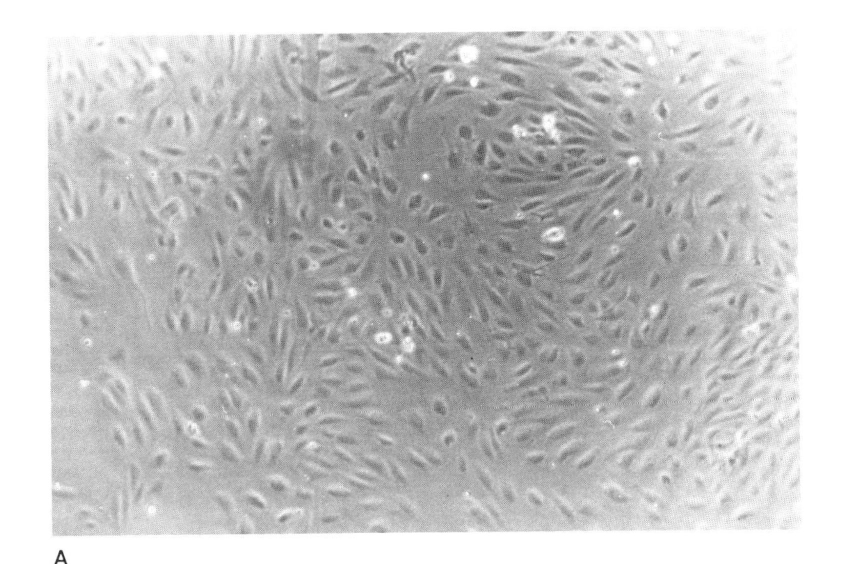

A

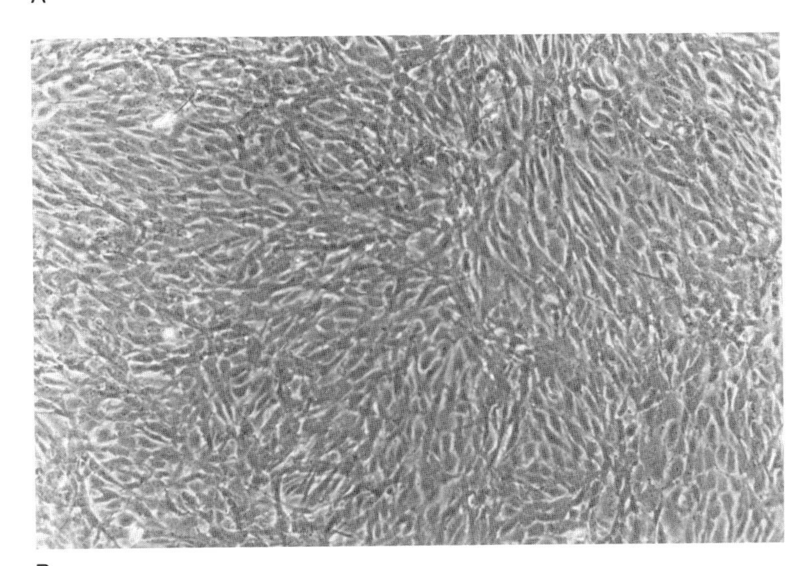

B

Figure 13-1. Endothelial cells were harvested from a human umbilical vein. A secondary culture was grown in the presence of 15% horse serum, ECGF (30 μg/ml) and heparin (6 μ/ml) for (*A*) 2 and (*B*) 5 days. Note the characteristic cobblestone appearance.

luminal surface is nonthrombogenic and is the surface exposed to flowing blood (or culture media). The endothelial cell also adheres to subendothelium (collagen, glycosaminoglycans, elastin, etc.) or, experimentally, to culture plates coated with fibronectin or collagen (gelatin). In vivo this would be the abluminal surface. The third surface is the endothelial–endothelial surface composed, in part, of "gap" or "tight" junctions.

Although a great deal is known about the platelet surface and the structure and function of its surface glycoproteins, the characterization of the endothelial cell surface is just beginning. Other sections of this book will consider the structure of the platelet surface glycoproteins and their function as receptors in modulation of complex hemostatic and immunologic reactions. Emerging knowledge suggests that endothelial cells may participate in similar thrombotic and antithrombotic reactions, as well as sharing surface glycoprotein antigens that may contribute to the clinical expression of autoimmune and alloimmune disorders.

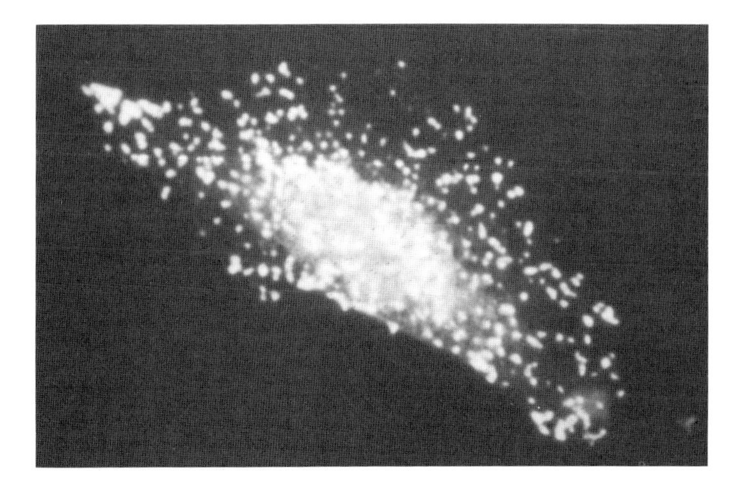

Figure 13-2. Human umbilical vein endothelial cells were first reacted with monoclonal antibody to human plasma von Willebrand's antigen II (vW AgII) and then a fluoresceinated rabbit antimouse immunoglobulin antibody. The Weibel-Palade bodies are then visualized by fluorescent microscopy, demonstrating the intracellular localization of vW AgII, the propolypeptide of von Willebrand factor. These secretory organelles also contain mature von Willebrand factor.

The large surface area of predominantly capillary endothelium and its anatomic location, juxtaposed between the vascular and extravascular tissue, provide a basis for the regulation of a variety of physiologic events that control hemorrhage, clotting, host defense and, through its interaction with smooth-muscle cells, the regulation of blood flow itself. Thus, the functional and structural characterization of its luminal surface is crucial to our understanding of these various mechanisms.

Glycoprotein IIIa

Glycoprotein IIIa is a transmembrane platelet glycoprotein that forms a heterodimer with GPIIb called the GPIIb-IIIa complex. On platelets this GPIIb-IIIa complex functions as a receptor for fibrinogen, fibronectin, and von Willebrand factor,[92,94,96] although the latter may only bind to GPIIb-IIIa when fibrinogen and other constituents are present in reduced amounts.[96] By using monoclonal antibodies to GPIIIa, investigators have identified a protein similar to GPIIIa on the surface of cultured human endothelial cells.[26,83,107] The DNA sequence of the platelet GPIIIa and endothelial cell GPIIIa (EC-GPIIIa) appear to be identical.[27] The implications of the presence of this glycoprotein for interactions with "platelet-specific" alloantibodies will be discussed later.

Glycoprotein IIb

Glycoprotein IIb is also a transmembrane platelet glycoprotein composed of disulfide-linked large and small subunits. In contrast to EC-GPIIIa, an analogue of platelet GPIIb appears not to be located on endothelial cells. Thiagarajan and coworkers[107] did not identify GPIIb on the surface of endothelium, although other laboratories did find that the EC-GPIIIa is part of one or two heterodimeric complexes with proteins that are slightly larger than GPIIb.[26,83] These have now been demonstrated to be the α chain of the vitronectin (VNR_{α}) and fibronectin (FNR_{α}) receptors.[33,88] This is discussed elsewhere in more detail by Newman (Chap. 9) and Fitzgerald (Chap. 2). Whether these heterodimeric complexes surve as receptors for luminal reactions is not known. These complexes might be more important in cell-cell interactions on the abluminal surface or at the site of lateral junctions.

Glycoprotein Ib

Glycoprotein Ib is the platelet glycoprotein surface receptor for von Willebrand factor in the presence of ristocetin.[92,94,96] Glycoprotein Ib (170 kDa) comprises a large α subunit (143 kDa) that is disulfide-linked to a smaller β subunit (22 kDa)—both subunits have transmembrane domains. It is exquisitely sensitive to cleavage by the calcium-activated neutral protease (calpain), yielding a large, soluble fragment termed glycocalicin.[54] Platelets contain calpain, but its presence in endothelial cells has not been determined. Platelet GPIb contains a binding site for plasma von Willebrand factor. The presence of this glycoprotein on the endothelial cell has been studied by several laboratories with somewhat conflicting results[1,103b,112] The specific isolation, characterization, and protein sequence of an "endothelial cell GPIb" has not yet been reported and will await confirmation by endothelial cell-derived cDNA sequencing because the cDNA sequence of platelet GPIb is now known from cloning in a HEL cell cDNA library.[61] At a functional level, however, several groups have identified ristocetin-induced binding of von Willebrand factor to endothelial cells[1,103b,112], suggesting there is at least a "functional" equivalent to platelet GPIb, although there are some differences between the binding of von Willebrand factor to endothelial cells and its binding to platelets (*see* following discussion).

Von Willebrand's Disease — A Syndrome Involving Plasma, Platelets, and Endothelium

Von Willebrand's disease is a common clinical syndrome that is associated with mild bleeding symptoms. It is the qualitative or quantitative deficiency of von Willebrand factor — a large multimeric (4×10^5 to $>2 \times 10^7$ Da) glycoprotein that is produced in endothelial cells and megakaryocytes/platelets. Most of the studies on this disorder that have focused on the platelet and plasma have been reviewed recently.[39,121] Three distinct plasma proteins (Table 13-1) are decreased, absent, or abnormal in von Willebrand's disease, including von Willebrand factor, factor VIII, and von Willebrand antigen II (vW AgII).[68,76,94] In severe von Willebrand's disease, plasma and platelet von Willebrand factor are undetectable.[39,93] Virtually all of the platelet von Willebrand factor is located in the α granules.[98,99] The multimeric structure of platelet von Willebrand factor is normal and contains multimers slightly larger than those seen in normal plasma.[54,60]

Our current understanding of von Willebrand's disease is that von Willebrand factor serves as the carrier protein for factor VIII (antihemophilic factor) and that the deficiency of factor VIII in von Willebrand's disease is secondary to the deficiency of von Willebrand factor.[39,94] The codeficiencies of von Willebrand factor and von Willebrand antigen II (vW AgII) were more difficult to understand until studies of the endothelial cell[72,73] and the cloning of the von Willebrand factor gene[32,66] demonstrated that both are derived from a common precursor[25,72] and that vW AgII is identical with a 100-kDa protein previously thought by other investigators to be factor VIIIC.[24] No immunologic relationship exists between plasma von Willebrand factor and plasma vW AgII,[76] but a precursor molecule containing antigenic epitopes of both von Willebrand factor and vW AgII was discovered in the endothelial cell.[72] This precursor molecule was proved to be pro-von Willebrand factor after the gene for von Willebrand factor was sequenced and the derived amino acid sequence obtained from the cDNA for the NH^2-terminal end of pro-von Willebrand factor was shown to be identical to the NH^2-terminal sequence of vW AgII.[25] A hereditary persistence of pro-von Willebrand factor has been identified in one family[74] in whose plasma the von Willebrand factor multimers appeared to be normal. In another coagulation protein — factor IX-Cambridge, the failure of cleavage of the propolypeptide may be due to a single amino acid substitution.[19] The proposed mechanism for the role of the vW AgII propolypeptide in intracellular von Willebrand factor processing and assembly will be reviewed later.

Table 13-1
Terminology

Von Willebrand factor is the large multimeric glycoprotein that binds to platelet GPIb and mediates platelet adhesion. It is deficient in severe von Willebrand's disease and appears to function as a carrier protein for factor VIII.

Von Willebrand antigen II (vW AgII) is the circulating propolypeptide of von Willebrand factor that is cleaved from pro-von Willebrand factor during normal intracellular processing. It is deficient in the plasma and platelets of patients with von Willebrand's disease, although its concentration may be normal in the plasma of patients with type II variants of von Willebrand's disease.

Pro-von Willebrand factor is the intracellular precursor of von Willebrand factor and vW AgII that is directed by the gene for von Willebrand factor. Intracellular processing results in glycosylation, sulfation, multimerization, and proteolytic cleavage of pro-von Willebrand factor into mature von Willebrand factor multimers and von Willebrand antigen II.

Factor VIII is the procoagulant protein that is a cofactor in the factor IXa activation of factor X. It is deficient in the plasma of patients with hemophilia A. Factor VIII circulates in plasma noncovalently attached to von Willebrand factor.

The Binding of Plasma von Willebrand Factor to Platelets

The binding of plasma von Willebrand factor to platelets has been the subject of investigation by numerous laboratories since the initial identification by Howard and coworkers that the antibiotic ristocetin induced platelet aggregation (and agglutination).[40] There appear to be at least two mechanisms by which von Willebrand factor binds to platelets.[96] Platelet adhesion to vessel wall endothelium or subendothelium, similarly to ristocetin-induced binding of von Willebrand factor, is mediated by binding of von Willebrand factor to the platelet GPIb. This binding can be blocked specifically by AP1, a monoclonal antibody that we have raised against GPIb, and AVW3, a monoclonal antibody to plasma von Willebrand factor. Other investigators have also demonstrated thrombin- or ADP/epinephrine-induced von Willebrand factor binding to the GPIIb-IIIa complex,[92,96] but this latter site is functional for plasma von Willebrand factor only if purified von Willebrand factor and washed platelets are used, or in the plasma milieu if the concentration of plasma fibrinogen is drastically reduced (<75 mg/dl).[96] In patients with afibrinogenemia, this von Willebrand factor-induced binding may serve as a physiologic backup to fibrinogen to support platelet aggregation. This latter binding site is blocked by AP2, a monoclonal antibody that blocks both von Willebrand factor and fibrinogen binding to GPIIb-IIIa when induced by thrombin or ADP/epinephrine.[96]

Identification of von Willebrand Factor in Endothelial Cells

Hoyer and coworkers first demonstrated von Willebrand antigen in endothelial cells by immunofluorescent microscopy.[41] Jaffe and coworkers[42] demonstrated that cultured endothelial cells synthesize von Willebrand factor. The demonstration of von Willebrand antigen within cultured vascular cells has become a specific marker of human endothelial cells. Platelets (and megakaryocytes) also contain von Willebrand antigen where it is found in the α granules,[79,99] and it is synthesized by the megakaryocyte.[80] The Weibel-Palade body, a specific subcellular organelle of endothelial cells, was found by Wagner and coworkers[113] to contain von Willebrand factor.[117] Desmopressin (DDAVP) releases endothelial cell von Willebrand factor in vivo, and this von Willebrand factor is presumed to be released from these Weibel-Palade bodies. More information concerning the endothelial cell processing of von Willebrand factor and vW AgII will be provided in the following.

Association of von Willebrand Factor with the Subendothelial Matrix

Studies have demonstrated von Willebrand factor in association with extracellular components of the subendothelium, including the basement membrane and the internal elastic lamina, where it is, in part, associated with collagen.[89] Native fibrillar collagen of several types (type I, III, IV, and V) binds von Willebrand factor in solution, with preference for high molecular mass multimers of von Willebrand factor.[39] Other components of the extracellular matrix may also bind von Willebrand factor.[23,118] In an attempt to study the physiologic mechanisms involved in this interaction, functional studies were developed and are discussed in the following sections.

In Vitro Studies on the Role of von Willebrand Factor and Blood Vessels

Several groups have investigated the role of von Willebrand factor in the interaction of platelets with the blood vessel wall, using perfusion chambers in which the blood, or platelet-rich plasma, is passed through chambers containing everted large vessels denuded of their endothelium. Baumgartner and coworkers and other groups have used this system to study both adhesion and thrombus formation by morphometry[4] or deposition of platelets after ^{51}Cr labeling.[95] In general, these studies are carried out using rabbit aortas that have had the endothelium removed by balloon injury or stripping. The adhesion and subsequent aggregation of platelets is, therefore, in response to the interaction of platelets and plasma with subendothelium. Although these studies have been done at different shear rates, most of the recent studies use low-shear rates that are more representative of those found in small capillaries. For maximal platelet binding of von Willebrand factor, the presence of normal platelets and normal von Willebrand factor is necessary. In the absence of von Willebrand factor, approximately 33% of the normal number of platelets are deposited. If the vessels are first perfused with von Willebrand factor, followed by the platelet suspension without von Willebrand factor, platelets still bind maximally. This suggests that von Willebrand factor can bind to subendothelium in a manner that permits the subsequent adhesion of platelets without any other stimulus (such as ristocetin). Because there was still significant binding of platelets when no von Willebrand factor was present, alternative backup systems may be operative. This might be due to normal von Willebrand factor adhering to the exposed subendothelium. The study of platelets by this approach, however, assumes that the only role for the endothelial cell is in covering the subendothelium. The other possibility for the formation of von Willebrand factor participation in platelet adhesion is that perturbed endothelial cells, themselves, might bind von Willebrand factor and, thereby, provide a cellular response and regulation of this biologic process. Data on this possibility will be presented later in this chapter.

Synthesis of von Willebrand Factor and Pro-von Willebrand Factor

Jaffe and coworkers initially identified von Willebrand factor synthesis by endothelial cells.[42] Studies by Lynch and coworkers[65] and Wagner and Marder[115] demonstrated a large precursor molecule termed "pro-von Willebrand factor" within endothelial cells. The apparent difference between the relative molecular mass of von Willebrand factor (225 kDa) and pro-von Willebrand factor (255 kDa) on sodium dodecyl sulfate (SDS) polyacrylamide gels was only 30 kDa, a molecular mass smaller than that observed for vW AgII (100 kDa). Results with pulse-labeling experiments demonstrated that [^{35}S] methionine is first incorporated into pro-von Willebrand factor and then into mature von Willebrand factor. These research groups further characterized the biosynthesis of von Willebrand factor and studied its intracellular processing through complex glycosylation and sulfation.[67,114,116,118] The protomeric form of intracellular von Willebrand factor is a dimer (COOH-terminal linked through a disulfide bond) that comprises two pro-von Willebrand factor molecules that are glycosylated, sulfated, assembled, and subsequently cleaved into mature von Willebrand factor. The mature multimers of von Willebrand factor are formed during the processing step that stores von Willebrand factor in the Weibel-Palade body. The vW AgII is also cleaved from the pro-von Willebrand factor upon packaging in the Weibel-Palade body, but this cleavage is not a prerequisite for multimer assembly, although the presence of vW AgII on pro-von Willebrand factor may be necessary to form the multimers. Recent studies by Verweij and coworkers[110] demonstrate the absence of multimer formation when the vW AgII portion of the cDNA is deleted from the von Willebrand factor gene. This, together with our demonstration of the self-association of vW AgII,[47] suggests that vW AgII assists in the formation of the NH^2-terminal disulfide bond and the subsequent high molecular mass multimers (Fig. 13-3).

Interaction of von Willebrand Factor with the Endothelial Surface

Recently, our laboratory and several other laboratories have investigated endothelial cells to determine whether they contain surface glycoproteins that are structural and functional analogues to counterparts on the platelet. In studies done in collaboration with Newman and Kunicki, we previously demonstrated surface glycoproteins analogous to platelet GPIIb–IIIa[83] and the endothelial synthesis and surface expression of both Pl^{A1} and Pen^{a} antigens on platelet GPIIIa, previously thought to be platelet-specific.[49,84]

Recently, ours and a number of other laboratories have studied von Willebrand factor binding to endothelial cells.[1,11a,103b,112] There is binding of von Willebrand factor to endothelial cells by means of the RGDS receptor described by Cheresh.[11a] This cell adhesion receptor comprises the α chain of the vitronectin receptor (VNR α) and GPIIIa. Our laboratory and others have also studied the ristocetin-induced binding of von Willebrand factor to endothelial cells through a receptor that may be similar to GPIb on platelets.[1,103b,112] Controversy remains over the identification of this receptor, although AP1, our monoclonal antibody to GPIb, has been used to isolate a protein similar to GPIb from endothelial cells.[103a] In studies performed in our laboratory, AP1

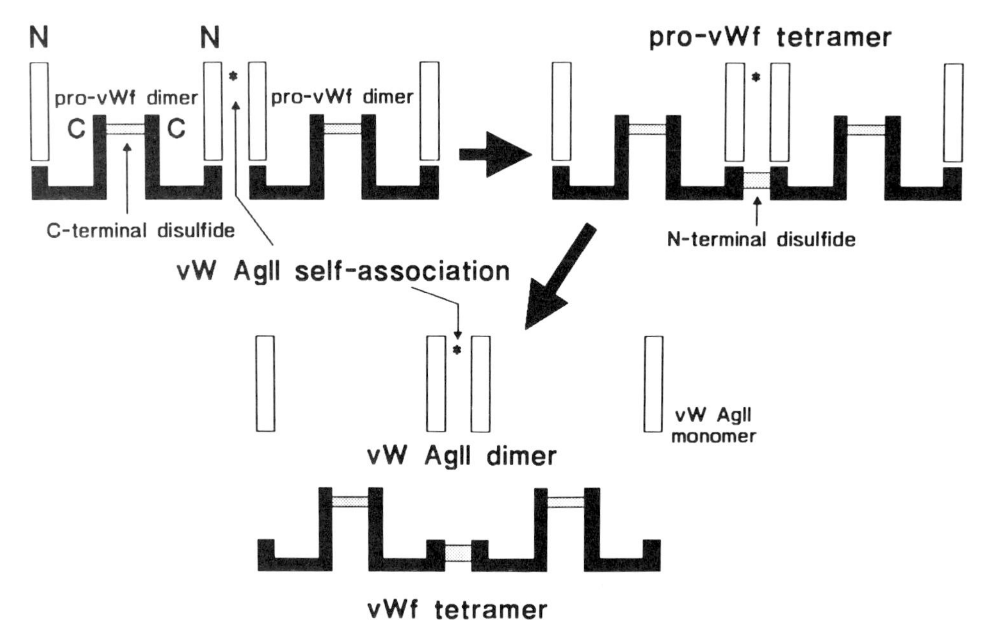

Figure 13-3. This figure demonstrates the possible role of the vW AgII portion of the pro-von Willebrand factor molecule in the assembly of higher molecular weight multimers of von Willebrand factor. The self-association of the vW AgII ends (N-terminal) could bring the N-terminal ends of the pro-von Willebrand factor C-terminal-linked dimers together and result in the correct orientation for the formation of the N-terminal disulfide-bonds. In plasma, vW AgII circulates as a noncovalent homodimer.

does not bind to endothelial cells in cultured monolayers. This raised the possibility that such a receptor may not be lumenally expressed and might have an interaction with the von Willebrand factor that is localized to the subendothelium. Now that the gene for GPIb has been isolated, the answer to the structural presence of GPIb in endothelial cells with the forthcoming, and further studies will be necessary to establish the physiologic function of the interaction of von Willebrand factor with the endothelial cell surface(s).

Secretion of von Willebrand Factor and von Willebrand Antigen II by Endothelial Cells

Because platelets do not release von Willebrand factor or VW AgII after in vitro exposure to DDAVP, the source of von Willebrand factor and vW AgII in plasma after DDAVP is presumed to be secreted from endothelial cells. Only recently have specific studies in vitro confirmed this. Reinders and coworkers found that calcium ionophore A23187 and phorbol myristate acetate (PMA) perturb the secretion of von Willebrand factor from cultured endothelial cells.[90] Studies by Wagner and coworkers also demonstrate release of von Willebrand factor by fibrin (in addition to ionophore A23187 and phorbol myristate acetate) and extended their studies to evaluate the binding of the synthesized von Willebrand factor to the extracellular matrix.[91,101,102,113]

Farquhar[22] and Kelly[50] have defined some of the important molecular and cellular events of protein secretion by eukaryotic cells. They have defined two pathways of protein secretion, termed *constitutive secretion* and *regulated secretion*. Constitutive secretion occurs as soon as the protein is synthesized and transported to the cell surface, whereas regulated secretion involves the formation of a secretory vesicle whose contents are subsequently released after an appropriate stimulus. These pathways are illustrated in Figure 13-4. With proteins, such as chymotrypsinogen, insulin, and ACTH, constitutive secretion results in the

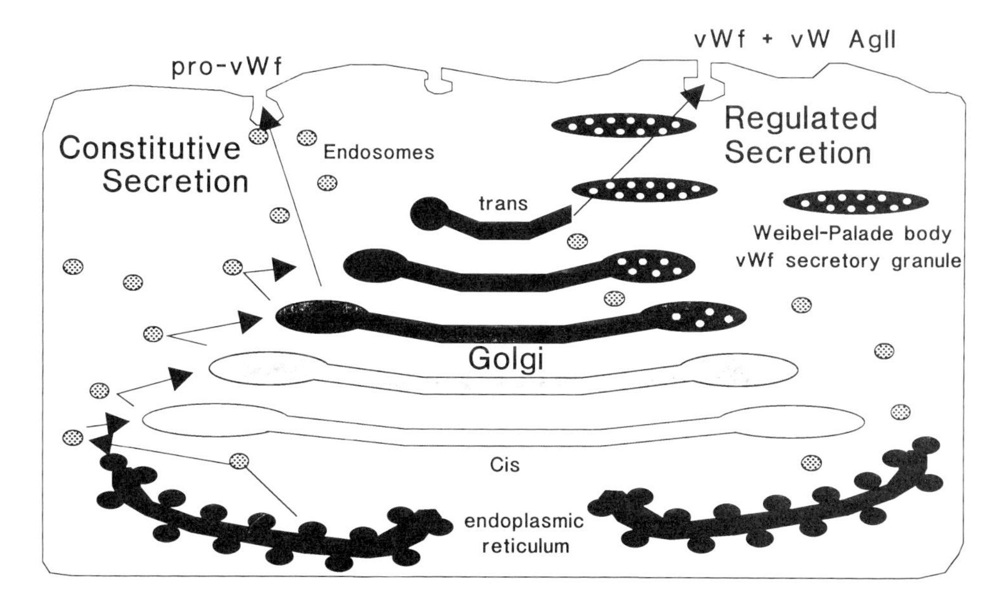

Figure 13-4. Endothelial cells may have both constitutive and regulated secretion of proteins. For von Willebrand factor, this would result in the constitutive secretion of pro-von Willebrand factor and the regulated secretion of von Willebrand factor and vW AgII. The Weibel-Palade body is the regulated secretory granule in endothelial cells.

secretion of the pro-form of the precursor protein, whereas regulated secretion results in the secretion of the mature protein. Sporn and coworkers[101,102] have demonstrated similar pathways for von Willebrand factor: the pro-von Willebrand factor in the cell culture supernates comes from constitutive release, and the von Willebrand factor released by thrombin or ionophore A23187 (regulated release) comprises mature von Willebrand factor multimers and vW AgII with no pro-von Willebrand factor. The understanding of these endothelial cell events should help to better delineate the biology of hemostasis. Release of von Willebrand factor and vW AgII following DDAVP may serve as an example of artificial stimulus inducing regulated release.

Procoagulant Events on the Endothelial Cell Surface

Although the endothelial cell surface participation in hemostatic events has not been as extensively studied as that of platelet surface, this cell surface has been preliminarily studied for its binding of important coagulation proteins and reviewed recently.[82] Although endothelial cells are generally nonthrombogenic,[119] recent studies have demonstrated binding of the factor IX–factor VIII complex,[27,105,109] the production of tissue factor,[64] synthesis of factor V,[11] and the synthesis of plasminogen activator inhibitor.[62] Cellular receptors for these coagulation events are beginning to be characterized.[105]

Anticoagulant Events on the Endothelial Cell Surface

Heparinlike molecules have been reported in association with the endothelial cell lumen,[17] where they can interact with antithrombin III and, thereby, provide a downstream inhibitor of activated clotting[71] and promote the clearance of thrombin.[59] Thrombin may also combine with a specific endothelial cell receptor, termed *thrombomodulin* to activate protein C, the important vitamin K-dependent plasma anticoagulant. This system has been extensively studied by Esmon and coworkers,[20,21] who demonstrated surface expression of thrombomodulin and subsequent activation of protein C in vivo after the infusion of thrombin into dogs. The surface-bound thrombin can still be inactivated by antithrombin III (AT III), thereby rendering it ineffective in the activation of protein C. How the balance between these two functions is determined is not known.

There are two forms of plasminogen activator synthesized by endothelial cells: tissue-type plasminogen activator and urokinase-type plasminogen activator.[62] In addition, plasminogen activator inhibitor is also synthesized by endothelial cells.[62] This system is made even more complex by the interaction of these fibrinolytic regulators with the protein C–protein S system. Currently, it is thought that activated protein C inactivates plasminogen activator inhibitor and, thereby, promotes the activity of plasminogen activator. Thus, protein C is profibrinolytic as well as anticoagulant.

Immune Recognition of Endothelial Cells

The surface immunology of the endothelial cell is currently under intense investigation but is not clearly understood. As mentioned earlier, endothelial cells contain similar or analogous cell surface glycoproteins when compared with platelets. The platelet's antigenic surface is extensively studied and reviewed elsewhere in this monograph. Some of these platelet alloantigen systems have been investigated on cultured human endothelial cells using antibodies to P1^{A1}, Bak^a, Bak^b, Lek^a, Pen^a, and an isoantibody from the plasma of a patient with Glanzmann's thrombasthenia,[46,48,49,55] and demonstrate cross-reactivity with endothelial cell surface antigens (Table 13-2). With use of [^{35}S]methionine, lysates of cultured umbilical vein endothelial cells were immunoprecipitated in the presence of EDTA with anti-P1^{A1} antibodies obtained from patients with posttransfusion purpura. Figure 13-5 demonstrates that these antibodies, in the presence of EDTA, immunoprecipitated two proteins from endothelial cells: one was 135 kDa (corresponding to the α chain of the vitronectin receptor) and the other was 110 kDa (corresponding to EC-GPIIIa). In contrast to platelets, from which the antibodies immunoprecipitated only GPIIIa (platelet GPIIb–IIIa is a calcium-dependent complex), the immunoprecipitates from endothelial cells suggest a calcium-independent complex between the two identified glycoproteins. Thus, the platelet alloantigens that have been identified on platelet GPIIIa are also present on endothelial cells, and the EC-GPIIIa is complexed to the VNR_α in a calcium-independent complex. As expected, the antigens of GPIIb are not expressed on endothelial cells.

Table 13-2
Alloantigens on Endothelial Cells

	Platelet		
Alloantigens	***GPIIb***	***GPIIIa***	**Endothelial Cells**
Pl^{A1}	0	+	+
Bak^a	+	0	0
Bak^b	+	0	0
Lek^a	+	0	0
Pen^a	0	+	+
GT isoAB*	0	+	+

*Acquired isoantibody to GPIIIa from the plasma of a patient with Glanzmann's thrombasthenia (GT).

Specific Antigens Expressed by Endothelial Cells

Numerous groups are currently studying the diversity of endothelial cells from various tissue origins. Some of these groups have studied this diversity using immunologic probes to surface proteins. Auerbach and coworkers have used monoclonal antibodies to angiotensin-converting enzyme, Thy 1 antigen, as well as other antigens, and hypothesize that organ-specific differences are found in endothelial cells.[2,3] It is not clear if these differences are due to the development of the endothelial cells in the specific tissue milieu or whether these surface antigens are due to tissue modification of these cell surface antigens.[2,3,108]

The Endothelial Cell in Autoimmune Disorders

Because endothelial cells line the interface between circulating blood and the other tissues and organ systems, they are in a unique position to be involved in the autoimmune process. As such, it is not surprising that studies have demonstrated antibody binding to endothelial

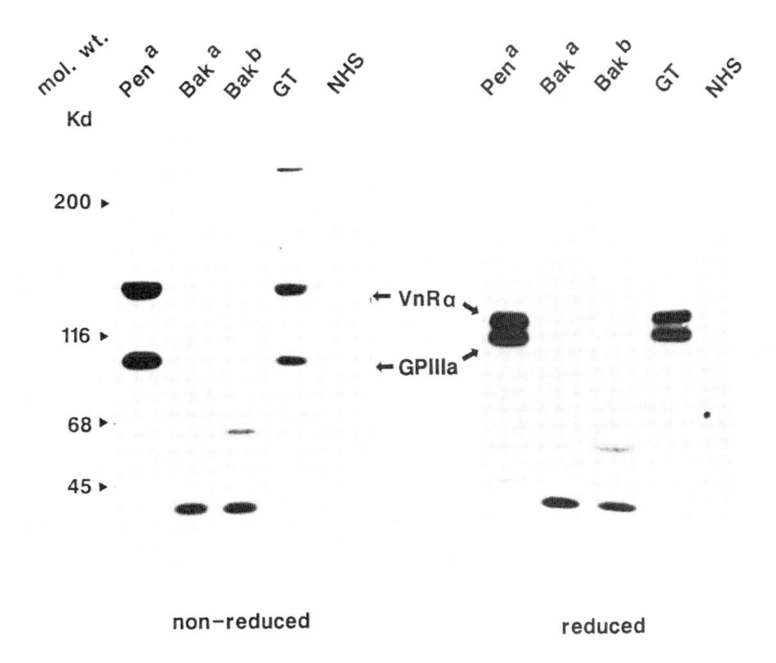

Figure 13-5. Endothelial cells were metabolically labeled with [^{35}S]methionine. Various antibodies to platelet alloantigens were used to immunoprecipitate the labeled endothelial cell lysates. These immunoprecipitates were subjected to polyacrylamide gel electrophoresis with and without reduction. Fluorography demonstrates the immunoprecipitation of both endothelial cell GPIIIa and the α chain of the vitronectin receptor (VnRα) by antibodies to PI^{A1}, Pen^a and an isoantibody to GPIIb-IIIa from a patient with Glanzmann's thrombasthenia (GT). Antibodies to Bak^a and Bak^b failed to immunoprecipitate this heterodimeric complex because they are directed against antigens on platelet GPIIb, a glycoprotein that is not made by endothelial cells. In endothelial cells the GPIIb in this heterodimeric complex is replaced by the α chain of the vitronectin receptor.

cells themselves or cytotoxicity of endothelial cells induced by sera from patients with autoimmune disorders. It would be much too simple to limit the participation of endothelial cells to isolated antigen-antibody interactions; their role may involve several arms of the immune response. The immune system is frequently dysregulated or activated in a number of these syndromes[100] in which the endothelial cell has a role both as an antigen-presenting cell[30,38] and as a cell that may undergo substantial alterations secondary to the influence of modulators of the immune response, such as interferon,[14] interleukins,[6] or other lymphokines. These mediators have been demonstrated to alter the expression of cell surface polypeptides by endothelial cells and to up-regulate or down-regulate the expression of other proteins and receptors. The functional role of these altered polypeptides is not well understood.[120] Studies in various laboratories have demonstrated alterations induced by γ-interferon, the interleukins, or tumor necrosis factor, resulting in increased procoagulant activity[5,6] leukocyte adhesion,[6] expression of class II histocompatibility antigens,[14] plasminogen activator inhibitor,[7a] and other activation antigens.[15,87] The identification of each of the induced proteins and determination of each of their functional roles will likely be vital to our understanding of these autoimmune disorders. One example of an inducible protein is a γ-interferon-regulated gene identified by Luster and coworkers in endothelial cells, which controlled the synthesis of a 12,400-Da molecule with homology to β-thromboglobulin and platelet factor 4.[63] Within 30 min of exposure to γ-interferon, the RNA for this protein is induced, and within 5 h a 30-fold increase in mRNA is found. The authors suggested that this protein may be a member of a family of proteins important in immune and inflammatory responses. One implication of these studies is that autoantibodies may not recognize endothelial cells in the resting state, but only after the endothelial cells are stimulated by lymphokines or monokines to produce previously unexpressed surface antigens.

As noted earlier, antibody-mediated endothelial cell damage likely plays a role in a number of known or suspected autoimmune diseases. After antibody binding, mechanisms by which hemostasis could be altered include (1) endothelial cell disruption, with exposure of subendothelial collagen and subsequent activation of hemostasis; (2) attraction and binding of effector cells to the antibody-coated endothelial cell with subsequent cellular cytotoxicity; (3) sublethal damage, inducing alterations in the anticoagulant function of endothelial cells as manifested by increased adherence of platelets, generation of procoagulant material (tissue factor or prothrombinase receptors), or loss of anticoagulant activity (thrombomodulin or antithrombin III). Many of these activities have already been demonstrated to be under immune modulation by lymphokines or monokines. Thus, the addition of an autoantibody in circumstances in which widespread activation of the immune response exists may have an even greater additive effect.

Antiendothelial Cell Antibodies in Clinical Disorders

Cines and coworkers demonstrated the presence of complement-fixing IgG antiendothelial cell antibodies in serum samples from patients with systemic lupus erythematosus (SLE).[13] Binding of IgG from the patient samples on the monolayer of umbilical vein endothelial cells was associated with the deposition of complement and eventual disruption of the monolayer. Endothelial cells treated with IgG from patients with SLE secreted prostacyclin upon stimulation but later demonstrated increased platelet adherence. The authors explain these paradoxic findings by speculating that antiendothelial cell antibody initially triggers release of prostacyclin, a potent inhibitor of platelet aggregation; however, persistent exposure to antibody results in exhaustion of endothelial cell prostacyclin synthesis and a subsequent increase in platelet adherence. Similar IgG binding to endothelial cells in SLE was reported by Leroux.[56] Hashemi and coworkers, utilizing an enzyme-linked immunosorbent assay (ELISA), found evidence for the binding of both IgG and IgM to human umbilical vein endothelial cells using serum samples from patients with SLE.[36] Tan and Pearson[106] demonstrated evidence for the deposition of IgG on endothelial cells by indirect immunofluorescence. The antigenic target(s) for these IgG and IgM antibodies has not been identified. Antibodies to endothelial cells may bind only after the stimulation of these cells with lymphokines or monokines. Leung and coworkers showed evidence of cytotoxic antibodies against human umbilical vein endothelial cells that were present in serum samples from patients with Kawasaki's syndrome.[57] These antibodies were cytotoxic only after exposure of the endothelial cells to γ-interferon,[57] interleukin,[58] or tumor necrosis factor.[58] This cytotoxicity was complement-mediated and did not appear to be HLA antigen-directed. Both IgM and IgG antibodies were implicated in this process.

In scleroderma, both IgG and IgM antibodies against the endothelial cell have been demonstrated by ELISA as well as by immunofluorescence.[36,86,106] Studies on patients with dermatomyositis have demonstrated serum antiendothelial cell antibodies[36] and microvascular deposition of the membrane attack complex of complement.[52] Further studies have also demonstrated an increase in the degradation products of complement in the plasma of patients with dermatomyositis.[97]

The role of antibodies against platelet and endothelial cells in thrombotic thrombocytopenic purpura (TTP) remains an area of debate. Plasma, and especially the IgG fraction of plasma, from three patients with TTP was cytotoxic to human umbilical vein endothelial cells.[8,81] By immunofluorescence, IgG was detected on the endothelial cell surface after treatment with TTP plasma but not after treatment with control plasma. Nakajima and coworkers demonstrated that a monoclonal antibody to platelet GPIIb–IIIa bound to endothelial cells and the binding of this antibody was inhibited by serum samples from three patients with TTP.[81] The characterization of this monoclonal antibody was not, however, provided but, presumably, it was directed to GPIIIa. Antiendothelial cell antibodies may participate in the functional abnormalities of glomerulonephritides. Immunoglobulin G and complement deposition are commonly identified by immunofluorescent examination of kidney in these disorders. In animal models, perfusion of the kidney with antibodies against antigens known to be present on endothelial cells results in clinical glomerulonephritis and deposition of IgG and C3.[106]

Cines and coworkers recently showed that incubation of endothelial cells with serum samples from 27 patients with heparin-associated thrombocytopenia yielded increased amounts of IgG, IgA, and IgM binding on endothelial cells and stimulated tissue factor expression by these cells.[12] Binding occurred only on samples obtained when heparin was being infused in the patient. They postulated that the immune injuries to both platelets and endothelial cells may occur as part of the heparin-associated thrombocytopenia syndrome and may play a role in the thrombosis that occurs in some patients after heparin treatment.[13]

In an attempt to explain renal allograft rejection in patients who were HLA-compatible, Moraes and Stastny described a new antigen system expressed in human endothelial cells.[77] These antigens appeared to be different from HLA and class II molecules. Interestingly, these antibodies could not be absorbed by lymphocytes but could be absorbed by monocytes. These antibodies were also cytotoxic to monocytes. Cerilli and coworkers tested whether or not cross-matching with monocytes could be a predictor of graft failure in otherwise well-matched renal transplant candidates.[10] An early study demonstrated that 76% of recipients who reject their HLA-identical living-related graft have cytotoxic antibodies to the non-HLA antigen(s) expressed on donor monocytes and venous endothelial cells. Patients with a positive monocyte cross-match with negative HLA and mixed lymphocyte culture (MLC) studies have a high incidence of renal allograft rejection.[9] The identity of this antigen system is unclear, but preliminary family segregation studies support a genetic linkage between the vascular endothelial antigen system and the major histocompatibility antigens.[10]

Thus, there exists a number of syndromes in which suggestive evidence can be found that a specific endothelial cell antibodies play an integral role in the pathogenesis of autoimmune diseases. Only a few of the antigens have now been identified, and the antigenic sites of attachment of the majority of antibodies are unknown. Identification of these antigens and understanding the mechanism of their expression will be a significant step in our understanding of the functional abnormalities of these diverse disorders.

SUMMARY

Endothelial cells, like platelets, are capable of interacting in diverse reactions involving procoagulant, anticoagulant, profibrinolytic, and immunologic specificities. Although much progress has been made on the characterization of the platelet in these processes, the study of the endothelial cell is only now coming to the forefront. The communication between the stationary phase (endothelial cell) and the circulating phase (platelets and plasma) in regulating the homeostasis of hemostasis remains to be fully delineated. Techniques and studies used in the other chapters of this book to characterize the platelet and its interactions should be helpful in determining the similarities and differences between the cell surface regulatory mechanisms of platelets and endothelial cells.

REFERENCES

1. Asch AS, Fujimoto M, Adelman B, Nachman RL: An endothelial cell GPIb like molecule mediates von Willebrand factor binding. Circulation (Supp II) 74:232, 1986.

2. Auerbach R, Alby L, Form D, Grieves J, Joseph J, Kubai L, Morrissey LFW, Sidky YA, Miao T: Proceedings of the 2nd International Conference on the Biology of the Vascular Endothelial Cell, p 19, 1981.

3. Auerbach R, Joseph J: Cell surface markers on endothelial cells: A developmental perspective. In Jaffe EA (ed.): Biology of Endothelial Cells. The Hague, Nijhoff, 1982

4. Baumgartner HR, Tschopp TB, Meyer D: Shear rate dependent inhibition of platelet adhesion

and aggregation on collagenous surfaces by antibodies to human factor VII/von Willebrand factor. Br J Haematol 44:127, 1980

5. Bevilacqua MP, Pober JS, Majeau GS, Fiers W, Cotran RS, Gimbrone MA: Recombinant tumor necrosis factor induces procoagulant activity in cultured human vascular endothelium: Characterization in comparison with the actions of interleukin-1. Proc Natl Acad Sci USA 83:4533, 1986

6. Bevilacqua MP, Pober JS, Wheeler MP, Gimbrone MA: Interleukin-1 activation of vascular endothelium: Effects on procoagulant activity and leukocyte adhesion. Am J Pathol 121:393, 1985

7. Brucke E: Uber die Ursache der Gerinnung des Blutes. Arch Pathol Anat 12:81, 1857

8. Burns ER, Zucker-Franklin D: Pathologic effects of plasma from patients with thrombotic thrombocytopenic purpura on platelets and cultured vascular endothelial cells. Blood 60:1032, 1982

9. Cerilli J, Brasile L, Galousiz T, Defrancis ME: Clinical significance of antimonocyte antibody in kidney transplant recipients. Transplantation 323:495, 1981

10. Cerilli J, Brasile L. Galousiz T, Lempert T, Clarke J: The vascular endothelial cell antigen system. Transplantation 139:286, 1985

11. Cerveny TJ, Fass DN, Mann KG: Synthesis of coagulation factor V by cultured aortic endothelium. Blood 63:1467, 1984

11a. Cheresh DA: Human endothelial cells synthesize and express an Arg-Gly-Asp-directed adhesion receptor involved in attachment to fibrinogen and von Willebrand factor. Proc Natl Acad Sci USA 84:6471, 1987

12. Cines DB, Cann CA, Tomaski T, Tannenbaum S: Immune endothelial cell injury in heparin-associated thrombocytopenia. N Engl J Med 316:581, 1987

13. Cines DB, Lyss AP, Reeber M, Bina M, Dehoratius RJ: Presence of complement fixing anti-endothelial cell antibodies in systemic lupus erythematosus. J Clin Invest 73:611, 1984

14. Collins T, Corman AJ, Wake CT, Boss JM, Kappes DJ, Fiers,W, Ault K, Gimbrone MA, Strominger JL, Pober JS: Immune interferon activates multiple class II major histocompatibility complex genes and the associated invariant chain gene in human endothelial cells and dermal fibroblasts. Proc Natl Acad Sci USA 81:4917, 1984

15. Cotran RS, Gimbrone MA, Bevilacqua MP, Mendrick DL: Induction and detection of a human endothelial cell activation antigen in vivo. J Exp Med 64:661, 1986

16. Cramer EM, Meyer D, le Menn R, Breton-Gorius J: Eccentric localization of von Willebrand factor in an internal structure of the platelet alpha-granule resembling that of Weibel-Palade bodies. Blood 66:710, 1985

17. Damus RL, Hicks M, Rosenberg RD: A generalized view of heparin's anticoagulant actions. Nature 246:355, 1973

18. Diglio CA, Grammas P, Giacomelli F, Wiener J: Primary culture of rat cerebral microvascular endothelial cells. Lab Invest 46:554, 1982

19. Diuguid DL, Rabiet MJ, Furie BC, Liebman HA, Furie B: Molecular basis of hemophilia B: A defective enzyme due to an unprocessed propeptide is caused by a point mutation in the factor IX precursor. Proc Natl Acad Sci 83:5803, 1986

20. Esmon CT: Protein C, Prog Hemost Throm 7:25, 1984

21. Esmon CT: Regulation of protein C activation by components of the endothelial cell surface. In Gimbrone MA (ed): Vascular Endothelium in Hemostasis and Thrombosis, pp 99–119, New York, Churchill Livingstone, 1986

22. Farquhar MG: Progress in unraveling pathways of Golgi traffic. Annu Rev Cell Biol 1:447, 1985

23. Fauvel F, Grant ME, Legrand YJ, Souchon H, Tobelem G, Jackson DS, Caen JP: Interaction of blood platelets with microfibrillar extract from adult bovine aorta: Requirement for von Willebrand factor. Proc Natl Acad Sci USA 80:551, 1983

24. Fay PJ, Chavin SI, Schroeder D, Young FE, Marder VJ: Purification and characterization of a highly purified human factor VIII consisting of a single type of polypeptide chain. Proc Natl Acad Sci 79:7200, 1982

25. Fay PJ, Kawai Y, Wagner D, Ginsburg D, Bonthron D, Ohlsson-Wilhelm BM, Chavin SI, Abraham GN, Handin RI, Orkin SH, Montgomery RR, Marder VJ: The propolypeptide of von Willebrand factor circulates in blood and is identical to von Willebrand antigen II. Science 232:995, 1986

26. Fitzgerald LA, Charo IF, Phillips DR: Human and bovine endothelial cells synthesize membrane proteins similar to human platelet glycoproteins IIb and IIIa. J Biol Chem 260:10893, 1985

27. Fitzgerald LA, Steiner B, Rall SC, Lo SS, Phillips DR: Protein sequence of endothelial cell glycoprotein IIIa derived from a cDNA clone. Identity with platelet glycoprotein IIIa and similarity to "integrin." J Biol Chem 262:3936, 1987

28. Florey HW: The endothelial cell. Br Med J 2:487, 1966

29. Fryer DG, Birnbaum G, Luttrell CN: Human endothelium in cell culture. J Atherosclerosis Res 6:151, 1966

30. Geppert TD, Lipsky PE: Antigen presentation by interferon gamma treated endothelial cells and fibroblasts: Differential ability to function as

antigen presenting cells despite comparable Ia expression. J Immunol 135:3750, 1985

31. Gimbrone MA, Cotran RS, Folkman J. Human vascular endothelial cells in culture. Growth and DNA synthesis. J Cell Biol 60:673, 1974

32. Ginsberg D, Handin RI, Bonthron DT, Donlon TA, Bruns GA, Latt SA, Orkin SH: Human von Willebrand factor (vWf): Isolation of complementary DNA (cDNA) clones and chromosomal localization. Science 228:1401, 1985

33. Ginsberg MH, Loftus J, Ryckwaert JJ, Pierschbacher M, Pytela R, Ruoslahti E, Plow EF: Immunochemical and amino-terminal comparison of two cytoadhesions indicates they contain similar or identical β subunits and distinct α subunits. J Biol Chem 262:5437, 1987

34. Green D, Potter EV: Platelet-bound ristocetin aggregating factor in normal subjects and patients with von Willebrand's disease. J Lab Clin Med 87:976, 1976

35. Hardin NJ, Minick CR, Murphy GE: Experimental induction of atherosclerosis by the synergy of allergic injury to arteries and lipid-rich diet. Am J Pathol 73:301, 1973

36. Hashemi S, Smith CD, Izaguirre CA: Anti-endothelial cell antibodies: Detection and characterization using a cellular enzyme-linked immunosorbent. J Lab Clin Med 109:434, 1987

37. Heimark RL, Schwartz SM: Binding of coagulation factors IX and X to the endothelial cell surface. Biochem Biophys Res Commun 111:723, 1983

38. Hirschberg H, Bergh OJ, Bethorsby E: Antigen presenting properties of human endothelial cells. J Exp Med 152:249, 1980

39. Holmberg L. Nilsson IM: von Willebrand's disease. Clin Haematol 14:461, 1985

40. Howard MA, Sawers RJ, Firkin BG: Ristocetin: A means of differentiating von Willebrand's disease into two groups. Blood 41:687, 1973

41. Hoyer LW, De los Santos RP, Hoyer JR: Antihemophilic factor antigen. Localization in endothelial cells by immunofluorescent microscopy. J Clin Invest 52:2737, 1973

42. Jaffe EA: Physiologic functions of normal endothelial cells. Ann NY Acad Sci 454:279, 1985

43. Jaffe EA, Hoyer LW, Nachman RL: Synthesis of antihemophilic factor antigen by cultured human endothelial cells. J Clin Invest 52:2757, 1973

44. Jaffe EA, Nachman RL, Becker CG, Minick CR. Culture of human endothelial cells derived from umbilical cord veins. Identification by morphologic and immunologic criteria. J Clin Invest 52:2745, 1973

45. Kaiser L, Sparks HV: Endothelial cells. Not just a cellophane wrapper. Arch Intern Med 147:569, 1987

46. Kawai Y, Montgomery RR, Furihata K, Kunicki TJ: Expression of platelet alloantigens on human endothelial cells and HEL cells. Thromb Haemostasis 58:4, 1987

47. Kawai Y, Mosesson MW, Schmidt W, Vokac E, Schullek J, Montgomery RR: The self-association of vW AgII in plasma, platelet releasate, and endothelial cell lysate. Circulation 74 (Suppl II):406, 1986

48. Kawai Y, Newman PJ, Furihata K, Kunicki TJ, Montgomery RR: The $P1^{A1}$ alloantigen is expressed on human endothelial cells. Clin Res 34:460a, 1986

49. Kawai Y, Newman PJ, Furihata K, Kunicki TJ, Montgomery RR: The $P1^{A1}$ alloantigen is expressed on cultured human endothelial cells. (in press, J Lab Clin Med)

50. Kelly RB: Pathways of protein secretion in eukaryotes. Science 230:25, 1985

51. Kern PA, Knedler A, Eckel RH: Isolation and culture of microvascular endothelium from human adipose tissue. J Clin Invest 71:1822, 1983

52. Kissel JT, Mendell JR, Rammohan KW: Microvascular deposition of complement membrane attack complex in dermatomyositis. N Engl J Med 314:329, 1986

53. Krough A: The Anatomy and Physiology of Capillaries. pp 22–46. New Haven, Yale University Press, 1929

54. Kunicki TJ, Montgomery RR, and Schullek J: Cleavage of human von Willebrand factor by platelet calcium-activated protease. Blood 65:352, 1985

55. Leeksma OC, Giltay JC, Zandbergen-Spaargaren J, Modderman PW, van Mourik JA, von dem Borne AEG: The platelet alloantigen Zw^{a} or $P1^{a1}$ is expressed by cultured endothelial cells. Br J Haematol 66:369, 1987

56. Leroux GL, Wautier MP, Wautier JL: IgG binding to endothelial cells in systemic lupus erythematosus. Thromb Haemostasis 56:144, 1986

57. Leung DYM, Collins T, Lapierre LA, Geha RS: IgM antibodies present antibodies in the acute phase of Kawasaki's syndrome lyse cultured vascular endothelial cells stimulated by gamma interferon. J Clin Invest 77:1428, 1986

58. Leung DYM, Geha RS, Newburger JW, Burns JC, Fiers W, Lapierre LA, Pober JS: Two monokines, interleukin-1 and tumor necrosis factor, render cultured vascular endothelial cells susceptible to lysis by antibodies circulating during Kawasaki's syndrome. J Exp Med 164:1958, 1986

59. Lollar P, Owen W: Clearance of thrombin from the circulation in rabbits by high-affinity bind-

ing sites on endothelium. J Clin Invest 66:1222, 1980

60. Lopez Fernandez MF, Ginsberg MN, Ruggeri ZM, Batille FJ, Zimmerman TS: Multimeric structure of platelet factor VIII/von Willebrand factor: The presence of larger multimers and their reassociation with thrombin-stimulated platelets. Blood 60:1132, 1982

61. Lopez JA, Chung DW, Fujikawa K, Hagen FS, Papayannopoulou T, Rother GJ: Cloning of the alpha chain of human platelet glycoprotein Ib: A transmembrane protein with homology to leucine-rich $alpha_2$-glycoprotein. Proc Natl Acad Sci USA 84:5615, 1987

62. Loskutoff DJ, Ny T, Sawdey M, Lawrence D: Fibrinolytic system of cultured endothelial cells: Regulation by plasminogen activator inhibitor. J Cell Biochem 32:273, 1986

63. Luster AD, Unkeless AD, Ravetch JV: Gamma interferon transcriptionally regulates and early response gene containing homology to platelet proteins. Nature 315:672, 1985

64. Lyberg T, Galdal KS, Evensen SA, Prydz H: Cellular cooperation in endothelial cell thromboplastin synthesis. Br J Haematol 53:85, 1983

65. Lynch DC, Williams R, Zimmerman TS, Kirby EP, Livingston DM: Biosynthesis of the subunits of factor VIIR by bovine aortic endothelial cells. Proc Natl Acad Sci USA 80:2738, 1983

66. Lynch DC, Zimmerman TS, Collins CJ, Brown M, Morin MJ, Ling EH, Livingston DM: Molecular cloning of cDNA for human von Willebrand factor: Authentication by a new method. Cell 41:49, 1985

67. Lynch DC, Zimmerman TS, Kirby EP, Livingston DM: Subunit composition of oligomeric human von Willebrand factor. J Biol Chem 258:1275, 1983

68. Lynch DC, Zimmerman TS, Ruggeri ZM: von Willebrand factor, now cloned. Br J Haematol 64:15, 1986

69. Madri JA, Williams SK: Capillary endothelial cell cultures: Phenotypic modulation by matrix components. J Cell Biol 97:153, 1983

70. Majno G, Joris I: Endothelium, 1977: A review. Adv Exp Med Biol 104:169, 1978

71. Marcum JA, Rosenberg JS, Bauer KA, Rosenberg RD: The heparin-antithrombin mechanism and vessel wall function. In Gimbrone MA (ed): Vascular Endothelium in Hemostasis and Thrombosis, pp 70–98. New York, Churchill-Livingstone, 1986

72. McCarroll DR, Levin EG, Montgomery RR: Endothelial cell synthesis of vW AgII, vWf, and vWf/vW AgII complex. J Clin Invest 75:1089, 1985

73. McCarroll DR, Ruggeri ZM, Montgomery RR: The effect of DDAVP on plasma levels of von Willebrand's antigen II in normal individuals and patients with von Willebrand's disease. Blood 63:532, 1984

74. Montgomery RR, Dent J, Schmidt W, Kyrle P, Niessner H, Ruggeri ZM, Zimmerman TS: Hereditary persistence of circulating pro von Willebrand factor (pro-vWf). Circulation 74 (Suppl II): 406, 1986

75. Montgomery RR, Kunicki TJ, Glode LM: Use of monoclonal antibody to increase the sensitivity and specificity of precipitating immunoassays and cell surface binding immunoassays. *Methods* Enzymol 121:702, 1986

76. Montgomery RR, Zimmerman TS: von Willebrand's disease antigen II—a new plasma and platelet antigen deficient in severe von Willebrand's disease. J Clin Invest 61:1498, 1978

77. Moraes JR, Stastny P: A new antigenic system expressed in human endothelial cells. J Clin Invest 60:449, 1977

78. Nachman RL, Hajjar KA, Silverstein RL, Dinarell CA: Interleukin-1 induces endothelial cell synthesis of plasminogen activator inhibitor. J Exp Med 163:1595, 1986

79. Nachman RL, Jaffe EA: Subcellular platelet factor VIII antigen and von Willebrand factor. J Exp Med 141:1101, 1975

80. Nachman RL, Levine R, Jaffe EA: Synthesis of factor VIII antigen by cultured guinea pig megakaryocytes. J Clin Invest 60:914, 1977

81. Nakajima T, Koyama T, Kakashita E, Nagai K: Inhibitory effects of TTP sera on binding of antiplatelet glycoprotein IIb–IIIa monoclonal antibodies to human vascular endothelial cells. Am J Hematol 25:115, 1987

82. Nawroth P, Kisiel W. Stern D: The role of endothelium in the homeostatic balance of haemostasis. Clin Haematol 14:531, 1985

83. Newman PJ, Kawai Y, Montgomery RR, Kunicki TJ: Synthesis by cultured human umbilical vein endothelial cells of two proteins structurally and immunologically related to platelet membrane glycoprotein IIb and IIIa. J Cell Biol 103:81, 1986

84. Newman PJ, Martin LS, Knipp MA, Kahn RA: Studies on the nature of the human platelet alloantigen, $P1^{A1}$. Localization to a 17,000 dalton polypeptide. Mol Immunol 22:719, 1985

85. Okumura T, Jamieson GA: Platelet glycocalicin. I. Orientation of glycoproteins of the human platelet surface. J Biol Chem 251:5944, 1976

86. Penning CA, Cunningham J, French MAH, Harrison G, Rowell NR, Hughes P: Antibody dependent cellular cytotoxicity of human vascular endothelium in systemic sclerosis. Clin Exp Immunol 58:548, 1984

87. Pober JS, Gimbrone MA, Lapierre LA, Mendrick DL, Fiers W, Rothlein R, Springer TA: Overlapping patterns of activation of human endothelial cells by interleukin-1, tumor necrosis factor, and immune interferon. J Immunol 137:1893, 1986

88. Poncz M. Eisman R, Heidenreich R, Silver S, Vilaire G, Surrey S, Schwartz E, Bennet JS: Structure of platelet membrane glycoprotein IIb. Homology to the alpha subunits of the vitronectin and fibronectin membrane receptors. J Biol Chem 262:8476, 1987

89. Rand JH, Gordon RE, Sussman II, Chu SV, Solomon V: Electron microscopic localization of factor VIII-related antigen in adult human blood vessels. Blood 60:627, 1982

90. Reinders JH, de Groot PG, Gonsalves MD, Zandbergen J, Loesberg C. Van Mourik JA: Isolation of a storage and secretory organelle containing von Willebrand protein from cultured human endothelial cells. Biochem Biophys Acta 804:361, 1984

91. Ribes JA, Francis CW, Wagner DD: Fibrin induces release of von Willebrand factor from endothelial cells. J Clin Invest 79:117, 1987

92. Ruggeri ZM, De Marco L, Gatti L, Bader R, Montgomery RR: Platelets have more than one binding site for von Willebrand factor. J Clin Invest 72:1, 1983

93. Ruggeri ZM, Mannucci PM, Bader R, Barbui T: Factor VIII-related properties in platelets from patients with von Willebrand's disease. J Lab Clin Med 91:132, 1978

94. Ruggeri ZM, Zimmerman TS: Platelets and von Willebrand's disease. Semin Hematol 22:203, 1985

95. Sakariassen KS, Bolhuis PA, Sixma JJ: Platelet adherence to subendothelium of human arteries in pulsatile and steady flow. Thromb Res 19:547, 1980

96. Schullek JR, Jordan J, Montgomery RR: Interaction of von Willebrand factor with human platelets in the plasma milieu. J Clin Invest 73:421, 1984

97. Scott JP, Arroyave CR: Activation of complement and coagulation in juvenile dermatomyositis. Arthritis Rheum 30:572, 1987

98. Scott JP, Montgomery RR: Platelet von Willebrand's antigen II: Active release by aggregating agents and a marker of platelet release reaction in vivo. Blood 58:1075, 1981

99. Slot JD, Bouma BN, Montgomery RR, Zimmerman TS: Platelet factor VIII-related antigen: Localization by immunofluorescence and demonstration of release by chymotrypsin. Thromb Res 13:871, 1978

100. Smith HR, Steinberg AD: Autoimmunity–A perspective. Annu Rev Immunol 1:175, 1983

101. Sporn LA, Marder VJ, Wagner DD: von Willebrand factor released from Weibel-Palade bodies binds more avidly to extracellular matrix than that secreted constitutively. Blood 69:1531, 1987

102. Sporn LA, Marder VJ, Wagner DD: Inducible secretion of large, biologically potent von Willebrand factor multimers. Cell 46:185, 1986

103a. Sprandio JD, Shapiro SS, Thiagarajan P, McCord S: Cultured human umbilical vein endothelial cells contain a membrane glycoprotein immunologically related to platelet glycoprotein Ib. Blood 71:234, 1988

103b. Sprandio JD, Thiagarajan P, Shapiro SS, Montgomery RR: Cultured human umbilical vein endothelial cells (HUVEC) contain a membrane glycoprotein (Gp) immunologically related to GpIb. Blood (Suppl 1) 68:357a, 1986

104. Stemerman MB, Colton C, Morell E: Perturbations of the endothelium. Prog Hemost Thromb 7:289, 1984

105. Stern DM, Drillings M, Nossel HL, Hurlet-Jensen A, LaGamma KS, Owen J: Binding of factors IX and IXa to cultured vascular endothelial cells. Proc Natl Acad Sci USA 80:4119, 1983

106. Tan EM, Pearson CM: Rheumatic sera reactive with capillaries in the mouse kidney. Arthritis Rheum 15:23, 1972

107. Thiagarajan P, Shapiro SS, Levine E, DeMarco L, Yalcin A: A monoclonal antibody to human platelet glycoprotein IIIa detects a related protein in cultured human endothelial cells. J Clin Invest 75:896, 1985

108. Thilo-Korner DGS, Heinrich D, Temme H: Endothelial cells in culture. In Thilo-Korner DGS, Freshney, RI (eds.): The Endothelial Cell—A Pluripotent Control Cell of the Vessel Wall, pp 158–202. New York, Karger, 1983

109. Varadi K, Elodi S: Formation and functioning of the factor IXa–VIII complex on the surface of endothelial cells. Blood 69:442, 1987

110. Virchow R: Phlogose ung Thrombose in Gefessystem. Gesammelte Abhandlungen zur wissenschaftlichen Medicine. pp 458–463. Frankfurt-am-Main, Meidinger Sohn and Company, 1856

111. Verweij CL, Hart M, Pannekoek H: Expression of variant von Willebrand factor cDNA in heterologous cells: Requirement of the pro-polypeptide in vWf multimer formation. EMBO J 6:2885, 1987

112. Vokac EA, Ferrara J, Montgomery RR: Ristocetin-induced endothelial cell binding of plasma von Willebrand factor. Thromb Haemostasis 58:31, 1987

113. Wagner DD, Fay PJ, Sporn LA, Sinha S, Lawrence SO, Marder VJ: Divergent fates of von

Willebrand factor and its propolypeptide (von Willebrand antigen II) after secretion from endothelial cells. Proc Natl Acad Sci USA 84:1955, 1987

114. Wagner DD, Marder VJ: Biosynthesis of von Willebrand protein by human endothelial cells: Processing steps and their intracellular localization. J Cell Biol 99:2123, 1984

115. Wagner DD, Marde VJ: Biosynthesis of von Willebrand protein by human endothelial cells. Identification of a large precursor polypeptide chain. J Biol Chem 258:2065, 1983

116. Wagner DD, Mayadas T, Urban-Pickering M, Lewis BH, Marder VJ: Inhibition of disulfide bonding of von Willebrand protein by monensin results in small, functionally defective multimers. J Cell Biol 101:112, 1985

117. Wagner DD, Olmsted JB, Marder VJ: Immunolocalization of von Willebrand protein in Weibel-Palade bodies of human endothelial cells. J Cell Biol 95:355, 1982

118. Wagner DD, Urban-Pickering M, Marder VJ: von Willebrand protein binds to extracellular matrices independently of collagen. Proc Natl Acad Sci USA 81:471, 1984

119. Wall RT, Harker LA: The endothelium and thrombosis. Annu Rev Med 31:361, 1980

120. Weil J, Epstein CJ, Epstein LB, Sedmak JJ, Sabrin JL, Grossberg SE: A unique set of polypeptides is induced with gamma interferon in addition to those induced in common with alpha and beta interferons. Nature 301:437, 1983

121. Zimmerman TS, Ruggeri ZM: von Willebrand's disease. Hum Pathol 18:140, 1987

14

Human Monoclonal Antibodies in the Characterization of Platelet Antigens

DIANE J. NUGENT

As a model of autoimmune disease in humans, we are studying antibody-mediated destruction of platelets. The disease state which results from these autoantibodies, known as idiopathic thrombocytopenic purpura (ITP), is seen in both children and adults who present with critically low platelet counts, increased bruising, and sometimes life-threatening bleeding. Although the role of "platelet-reactive" antibodies in the etiology of this autoimmune disease was well documented over two decades ago, we are only now beginning to understand the nature and origin of the responsible autoantibodies, the role of the platelet target antigen in triggering sensitization, and the possible factors that predispose certain individuals or families to this form of autoimmune disease. Idiopathic thrombocytopenic purpura is an excellent model to study autoimmunity because it is one of the most common forms of autoimmune disease in adults and children; the B-lymphocytes, which produce the autoantibody, are readily harvested; and the target antigens, the platelet membrane glycoproteins, are readily isolated, identified, and characterized biochemically.

Although murine monoclonal antibodies have proved invaluable in the characterization and purification of platelet membrane proteins, human antiplatelet antibodies must be used to identify platelet autoantigens or to further define activation and senescence epitopes that might trigger clearance of aged cells from circulation. The production of murine monoclonal antibodies is based on interspecies differences on the platelet membrane and, thus, few murine monoclonal antibodies recognize the more-subtle receptor changes that may occur when platelets age or become activated.

This chapter will review the production of human monoclonal antibodies, the use these reagents to identify platelet antigens and to characterize membrane changes following thrombin activation, and the role of human monoclonal autoantibodies in understanding the nature of the autoantigen and the origin of antiplatelet antibodies in ITP. Concluding remarks will cover the potential use of these reagents in the diagnosis and treatment of conditions involving increased platelet destruction.

PRODUCTION OF HUMAN MONOCLONAL ANTIBODIES

The isolation of human B-cell lines that secrete monoclonal autoantibody, by using Epstein-Barr virus (EBV) transformation or by somatic cell hybridization, has greatly facilitated the identification of autoantigens and their tissue distribution. Although the production of human monoclonal antibodies began over 10 years ago,[69] there are still few laboratories that have used this technique for the routine isolation of immunoglobulin-secreting cell lines. One of the reasons for this lack of success is that few human myeloma lines can attain the fusing and cloning efficiency seen in murine somatic cell hybridization. Second, human monoclonal methodology must rely on "natural" immunization, such as viral infections or, as in ITP, the spontaneous occurrence of platelet-reactive autoantibody, to generate the antibody specificities of interest. However, the unique specificities expressed in the human immunoglobulin repertoire, and the potential usefulness of these reagents in diagnosis and treatment of autoimmune disease and cancer, provide substantial rewards to those who are willing to accept such delayed gratification.

Over the past 10 years, three modalities have predominated in the production of human monoclonal antibodies, namely, EBV transformation, somatic cell hybridization of B-lymphocytes with human or murine myeloma fusing lines, or a combination of the two techniques. The methodology inherent in each of these approaches, together with the results obtained using each, will be discussed in the following:

Epstein-Barr Virus Transformation

An EBV infection of human mononuclear cells, derived from bone marrow, spleen, or peripheral blood, has been used to generate B-cell lines that secrete antibody against a wide variety of antigens, including bacterial proteins,[37,60,70,72] red cell Rh antigens,[91,40] tetanus toxoid,[84] rheumatoid factor,[1] and IgG.[71] This method of cellular transformation has also been used to create autoantibody-secreting B-cell lymphoblastoid lines from patients with myasthenia gravis[31] and Graves disease.[21,74] We have also applied this approach to the generation of cell lines secreting platelet-reactive autoantibodies.[49]

Epstein-Barr virus is a lymphotrophic herpes virus that can infect and transform human B cells in vitro, thus, creating a lymphoblastoid cell line that will grow in continuous cell culture.[56] Infection of B cells with this virus results in polyclonal activation, with synthesis and secretion of immunoglobulin.[59] This process does require true infection of the cells with viable virus, because UV-irradiated EBV does not induce antibody synthesis.[13] Apparently, almost all peripheral B cells may be infected by EBV, but only 20% are actually immortalized in vitro,[34] and only about 1% secrete immunoglobulin in long-term culture.[82] The ability to infect B cells may vary according to B-cell maturation, the smaller, less-mature B cells are more easily transformed, whereas activated B cells have a lower rate of infection. Plasma cells, which lack the receptor for EBV, are virtually impossible to infect under standard conditions.[2]

The B-lymphoblastoid cell lines are generated following incubation of B cells in supernatant containing EBV, or coincubation with EBV-secreting cell lines, a process known as cell-driven transformation. The most commonly used cell line for obtaining EBV-containing supernatant is called B95-8 and is derived from marmoset peripheral blood mononuclear cells that were infected with wild-type virus from a patient with infectious mononucleosis.[47] The rate of virus secretion by these cells may be enhanced from 20% to 80% by certain agents such as phorbol esters,[81] *n*-butyrate,[43] and bromodeoxyuridine.[21] The B95-8 cells are grown at a density of 10^6 cells/ml. Viral particles are obtained by first centrifuging the supernatant at 400 *g* and then passing the supernatant through a 0.45-μm filter, to remove cellular debris. The viral particles, which pass easily through the filter, may then be concentrated by centrifuging the filtered supernatant at 13,000 for 2 hr at 4°C. The pellet is then resuspended and stored in 1 ml of sterile culture medium at −70°C.[13] Filtered supernatant from those B95-8 cells that are not treated with inducing agents and are grown at 10^6/ml will transform approximately 1 in 1000 B cells. Concentrating the viral particles will increase the transforming titer proportionately,[83] but we have found it useful to confirm the titer for each batch after freezing at −70°C. If stored above −70°C, the infectivity of frozen preparations is strikingly decreased. Some laboratories have reported contamination of the B95-8 cell line with mycoplasmas that have been isolated with the EBV particles.[17] If the efficiency of transformation and cloning of B-cell lines is poor, one should screen for mycoplasma in both the B95-8 and human lymphoblastoid lines.

Because EBV is an ubiquitous pathogen, most older children and 90% of adults show serologic evidence of past infection with this virus. Individuals that have had previous infections with EBV develop a subpopulation of memory T cells that can be cytotoxic for EBV-transformed autologous B cells.[57] Therefore, when preparing to maintain immunoglobulin-secreting, B-lymphoblastoid lines in long-term culture, something must be done to prevent the emergence of cytotoxic T cells, which will destroy the B-cell lines after 3 to 4 weeks in culture. In our laboratory the T cells are removed from the mononuclear fraction before infection with EBV, using a rosetting technique described by Kaplan.[33] Other successful techniques include culturing the infected mononuclear cells at very low cell density, 5×10^4 to 1×10^5/ml,[57] or culturing the transformed cells in the presence of 1 μg/ml cyclosporin A, which inhibits the cytotoxic T cells.[12] Once the T cells have been removed, the remaining mononuclear cells are incubated at 37°C in the supernatant containing EBV particles. After establishing the infectious titer of each batch of EBV concentrate we try to infect between 1:250 and 1:500 B cells. In our laboratory, the cells are incubated on a gently rocking platform overnight with the EBV supernatant; however, the process of vital attachment and entry into the cell has been reported to occur within 1 hr under these conditions in other centers.[13] This procedure is summarized in the diagram depicted in Figure 14-1.

Feeder layers of irradiated thymic lymphocytes, allogenic peripheral blood mononuclear cells (PBM), or even cord blood PBM have been used successfully in our laboratory to support the growth of transformed B-lymphocytes. No feeder layer is necessary if the cells are plated at a density of 5×10^6 cells/ml after T-cell depletion. However, if the B cells are preselected based on antigen specificity or idiotype by use of panning techniques or flow cytofluorimetry, then there will be no accessory cells to support cell growth, and a feeder layer must be supplied. Because the frequency of any given B-cell idiotype may be as low as 1–2:1000 B cells, and the rate of infection with EBV may be as low as 1:500 B cells, we have tried to culture the infected mononuclear cell fraction at the lowest cell density possible so that a transformed cell with the antigen specificity of interest will have less competition with other, perhaps more rapidly growing, B-lymphoblastoid cell lines in the same well. By seeding each well at 200 to 500 infected mononuclear or preselected B cells per well, we have between 20 and 50 wells containing transformants per 96-well plate. This rate is quite variable, based on the tissue source of B cells (bone marrow, spleen, or PBM) and the individual from whom the tissue was obtained.

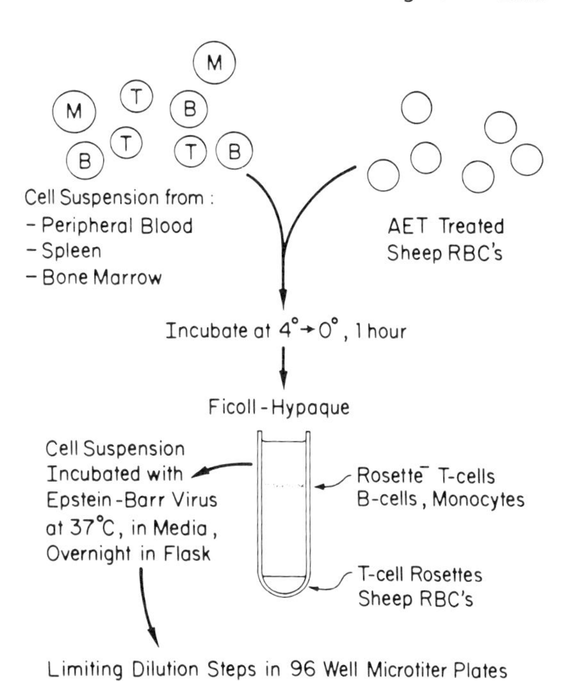

Figure 14-1. Diagram of EBV transformation. The mononuclear cell suspension from peripheral blood, spleen, or bone marrow is depleted of T cells by a standard rosetting technique. The remaining cells are then coincubated with supernatant containing EBV overnight at 37°C and, then, are transferred to 96-well microtiter plates, with or without a feeder layer. (*See* text for details.)

Cocultivation of a 6-thioguanine (6-TG)-resistant cell line, such as 1A2,[66] which secretes EBV, can be used to promote transformation of B-lymphocytes, thus inducing the secretion of immunoglobulin in culture. This process is known as *cell-driven viral transformation* and is described in detail in an excellent review by Siadek and Lostrum.[66] We have applied this technique to the isolation of platelet-reactive human monoclonal antibodies from an individual with ITP.[50] The benefit of this approach includes a higher rate of transformation of B cells and, therefore, a greater possibility of obtaining a lymphoblastoid line secreting an antibody specific for the antigen of interest. In this procedure, donor mononuclear cells are cocultured with a 6-TG-resistant cell line infected with EBV. To eliminate the EBV-secreting cell line, 1A2, the cell mixture is cultured in medium containing HAT for the first 2 weeks leaving only those transformed B-lymphoblastoid lines from the donor cells. Cell-driven transformation has a very high rate of infectivity, with transformation of 1:50 to 1:100 B cells to an immunoglobulin-secreting lymphoblastoid line. Furthermore, with this system, cell lines are routinely isolated that produce IgM, IgG, or IgA, depending on the frequency of the various isotypes in the mononuclear fraction.[66]

With either routine EBV transformation or cell driven transformation, after 2 to 4 weeks in culture the supernatants from wells with transformed B cells, should be screened for the presence of immunoglobulin that is reactive with the target antigen of interest. It is essential to screen as soon as possible because those transformed B-cell lines that are producing antibody may either lose the capacity to produce immunoglobulin or may have a selective disadvantage, compared with faster-growing nonimmunoglobulin-producing cell lines in the same well.

With this approach, we evaluated the effectiveness of EBV transformation and isolated over 30 B-lymphoblastoid cell lines that produce human monoclonal antiplatelet antibody that is reactive with platelet surface antigens. As an illustration of this process, we describe the standard procedure to transform T-cell-depleted splenic lymphocytes from six different patients with ITP. These cells were infected with EBV overnight at a concentration of 2×106 cells/ml and then plated into round-bottomed, 96-well microtiter plates at 400 to 500 cells per well. There were 200 to 300 colonies on each plate after 2 weeks in culture. Table 14-1 summarizes the frequency of wells containing antiplatelet antibody 2 to 3 weeks after infection with EBV in 12 successive transformations, from six of these patients, over a 15 month period.

By using such B lymphoblastoid lines secreting antiplatelet antibody, the levels of antibody attained are high enough that the tissue-specificity of each autoantibody may be assessed and the biochemical nature of its target antigen evaluated. An indirect solid-phase radioimmunoassay detected antiplatelet antibody in 1.1% to 8.1% of the wells containing transformed cells. All of the antiplatelet antibodies in this transformation were found to be of the IgM isotype, and approximately 50% of these bound staphylococcal protein A directly. Surface reactivity of these antiplatelet antibodies was analyzed by indirect immunofluorescent staining and flow cytofluorimetry. This method not only enables us to establish platelet specificity but, also, to determine whether the monoclonal autoantibodies react uniformly with all platelets, or whether they recognize only a subset of circulating platelets. The B-lymphoblastoid cells from wells containing antiplatelet antibody were expanded, cloned by a limiting-dilution technique, and those cultures that continued to secrete high levels of antiplatelet antibody were selected for further characterization and evaluation of the platelet membrane target antigens.

With use of the Western blot technique, the supernatants from eight B-lymphoblastoid cell

Table 14-1
Frequency of Wells Producing Antibody After EBV Transformation

Transformation Designation	Number of Wells Containing Antiplatelet Antibody	Percentage
JTt6.15.83	10:864	1.1
SBt9.14.83	9:796	1.1
SFt6.3.83	15:57	2.6
SFt9.27.83	38:672	5.6
SFt11.7.83	28:384	7.2
SFt11.17.83	3:70	4.2
BBt1.84	12:480	2.5
BBt3.14.84	30:496	6.0
GGt3.13.84	24:960	2.5
GGt5.9.84	13:248	5.2
DUt4.15.84	19:672	2.8
DUt8.20.84	94:1152	8.1

cultures containing the antiplatelet autoantibody were incubated with platelet proteins that had been separated in an 8% sodium dodecyl sulfate (SDS) polyacrylamide gel and transferred to nitrocellulose paper. The reactivity of nine monoclonal autoantibodies with platelet proteins is illustrated in Figure 14-2. HM-1 (lane 2), an isotype-identical human monoclonal antibody that does not bind to platelets, was used in this study as a negative control. In some instances, binding to a limited range of platelet proteins was observed, as illustrated in lanes 3 and 7 (designated 1A3 and 1C6). In both instances, a protein with a relative molecular mass (M_r) of 97,000 was detected. In other instances, the autoantibodies bound to multiple proteins in the platelet preparation, for example, lanes 1, 4, and 8 (designated 1D9, 1B3, and 2E10).

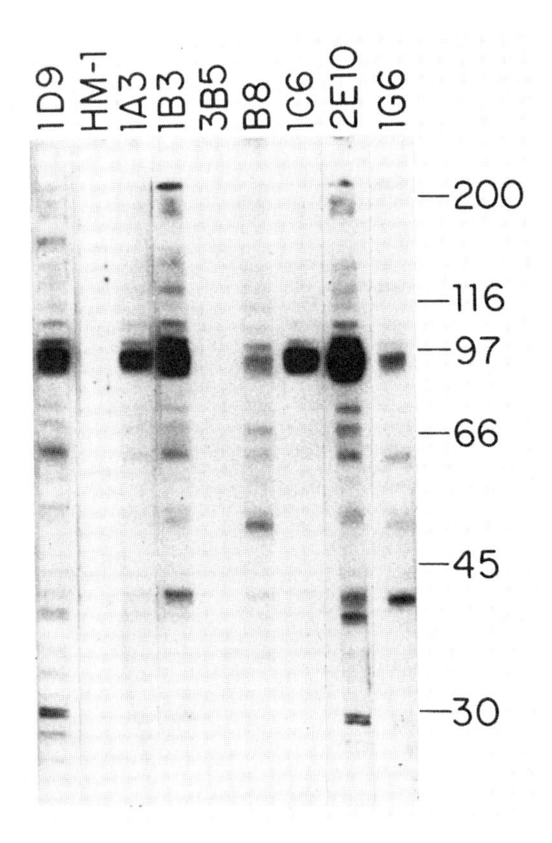

Figure 14-2. Immunoblot of nine human monoclonal, platelet-reactive, antibodies. Platelet proteins from a whole-platelet lysate, prepared with 1% Triton X, 10 mM NEM, 10 mM leupeptin, and 5 mM EDTA, were separated under nonreducing conditions, using SDS-PAGE and then transferred to nitrocellulose membrane using the Transblot apparatus (BioRad, Richmond, Calif.) The monoclonal antibodies were then incubated with individual strips, washed, and immunoreactivity was assessed with radiolabeled rabbit antihuman IgM, followed by autoradiography.

This pattern of reactivity suggests that these antibodies recognize an epitope shared by many platelet proteins. We have also observed that some human B-lymphoblastoid cell lines secrete antiplatelet antibodies that bind to cytoskeletal elements of platelets. Five of the antibodies used in this Western blot (1D9, 1B3, 2E10, 3B5, 1G6) were also screened, by indirect immunofluorescence, for binding to cytoskeletal elements on fixed and permeabilized rat fibroblasts. Antibodies 1G6 and 1D9 demonstrated binding that was characteristic of vimentin in the fibroblast. The other three antibodies bound to strands, within the cells, that appear to be associated with substrate attachment sites and may, in some, be associated with the actin subunits. This is reminiscent of studies by Winger,[80] and Houghton,[27] which describe the hybridization of human lymph node B-lymphocytes, isolated from patients with malignant melanoma, to either a human myeloma line (LICR-2) or to murine myeloma lines (NS-1 or SKO-007). With these techniques, Houghton[27] found that 24:771 immunoglobulin-producing cell cultures (4%) contained antibody reactive with intracellular antigens, such as nuclei, nucleoli, Golgi complex, cytoskeletal, and other cytoplasmic elements, as well as binding to melanoma cells. Andre-Schwartz et al.[3] describe human hybrid cell lines resulting from the fusion of B-lymphocytes of patients with systemic lupus erythematosus (SLE) to a human myeloma line (GM1600), which secrete monoclonal anti-DNA antibodies that also recognize cytoskeletal elements in fibroblasts. Thus, whether or not the antiplatelet autoantibodies that we have described recognize a specific epitope, which is represented on cytoskeleton or polynucleotides, as well as platelet membrane proteins, is currently under investigation.

Somatic Cell Hybridization

Prior to 1980, when Croce[14] and Kaplan[53] each reported the development of a human B-cell-fusing line, somatic cell hybridization was primarily restricted to the production of murine monoclonal antibodies. With the advent of a human fusion line, many laboratories attempted similar fusion procedures to isolate human monoclonal antibodies for diagnostic and therapeutic purposes. However, difficulties in achieving a high fusion rate and in maintaining adequate cloning efficiency have presented obstacles to human hybridoma production not previously encountered in the preparation of murine monoclonal antibodies. The methodology described in the following discussions will incorporate the experience reported from many laboratories in the preparation of human-human hybridomas. For additional resource material on this topic, there have been excellent reviews recently published.[32]

Fusion Partners

The development of a stable human B-cell line, with a high fusion frequency and cloning efficiency, continues to be the focus of several laboratories across the country. Fusion lines have been derived from either human myeloma or lymphoblastoid cell lines.[32,38,54] At least nine myeloma or plasmacytoma cell lines have been described and have been isolated from multiple myeloma patients with very advanced disease. Although the rate of immunoglobulin production by these cell lines may be very high, their doubling time in culture is extended and often requires a conditioned medium to proliferate in vitro. Therefore, very few of these lines can be maintained in long-term culture. Furthermore, the production of immunoglobulin by the fusing line itself will often result in the production of a hybridoma that secretes an antibody composed of heavy chains from the immunized B-cell donor and light chains from the parent myeloma cell line, or vise versa. These hybrid antibodies are often of lower affinity, and they may not even bind to the antigen of interest.

Therefore, to circumvent these difficulties, many laboratories have derived human fusing lines from lymphoblastoid cell lines (LCL) rather than plasmacytomas.[54] The LCL have a short doubling time and, in general, grow well in vitro without a conditioned medium. Many of these cell lines do not secrete any immunoglobulin of their own. They also have a very high fusing frequency (10^{-6} as compared with $25-35 \times 10^{-7}$ for plasmacytomas). Two problems plague researchers who are using LCL to produce large quantities of human monoclonal antibodies for diagnosis or treatment. All of these lines appear to demonstrate EBV in their genome, which may contaminate immunoglobulin preparations to be administered to patients. Given the recent success in eliminating virus from certain blood product derivatives, this may not be a problem for large biotechnical or pharmacologic firms in the future. However, a second problem associated with EBV contamination is the instability of antibody production in these hybridomas, which must be constantly cloned to select for increased immunoglobulin secretion.

One method to improve cloning efficiency and shorten the doubling time of human lymphoblastoid cell lines is described by Olsson et al.[52] By using the demethylating agent, 5-azacytidine, Olsson was able to induce changes in cell growth. After 5-azacytidine treatment for 3 days, subclones isolated from the parent fusing line, RH-L4, demonstrated improved cloning efficiency and immunoglobulin production following fusion with donor B-lymphocytes. One of these subclones, RH-L4-14, has remained stable for over 1 year in culture. This technique may also be used on the hybridomas to induce a higher rate of immunoglobulin production.

Fusion Procedure

The fusion procedure is summarized in Figure 14-3. With the use of Ficoll-Hypaque density gradient centrifugation, the mononuclear leukocyte fraction is obtained from human spleen, peripheral blood, bone marrow, tonsillar tissue, and lymph node. These cells are mixed, at a 1 : 1 to 1 : 5 ratio, with 6-thioguanine (6-TG)- or 8-azaguanine (8-AG)-resistant LCL or plasmacytomas in RPMI (Gibco) medium or Iscove's medium with 10 mM Hepes buffer (Gibco). The cells (no more than 5×10^7/vial) are then pelleted together in a capped round-bottom 40-ml glass vial at 300 g for 10 min. The cells are gently resuspended in 4 ml of 37% to 45% (w/v) polyethylene glycol (PEG; J. T. Baker 1300-1600, Phillipsburg, N.J.) in RPMI. We have found that maintaining the PEG/RPMI at 37°C and slightly alkaline (*p*H 8.0—8.5) improves fusion frequency. After a 3 to 5 min centrifugation at 300 *g* the supernatant is gently removed and 10 ml of fresh medium, either RPMI or Iscove's is quickly added to resuspend the cells and dilute the continued toxic effect of the PEG. Only experience can dictate the fine line between resuspension of these cells for washing and, at the same time,

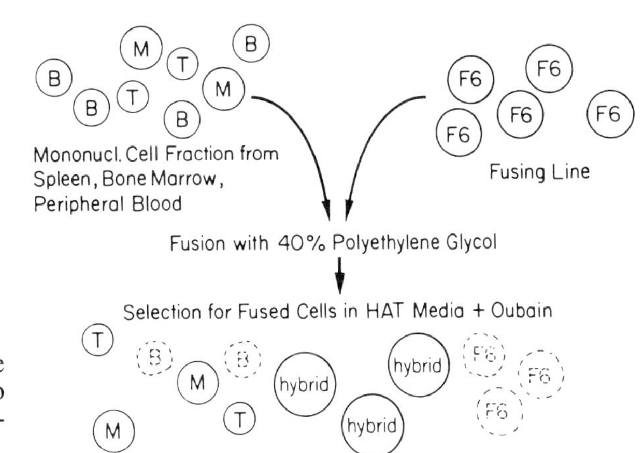

Figure 14-3. Diagram of cell fusion technique using F6, mouse–human heteromyeloma, to hybridize with human B-lymphocytes or transformed B-lymphoblastoid lines.

avoiding disruption of two cells in the process of membrane fusion. We first add a small amount of the medium and gently swirl the cells pelleted at the bottom of the vial. The remaining portion of the 10 ml is added and, if large clumps of cells are visible, the suspension is slowly aspirated once or twice into a 10-ml pipette before the final centrifugation at 300 *g* for 10 min. These cells are then gently resuspended in tissue culture medium, either RPMI or Iscove's modified Dulbecco, with 10 mM Hepes containing 15% fetal calf serum, 1 mM sodium pyruvate, 2 mM L-glutamine, 100 U/ml penicillin, and 100 μg/ml streptomycin; and incubated in a flask at 5×10^5 to 1.0×10^6 cells/ml for 14 to 24 hr at 37°C and 6% CO_2. This period allows stabilization of fusing cell membranes, thus improving the frequency of hybrid generation in our hands. The following day the cells are transferred to round-bottom, 96-well microtiter plates ($1-2 \times 10^4$ cells per well). At this point, HAT (1×10^{-4} M hypoxanthine, 4×10^{-7} M aminopterin, and 1.6×10^{-5} M thymidine, final concentrations) is also added to the medium to eliminate unfused LCL or plasmacytoma cells. The cells are fed with HAT-containing medium for the first 10 to 14 days. If the whole mononuclear leukocyte cell fraction is used, a feeder layer may not be necessary. However, if the B cells are preselected using a panning technique or flow cytofluorimetry, then irradiated PBL or thymocytes should be added to support proliferation of the hybridomas. Optimal conditions for plating cell density, for medium, for feeder layer, and for PEG concentration, may vary considerably between LCL and plasmacytomas and should be established for each fusing line.

The screening for antibody production, as described in the earlier section on EBV transformation, is performed after 18 to 21 days in culture, when hybridomas are easily seen and occupy approximately 20% to 30% of the cell population in each well. After identifying those wells that contain hybridomas producing antibody directed against platelets or the antigen of interest, the cells from each well are expanded and cloned using limiting dilution.

With either plasmacytomas or LCL as fusion partners, the antibodies produced by these human hybridomas express unique specificities that enable researchers to identify epitopes and characterize receptor structures not previously defined by murine monoclonal antibodies. Shoenfeld et al.[64] were among the first to use somatic cell hybridization to isolate human monoclonal autoantibody from patients with systemic lupus erythematosus (SLE). Certain of these human monoclonal antibodies not only reacted with single- or double-stranded DNA, RNA, and other polynucleotides, but also, in varying degrees, reacted to cardiolipin, erythrocytes, and platelets, depending on the monoclonal antibody screened. In 1983, Shoenfeld et al.,[65] using three anti-idiotypic antibodies raised against autoantibodies from two patients with SLE, demonstrated that there was considerable idiotypic relatedness between 60 human anti-DNA monoclonal antibodies isolated from patients with SLE, and that those anti-DNA autoantibodies that also bound to platelets fell within the idiotypic group designated 16/6. Four of these idiotypically related (16/6) monoclonal autoantibodies, derived from two different SLE patients, were sequenced by use of automated Edman degradation of the heavy and light chains.[5] The light chains had identical NH_2-terminal amino acid sequences from residues 1 through 40, and the framework structures were typical of the VKI (K-variable region, family or cluster III) subgroup. The heavy chain NH_2-terminal amino acid sequences were nearly identical from residue 1 through residue 40, and the framework structures were characteristic of the VHIII (heavy-chain variable region, family III) subgroup. This high degree of homology within the variable regions of the 16/6 idiotype heavy and light chains suggests that these sequences are encoded by a single germ-line gene.

Further characterization of the antiplatelet properties of the 16/6 monoclonal lupus antibodies was presented in an excellent paper by Asano et al., in 1985.[4] By use of competitive inhibition studies, they demonstrated that the 16/6 antiplatelet activity could be blocked by single-stranded DNA. Furthermore, the surface binding of these polyspecific autoantibodies was not affected by treatment of the platelets with nuclease I, trypsin, chymotrypsin, or neuraminidase. Thus, although the 16/6 autoantibodies appear to cross-react with platelets and single-stranded DNA, the platelet epitope does not seem to contain DNA, protein, or sialic acid susceptible to enzymatic degradation. Similar results have been obtained with a murine monoclonal anti-DNA antibody, spontaneously produced in the autoimmune B/W mouse strain.[29] As described by Asano et al.,[4] this murine monoclonal anti-DNA autoantibody binds to a common epitope expressed on platelets, erythrocytes, T and B cells, neuronal tissue, and glomeruli and may account, in part, for the multiple-organ involvement characteristic SLE.

It is the purpose of this chapter to focus upon those human monoclonal autoantibodies that recognize platelet antigens. However, excellent reviews have been published summarizing the use of this technique to characterize rheumatoid factors, thyroglobulin and thyroid antigens, acetylcholine receptors in myasthenia gravis, β-cell antigens, insulin, and human spermatocyte antigens.[15,18,24–26,61,68]

Combination of Techniques: Somatic Cell Hybridization of Transformed Cells

The EBV-transformed B cells can be difficult to clone, and a progressive decline in antibody production has been reported.[58] Kozbor et al.[36] were able to overcome these difficulties by fusing a cloned B-lymphoblastoid line secreting human antitetanus antibody with a 6-TG resistant, human lymphoblastoid line selected for ouabain resistance. The hybrid cells produced from this fusion were more stable than the lymphoblastoid line from which they were derived, and they secreted an eightfold greater amount of antibody.

Therefore, we have investigated the value of somatic cell hybridization as a means of rescuing and maintaining antibody production. Some of the human B-lymphoblastoid lines secreting antiplatelet autoantibody, described earlier, were selected for fusion with a 6-TG-resistant mouse myeloma (NS-1)–human B-lymphoblastoid heterohybrid fusing line, F6.[8] This approach was based upon the premise that inclusion of human genetic material in the mouse myeloma fusion line would produce more stable hybrids. This line, F6, was originally generated during earlier studies in which we cloned a human lymphocyte–NS-1 myeloma hybrid cell that secreted human IgM reactive with the Forssman glycolipid.[48] F6, a nonsecretor of immunoglobulin, was subsequently subcloned until a 6-TG-resistant subline was selected. F6 has 125 chromosomes, including a large metacentric aberrant mouse chromosome typical of NS-1, ten of these are human chromosomes, and there are two pairs of double minutes. This chromosomal pattern has remained intact for over 1 year in continuous culture. Thus far, there are no measurable human or murine light or heavy immunoglobulin chains spontaneously secreted by F6, as detected by two-dimensional gel electrophoresis.*

After the fusion of F6 with B-lymphoblastoid cell lines, a double-selection step is required. Cells are plated, using the limiting dilution technique, in medium containing HAT, to eliminate nonfused F6 cells, and also containing 10^{-6}M ouabain, to eliminate nonfused transformed lymphocytes.

To compare F6 and murine NS-1 cells as fusion partners for the B-lymphoblastoid cells, we hybridized nontransformed splenic lymphocytes to both F6 and NS1 and screened for frequency of hybrid cells in culture, for immunoglobulin production, and for cloning efficiency. The percentage of wells containing hybrids (cells plated at 2×105 per well) was

*Nepom, J.: Personal communication.

essentially the same, 75% versus 72%. After 15 days in culture, the proportion of hybrids secreting antibody was also similar, with those hybrids established from F6 cells having a slightly higher fraction of antibody-producing cells (31%, as compared with 20% for NS-1). However, the most striking difference between the two fusing lines was observed when the stability of antibody secretion was compared. As seen in Figure 14-4, the percentage of wells which contained heterohybrid cells secreting antibody after subcloning, was considerably higher after fusion with F6. We, therefore, have hybridized lymphoblastoid cells with F6 cells, rather than with NS-1, to more efficiently establish stable lines and circumvent some of the problems encountered with the low antibody production and cloning instability that is seen with transformed cell lines. Nonetheless, it should be emphasized that recloning at intervals of 2 to 3 months is necessary to select clones maintaining a high level of antibody secretion. In our experience, however, these hybrid cells grow readily and, with careful cultivation, yield up to 10 to 50 μg of immunoglobulin per milliliter of culture supernatant.

Future efforts in the production of monoclonal human antibodies will focus upon improved methods to isolate high-affinity antibodies that more closely resemble serum alloantibodies and autoantibodies. This is critical, not only for the isolation and characterization of target antigens, but also for the development of reagents that might be used therapeutically as immunoglobulin infusions in patients with tumors, with autoimmune disease, or with an immune-compromised state. Human monoclonal antibodies, like commercial pooled immunoglobulin preparations, have a longer half-life in vivo because their protein sequence and carbohydrate composition are species-compatible, compared with that of rat, horse, or mouse immunoglobulin. The human immune response to repeated injections of horse or mouse immunoglobulin has limited the frequency and number of xenogeneic antibody infusions in the clinical setting. This is largely due to the emergence of host antimouse or antihorse antibodies, even in immunocompromised patients.[30,62] Human monoclonal antibodies are now emerging as promising therapeutic reagents. Specifically, human monoclonal antibodies have been used for radiolocalization of glioma and bronchial carcinomas and have been administered therapeutically through a subcutaneous chamber.[67,79] Thus far, little is known about sensitization to idiotypic regions on these antibodies, but there have not been any reports of the type of anaphylaxis seen with xenogeneic immunoglobulin infusions.

Preselection, or enrichment, of B-lymphocytes with a desired specificity before EBV transformation or before direct fusion to a human myeloma fusing line should increase the likelihood of isolating monoclonal antibodies against a particular target antigen. Rosetting and panning techniques, using purified proteins or target cells, have been used to enrich for B-cell populations, which are then directly fused to murine or human myeloma lines.[39] Fluorescent activated cell sorting, with FITC-conjugated target antigen, or with anti-idiotypic reagents has also been tested for preselection of B cells before transformation or fusion.[55] In vitro immunostimulation with pu-

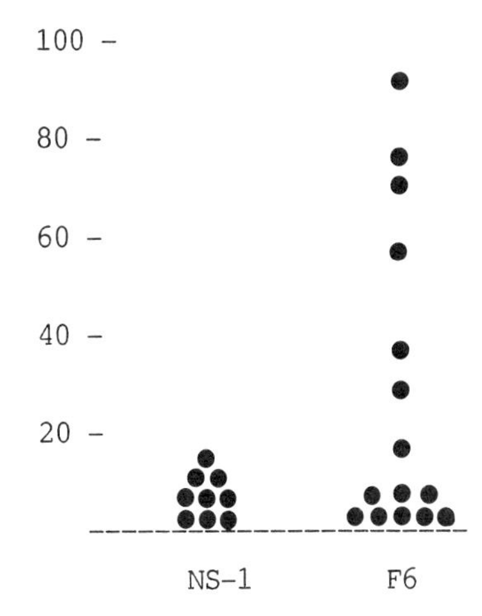

% Wells Containing Antibody Producing Hybrids With Subcloning

Figure 14-4. A comparison of the relative cloning efficiency of NS-1 versus F6. After fusion with human B-lymphocytes, those hybridomas produced with F6 demonstrated a marked improvement in antibody production and stability during cloning steps, compared with those hybridomas produced with S-1 using B-lymphocytes from the same preparation used with F6.

rified antigen, to expand the antigen-specific B-cell response and, thereby, the absolute number of lymphocytes available for fusion, has been used for the generation of human monoclonal antibodies to both foreign antigens and autoantigens.[41,42] These preselection or enrichment protocols point to the general usefulness of this approach.

HUMAN MONOCLONAL ANTIBODIES TO CHARACTERIZE PLATELET ANTIGENS

Human monoclonal antibodies that react selectively with only activated or aged platelets would greatly facilitate the isolation and characterization of membrane epitopes responsible for clearance of these cells. In both the murine and human systems, monoclonal autoantibodies have been isolated that react with a broad spectrum of antigens, including cytoskeletal proteins, polynucleotides, thyroglobulin, immunoglobulin, platelets, and erythrocytes.[3-5,18,65] All of the monoclonal antibodies characterized thus far are of the IgM isotype, and these are found in both normal individuals and patients with autoimmune disease upon idiotypic analysis of many individual sera. Included in this group of naturally occurring autoantibodies are the 16/6 anti-DNA and antiplatelet human monoclonal autoantibodies described in the first section of this chapter.[4,5,65] It is interesting that these monoclonal antibodies, particularly HF 2-1/17, react strongly with thrombin-activated platelets, whereas other antibodies, such as HF2-18/2, preferentially bind to glutaraldehyde-fixed platelets.[4] In the previous section, techniques to isolate human monoclonal autoantibody were described. In the following section, I will describe how this technology is used successfully in our laboratory to characterize a platelet antigen, recognized by human monoclonal antibody 5E5, that is expressed on thrombin-activated platelets and may, thus, represent a prototype of the naturally occurring autoantibodies found in normal sera.

Collective evidence suggests that specific membrane changes occur that are unique to aged or activated platelets.[11,19,23,45,50] Neoantigens, generated thereby, may play a role in the selective removal of aged or thrombin-activated cells from circulation. There are scattered reports of naturally occuring immunoglobulins, primarily of the IgM isotype, that specifically react with "cryptantigens" expressed under various conditions on the platelet surface, for example, after thrombin or papain treatment,[22] exposure to EDTA,[76] or fixation with paraformaldehyde.[78] Very little is now known about the expression of platelet senescence or activation antigens, or about the role these play in disease states associated with shortened platelet survival.

From our laboratory, we have reported the characterization of the human IgM monoclonal autoantibody, 5E5, that recognizes an antigen found on thrombin-activated or stored platelets.[50] The surface expression of the 5E5 epitope increases with time, as platelets age in vitro (Fig. 14-5), suggesting that it may represent a senescence or activation-specific antigen. Further testing has demonstrated that 5E5 binds to a component of the purified platelet membrane glycoprotein (GP) IIb–IIIa complex in an antigen-specific enzyme-linked immunosorbent assay (ELISA). By immunoblot technique, 5E5 binds to a protein with a relative molecular mass (M_r) of 95,000. That this protein is GPIIIa was confirmed by its M_r being identical with that of GPIIIa, identified

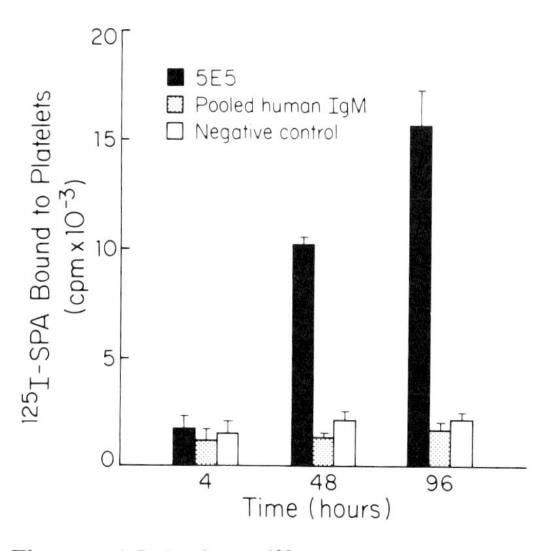

Figure 14-5. Indirect ^{125}I-labeled staphylococcal protein A platelet-binding assay demonstrating reactivity of 5E5 as platelets age in vitro. The increase in expression of the epitope recognized by 5E5 is progressive as platelets age or become activated with storage, compared with pooled human IgM or an isotype-identical, negative control human IgM monoclonal antibody. The results are mean values ±SD for five separate experiments.

by its reactivity with anti-P1^{A1} antibody on the same immunoblot preparation (Fig. 14-6). In crossed-immunoelectrophoresis (CIE; Fig. 14-7), the predominant antigen recognized by 5E5 is shown to be contained in the GPIIb–IIIa precipitin arc. An additional precipitin arc recognized by 5E5 is often seen only on gels derived from lysates of platelets that have been stored under blood bank conditions for longer than 3 days. In collaboration with Dr. June Wencel-Drake, immunofluorescence microscopy was used to localize the 5E5 epitope on both resting and activated, permeabilized platelets. These studies revealed that, in resting, fixed, nonpermeabilized platelets, there is no expression of the 5E5 epitope on the platelet surface. However, in resting permeabilized platelets, this epitope is found in an internal pool of GPIIIa which does not colocalize with the α-granule marker, fibrinogen. In contrast, with thrombin activation, the 5E5 epitope is expressed on the platelet surface, as demonstrated using flow cytofluorimetry (Fig. 14-8). These findings illustrate the usefulness of human monoclonal antibodies for the identification and study of membrane neoantigens that are expressed on the platelet surface as a result of activation or as platelets age in vitro.

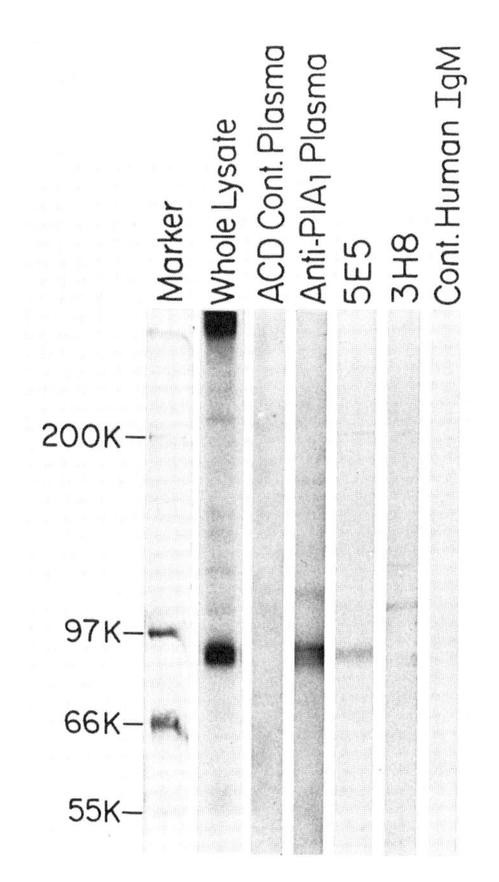

Figure 14-6. Immunoblot of platelet proteins. Under nonreducing conditions, 5E5 bound to a protein of 95,000 M_r, as seen in lane 4. A nonplatelet-binding human IgM monoclonal antibody isolated from an EBV-transformed cell line was used as a negative control (lane 6). Antibody 3H8, a platelet-reactive human monoclonal autoantibody used in the crossed-electroimmunophoresis studies, is shown in lane 5. Simultaneously, a normal plasma in lane 2 and a plasma containing anti-Pl^{A1} antibodies in lane 3 were screened for reactivity with immunoblotted platelet proteins. As is apparent in lane 3, the anti-Pl^{A1} antibodies reacted with a protein that comigrated with the protein recognized by 5E5.

Further understanding of the nature of immune-mediated removal of aged or activated platelets will provide insight into the mechanisms of clearance in other cell lines, as well as provide a foundation for more effective treatment in disease states associated with increased platelet activation and rapid platelet turnover.

HUMAN MONOCLONAL ANTIBODIES IN THE CHARACTERIZATION OF AUTOANTIGENS

Increasingly sensitive assays have been developed to document platelet reactive autoantibody in the plasma or bound to the surface of platelets from patients with idiopathic thrombocytopenic purpura.[35,46] However, it has been difficult to determine which proteins, or glycoproteins, carry the target antigens, because of low titers of circulating autoantibody and the polyclonal nature of patient sera. Finally, in the early 1980s several groups published reports suggesting that a number of patients with chronic ITP had a antiplatelet autoantibody that reacted with GPIIb–IIIa.[7,75,81] In the first study, van Leeuwen et al.[75] demonstrated that platelet eluates from patients with immune-mediated thrombocytopenia would bind to normal platelets, but they did not react with platelets from patients with Glanzmann's thrombasthenia. This report was followed, 2 years later, by two studies that confirmed the increased frequency of anti-GPIIb–IIIa antibodies in chronic ITP, by use of sensitive immunoblot assay[7] and an antigen-capture indirect immunoassay.[81] Antibodies to GPIb were also described, but at a much lower frequency

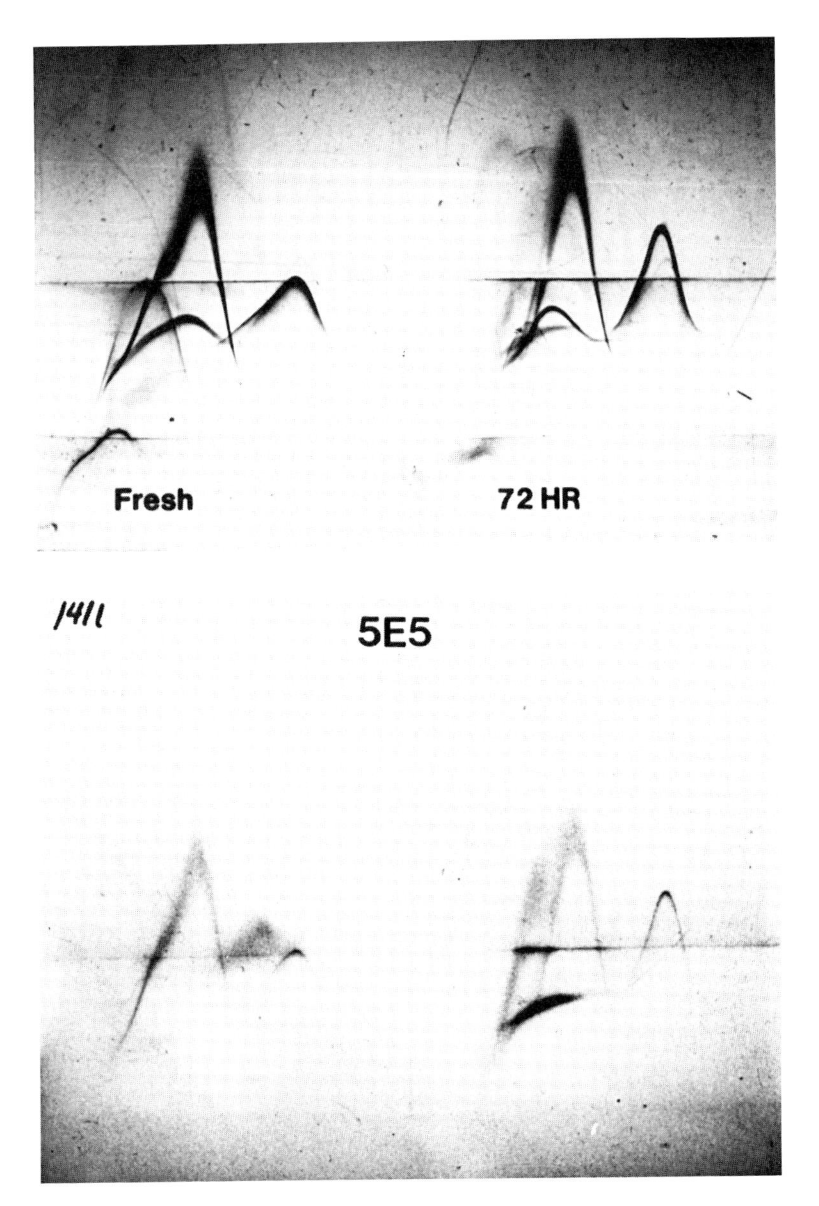

Figure 14-7. Crossed-immunoelectrophoresis of platelet proteins. The 5E5 antibody reacted with the GPIIb-IIIa precipitin arc from both fresh and aged platelet preparations. 5E5 also bound to an, as yet, unidentified precipitin arc present only in lysates prepared from stored platelets.

than anti-GPIIb-IIIa.[16,73,81] Over the past 3 to 4 years, larger groups of ITP patients have been studied, with even more sensitive assays, and collective evidence now suggests that in chronic ITP patients, 40% to 60% of plasmas screened contain anti-GPIIb-IIIa antibodies and 10% to 20% contain anti-GPIb-IX.[46] A subset of acute ITP patients, particularly those with an associated viral illness, have an antibody in their plasma that reacts, on immunoblot analysis, with an 80,000-85,000 Da protein, which appears to be sensitive to thrombin degradation.[6] This finding, along with the protein's absence from Bernard-Soulier patients, suggests that this glycoprotein may be GPV.

To further define the nature of antiplatelet autoantibodies and characterize the membrane target antigens, we are isolating human monoclonal antibodies directed against specific membrane glycoproteins. Antiplatelet antibodies directed against GPIb appear to be associated with a particularly severe form of ITP. Identification of the primary platelet target antigen in patient plasma can be demonstrated with CIE of solubilized, nondenatured platelet proteins (Fig. 14-9). To focus upon those au-

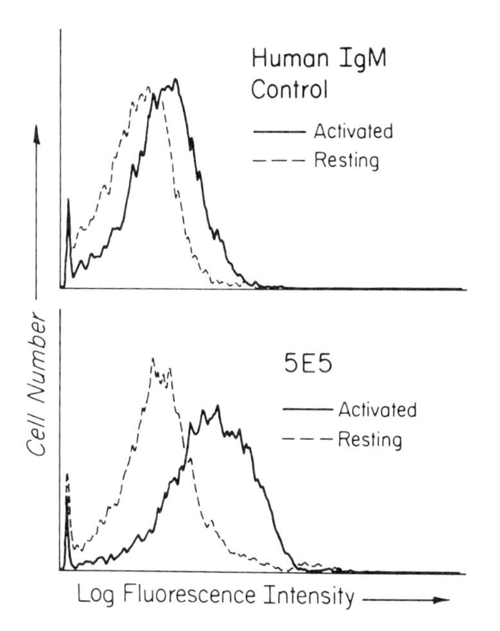

Figure 14-8. Indirect immunofluorescent analysis of antibody 5E5 binding to fresh, resting versus thrombin-activated platelets. As observed in stored platelets, a subset of thrombin-activated, fresh platelets (60%) demonstrates increased expression of the epitope recognized by 5E5 when compared with human IgM, the negative control antibody.

toantibodies that are responsible for the patient's thrombocytopenia, and to avoid other naturally occurring antiplatelet antibodies, we have elected to screen the EBV-transformed B-cell lines derived from ITP patients not only for production of antiplatelet antibody, but also for reactivity with this specific platelet membrane target antigen, GPIb. By using ELISA as the screening technique,[20] we can detect and distinguish autoantibodies, in tissue culture supernatants or patient plasma, that are directed against either GPIIb-IIIa or GPIb-GPIX. With this approach in one particular fusion, we identified 10:1078 wells that contained B-lymphoblastoid lines producing anti-GPIb autoantibody. On the basis of stability and continued antibody production, two lines were selected for further characterization, 5D5 and PBL6 (Fig. 14-10). These human monoclonal autoantibodies have been biotinylated and used in competitive inhibition assays to demonstrate that patient plasma antiplatelet antibodies specifically block the human monoclonal anti-GPIb antibodies (*see* Fig. 14-9). With use of a panel of these reagents directed at different epitopes on the GPIb molecule, we can ultimately determine whether the patient's antibodies are polyclonal or oligoclonal in their anti-GPIb reactivity. Importantly, we are now using these monoclonal antiplatelet autoantibodies to map specific regions on the autoantigen, GPIb and, thus hope to ascertain the identity and size of the immunogenic region of this molecule.

By using GPIb-specific autoantibodies, isolated from the plasma of a patient with this form of ITP, we have also produced a number of rabbit polyclonal and murine monoclonal anti-idiotypic antibodies. These antibodies recognize an idiotypic region expressed on the IgM antibody of this patient, as well as IgG or IgM antibodies from several other patients with ITP, almost all of which can be shown to bind specifically to GPIb. The Fisher's exact χ^2 analysis was used to evaluate the correlation between anti-GPIb reactivity and the presence of idiotypic antibodies in the plasma of several patients with ITP. The results for the first 72 plasmas tested are shown in Table 14-2 and represent the results obtained from duplicate experiments performed in two separate laboratories. The p-values obtained when all plasmas are included in the analysis, and when only plasmas with reactivity with GP IIb-IIIa or GPIb-IX are included, are shown below the grid. Additional testing and statistical analysis of 60 age-matched *normal* individuals and 258 thrombocytopenic patients continue to demonstrate a very strong correlation between the presence of this idiotype and GPIb reactivity ($p < 0.00001$).

Of note, there are some plasmas that demonstrate low levels of idiotypic antibody in the absence of detectable anti-GPIb reactivity. There are two possible explanations for this discrepancy. First, the rabbit polyclonal anti-idiotypic antibody was isolated after repeated immunizations with human anti-GPIb plasma antibody eluted from platelets. Consequently, high-affinity polyclonal antibodies to "foreign protein" were produced in these rabbits. Plasma autoantibody, on the other hand, is usually low titered and, generally, has a lower affinity for its target antigen when compared with polyclonal antibodies raised to foreign protein, such as alloantigens. Thus, the antigen-specific ELISA might not be sensitive enough to detect all anti-GPIb antibodies. Second, because the rabbit antibody is polyclonal, there may be many epitopes on the anti-GPIb

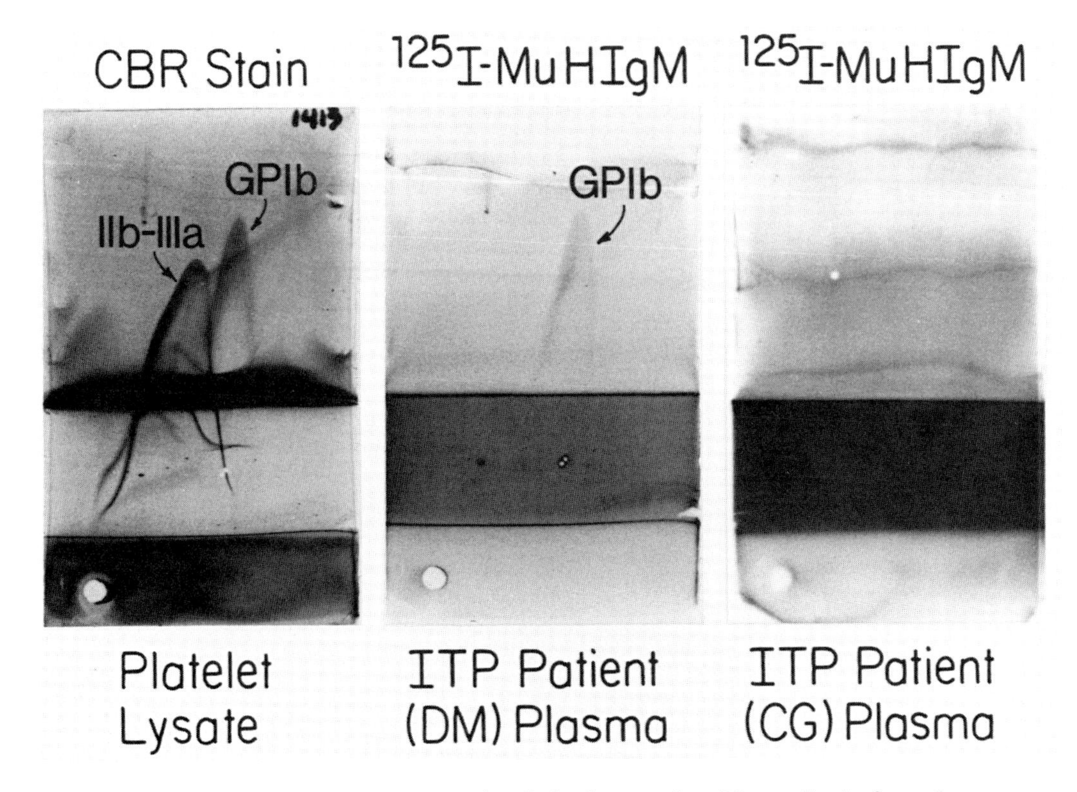

Figure 14-9. Crossed-immunoelectrophoresis of platelet proteins. The antibody from the ITP patient DM, binds to the GPIb precipitin arc. The platelet lysate used in the CIE was identical in all three panels. A control plasma from another ITP patient was not reactive with GPIb in this assay.

antibody that are immunogenic, but they do not bind to a site that directly blocks binding to GPIb. Upon examination of idiotypic antibodies raised in inbred mice, it has been shown that there are idiotype-positive, azobenzenearsonate-binding antibodies (Id+/Ars+) that differ in their hypervariable, antigen-binding region, by only one or two amino acid substitutions, from those antibodies that are Id+/Ars−.[44,63] This observation would support the hypothesis that certain germ-line, Id+/GPIb−, variable gene sequences, might produce, under the influence of a viral or bacterial stimulus, an Id+/GPIb+ antibody through normal somatic mutation, resulting in immune-mediated thrombocytopenia. Thus, we are using these anti-idiotypic reagents to select B-cell lines that produce an autoantibody that is idiotype-positive and reactive with GPIb, as opposed to those cell lines that are idiotypic-positive but are not reactive with GPIb. In this manner, it may be possible to determine the degree of somatic mutation required, within the variable gene region, to encode for autoantigen specificity. To this end, we have sequenced our first variable region gene from a cell line that is anti-GPIb reactive (in collaboration with Dr. E. Milner, Seattle, Wash.). Theoretically, it may be possible to infuse patients with Id+/GPIb− human monoclonal antibody to induce endogenous production of anti-idiotypic antibody that would then suppress the Id+/GPIb+ antibody-producing clone, as has been described with mice.[77] It has been proposed that this mechanism may account for the success of pooled immunoglobulin infusions in the treatment of some chronic ITP patients for whom long-term resolution of thrombocytopenia cannot be explained by Fc blockade alone.[10,28] We are currently screening commercial, pooled immunoglobulin preparations for the presence, or absence, of idiopathic antibod-

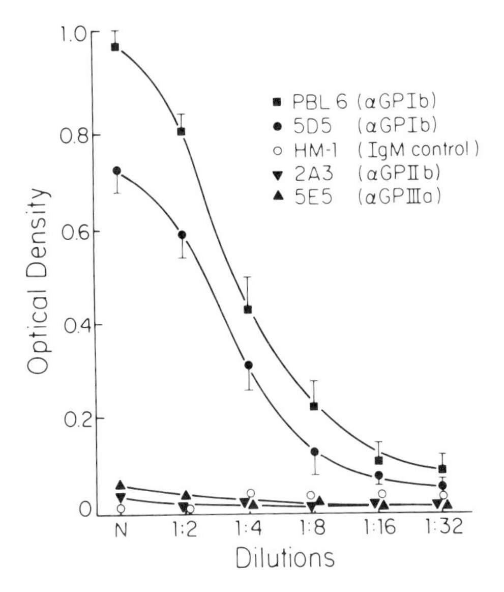

Figure 14-10. Platelet glycoprotein specific ELISA. In this assay, purified GPIb-IX complex is adsorbed to the bottom of a 96-well microtiter plate. Various human monoclonal autoantibodies are screened for their reactivity to this platelet membrane glycoprotein. PBL and 5D5 bind specifically to GPIb-IX complex. Antibodies 2A3 (anti-GPIIb) and 5E5 (anti-GPIIIa) are nonreactive, as is the negative control, an isotype-identical antibody, HM-1.

ies so that we can correlate clinical response with the emergence of anti-idiotypic antibodies in the patient's plasma.

The use of these reagents and the development of human B-lymphoblastoid cell lines producing monoclonal anti-GPIb antibodies will serve to elucidate the clonal origin and cellular regulation of autoantibody production in this disease. Anti-idiotypic antibodies may prove useful for the detection and characterization of GPIb-specific antibodies in the sera of patients with ITP, as well as in the identification of those individuals in whom more aggressive therapeutic regimens may be indicated from the outset of their disease. It is hoped that information obtained from these studies will serve to define the events triggering immune-mediated platelet clearance in humans and will lead to the development of strategies to prolong platelet survival in disease states wherein increased platelet destruction is a major pathologic mechanism.

Table 14-2
Statistical Evaluation: Fisher's Exact χ^2 Analysis

	Anti-GPIb Antibody +	Anti-GPIb Antibody −
Idiotype present*	18	4
Idiotype absent*	5	47
Idiotype present†	18	0
Idiotype absent†	5	15

*All plasma samples from ITP patients included. Correlation of anti-GPIb antibody and presence of idiotype ($n = 74$), $p = 2 \times 10^{-9}$ ($p < 0.0002$)
†Only those plasmas in which specific anti-GPIIb–IIIa +r anti-GPIb complex can be demonstrated were evaluated ($n = 38$ of 74), Correlation of anti-GPIb antibody and presence of idiotype, $p = 10^{-6}$ ($p < 0.0001$).

This work was supported in part by the National Heart, Lung, and Blood Institute Clinical Investigator Award HL 01649.

REFERENCES

1. Agnello V, Arbetter A, Ibanez de Kasep G, Powell R, Tan E, Joslin F: Evidence for a subset of rheumatoid factor populations. Scand J Immunol 9:281, 1979

2. Aman P, Ehlin-Henriksson B, Klein G: Epstein-Barr virus susceptibility of normal human B lymphocyte populations. J Exp Med 159:208, 1984

3. Andre-Schwartz J, Satta SK, Shoenfeld Y, Isenberg DA, Stollar BD, Schwartz RS: Binding of cytoskeletal proteins by monoclonal anti-DNA lupus autoantibodies. Clin Immunol Immunopathol 31:261, 1984

4. Asano T, Furie BC, Furie B: Platelet binding properties of monoclonal lupus autoantibodies produced by human hybridomas. Blood 66:1254, 1985

5. Atkinson PM, Lampman GW, Furie BC, Naparstek Y, Schwartz RS, Stollar BD, Furie B: Homology of the NH_2 terminal amino acid sequences of the heavy and light chains of human monoclonal lupus autoantibodies containing the 16/6 idiotype. J Clin Invest 75:1138, 1985

6. Beardsley D, Ho JS, Beyer EC: Varicella associated thrombocytopenia: Antibodies against an 85 kD thrombin sensitive protein (GP V?). Blood 66(suppl 1):286a, 1985

7. Beardsley DS, Spiegel JE, Jacobs MM: Platelet membrane glycoprotein IIIa contains target antigens that bind anti-platelet antibodies in immune thrombocytopenias. J Clin Invest 74:1701, 1984

8. Berglund C, Bernstein I, Nowinski RC, Wright P: Fed Proc 134:256, 1981

9. Bloy C, Blanchard D, Lambin P, Goossens D, Rouger P, Salmon C, Cartron JP: Human monoclonal antibody against Rh(D) antigen: Partial characterization of the Rh(D) polypeptide from human erythrocytes. Blood 69:1491, 1987

10. Bussel JB, Kimberly RP, Inman RD: Intravenous gammaglobulin treatment of chronic idiopathic thrombocytopenic purpura, Blood 62:480, 1983

11. Coller BS, Kalomiris E, Steinberg M, Scudder LE: Evidence that glycocalicin circulates in normal plasma. J Clin Invest 73:794, 1984

12. Crawford DH: Lymphoma after cyclosporin A treatment. In Tourain, JT, Traeger J, Bertrul H (eds): Transplantation and Clinical Immunology XIII pp 48-52. Amsterdam, Excerpta Medica, 1981

13. Crawford DH: Human monoclonal antibodies using Epstein-Barr virus In Engleman EG, Foung SKH (eds): Human Hybridomas and Monoclonal Antibodies, pp 37-53. New York, Plenum Press, 1985

14. Croce CM, Linnenback A, Hall W, Steplewski Z, Koprowski H: Production of human hybridomas secreting antibodies to measles virus. Nature 288:488, 1980

15. De Bernardo E, Davis TF: A Study of human-human hybridomas from patients with autoimmune thyroid disease. J Clin Immunol 7:71, 1987

16. Devine DV, Currie MS, Rosse WF: Pseudo-Bernard-Soulier syndrome caused by autoantibody to platelet glycoprotein Ib. Blood 68(Suppl 1):106a, 1986

17. Doyle A, Jones T, Bidwell J, Bradley B: In vitro production of human monoclonal antibody producing plasmacytoma. Hum Immunol 6:101, 1985

18. Essani K, Srinivasappa J, McClintock PR, Prabhaker BS, Nokins AL: Multiple organ reactive IgG antibody induced by an anti-idiotypic antibody to a human monoclonal IgM autoantibody. J Exp Med 163:1355, 1986

19. Fox JEB, Reynolds CC, Phillips DR: Calcium dependent proteolysis occurs during platelet aggregation. J Biol Chem 258:9973, 1983

20. Furihata K, Nugent DJ, Bissonette A, Aster RH, Kunicki TJ: On the association of platelet-specific alloantigen, Pen[a] with GP IIIa. J Clin Invest 80:1624, 1987

21. Gerber P: Activation of Epstein-Barr virus by *S* bromodeoxyuridine in virus-free human cells. Proc Natl Acad Sci USA 69:83, 1972

22. Gill JC, Carlson P, Kunicki TJ, Aster RH: A naturally occurring, warm reactive macroglobulin specific for papain-treated human platelets: Preliminary characterization. Am J Hematol 21:189, 1986

23. Ginsberg MH, Painter RG, Forsyth J, Birdwell C, Plow EF: Thrombin increases the expression of fibronectin antigen on the platelet surface. Proc Natl Acad Sci USA 77:1049, 1980

24. Harcourt G, Jermy A: Mapping the autoimmunizing epitopes on acetylcholine receptors. Immunol Today 8:319, 1987

25. Haskard DO, Archer JR: The production of human monoclonal autoantibodies from patients with rheumatoid arthritis by the EBV-hybridoma technique. J Immunol Methods 74:361, 1984

26. Herr JC, Fowler JE Jr, Howards SS, Sigman M, Sutherland WM, Koons DJ: Human antisperm monoclonal antibodies constructed postvasectomy. Biol Reprod 32:695, 1985

27. Houghton AN, Brooks H, Cote RJ, Taormina MC, Oettgen HF, Old LJ: Detection of cell surface and intracellular antigens by human monoclonal antibodies. J Exp Med 160:255, 1984

28. Imbach P, Jungi TW: Possible mechanisms of intravenous immunoglobulin treatment in childhood idiopathic thrombocytopenic purpura (ITP). Blut 46:117, 1983

29. Jacob L, Lety MA, Louvard D, Bach JF: Binding of monoclonal anti-DNA autoantibody to identical protein(s) present at the surface of several human cell types involved in lupus pathogenesis. J Clin Invest 75:315, 1985

30. Jaffers GJ, Fuller TC, Cosimi AB, Russell PS, Winn HJ, Colvin RB: Monoclonal antibody therapy. Anti-idiotypic antibodies to OKT3 arising despite intense immunosuppression. Transplantation 41:572, 1986

31. Kamo I, Furakawa S, Tada A: Monoclonal antibody to acetylcholine receptor: Cell line established from thymus of patient with myasthenia gravis. Science 215:995, 1982

32. Kaplan HS, Olsson L, Raubitschek A: Monoclonal human antibodies: A recent development with wide ranging clinical potential. In McMichael AD, Fabre JW (eds): Monoclonal Antibodies in Clinical Medicine, pp 17-35. London, Academic Press, 1982

33. Kaplan ME, Clark C: An improved rosetting assay for detection of human T lymphocytes. J Immunol Methods 5:131, 1974

34. Katsuki T, Hiruma Y, Yamanoto N, Abo T, Kumagai K: Identification of the target cells in human B lymphocytes for transformation by Epstein-Barr virus. Virology 83:287, 1977

35. Kiefel V, Santoso S, Weisheit M, Mueller-Eckhardt C: Monoclonal antibody-specific immobilization of platelet antigens (MAIPA): A new tool for the identification of platelet reactive antibodies. Blood 70:1722, 1987

36. Kozbor D, Lagarde AE, Roder JC: Human

hybridomas constructed with antigen specific Epstein-Barr virus-transformed cell lines. Proc Natl Acad Sci USA 79:6651, 1982

37. Kozbor D, Roder JC: Requirements for the establishment of high-titered human monoclonal antibodies against tetanus toxoid using the Epstein Barr technique. J Immunol 127:1275, 1981

38. Kozbor D, Roder JC: The production of human monoclonal antibodies from human lymphocytes. Immunol Today 4:72, 1983

39. Kozbor D, Steinitz M, Klein G, Koskimies S, Makela O: Establishment of anti-TNP antibody-producing human lymphoid lines by preselection for hapten binding followed by EBV transformation. Scand J Immunol 10:187, 1979

40. Koskimeis S: Human lymphoblastoid cell line producing specific antibody against Rh antigen. Scand J Immunol 11:73, 1980

41. Logtenberg T, Kroon A, Gmelig-Meyling FH, Ballieux RE: Antigen-specific activation of autoreactive B cells in normal human individuals. Eur J Immunol 16:1497, 1986

42. Logtenberg T, Kroon A, Gmelig-Meyling FH, Ballieux RE: Production of anti-thyroglobulin antibody by blood lymphocytes from patients with autoimmune thyroiditis, induced by the insolubilized autoantigen. J Immunol 136:1236, 1986

43. Luker J, Kallin B, Klein G: Induction of the Epstein-Barr virus (EBV) cycle in latently infected cells by *n*-butyrate. Virology 94:228, 1979

44. Manser T, Gefter ML: The molecular evolution of the immune response: Idiotope-specific suppression indicates that B cells express germ-line encoded V genes prior to antigenic stimulation. Eur J Immunol 16:1439, 1986

45. McEver RP, Martin MN, A monoclonal antibody to a membrane glycoprotein binds only to activated platelets. J Biol Chem 259:9799, 1984

46. McMillan R, Tani P, Millard F, Berchtold P, Renshaw L, Woods VL Jr: Platelet associated and plasma anti-glycoprotein autoantibodies in chronic ITP. Blood 70:1040, 1987

47. Miller G, Shope T, Lisco H, Stitt D, Lipman M: Epstein-Barr virus: Transformation cytopathic changes and viral antigens in squirrel, monkey and marmoset leucocytes. Proc Natl Acad Sci USA 69:383, 1972

48. Nowinski R, Berglund C, Lane J, Berstein I, Hakamori SI: Human monoclonal antibody against Forssman antigen. Science 210:537, 1980

49. Nugent DJ, Berglund C, Bernstein ID: Isolation of platelet specific human monoclonal antibodies using cell hybridization. In McGregor JL (ed): Monoclonal Antibodies and Human Blood Platelets, pp 307–317. Inserm Symposium No. 27, 1986

50. Nugent DJ, Kunicki TJ, Berglund C, Berstein ID: A human monoclonal autoantibody recognizes a neoantigen on glycoprotein IIIa expressed on stored and activated platelets. Blood 70:16, 1987

51. Olsson L: Human monoclonal antibodies: Methods of production and some aspects of their application in oncology. Med Oncol Tumour Pharmacother 4:235, 1984

52. Olsson L, Due C, Dianant M: Treatment of human cell lines with 5-azacytidine may result in profound alterations in clonogenicity and growth rate. J Cell Biol 100:508, 1985

53. Olsson L, Kaplan HS: Human–human hybridomas producing monoclonal antibodies of predefined specificity. Proc Natl Acad Sci USA 77:5429, 1980

54. Olsson L, Kaplan HS: Human–human monoclonal antibody producing hybridomas. Technical aspects. Methods Enzymol 92:3, 1983

55. Parks DR, Bryan VM, Oi VT, Herzenberg LA: Antigen-specific identification and cloning of hybridomas with a fluorescence-activated cell sorter. Proc Natl Acad Sci USA 76:1962, 1979

56. Pattengale PK, Smith RW, Gerber P: Selective transformation of B lymphocytes by EB-virus, Lancet 2:93, 1973

57. Rickinson AB, Moss DJ, Pope JH: Long term T-cell mediated immunity to Epstein-Barr virus in man. Int J Cancer 23:610, 1979

58. Roome AJ, Reading CL: The use of Epstein-Barr virus transformation for the production of human monoclonal antibodies. Exp Biol 43:35, 1984

59. Rosen A, Gergely P, Jondal M, Klein G, Britton S: Blyclonal Ig production after Epstein-Barr virus infection of human lymphocytes, in vitro. Nature 267:52, 1977

60. Rosen A, Persson K, Klein G: Human monoclonal antibodies to a genus-specific chlamydial antigen produced by EBV-transformed B-cells. J Immunol 130:2899, 1983

61. Satoh J, Prabhakar BS, Haspel MV, Ginsberg-Fellner F, Notkins AL: Human monoclonal autoantibodies that react with multiple endocrine organs. N Engl J Med 309:217, 1983

62. Schroff RW, Foon KA, Beatty SM, Oldham RK, Morgan AC: Human anti-murine immunoglobulin responses in patients receiving monoclonal antibody therapy. Cancer Res 45:879, 1985

63. Sharon J, Gefter ML, Manser T, Ptashne M: Site directed mutagenesis of an invariant amino acid residue at the variable-diversity segments junction of an antibody. Proc Natl Acad Sci USA 83:2628, 1986

64. Shoenfeld Y, Hsu-lin SC, Gabriels JE, Stollar BD, Schwartz RS: Production of human monoclonal autoantibodies. J Clin Invest 70:205, 1982

65. Shoenfeld Y, Isenberg DA, Rauch J, Madaio MP, Stollar BD, Schwartz RS: Idiotypic cross-reactions of monoclonal human lupus autoantibodies. J Exp Med 158:718, 1983

66. Siadek AW, Lostrum ME: Cell-driven viral transformation. In Engleman EG, Foung SKH (eds): Human Hybridomas and Monoclonal Antibodies, pp 167–185. New York, Plenum Press, 1985

67. Sikora K, Alderson T, Nethersell A, Smedley H: Tumour localization by human monoclonal antibodies. Med Oncol Tumour Pharmacother 2:77, 1985

68. Sklenar I, Wilkin TJ, Diaz JL, Erb P, Kellar U: Spontaneous hypoglycemia associated with autoimmunity specific to human insulin. Diabetes Care 10:152, 1987

69. Steinitz M, Klein G, Koskinies A, Makela D: EB-virus induced B lymphocyte cell lines producing specific antibody. Nature 269:420, 1977

70. Steinitz M, Seppala F, Eichman K, Klein G: Establishment of a human lymphoblastoid cell line with specific antibody production against group A streptococcal carbohydrate. Immunobiology 156:41, 1979

71. Steinitz M, Tamir S: Human monoclonal autoimmune antibody produced in vitro: Rheumatoid factor generated by Epstein-Barr virus transformed cell line. Eur J Immunol 12:126, 1982

72. Steinitz M, Tamir S, Goldfarb A: Human auto-pneumococci antibody produced by an Epstein-Barr virus (EBV)-immortalized cell line. J Immunol 132:877, 1982

73. Szatkowski NS, Kunicki TJ, Aster RH: Identification of glycoprotein Ib as a target for autoantibody in idiopathic (autoimmune) thrombocytopenic purpura. Blood 67:310, 1986

74. Valente WA, Vitti P, Yavin Z: Monoclonal antibodies to the thyrotropin receptor. Stimulating and blocking antibodies derived from lymphocytes of a patient with Graves' disease. Proc Natl Acad Sci USA 79:6680, 1982

75. van Leeuwen EF, van der Ven JTM, Engelfriet CP: Specificity of autoantibodies in autoimmune thrombocytopenia. Blood 59:23, 1982

76. van Vliet H, Kappers-Klunne MC, Abels J: Pseudothrombocytopenia: A cold autoantibody against platelet glycoprotein IIb. Br J Haematol 62:501, 1986

77. Victor-Kobrin C, Manser T, Moran TM, Imanishi-Kari T, Gefter M, Bona CA: Shared idiotopes among antibodies by heavy chain variable region (VH) gene members of the J558 VH family as basis for cross reactive regulation of clones with different antigen specificity. Proc Natl Acad Sci USA 82:769, 1985

78. Von dem borne AE, Vos JJ, Pegels HG: Cryptantigens. Curr Stud Hematol Blood Transfusion 52:33, 1986

79. Watson J, Alderson T, Sikora K, Phillips J: Subcutaneous culture chamber for continuous administration of monoclonal antibodies. Lancet 1:99, 1983

80. Winger L, Winger C, Shastry P, Russell A, Longinecker M: Efficient generation in vitro, from human peripheral blood cells, of monoclonal Epstein-Barr virus transformants producing specific antibody to a variety of antigens without prior deliberate immunization. Proc Natl Acad Sci USA 80:4484, 1983

81. Woods VL, Kurata Y, Montgomery RR: Autoantibodies against platelet glycoprotein Ib in patients with chronic immune thrombocytopenic purpura. Blood 64:156, 1984

82. Yarchoan R, Tosato G, Blaese RA, Simon RM, Nelson DC: Limiting dilution analysis of Epstein-Barr virus-induced immunoglobulin production by human B cells. J Exp Med 157:1, 1983

83. Zerbini M, Emberg I: Can Epstein-Barr virus infect and transform all the B-lymphocytes of human cord blood? J Gen Virol 64:539, 1983

84. Zurawski VR, Haber E, Black PH: Production of antibodies to tetanus toxoid by continuous human lymphoblastoid lines. Science 199:1439, 1978

85. Zur Hausen H, O'Neill FJ, Freese UK, Hecker E: Persisting oncogenic herpes virus induced by the tumor promoter TPA. Nature 272:373, 1978

15

Molecular Characterization of the Antigenic Sites of Antiplatelet Antibodies

MARK H. GINSBERG · JOSEPH C. LOFTUS · EDWARD F. PLOW

Major goals of platelet immunology include development of assays to assist in platelet transfusion and in diagnosis and therapy of patients with immune-mediated platelet destruction. A second goal is to develop novel therapeutic approaches for the management of such patients. Achievement of these goals would be facilitated by chemical characterization of the antigens recognized by antiplatelet antibodies. While much work has gone into the identification of the macromolecules that bear these antigens, we are at the beginning of a time in which the precise chemical nature of certain antigenic sites may be readily defined. Furthermore, for some, those sites may then be synthesized either chemically or by recombinant DNA technology. The ready availability of such synthetic antigens will have important practical consequences. For example, synthetic antigens would provide a simple method for establishment of automated immunoassays for platelet allo- and autoantibodies. In addition, such synthetic antigens could be used to block auto- and alloantibodies or as immunoabsorbants for the in vivo depletion of these antibodies.[17] Finally, the characterization of such antigenic sites may provide important clues to the etiology of certain autoimmune reactions by the discovery of unexpected molecular "mimicries."[8] In this review, we will discuss an approach to the delineation of antigenic sites utilizing a combination of recombinant DNA technology, computerized antigen prediction algorithms, and peptide synthesis.

FUNDAMENTAL CONSIDERATIONS

The structure recognized by an antibody is an *antigenic site*, also referred to as an *epitope* or *antigenic determinant*. Within proteins, antigenic sites may be residue within the polypeptide moiety, or be partially or totally dependent upon nonpeptide constituents, e.g., carbohydrates. We will treat only the former situation here. Polypeptide determinants may be *continuous* (synonym = segmental) in which the epitope is defined by a continuous amino acid sequence. Alternatively, they may be *discontinuous* (synonym = assembled topographic) determinants in which residues far apart in the primary sequence are brought together within the three-dimensional structure of the protein to form the epitope.[3] Discontinuous epitopes are obviously dependent upon protein conformation, but the binding of antibodies to continuous epitopes may also be influenced by protein conformation. This may occur because the antibodies recognize a preferred conformation of a given peptide sequence[3] or because the conformation of the macromolecule may influence the accessibility of the antibody to the target sequence. The strategy to be discussed here is directed toward the definition of continuous epitopes.

For most proteins, roughly one-third of antibodies arising from immunization with the native protein will react solely with discontinuous epitopes,[3] but this figure will probably vary depending on the protein and the sensitivity of the assay used for detection of antibody binding. For example, Mehra et al.[28] were able to place epitopes for each of six monoclonal antibodies against the *Mycobacterium leprae* 65-kDa antigen within specific peptide sequences. Barlow et al.[2] utilized the dimensions of the recognition zone of a single antibody–discontinuous lysozyme epitope complex[1] and the crystal structure of lysozyme to derive a theoretical analysis of the frequency of continuous epitopes in the protein. It was found that less than 10% of the surface area of the protein was occupied by potential continuous epitopes. Nevertheless, it was also realized that synthetic peptides might contain parts of discontinuous epitopes and might be predicted to bind to the target antibodies, albeit with lower affinities than that of the native protein. The potential to prepare peptides that partially mimic discontinuous epitopes has been experimentally validated by Lerner and his coworkers.[10] It thus seems that this approach will be useful for a large number of antibodies. Moreover, it is possible to decide a priori, which antibodies are potential candidates for this approach based on their reactivity with the denatured protein.

EXPRESSION CLONING FOR THE MAPPING OF ANTIGENIC DETERMINANTS

The phage λ *gt*11 expression cloning vector introduced by Young and Davis[44] has proved valuable in the isolation of cDNA clones by antibody screening. This vector can accommodate up to 8 kb of insert DNA and permits the construction and maintenance of libraries of 10^5 to 10^7 recombinants. The vector contains the *lacZ* gene that encodes for inducible β-galactosidase and there is an *Eco*R1 restriction site near the 3′-end of the β-galactosidase-coding sequence. Thus, insert-coded polypeptides are produced as a portion of fusion proteins with β-galactosidase; they are produced at high concentrations following induction with activators of the *lacZ* transcriptional unit (e.g., isopropyl thioglucose). In addition, the production of fusion proteins increases the stability[44] of the insert-coded polypeptides and provides a convenient "handle" for their purification. Furthermore, because insertions at this *Eco*R1 site inactivate the β-galactosidase, a blue–clear color selection can be used to identify phage containing inserts.[44] The widespread employment of this system in cDNA cloning[4,11,22,34,36] attests to its usefulness. Indeed, it is possible to clone antigens in the absence of protein sequence information[41] with this vector. Here, the authenticity of the clones remains a concern; however, several immunologic criteria may assuage (but not fully remove) these concerns.

- *Epitope selection.*[43] In this process, the antibody used in the cloning is affinity purified by use of the expressed, insert-coded polypeptide, and the affinity-purified antibody is then shown to react with the desired protein. This criterion is valid only if the initial antibody reacts with multiple polypeptides and reactivity with only one is selected. For example, we[25] employed a polyclonal anti-GPIIb–IIIa that reacted with both subunits to select clones whose expressed polypeptides could be used to affinity-purify anti-GPIIb selectively.
- *Appropriate reactivity of antibodies raised against the insert-coded polypeptide.* Here, an antibody is raised against the expressed fusion protein and shown to react with the desired protein. Both this criterion and epitope selection are susceptible to the dreaded complication of immunologic cross-reactivity between what has been cloned and the desired protein. In this event, one can increase certainty by demonstrating that the fusion protein antibody reacts independently with several regions of the protein by blotting immunologically non–cross-reactive fragments of the target protein. Alternatively, antibodies can be raised against fusion proteins specified by subclones of different regions of the protein.
- *Antipeptide antibodies.* Once the insert is sequenced, antibodies can be made against synthetic peptides from several portions of the predicted protein sequence. Reactivity of several of these antibodies with the target protein is a reassuring result.

Whatever the results of the foregoing immunologic tests, the most stringent criterion for clone authenticity is identity between its predicted peptide sequence and the determined amino acid sequence of the protein. In our laboratory, this criterion is the only basis for the popping of champagne corks, although satisfaction of the immunologic criteria may justify an indulgence in a domestic sparkling wine.

The *gt*11 phage cloning system just discussed will generally express authentic protein in a maximum of one-sixth of recombinants containing a coding sequence, because the true coding sequence will be expressed only when it is in frame with β-galactosidase (with an occasional[28,44] exception). Moreover, because vector translation initiation sites are used, small fragments of the protein are readily expressed. This implies that "nonsense" polypeptides will be expressed the remaining five-sixths of the time, and one of these neoproteins might react with the screening antibody. In a random DNA sequence (with the proportion of each nucleotide being equal), 3 out of 64 possible codons represent stop codons. Thus, such "nonsense" polypeptides are likely to be short. Because the length of the insert-coded polypeptide can be readily estimated by Western blotting, a major disparity between the size of the fusion protein predicted from the known insert size and the determined size of the fusion protein should suggest this possibility. Other possible causes of an unexpectedly short fusion protein are a clone containing a large 3′ untranslated region, an insert-coded polypeptide expressed without β-galactosidase, or intervening sequences in the cDNA.

The capacity of the *gt*11 system to express short fragments of proteins has been exploited for the construction of epitope libraries.[28,29,33] This approach permits the precise delineation of continuous epitopes and involves randomly fragmenting the cDNA and reinserting the size-selected fragments into the *gt*11 vector. This sublibrary may then be rescreened with the antibody in question, and short inserts coding for the epitope may be isolated. The sequences of those inserts that code for the epitope can then serve to precisely map it. Mehra et al.[28] have used this approach to map six monoclonal antibodies to the same polypeptide. Those workers also employed direct sequencing within the λ phage to rapidly define the limits of each antibody-positive insert. Because the sequence of the whole parent insert was known, this permitted an efficient, precise mapping of each determinant. It must be stressed that these approaches are probably only applicable to continuous epitopes. Thus, identification of discontinuous epitopes, such as Pl^{A1}[20], may require expression in vectors that process and fold eukaryotic polypeptides appropriately. One such system for membrane antigens employing a *COS* cell expression system and immunoselection by cell "panning" has been described by Seed and Aruffo.[37]

USE OF EXPRESSION CLONING AND PEPTIDE SYNTHESIS TO DEFINE A REGION OF PLATELET MEMBRANE GLYCOPROTEIN IIb INVOLVED IN ADHESIVE FUNCTION

A recent example of the potential utility of expression cloning in the definition of continuous epitopes was provided by our recent success in defining the epitope for a monoclonal antibody, PMI-1.[25] Several observations had suggested that a functionally significant site on GPIIb–IIIa is near the epitope defined by this monoclonal antibody. This antibody binds to the heavy chain of GPIIb[38] and defines a region of GPIIb that is associated with four distinct functional activities. First, PMI-1 inhibits platelet adhesion to collagen.[38] Second, the surface orientation of this region is regulated by divalent cations, as millimolar concentrations of calcium or magnesium suppress expression of the PMI-1 epitope.[12] Third, abnormal divalent cation regulation of the conformation of this site is associated with a functional thrombasthenic state.[21] Finally, the interaction of Arg-Gly-Asp (RGD)-containing ligands with GPIIb–IIIa alters the conformation of this region, resulting in increased exposure of the PMI-1 epitope.[7]

Given the reactivity of this antibody in Western blotting of reduced GPIIb,[38] it seemed that expression cloning might offer a means of defining its antigenic site. In our initial screening of 200,000 λ *gt*11 recombinants from a human erythroleukemia (HEL) cell cDNA library with rabbit polyclonal GPIIb-IIIa antiserum, we identified six immunoreactive clones. One of these clones, HEL41, contained a 1.1-kDa insert that directed the synthesis of a bacterial fusion protein of approximately M_r 140 kDa, with characteristics that would be consistent with it possessing GPIIb epitopes. These characteristics included (1) reactivity of the polyclonal serum with the fusion protein encoded by this clone was blocked by prior absorption with purified GPIIb–IIIa; (2) antibodies affinity-purified on the fusion protein reacted specifically with GPIIb in immunoblots of platelet lysates and purified GPIIb–IIIa; and (3) GPIIb–IIIa was immunoprecipitated from surface-labeled platelet proteins by the affinity-purified antiserum. The affinity-purified antibody failed to react with the α subunit of the vitronectin receptor by Western blotting, and it failed to immunoprecipitate the related endothelial cell cytoadhesin.[26] The fusion protein encoded by HEL41 was immunoreactive with the monoclonal antibody PMI-1 (Fig. 15-1), and the size of the fusion protein suggested an insert-coded polypeptide of 23 kDa, indicating that a long open-reading frame was present in the clone.

The cDNA sequence (Fig. 15-2) had an open-reading frame of 682 bases with a TAG termination codon at position 683 followed by 419 bases of 3′ untranslated sequence. The first 120 nucleotides at the 5′-end of the clone possess the characteristics of the consensus Alu repetitive sequence,[35] indicating that this clone may have been derived from an incompletely processed mRNA. Computer search revealed no significant identity between the HEL41 coding sequence and other nucleotide sequences present in the GENBANK and EMBL databases as of March 1987. The cDNA sequence of clone HEL41 encoded an open-reading frame of 227 amino acids (*see* Fig. 15-2). The determined NH_2-terminal sequence for the light chain of GPIIb, as reported by Charo et al.,[5] was identified within the clone as the sequence between L-157 and T-171. The consensus Alu repetitive sequence translated in frame and accounts for the first 40 amino acids encoded by HEL41. To investigate whether or not this sequence was present in mature GPIIb, the reactivity of antibodies to peptides from within this region with GPIIb was determined by immunoblotting. Two peptides—W(19)–S(34), which is encoded by the repetitive sequence, and R(53)–K(64), which lies outside this region—were synthesized and antipeptide antibodies were produced. Antibodies to

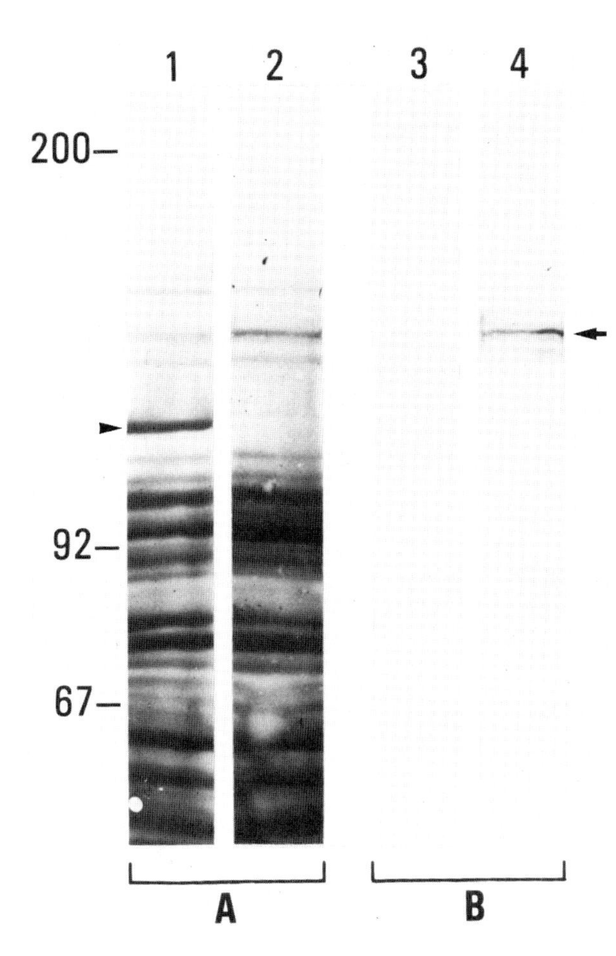

Figure 15-1. Characterization of HEL41 β-galactosidase fusion protein. Bacterial lysates were prepared from the lysogens Y1089/*gt*11 (lanes 1 and 3) and Y1089/HEL41 (lanes 2 and 4) after induction with isopropyl thiogalactoside (IPTG). All samples were reduced, resolved on a 6% SDS polyacrylamide gel, and transferred to nitrocellulose. (*A*) Amido black staining. β-Galactosidase (arrowhead) and fusion protein (arrow) are indicated; (*B*) immunoblot with PMI-1.

```
   1  CGAGAATATGACCTTGGTCAGGTGCAGTGGCTCACGCCTGTAATCCCAGTACTTTGGGAG    60
      R  E  Y  D  L  G  Q  V  Q  W  L  T  P  V  I  P  V  L  W  E

  61  GCCAAGGCAGGCAGATCACCTGAGGTCAGGAGTTCGAGGTCAGCCTTGCCGAACCCCTTT   120
      A  K  A  G  R  S  P  E  V  R  S  S  R  S  A  L  P  N  P  F

 121  CCAGCCTCCCTGGTGGTGGCAGCAGAAGAAGGTGAGAGGGAGCAGAACAGCTTGGACAGC   180
      P  A  S  L  V  V  A  A  E  E  G  E  R  E  Q  N  S  L  D  S

 181  TGGGGACCCAAAGTGGAGCACACCTATGAGCTCCACAACACTGGCCCTGGGACTGTGAAT   240
      W  G  P  K  V  E  H  T  Y  E  L  H  N  T  G  P  G  T  V  N

 241  GGTCTTCACCTCAGCATCCACCTTCCGGGACAGTCCCAGCCCTCCGACCTGCTCTACATC   300
      G  L  H  L  S  I  H  L  P  G  Q  S  Q  P  S  D  L  L  Y  I

 301  CTGGATATACAGCCCCAGGGGGCGCTTCAGTGCTTCCCACAGCCTCCTGTCAATCCTCTC   360
      L  D  I  Q  P  Q  G  A  L  Q  C  F  P  Q  P  P  V  N  P  L

 361  AAGGTGGACTGGGGGCTGCCCATCCCCAGCCCCTCCCCCATTCACCCGGCCCATCACAAG   420
      K  V  D  W  G  L  P  I  P  S  P  S  P  I  H  P  A  H  H  K

 421  CGGGATCGCAGACAGATCTTCCTGCCAGAGCCCGAGCAGCCCTCGAGGCTTCAGGATCCA   480
      R  D  R  R  Q  I  F  L  P  E  P  E  Q  P  S  R  L  Q  D  P

 481  GTTCTCGTAAGCTGCGACTCGGCGCCCTGTACTGTGGTGCAGTGTGACCTGCAGGAGATG   540
      V  L  V  S  C  D  S  A  P  C  T  V  V  Q  C  D  L  Q  E  M

 541  GCGCGCGGGCAGCGGGCCATGGTCACGGTGCTGGCCTTCCTGTGGCTGCCCAGCCTCTAC   600
      A  R  G  Q  R  A  M  V  T  V  L  A  F  L  W  L  P  S  L  Y

 601  CAGAGGCCTCTGGATCAGTTTGTGCTGCAGTCGCACGCATGGTTCAACGTGTCGTTTGAG   660
      Q  R  P  L  D  Q  F  V  L  Q  S  H  A  W  F  N  V  S  F  E

 661  GAAGAAGCAAAGTGTAGTAGTTAGAATGGTGATTTCTGAGCAAGAAGATGGGGGCTCTGT   720
      E  E  A  K  C  S  S  *

 721  ATTCCTGGCCAAGTAGCTTGGCTTCTCTGGGTCTCAGTTTGCTGCCAAAGCAAACGAGGA   780

 781  TAATACTGATCCTACCTGTAATAGGACCATTGAAAGGATTTCACAGGATGAGGTTTATGA   840

 841  AAATACTTTATAGTTAATAATTCTACATCATATACCTGAAATTTGCTAAGAGAGAAAAAT   900

 901  CTTAAAACGTTCTCACCACAAAAGATAACTATGTGAGGTGATACATACGCTAATTAGCTT   960

 961  GATTGTGGTAATCCTTTCACAATGTATACATATACCAAAACATCATATTGCACACTGTGA  1020

1021  ATATATACAATTTATTTGTCAATTATACCTCAATACAGCTGGAAATACATAAATTTTCAT  1080

1081  GCACTGTGTAAATATGAGAGATGG  1104
```

Figure 15-2. DNA sequence and deduced amino acid sequence of cDNA clone HEL41. Amino acid sequence is given in the *single letter code.* Potential cleavage site of light and heavy chains of GPIIb is marked by the arrowhead. Determined NH_2-terminal amino acid sequence of GPIIb light chain is indicated by a dashed line. Synthetic peptides, corresponding to predicted antigenic region are boxed. V43, large box; V41, small box. Synthetic peptides corresponding to the translatable Alu sequence (double lines) and adjacent region (single line) are marked.

Single letter code: A, alanine; C, cysteine; D, aspartic acid; E, glutamic acid; F, phenylalanine; G, glycine; H, histidine; I, isoleucine; K, lysine; L, leucine; M, methionine; N, asparagine; P, proline; Q, glutamine; R, arginine; S, serine; T, threonine; V, valine; W, tryptophan; Y, tyrosine.

W(19)-S(34) failed to blot to GPIIb, whereas antibodies to R(53)-K(64) were reactive with GPIIb heavy chain in immunoblot analyses (not shown).

At this point, the next logical step would have been to proceed to construction of an epitope library derived from subclones of this clone. Nevertheless, we had performed preliminary experiments that indicated that a 9-kDa staphylococcal V8 protease fragment of GPIIb contained the PMI-1 epitope. Inspection of the deduced amino acid sequence of clone HEL41 identified a single predicted V8 fragment of appropriate size between L-71 and E-150 and this fragment lay within the predicted heavy chain sequence. We next reasoned that if this antibody recognized a segmental epitope, then it should react with the appropriate small synthetic peptide derived from this V8 protease fragment of the GPIIb heavy chain. In recent years, there has been a lively effort to establish rules for identification of protein sequences likely to function as continuous epitopes, i.e., for synthetic peptides, which will elicit antibodies that react with the native protein. Indeed, several highly informative studies and reviews of this subject have been published.[6,14,23,42] Initial efforts focused on simple algorithms to predict hydrophilic segments of proteins, based on the logic that such sequences are more likely to be surface exposed.[14] Subsequent studies have suggested that additional considerations, such as secondary structure, local protein mobility,[40] charge, and protein shape[10] may also enter into the equation. Accordingly, we utilized the algorithm of Jameson and Wolf[18] to analyze for potential continuous epitope within this predicted V8 fragment. This algorithm estimates antigenicity based on predictions of secondary structure, flexibility, and surface accessibility, as well as hydrophilicity. The results of such an analysis appear in Figure 15-3, and it identified a single, continuous region with a high predicted value for an antigenic site. Two peptides, one flanking and containing this region (V-43) and one immediately carboxy-terminal to it (V-41), were synthesized and their ability to inhibit the binding of PMI-1 to platelets was examined. Peptide V-43 [P-(129)-Q(145)] inhibited the binding of PMI-1 in a dose-dependent manner (Fig. 15-4). As 50% inhibition was achieved at 1.6 μM peptide when the antibody was present at 1 μM, the approximate K^d of the peptide-PMI-1 interaction is 1.2 μM. Conversely, peptide V-41 [R(144)-R(156)] had no effect on the binding of PMI-1. In control experiments, neither peptide had any effect on the binding of a monoclonal anti-GPIIIa antibody, 22C4,[31] to platelets (not shown).

Direct binding of PMI-1 to peptide V-43 was demonstrated by enzyme-linked immunosorbent assay (ELISA) (Table 15-1). PMI-1 bound to purified GPIIb-IIIa and peptide V-43, but failed to react with peptide V-41. The monoclonal antibody, Tab,[27] bound to purified GPIIb-IIIa but failed to bind to either peptide. In a competitive assay, peptide V-43 (20 μM) completely inhibited the binding of PMI-1 to purified GPIIb-IIIa but had no effect on Tab binding to GPIIb-IIIa. Peptide V-41 had no effect on the binding of either antibody.

These data have permitted the assignment of this epitope to a 17-residue peptide sequence near the carboxyl-terminus of GPIIb heavy chain. One may ask what are the potential implications of these results?

- We know that the PMI-1 antibody inhibits platelet spreading[38] on collagenous surfaces. Is this because the region of GPIIb recognized by the antibody is involved in events that lead to spreading and stabilization of attachment? Obviously, synthetic peptides that are based on this sequence should prove most useful in experimental evaluation of this possibility.
- This region of GPIIb undergoes a change in its microenvironment or structure after the binding of fibrinogen or Arg-Gly-Asp-containing peptides to platelets.[7] These binding events are also associated with self-association of GPIIb-IIIa within the plane of the plasma membrane.[16,24] Again, these synthetic peptides should prove valuable in testing the hypothesis that the change in the carboxy-terminus of the GPIIb heavy chain mediates this self-association or other postoccupancy events involving GPIIb-IIIa.
- There has been considerable interest in the identification of synthetic peptides that inhibit platelet function as inhibitors of adhesive protein binding.[13,19,32] Peptides based on the V-43 sequence may offer a novel class of such inhibitors that block selected postoccupancy events. As such, they may prove more cell type- or response-specific than the previous peptides.
- Antibodies that are selective for activated

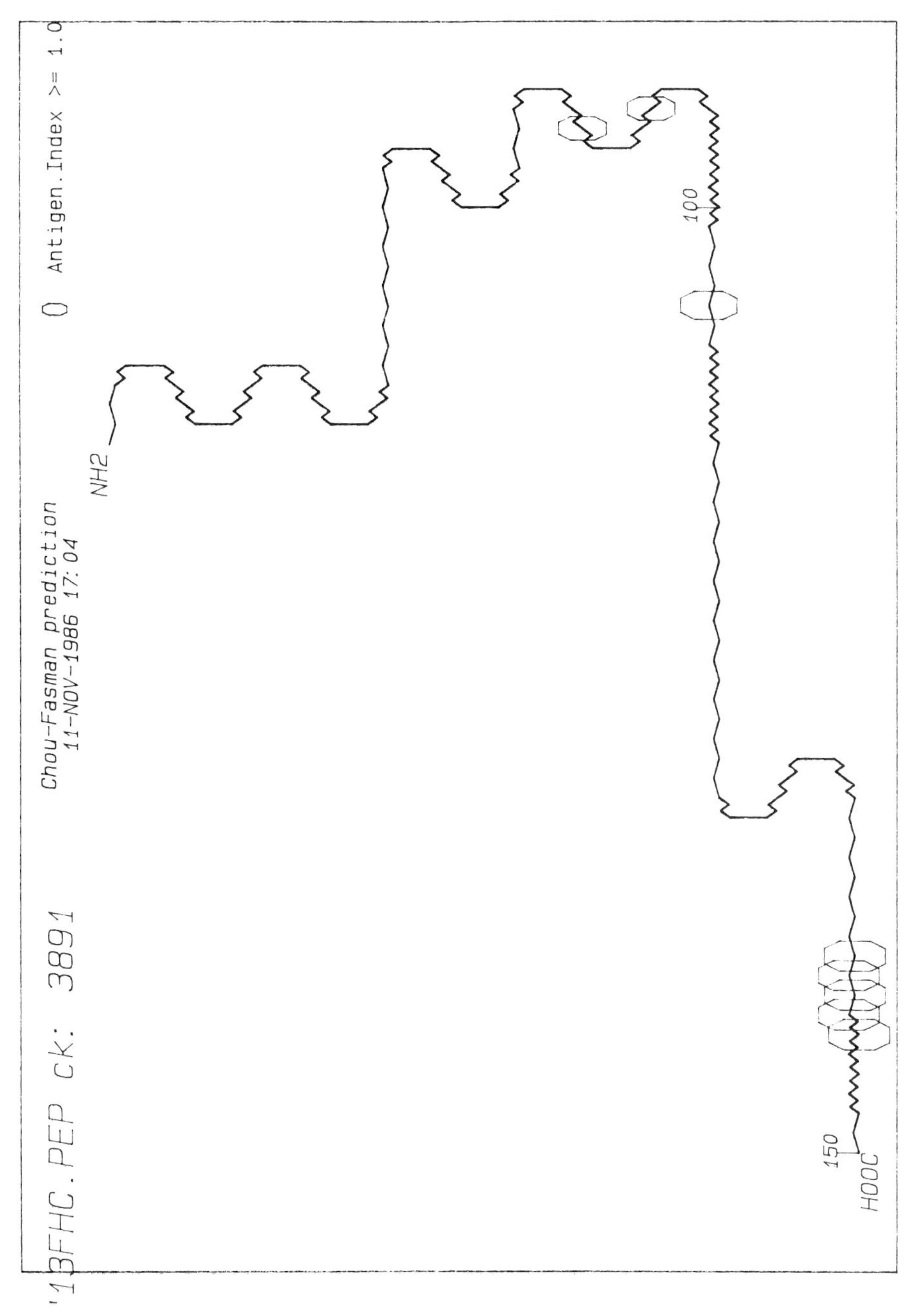

Figure 15-3. Plot of the secondary structure of the predicted V8 fragment of the GPIIb heavy chain with predicted antigenicity superimposed. The plot shows predictions according to Chou and Fasman.[5a] Predicted antigenic sites according to Jameson and Wolf[18] are circled. Note a single area containing a continuous series of predicted sites.

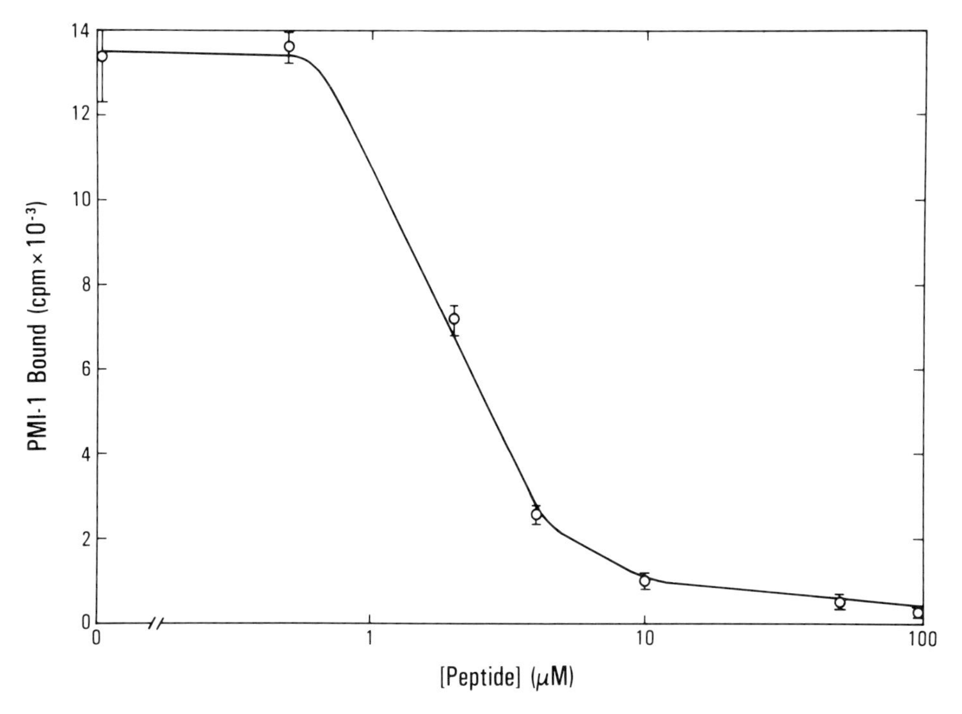

Figure 15-4. Effect of 17-amino acid peptide (V-43) on PMI-1 binding to platelets. Platelets (2×10^8/ml) in Tyrode's 1% albumin buffer were preincubated in the presence of 5 mM EDTA at 37°C for 30 min to ensure full exposure of the PMI-1 epitope. ^{125}I-labeled PMI-1 (1 μM) binding was then assayed in the presence of the indicated input concentration of V-43 peptide at 22°C for 30 min.

Table 15-1
A 17-Residue Peptide Binds to PMI-1 and Blocks Its Binding to GPIIb–IIIa

Parameter		Antibody Added	
		PMI-1	*Tab*
Capacity of soluble peptides to compete for PMI-1 binding to GPIIb–IIIa*			
	V-43	0.067 ± 0.002	1.002 ± 0.026
Competitor	V-41	0.814 ± 0.012	1.117 ± 0.024
	None	0.804 ± 0.002	1.040 ± 0.05
	GPIIb–IIIa	0.433 ± 0.013	0.134 ± 0.010
Detection of direct binding of PMI-1 to peptide V-43†			
Coating material	V-43	1.310 ± 0.013	0.068 ± 0.009
	V-41	0.069 ± 0.005	0.061 ± 0.005
	GPIIb–IIIa	0.389 ± 0.006	1.015 ± 0.035
	BSA	0.068 ± 0.005	0.060 ± 0.004

*Antibody (1.5 nM PMI-1 purified IgG or a 1 : 320,000 dilution of Tab ascites) binding to GPIIb–IIIa-coated microtiter wells was assessed in the absence of soluble competitor or in the presence of detergent-solubilized, purified GPIIb–IIIa (0.73 μM) or synthetic peptides from GPIIb (25 μM). V-43 = P(129)–Q(145); V-41 = R(144)–R(156). Values given are in the presence of 5 mM EDTA and are the average A_{490} readings of triplicate determinations ± SD

†Microtiter wells were coated with either GPIIb–IIIa (20 μg/ml) or peptides V-41 or V-43 (20 μM) then reacted with the indicated antibody. Values determined in the presence of 5 mM EDTA and are averages of triplicate determinations ± SD.

platelets may prove useful in detection of such cells in the circulation[9,15,39] or in imaging thrombi. The PMI-1 antibody represents a novel group of such reagents that recognize occupied fibrinogen receptors. Thus, antibody, or antibodies, directed against its synthetic epitope may prove useful for detection of platelet activation in vitro and in vivo.

- Patients with pseudothrombocytopenia often have antibodies that react with GPIIb–IIIa in the presence of EDTA, but not at physiologic divalent cation concentrations.[30] The PMI-1 epitope is an obvious target[12] for such antibodies, and the V-43 peptide would seem to offer a suitable reagent for assaying for PMI-1-like antibodies in these patients.

CONCLUSION

In this review, we have briefly discussed strategies for delineation of continuous epitopes within proteins. Moreover, we have presented a specific example in which this was done for a platelet antigen and indicated how this may open new doors of theoretical and practical significance. There has been explosive growth in biotechnology, and a growing number of platelet proteins have been cloned. Thus, it seems certain that there will be a release of much new data defining platelet epitopes and a resulting irreversible increase in aggregate knowledge concerning the immunology of this cell.

This work was supported by NIH Grants HL16411, AR27214, GM37696, and HL28235. This is publication #5061-IMM of the Research Institute of Scripps Clinic.

REFERENCES

1. Amit AG, Mariuzza RA, Phillips SE, Poljak RJ: Three-dimensional structure of an antigen–antibody complex at 6 A resolution. Nature 313: 156, 1985

2. Barlow DJ, Edwards MS, Thornton JM: Continuous and discontinuous protein antigenic determinants. Nature 322:747, 1986

3. Berzofsky JA: Intrinsic and extrinsic factors in protein antigenic structure. Science 229:932, 1985

4. Chambers JC, Keene JD: Isolation and analysis of cDNA clones expressing human lupus La antigen. Proc Natl Acad Sci USA 82:2115, 1985

5. Charo IF, Fitzgerald LA, Steiner B, Rall SC Jr, Bekeart LS, Phillips DR: Platelet glycoproteins IIb and IIIa: Evidence for a family of immunologically and structurally related glycoproteins in mammalian cells. Proc Natl Acad Sci USA 83:8351, 1986

5a. Chou PY, Fasman GD: Prediction of the secondary structure of proteins from their amino acid sequence. Adv Enzymol 47:45, 1978

6. Doolittle RF: Rapid Immunoselection Procedure: Of urfs and orfs. Mill Valley, University Science Books, 1986

7. Frelinger AL III, Lam SC-T, Smith MA, Plow EF, Ginsberg MH: Arg-Gly-Asp peptides induce changes in platelet membrane glycoproteins IIb–IIIa associated with loss of adhesive protein binding function. Clin Res 35:598A, 1987

8. Fujinami RS, Oldstone MB: Amino acid homology between the encephalitogenic site of myelin basic protein and virus: Mechanism for autoimmunity. Science 230:1043, 1985

9. George JN, Pickett EB, Saucerman S, McEver RP, Kunicki TJ, Kieffer N, Newman PJ: Platelet surface glycoproteins. Studies on resting and activated platelets and platelet membrane microparticles in normal subjects, and observations in patients during adult respiratory distress syndrome and cardiac surgery. J Clin Invest 78:340, 1986

10. Geysen HM, Tainer JA, Rodda SJ, Mason TJ, Alexander H, Getzoff ED, Lerner RA: Chemistry of antibody binding to a protein. Science 235:1184, 1987

11. Ginsberg D, Handin RI, Bonthron D, Donlon TA, Bruns GAP, Latt SA, Orkin SH: Human von Willebrand Factor (vWF): Isolation of complementary DNA (cDNA) clones and chromosomal localization. Science 228:1401, 1985

12. Ginsberg MH, Lightsey A, Kunicki TJ, Kaufman A, Marguerie G, Plow EF: Divalent cation regulation of the surface orientation of platelet membrane glycoprotein IIb: Correlation with fibrinogen binding function and definition of a novel variant of Glanzman's thrombasthenia. J Clin Invest 78:1103, 1986

13. Ginsberg M, Pierschbacher MD, Ruoslahti E, Marguerie G, Plow E: Inhibition of fibronectin binding to platelets by proteolytic fragments and synthetic peptides which support fibroblast adhesion. J Biol Chem 260:3931, 1985

14. Hopp TP, Woods KR: Prediction of protein antigenic determinants from amino acid sequences. Proc Natl Acad Sci USA 78:3824, 1981

15. Hsu-Lin S-C, Berman CL, Furie BC, August D, Furie B: A platelet membrane protein expressed during platelet activation and secretion. Studies

using a monoclonal antibody specific for thrombin-activated platelets. J Biol Chem 259:9121, 1984

16. Isenberg WM, McEver RP, Phillips DR, Shuman MA, Bainton DF: The platelet fibrinogen receptor: An immunogold-surface replica study of agonist-induced ligand binding and receptor clustering. J Cell Biol 104:1655, 1987

17. Iverson GM, Eardley DD, Janeway CA, Gershon RK: Use of anti-idiotype immunosorbents to isolate circulating antigen-specific T cell-derived molecules from hyperimmune sera (idiotype). Proc Natl Acad Sci USA 80:1435, 1983

18. Jameson BA, Wolf H: Predicting antigenicity from protein primary structure. A new algorithm for the prediction of antigenic sites. CABIOS (in press) 1988

19. Kloczewiak M, Timmons S, Hawiger J: Localization of a site interacting with human platelet receptor on carboxy-terminal segment of human fibrinogen gamma chain. Biochem Biophys Res Commun 107:181, 1982

20. Kunicki TJ, Aster RH: Isolation and immunologic characterization of the human platelet alloantigen, Pl^{A1}. Mol Immunol 16:353, 1979

21. Laterra J, Silbert JE, Culp LA: Cell surface heparan sulfate mediates some adhesive responses to glycosaminoglycan-binding matrices, including fibronectin. J Cell Biol 96:112, 1983

22. Lawler J, Hynes RO: The structure of human thrombospondin, an adhesive glycoprotein with multiple calcium-binding sites and homologies with several different proteins. J Cell Biol 103:1635, 1986

23. Lerner RA, Green N, Alexander H, Liu F-T, Sutcliffe JG, Shinnick TM: Chemically synthesized peptides predicted from the nucleotide sequence of the hepatitis B virus genome elicit antibodies reactive with the native envelope protein of Dane particles. Proc Natl Acad Sci USA 78:3403, 1981

24. Loftus JC, Albrecht RM: Redistribution of the fibrinogen receptor of human platelets after surface activation. J Cell Biol 99:822, 1984

25. Loftus JC, Plow EF, Frelinger AL III, D'Souza SE, Dixon D, Lacy J, Sorge J, Ginsberg MH: Molecular cloning and chemical synthesis of a region of platelet GPIIb involved in adhesive function. Proc Natl Acad Sci USA 84:7114, 1987

26. Loftus J, Sorge J, Plow EF, Marguerie GA, Ginsberg MH: Molecular cloning of cDNA coding for a divalent cation regulated epitope in platelet membrane GPIIb. Clin Res 34:660A, 1986

27. McEver RP, Baenziger NL, Majerus PW: Isolation and quantitation of the platelet membrane glycoprotein deficient in thrombasthenia using a monoclonal hybridoma antibody. J Clin Invest 66:1311, 1980

28. Mehra V, Sweetser D, Young RA: Efficient mapping of protein antigenic determinants. Proc Natl Acad Sci USA 83:7013, 1986

29. Nunberg JH, Rodgers G, Gilbert JH, Snead RM: Method to map antigenic determinants recognized by monoclonal antibodies: Localization of a determinant of virus neutralization on the feline leukemia virus envelope protein gp70. Proc Natl Acad Sci USA 81:3675, 1984

30. Pegels JG, Bruynes ECE, Engelfriet CP, von dem Borne AEG Kr: Pseudothrombocytopenia: An immunologic study on platelet antibodies dependent on ethylene diamine tetra-acetate. Blood 59:157, 1982

31. Plow EF, Loftus J, Levin E, Fair D, Dixon D, Forsyth J, Ginsberg MH: Immunologic relationship between platelet membrane glycoprotein GPIIb/IIIa and cell surface molecules expressed by a variety of cells. Proc Natl Acad Sci USA 83:6002, 1986

32. Plow EF, Marguerie G: Inhibition of fibrinogen binding to human platelets by the tetrapeptide glycyl-L-prolyl-L-arginyl-L-proline. Proc Natl Acad Sci USA 79:3711, 1982

33. Reinach FC, Fischman DA: Recombinant DNA approach for defining the primary structure of monoclonal antibody epitopes. The analysis of a conformation-specific antibody to myosin light chain 2. J Mol Biol 181:411, 1985

34. Sadler JE, Shelton-Inloes BB, Sorace JM, Harlan JM, Titani K, Davie EW: Cloning and characterization to two cDNAs coding for human von Willebrand factor. Proc Natl Acad Sci USA 82:6394, 1985

35. Schmid CW, Jelinek WR: The Alu family of dispersed repetitive sequences. Science 216:1065, 1982

36. Schwarzbauer JE, Tamkun JW, Lemischka IR, Hynes RO: Three different fibronectin mRNAs arise by alternative splicing within the coding region. Cell 35:421, 1983

37. Seed B, Aruffo A: Molecular cloning of the CD2 antigen, the T-cell erythrocyte receptor, by a rapid immunoselection procedure. Proc Natl Acad Sci USA 84:3365, 1987

38. Shadle PJ, Ginsberg MH, Plow EF, Barondes SH: Platelet-collagen adhesion: Inhibition by a monoclonal antibody that binds glycoprotein IIb. J Cell Biol 99:2056, 1984

39. Shattil SJ, Hoxie JA, Cunningham M, Brass LF: Changes in the platelet membrane glycoprotein IIb–IIIa complex during platelet activation. J Biol Chem 260:11107, 1985

40. Tainer JA, Getzoff ED, Alexander H, Houghton RA, Olson AJ, Lerner RA, Hendrickson WA: The reactivity of anti-peptide antibodies is a function of the atomic mobility of sites in a protein. Nature 312:127, 1984

41. Tamkun JW, DeSimone DW, Fonda D, Patel RS, Buck C, Horwitz AF, Hynes RO: Structure of integrin, a glycoprotein involved in transmembrane linkage between fibronectin and actin. Cell 46:271, 1986

42. Tanaka T: Efficient generation of antibodies to oncoproteins by using synthetic peptide antigens. Proc Natl Acad Sci USA 82:3400, 1985

43. Weinberger C, Hollenberg SM, Ong ES, Harmon J, Brower ST, Cidlowski J, Thompson EB, Rosenfeld MG, Evans RM: Identification of human glucocorticoid receptor complementary DNA clones by epitope selection. Science 228:740, 1985

44. Young RA, Davis RW: Efficient isolation of genes by using antibody probes. Proc Natl Acad Sci USA 80:1194, 1983

Part Five Platelet-Associated IgG and Complement

16

The Origin and Significance of Platelet IgG

JAMES N. GEORGE

Platelets were first shown to contain IgG by Salmon in 1958.[81] Using the newly described technique of immunoelectrophoresis, he demonstrated that antibodies raised against human serum produced multiple immunoprecipitin arcs when tested against platelet lysates. One of these arcs was identified as IgG. In 1966, Davy and Lüscher next noted the presence of IgG in platelets and showed that it was present in a particulate fraction containing the platelet granules and that it was secreted from platelets stimulated by thrombin. Albumin was also noted to be present in the platelet particulate fraction and to be secreted following thrombin stimulation.[12,13] Thus, early in the development of knowledge about platelet structure and function, the two most abundant plasma proteins were recognized as platelet secretory proteins. These observations lay dormant for 20 years. When the concentration of platelet IgG was found to be higher in patients with idiopathic thrombocytopenic purpura (ITP),[15] a disease presumed to be mediated by immunologic platelet destruction,[29] an implicit assumption was made that platelet IgG was antiplatelet antibody. This immediately focused attention on the possible clinical utility of assays of platelet IgG. In spite of a recurrent concern that not all platelet IgG could reasonably be antiplatelet antibody,[32,62,74,83] the subcellular location of platelet IgG and its relationship to plasma IgG was not adequately addressed. Based on more recent findings, it now seems clear that almost all platelet IgG is located within the α granules, probably originating through endocytosis of plasma IgG by megakaryocytes.[22,23,26] Normal platelets also express a small amount of IgG, less than 1% of the total amount, on their plasma membrane surface.[22,50,54,82] The origin of this surface IgG on normal platelets and the mechanism of its binding to the platelet surface, whether by Fab or Fc association or both, remains unknown.

The goals of this chapter are to summarize our current knowledge of the origin and significance of platelet IgG. First, in the traditional format of a research publication, the methods of measuring IgG will be reviewed because an understanding of the different methods that have been used to quantitate platelet IgG is essential for correct interpretation of past reports. Current data will then be reviewed that now allow a clear definition of the distribution of IgG within the platelet, its relationship to the platelet content of other abundant plasma proteins, and the development of hypotheses for how platelets acquire IgG. Finally, abnormalities of total platelet IgG and platelet surface IgG in disease states will be discussed. The data in this final section emphasize the limitations of platelet IgG assays in the evaluation of thrombocytopenia and the importance of an understanding of the equilibration of plasma proteins with platelet α granules.

MEASUREMENT OF PLATELET IMMUNOGLOBULIN G

Assays for IgG can be performed in several ways, as diagrammed in Figure 16-1. The total content of IgG, measured in platelets solubilized with detergent or disrupted by a mechanical means, such as freezing and thawing, is approximately 5 fg, or 20,000 molecules per platelet. Secreted, α-granule IgG is measured in the supernatant fluid following its treatment with thrombin, the most effective stimulus for activation of washed platelets. In Figure 16-1, secreted IgG is conservatively illustrated as being over 90% of the total IgG, but essentially all platelet IgG is recovered in the supernatant fluid after thrombin stimulation.[22,23] Less than 1% of IgG is actually found on the platelet surface when adequate precautions are taken to prevent interference by intracellular IgG. With this knowledge, the past literature concerning measurements of platelet IgG can be interpreted in a new light, allowing a clearer understanding of the nature and significance of IgG in platelets from normal subjects and from patients with a variety of diseases.

Measurement of Total Platelet Immunoglobulin G

Table 16-1 presents a summary of previous reports in which quantitative results in femtograms (fg) of IgG per platelet were presented. Some studies clearly measured total IgG by assays of solubilized or mechanically disrupted platelets. Other studies are included in Table 16-1 in which total platelet IgG was obviously measured, as indicated by the quantity reported, even though the original method was interpreted as determining "surface" or "membrane-bound" IgG. The probable reasons for these discrepancies will be discussed later. Because two of the earlier methods were so influential in subsequent studies, they will be reviewed in detail.

The first method to measure platelet IgG was the ^{125}I-labeled Fab–anti-Fab technique described by McMillan et al.[58] In this method, rabbit antibody against human IgG Fab fragments is added to platelet (or standard IgG) samples for 24 hr at 4°C, then ^{125}I-labeled human Fab fragments are added to the incubation mixture for another 24 hr and, finally,

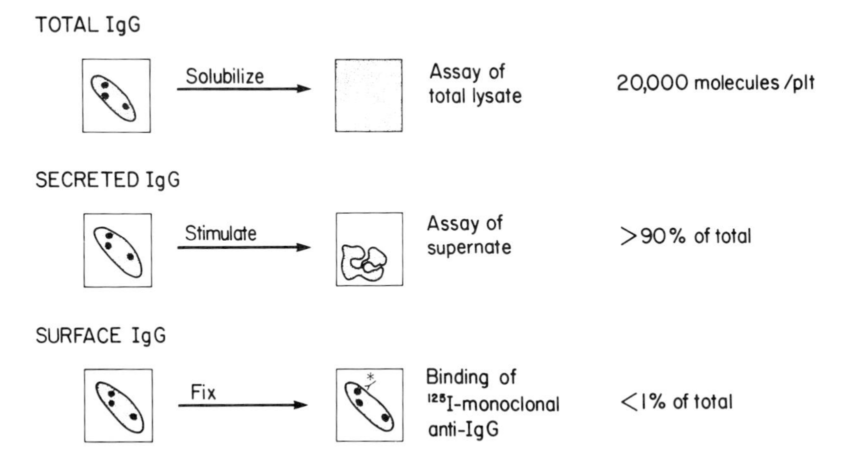

Figure 16-1. Measurement of platelet IgG. Three ways of measuring platelet IgG are illustrated. Total IgG is measured in solubilized platelets. In our laboratory, the normal total IgG equals 5 fg/platelet, equivalent to 20,000 molecules per platelet. Intracellular IgG that is secreted from α granules is measured in supernatant fluid after thrombin stimulation. In our laboratory, 90% to 100% of total platelet IgG is secreted in response to thrombin, 0.5 U/ml. Surface IgG is measured on fixed platelets by the binding of an ^{125}I-labeled monoclonal anti-IgG. In our laboratory, normal surface IgG equals 79 molecules per platelet, 0.4% of the total platelet IgG (George JN, Saucerman S: Blood 72:362, 1988, with permission).

Table 16-1
Total Platelet IgG. A Summary of Published Data on Normal Subjects and Patients with Idiopathic Thrombocytopenic Purpura (ITP)

Ref.	Method of Platelet Lysis	Method of IgG Assay	Normal Platelets (fg/platelet)	ITP Platelets Mean (fg/platelet)	ITP Platelets Highest Value (fg/platelet)
Luiken (55)	Freeze-thaw	^{125}I-labeled Fab-anti-Fab	1.2	5	17*
				19	56†
Hegde (30)	Unintentional	Anti-IgG consumption, C′ lysis	4.5	28	17*
Hymes (34)	Freeze-thaw	RIA	11.4	150	600
McGrath (57)	Unintentional	Anti-IgG consumption, C′ lysis	5.0		
Kelton (42)	Unintentional	Anti-IgG consumption, C′ lysis	4.7	42	81
Nel (69)	Unintentional	Anti-IgG consumption, ELISA	8.4	152	400
Rosse (79)	Unintentional	Anti-IgG consumption, C′ lysis	3.8		
Hegde (31)	Freeze-thaw	ELISA	10.0	33	82
Barrison (1)	Unintentional	Anti-IgG consumption, C′ lysis	2.8		
Pfueller (74)	Detergent	^{125}I-labeled Fab-anti-Fab	4.4		160
Morse (59)	Detergent	Immunodiffusion	3.8	20	71
Morse (60)	Detergent	Nephelometry	4.8		43
Kunicki (48)	Detergent	Electroimmunoassay	4.3		102
Cheung (6)	Sonication	RIA	3.3	12	113
Kelton (40)	Detergent	RIA	5.1		65
George (23)	Detergent	ELISA	5.4		
Blumberg (3)	Detergent	ELISA	5.3		
Court (11)	Freeze-thaw	RIA	9.9		
Hotchkiss (32)	Acid elution	RIA	1.4	104	750
Mean			5.2	57	187

References were included in which the total platelet content of IgG was measured. In six studies, the intention was to measure platelet surface IgG but the results indicated that total IgG was measured, presumably because the isolation and storage of platelets allowed α-granule secretion, and the secreted soluble IgG consumed the test antibody. When one author has reported multiple studies using the same method, a representative publication was selected.
Abbreviation used: RIA, radioimmunoassay; ELISA, enzyme-linked immunosorbant assay; C′, complement.
One femtogram of IgG = 4000 molecules.
*Data on 31 adults and children with chronic ITP.
†Data on six children with acute ITP.

ammonium sulfate is added to the mixture to achieve 50% saturation. More IgG in the sample binds more rabbit antihuman Fab, making less antihuman Fab available to subsequently bind to the ^{125}I-labeled human Fab added on day 2. Fifty percent saturated ammonium sulfate precipitates ^{125}I-labeled Fab bound to anti-Fab, whereas unbound ^{125}I-labeled Fab remains soluble. Therefore, with more IgG in the sample, more soluble ^{125}I-labeled Fab will be measured. The original report of 1.2 fg of IgG per platelet for "intact" platelets and 2.0 fg/platelet for lysed platelets was interpreted to indicate that 60% of IgG was on the platelet surface.[58] In their subsequent study,[55] only lysed platelets were used, and their normal value was 1.2 fg/platelet (*see* Table 16-1). It is clear that in the original report, lysis occurred in the "intact platelet" samples. Even though platelets were washed and, presumably, also resuspended in a buffer containing 10% rabbit serum, a procedure that should provide substantial protection against platelet lysis and secretion,[24] some α-granule secretion must have occurred during the 48-hr incubation.[21] Therefore, secreted α-granule IgG would become available to neutralize the rabbit antihuman Fab and create the impression of a high surface concentration of IgG on platelets that were assumed to be "intact." McMillan also demonstrated that IgG was removed from platelets by treatment with trypsin (1 mg/ml for 15 min at 37°C),[58] confirming an earlier observation of Nachman.[66] This result was also interpreted to support a surface location for platelet IgG. However, Davy and Lüscher had earlier demonstrated that trypsin, like thrombin, stimulates platelet secretion, and they demonstrated that complete secretion occurred with as little as 0.1 mg/ml trypsin for 15 min at 37°C.[13] Therefore, α-granule IgG would have been secreted and lost during trypsin treatment, causing the misinterpretation about the location of the platelet IgG measured.

With their report that platelet IgG was abnormally high in patients with ITP, Dixon et al.[15] were the first group to promote the measurement of platelet IgG as a clinical tool in the evaluation of thrombocytopenic patients. Their method was subsequently used by many other laboratories (*see* Table 16-1). Platelets (or standard IgG preparations) were incubated with rabbit antihuman IgG for 60 min at 37°C, then complement and human IgG-coated sheep red cells were added and hemolysis measured. Similarly to the assay described previously, greater amounts of IgG in the platelet or standard samples will consume more rabbit antihuman IgG antibody, making less of this rabbit antibody available for the subsequent red cell lysis. This method will measure all IgG present in the incubation mixture, whether or not it is platelet associated, because secreted, soluble IgG will also bind to and neutralize (or "consume") the anti-IgG antibody. Therefore, the technique of platelet isolation and incubation is critical. In the method of Dixon et al.,[15] "platelets were washed at least 5 times in isotonic (EDTA) and resuspended in isotonic sodium chloride," without buffer, protein, or colloid, and without reagents to prevent platelet activation. With these conditions, significant platelet lysis and secretion would be expected. However, Dixon et al. interpreted their data as demonstrating that platelet IgG was on the membrane surface.[15] As McMillan[58] had done previously, Dixon and co-workers also demonstrated the loss of platelet IgG following trypsin treatment (1 mg/ml for 60 min at 37°C), and interpreted this experiment as showing that IgG is on the platelet surface. The observation that platelet IgG is increased in ITP, together with the implicit assumption that platelet IgG is antiplatelet antibody, further supported the idea that the IgG was on the platelet surface. Dixon et al. gave the unrealistically high value for normal platelet IgG of 300 fg/platelet.[15] It must be assumed that this figure represents a calculation error, because in 1980, the same group, using the same method, published their value for normal platelets as 3.8 fg/platelet (*see* Table 16-1).[79] Five other groups have published data for normal platelet IgG using the method of Dixon et al.[1,30,42,57,69] In each report, anti-IgG consumption by complement-mediated hemolysis [or by enzyme-linked immunosorbent assay (ELISA) in one study] was measured (*see* Table 16-1). The average value for these six studies is 4.9 fg/platelet (SD = 1.7). This figure is no different than the average value for the 13 other studies presented in Table 16-1 in which the platelets were intentionally lysed to measure total IgG: 5.4 fg/platelet (SD = 3.0). Therefore, it can reasonably be assumed that these studies were unintentionally measuring total platelet IgG rather than surface IgG.

The preceding review of these previously published results emphasizes the technical problems that must be considered when developing an assay for the platelet IgG. Because total platelet IgG is essentially all contained within α-granules,[23] care must be taken to prevent α-granule secretion during blood collection and platelet isolation from plasma. The study of other α-granule proteins, such as platelet factor 4, has provided a basis for appreciating the importance of venipuncture technique and the inclusion of agents, such as prostaglandin E_1, (PGE_1), in the anticoagulant mixture to prevent platelet secretion.[51,52] Because plasma contains about 5000-fold as much IgG as the platelets in a given volume of whole blood, platelet washing must be effective in removing the preponderant amount of plasma IgG. In our initial study, we used platelets washed only twice.[23] Subsequently, we found that further washes remove additional plasma IgG and albumin, but even more plasma IgA (Table 16-2). Therefore, our current method involves four washes.[22] This change of methods resulted in a slight decrease

Table 16-2
Effect of the Number of Platelet Washes on the Total Platelet Content of IgG, IgA, and Albumin

Protein	Percent Remaining After Wash Number				
	2	3	4	5	6
IgG	100	92	89	86	85
IgA	100	82	77	71	69
Albumin	100	94	90	88	87

The data are the mean values for five experiments with IgG and IgA, three experiments with albumin. The value after two washes is arbitrarily assigned to be 100%.

in our normal IgG value from 5.4 to 5.0 fg/platelet. A compromise must be made between sufficient washing to remove plasma IgG and excessive in vitro manipulation that may cause α-granule secretion loss of platelet IgG. Another important variable is the completeness of IgG release from internal α-granule stores by platelet solubilization. In Figure 16-2 we have used Western blot analysis to assess our Lubrol solubilization method. All platelet IgG was in the Lubrol extract and none remained in the Lubrol-insoluble pellet. Comparison with our standard of purified IgG demonstrated that the extracted platelet IgG had an electrophoretic mobility identical with serum IgG. The apparent molecular mass (M_r) of IgG in this sodium dodecyl sulfate–polyacrylamide gel electrophoresis (SDS-PAGE) system (approximately 200 kD) is consistent with the aberrantly slow mobility of IgG noted by others.[47,71] Figure 16-2 also demonstrates the completeness of IgG secretion by thrombin; almost all of the platelet IgG was recovered in the supernatant fluid after thrombin stimulation and minimal IgG remained in the platelets. The platelet concentration of IgA is only 10% of the IgG concentration[22] and, therefore, the IgA band on the Western blot in Figure 16-2 was less intense than the IgG band. The behavior of IgA was the same as IgG: platelet IgA is totally extracted by Lubrol and totally secreted in response to thrombin stimulation.

Another potential technical difficulty in any IgG assay is the accuracy of the standard curve. Rosse et al. have addressed this problem and demonstrated that, for unknown reasons, the reaction of anti-IgG antibodies with fluid-phase IgG is stoichiometrically different from the reaction of the same antibodies with IgG bound to plastic wells.[80] This artifact can result in a ten-fold difference in assay results, depending upon the type of reference standard used. Immunoglobulin G also seems to be inherently unstable when stored in pure solutions. Although storage in the presence of albumin or in a glycine buffer may reduce aggregate formation, IgG aggregates inevitably form, and IgG solutions must be centrifuged immediately before each use. Repeated freezing and thawing seems to increase the potential for aggregate formation. In our initial studies, we used IgG purified from human serum by Rivanol-ammonium sulfate precipitation as our standard, documenting the purity by SDS-PAGE analysis (*see* Fig. 16-2).[23] The IgG was stored in aliquots in a glycine buffer containing 0.35% bovine serum albumin (BSA) at −70°C and, once thawed, never refrozen. Over the course of 2 years, however, we noted some variability in our values for normal total platelet IgG, attributable to variability in our standard curve. We suspect that even frozen samples of pure IgG may lose measurable antigen reactivity, with time, through aggregate formation and precipitation. Therefore, we changed our IgG standard to whole serum, stored in aliquots at −70°C with 0.1% Lubrol. The IgG concentration of these standards was determined by a standard nephelometric assay. The IgG antigen activity, assayed by ELISA, has remained stable in the frozen serum for over 1 year.

Our current method for measuring total platelet IgG, based upon the preceding considerations, is summarized in Table 16-3.

Measurement of Platelet Surface Immunoglobulin G

As noted in the previous section, a number of reports have purported to measure platelet surface IgG when, in fact, total IgG was measured.

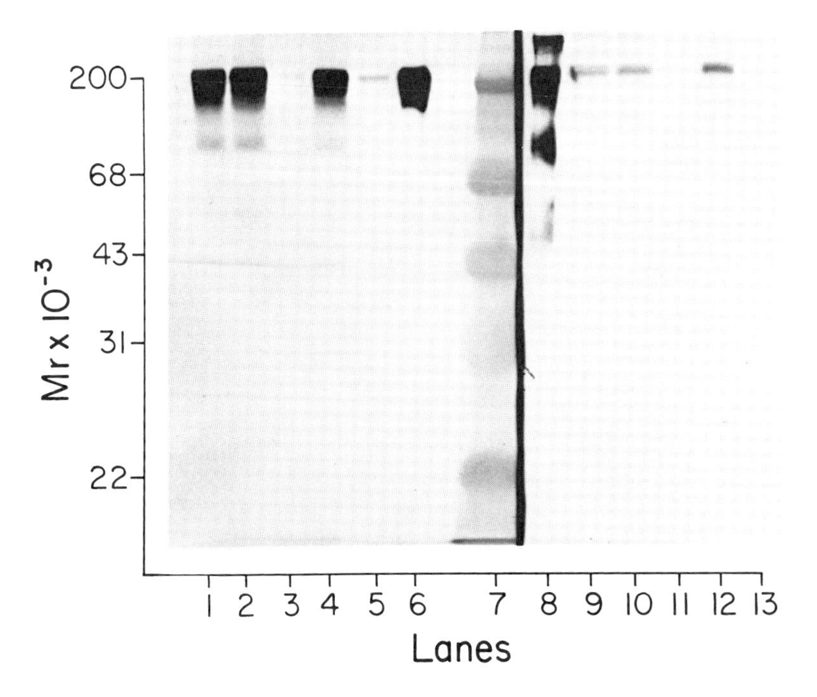

Figure 16-2. Platelet IgG and IgA: extraction by Lubrol detergent and secretion by thrombin. Samples are: Lanes 1 and 9: SDS-solubilized whole platelets; Lanes 2 and 10: Lubrol extract of platelets; Lanes 3 and 11: Lubrol-insoluble platelet pellet; Lanes 4 and 12: supernatant fluid after thrombin-induced platelet secretion; Lanes 5 and 13: platelets after thrombin-induced secretion; Lane 6: IgG standard; Lane 7: prestained M_r standards (Bethesda Research Laboratories): myosin, M_r, 200,000; β-galactosidase, M_r, 116,250; phosphorylase b, M_r, 97,400; bovine serum albumin, M_r, 68.000; ovalbumin, M_r, 43,000; carbonic anhydrase, M_r, 31,000; and soybean trypsin inhibitor, M_r, 22,000; and Lane 8: IgA standard (chromatographically purified human serum IgA, Cappel Scientific Division, Cooper Biomedical, Inc., Malvern, Pa.). The nitrocellulose, containing Lanes 1—6, was reacted with antihuman IgG; Lanes 8–13 with antihuman IgA.

Platelets were isolated from ACD-anticoagulated blood and washed four times in Tyrode's buffer, *p*H 6.5, containing 0.35% BSA and 50 ng/ml PGE_1, and resuspended to 8×10^8/ml in Tyrode's-BSA-PGE_1, *p*H 7.4, with 2mM Ca^{2+} and 1 mM Mg^{2+}. A 1-ml aliquot of platelets was incubated with human thrombin, 2 U/ml, at 37° C for 10 min, then the tube centrifuged at 1500 *g* for 10 min and the supernatant fluid removed and frozen. The platelet pellet was dispersed in 1 ml of Tyrode's resuspension buffer by sonication, solubilized in 0.5% Lubrol at 37° for 30 min, centrifuged at 12,000 *g* for 5 min, and the supernatant fluid removed and frozen for assay. Washed control platelets (1 ml at 8×10^8/ml) were similarly solubilized in 0.5% Lubrol and the Lubrol-insoluble pellet was obtained by centrifugation at 12,000 *g* for 5 min. The pellet was dispersed and solubilized as described above. The IgG standard was prepared by Rivanol and ammonium sulfate precipitation as previously described.[23] Samples were analyzed by the discontinuous SDS slab gel system of Laemmli,[45] with a stacking gel of 4% acrylamide and a separation gel containing a 7% to 12% exponential gradient of acrylamide. Samples contained 2×10^7 platelets for analysis of IgG, 6×10^7 platelets for IgA, or the volume of a supernatant or pellet fraction equivalent to these platelet numbers. Samples were solubilized in 2% SDS at 100° C for 5 min without disulfide reduction. After electrophoresis, proteins were transferred from the slab gel to nitrocellulose (0.45-μm pore size) using a Hoefer TE-42 "Transphor" electrophoresis cell (Hoefer Scientific Instruments, San Francisco, Calif.), following the manufacturer's instructions. After transfer, the nitrocellulose was blocked by incubation in 0.05% Tween 20 in PBS, pH 7.4, then incubated with either biotinylated affinity-purified goat antihuman IgG or IgA (Vector Laboratories, Burlingame, Calif.), 6.75 μg/ml, for 30 min. The membrane was washed in Tween-PBS and then the biotinylated antibodies were detected by the Vectastain avidin-biotin complex kit (Vector).

Table 16-3
Measurement of Total Platelet IgG in Solubilized Platelets by ELISA

1. Blood anticoagulated with 0.1 volume of 3.8% sodium citrate and 0.001 volume of 50 μg/ml PGE_1.
2. Platelet-rich plasma isolated and platelets washed four times in Tyrode's buffer, *p*H 6.5, containing 0.1% glucose, 0.35% BSA, and 50 ng/ml PGE_1.
3. Platelets resuspended to 10^8/ml in Tyrode's buffer, *p*H 7.4, containing glucose, BSA, PGE_1, plus 2 mM $CaCl_2$, and 1 mM $MgCl_2$.
4. Platelets solubilized by the addition of 0.05 volumes of 10% Lubrol at 37°C for 30 min. Centrifuged at 12,000 *g* for 5 min. Supernatant frozen.
5. Microtiter plate wells coated with 50 μl (10 μg/ml) of affinity-purified goat antihuman IgG in 0.05 M carbonate buffer, *p*H 9.6, overnight at 4°C.
6. Empty wells, fill with 1% gelatin in PBS for 15 min, wash twice with PBS containing 0.02% normal goat serum (NGS).
7. Add 50 μ of sample or standard. Samples, diluted five-fold in PBS, equivalent to 10^6 platelets in 0.1% Lubrol. Standard IgG: aliquots of standard human serum diluted to 0.5–8 ng of IgG/50 μl in PBS, 0.1% Lubrol. Incubate at 22°C for 60 min, then wash three times in PBS-NGS.
8. Add 50 μl containing 0.125 μg of biotinylated affinity-purified goat antihuman IgG in PBS, 1% gelatin. Incubate at 22°C for 30 min, then wash three times in PBS-NGS.
9. Add 50 μl avidin D-biotinylated horseradish peroxidase reagent. Incubate at 22°C for 30 min, then wash six times in PBS-NGS.
10. Add 50 μl *o*-phenylenediamine reagent in citrate buffer, *p*H 4.5, containing 0.03% H_2O_2. Incubate in dark at 22°C for 30 min, then measure color development at 450 nm.

The method is summarized from George et al.[23] The method of assay of IgA, IgM, and albumin is identical except for antibody specificity and the number of platelets contained in the sample. Abbreviations used are: PGE_1, prostaglandin E_1; BSA, bovine serum albumin; NGS, normal goat serum; PBS, phosphate-buffered saline.

Several investigators have attempted to specifically compare platelet surface IgG with total platelet IgG, reporting that the platelet surface IgG concentration is 1.3 to 1.8 fg/platelet (5200 to 7200 molecules per platelet), representing 35% to 45% of the total platelet IgG.[6,40,73] The total platelet IgG measured in each study was consistent with other reported data, presented in Table 16-1 (3.3–5.1 fg/platelet). However, the amount of IgG designated as being on the platelet surface is 50- to 100-fold greater than that measured by direct ^{125}I-labeled anti–IgG-binding assays (Table 16-4). As discussed earlier, the reason for this discrepancy seems to be that assays based on the principle of anti-IgG consumption are sensitive to leaked or to secreted soluble IgG, as well as to IgG actually associated with the platelet surface. In each of the three foregoing studies,[6,40,73] IgG was considered to be on the cell surface when intact platelets were assayed by an IgG-consumption method. However, in none of the assays were agents incorporated into the buffer to inhibit secretion. In two reports platelets were incubated in microtiter wells coated with IgG in the presence of labeled anti-IgG for either 2 hr or 12 to 24 hr.[6,73] It seems probable that platelet secretion occurred during this incubation, consuming some of the anti-IgG and competing with the solid-phase IgG. It may even be possible that IgG coated onto the surface of the well has platelet stimulatory properties similar to those of aggregated IgG[74], and thus it can accentuate platelet secretion. In the study by Kelton et al., intact platelets were incubated with ^{125}I-labeled anti-IgG for 30 min at 37°C in phosphate-buffered saline (PBS), then the unbound ^{125}I-labeled anti-IgG was measured by adding IgG-coated beads to the suspension for another 30 min.[40] Again, with no protein or platelet secretion-inhibiting agents in the incubation buffer, platelet secretion may have occurred and some ^{125}I-labeled anti-IgG may have reacted with soluble secreted IgG, as well as with platelet surface IgG. Again, the potential for stimulation of platelet secretion by IgG-coated beads must also be considered.

Therefore, accurate assessment of the surface concentration of IgG on platelets requires a direct-binding assay, in which platelets are documented to be intact, and only surface-bound anti-IgG is measured.

"Direct" Measurement of Platelet Surface Immunoglobulin G

Data from eight reports that measured only platelet surface IgG are presented in Table 16-4. The first reports of this nature, in 1979, were by Cines et al.[7] and Leporrier et al.[50] In both methods, polyclonal anti-IgG preparations were used as detection reagents so that a 1:1 ratio of bound anti-IgG/platelet surface IgG antigen could not be assumed. Previous

Table 16-4
Platelet Surface IgG. A Summary of Published Data on Normal Subjects, Patients with Idiopathic Thrombocytopenic Purpura (ITP), and Patients with Nonimmune Thrombocytopenia

Ref.	Platelet Preparation	Method of IgG Assay	Normal Platelets (molecules/platelet)	ITP Platelets (molecules/platelet)	Nonimmune Thrombocytopenia Platelets (molecules/platelet)
Cines (7)	Wash × 3	^{125}I-labeled polyclonal IgG	170* (70–350)	2000–48,000 (mean= approx 14,000)	1000–5000
Leporrier (50)	Wash × 6	Polyclonal anti-IgG-peroxidase	235 ± 74	800–21,000 (mean = 3800)	395 ± 200
LoBuglio (54)	Wash × 2	^{125}I-labeled monoclonal anti-IgG (HB-43)	169 ± 79	790–13,095 (mean= approx 2800)	246 ± 156
Rosse (80)	Wash × 3	^{125}I-labeled monoclonal anti-IgG (HB-43)	1060		
Shaw (82)	Wash × 2	^{125}I-labeled staphylococcal protein A	146 ± 112	approx 100–9645	<700
Janson (35)	Wash × 3	^{125}I-labeled monoclonal anti-IgG (HB-43)	400–1200		
Court (10)	Wash × 3	^{125}I-labeled monoclonal anti-IgG (HB-43)	122 ± 81	4120 ± 4043	338 ± 274
George (22)	Wash × 4, fix	^{125}I-labeled monoclonal anti-IgG (HB-43)	79 ± 27	1105 ± 1067 (range: 133–3982)	360–255 (range: 53–895)

Data are given as the mean ±1 SD. The normal data reported by Rosse et al.[80] represent only four values and were not intended to be a sample of normal subjects. The normal data reported by Janson et al.[35] were given only as the range. In some patient studies, data for this table had to be estimated from figures and are given as approximate values. 4000 molecules of IgG = 1 femtogram (fg).
*This is an estimate based on the assumptions of 50% specific binding of the antibody and a 7:1 ratio of polyclonal antibody molecules binding to platelet surface IgG (Cines, personal communication). The original reference reported 2400 "IgG combining sites per paletet."[7]

studies, in which polyclonal anti-IgG antibodies have been bound by red cells coated with a known concentration of alloantibodies or autoantibodies, have demonstrated an anti-IgG/cell surface IgG ratio as high as 7:1.[8,76] Cines et al. attempted to overcome this problem by relating anti-IgG binding to a standard curve derived from D-positive red cells coated with a known number of anti-D molecules.[7] One "anti–IgG-combining site" was defined as the amount of ^{125}I-labeled anti-IgG bound to one molecule of anti-D IgG antibody on red cells. By using this calculation, Cines et al. reported 2400 ± 1250 IgG combining sites per platelet in normal subjects.[7] In subsequent experiments, it was determined that on 50% of the rabbit polyclonal anti-IgG bound specifically to platelet surface IgG.* If one assumes that

*Cines, DB: Personal communication.

Cines' original figure of 2400 actually represented the number of anti-IgG molecules bound per platelet, and that one-half of these were specifically bound to platelet IgG, 1200 molecules of the polyclonal anti-IgG were reacting with platelet surface IgG. By further assuming that seven molecules of polyclonal anti-IgG bound molecules to each cell surface-bound IgG molecule, a figure of 170 ± 90 molecules of surface IgG per platelet is obtained. Therefore, this assay can be considered to be comparable with the assays using monoclonal anti-IgG reagents.

The assay of Leporrier et al. measured platelet IgG with peroxidase-conjugated polyclonal anti-IgG.[50] Their normal values of 235 ± 74 sites per platelet (*see* Table 16-4) were the first indication that only a small fraction of total platelet IgG exists on the membrane surface. This method had to assume a 1 : 1 molecular ratio both for the conjugation of peroxidase to anti-IgG, as well as for the binding of anti-IgG to platelet surface IgG. These assumptions were probably incorrect, for the reasons discussed earlier. Fortuitously, a peroxidase/antibody ratio of <1 must have compensated for an antibody/surface IgG ratio of >1.

In one report that did not use an anti-IgG antibody, Shaw et al. employed ^{125}I-labeled staphylococcal protein A and obtained results that were identical with those of studies using ^{125}I-labeled monoclonal anti-IgG antibodies.[82] Staphylococcal protein A binds to the Fc portion of IgG1, IgG2, and IgG4 molecules with an approximate stoichiometry of 1 : 1. A potential limitation of this method is the inability of staphylococcal protein A to bind to IgG3 molecules.

The remainder of the reports that have quantitated platelet surface IgG, presented in Table 16-4, have used the same murine monoclonal antibody as a detection reagent. This antibody, originally designated 1410KG7, was produced by J.D. Capra* and subsequently marketed by Bethesda Research Laboratories. The hybridoma producing this antibody is now available from the American Type Culture Collection (Rockville, Md.) under the designation ATCC HB-43. Murine ascites fluid containing HB-43 and the purified murine/HB-43 antibody are commercially available (Southern Biotechnology Associates, Birmingham, Ala.). Initial characterization of HB-43 by Capra demonstrated that it reacts with all IgG subclasses: with 16 different monoclonal IgG1 molecules, 8 IgG2 molecules, 8 IgG3 molecules, and 4 IgG4 molecules. Two-thirds of these contained κ light chains and one-third had λ light chains. HB-43 did not react with 17 IgA molecules, 12 IgM molecules, 3 IgD molecules, and 4 IgE molecules, nor did it react with 36 light chain isolates (urinary Bence-Jones proteins) of either κ or λ types.† Court et al.[11] and Rosse et al.[80] have confirmed these observations, demonstrating that HB-43 reacts equally with IgG1, IgG2, IgG3, and IgG4, that contain either κ or λ light chains, but not with IgA and IgM. Rosse et al. presented data suggesting that ^{125}I-labeled HB-43 detected only 53% of platelet surface IgG (quantified independently as bound anti-Pl^{A1} antibody molecules), that the binding was not saturable, and that binding was largely nonspecific because a 100-fold excess of nonradioactive antibody inhibited ^{125}I-labeled HB-43 binding by only 30%.[80] However, court et al. demonstrated that ^{125}I-labeled HB-43 bound to 91% of a known concentration of anti-D antibody molecules coated to D-positive red cells and also documented the specificity of ^{125}I-labeled HB-43 binding by demonstrating over 99% inhibition of binding by a 100-fold excess concentration of nonradioactive HB-43.[11] Our data on the specificity of ^{125}I-labeled HB-43 binding to normal platelets support the observations of Court et al.[11]

The reason why two of the studies in Table 16-4 that used ^{125}I-labeled HB-43 report higher values of platelet surface IgG[35,80] than those of the remaining six studies is unknown. One can speculate that a portion of the anti-IgG may have become altered or aggregated, or both, during iodination and storage, and that aggregates of ^{125}I-labeled anti-IgG bound to platelet surface Fc receptors. Karas et al. demonstrated that a 40-fold excess of IgG monomer inhibited only 50% of the binding of IgG dimers to the platelet Fc receptor[38] and, in the studies of Rosse et al.,[80] this could have been considered as "nonspecific" binding.

We have studied the binding of ^{125}I-labeled HB-43 to both normal platelets and to anti-Pl^{A1}-sensitized platelets. Our method is summarized in Table 16-5. Figure 16-3 demonstrates that the binding of HB-43 to normal

*Department of Microbiology, University of Texas Health Sciences Center at Dallas.

†Capra, J.D.: Personal communication.

Table 16-5
Measurement of Platelet Surface IgG Using ^{125}I-labeled HB-43, a Mouse Monoclonal Antibody to Human IgG

1. Blood anticoagulated with 0.1 volume of 3.8% sodium citrate and 0.001 volume of 50 μg/ml PGE_1.
2. Platelet-rich plasma isolated and platelets washed four times in Tyrode's buffer, *p*H 6.5, containing 0.1% glucose, 0.35% BSA, and 50 ng/ml PGE_1.
3. Platelets resuspended to 4×10^8/ml in Tyrode's buffer, *p*H 7.4, containing glucose, BSA, PGE_1, plus 2 mM EDTA.
4. Platelets were fixed by adding an equal volume of freshly prepared 3% paraformaldehyde in PBS, *p*H 7.2, and incubating at 22°C for 5 min.
5. ^{125}I-labeled HB-43 prepared by radioiodination, using lactoperoxidase/glucose oxidase beads, to achieve a specific activity of 1000–3000 cpm/ng. ^{125}I-labeled HB-43 was stored at 4°C in 0.05 M TRIS, 0.10 M glycine, *p*H 7.4, containing 0.35% BSA and 0.02% sodium azide. The antibody was centrifuged at 12,000 *g* at 4°C for 10 min immediately before each use.
6. 250 μl of fixed platelets were mixed in a capped microfuge tube with 1 μg ^{125}I-labeled HB-43 (approximately 5 μl) and the volume brought to 500 μl with TRIS-glycine-BSA, *p*H 7.4. Incubate with rotation at 22°C for 30 min.
7. Sample centrifuged at 12,000 *g* at 4°C for 5 min, and the undisturbed platelet pellet washed twice with centrifugation at 12,000 *g* at 4°C for 5 min. Supernatant fluid was aspirated and the tube tip cut off and cpm measured.

Abbreviations used are: PGE_1, prostaglandin E_1; BSA, bovine serum albumin.
(The method is summarized from George and Saucerman.[22])

platelets is saturable and specific. Two classes of binding sites were observed when the data were analyzed by the LIGAND computer program.[64] Although the number of binding sites on normal platelets was low, the conditions of the binding assay, as described in Table 16-5, allowed adequate counts per minute (cpm) to be measured in the platelet pellet. In our standard incubation of 1 μg of ^{125}I-labeled HB-43 (specific activity of 1000 to 3000 cpm/ng) with 2.5×10^7 platelets, normal platelets bound an average of 79 molecules per cell, represented by 1000 to 2000 cpm in the platelet pellet.[22]

The reason for two apparently distinct binding sites is unknown. They appeared to be independent, with no indication of cooperativity, as suggested by the observation that the slopes of Hill plots in each experiment were approximately 1.0. The higher-affinity sites had a K_d comparable after the K_d of ^{125}I-labeled HB-43 bound to anti-Pl^{A1}-coated platelets (Fig. 16-4). Therefore, the higher-affinity sites may represent IgG molecules bound to normal platelets by their Fab site, oriented in the same position as anti-Pl^{A1} antibody molecules bound to the platelet Pl^{A1} antigen.

The identity of the lower-affinity HB-43 binding sites is unknown. These are probably not simply "nonspecific" binding sites, because they appear to be saturable and are displaced by excess nonradioactive HB-43. In Figure 16-3, the nonspecific binding in the presence of 100-fold excess of nonradioactive HB-43 averaged 8.6% for the eight experimental points. To investigate the nature of the low-affinity HB-43-binding sites, we studied the effect of binding conditions (Table 16-6). Two independent binding sites were observed in all experiments. The use of an EDTA-containing buffer greatly reduced the number of low-affinity sites, and the remaining sites had a higher binding affinity. Two independent sites were also present when ^{125}I-labeled Fab fragments of HB-43 were used. The number of binding sites for Fab fragments was no different than that for intact HB-43 molecules, but their binding affinity was less. Because we suspected that the low-affinity binding sites may represent partially hidden IgG molecules with limited access to HB-43, we studied binding to thrombin-treated platelets. Thrombin treatment alters the display of platelet membrane surface antigens, allowing increased access of antibody to the surface-connected canalicular system.[21] Two distinct, independent binding sites persisted after thrombin treatment. The number of high-affinity binding sites may be slightly greater after thrombin treatment, but otherwise the data were similar to those obtained with unstimulated platelets. The possibility that the low-affinity sites represent platelet surface IgG buried within the surface-connected canalicular system thus seems unlikely. Additional evidence against this possibility is that the surface-connected, canalicular membrane system of untreated platelets is apparently accessible to Fab fragments of antibody.[91]

An alternative explanation for the low-affinity sites is that they represent IgG multimers that are oriented differently from specific antibody on the platelet surface, for example, by

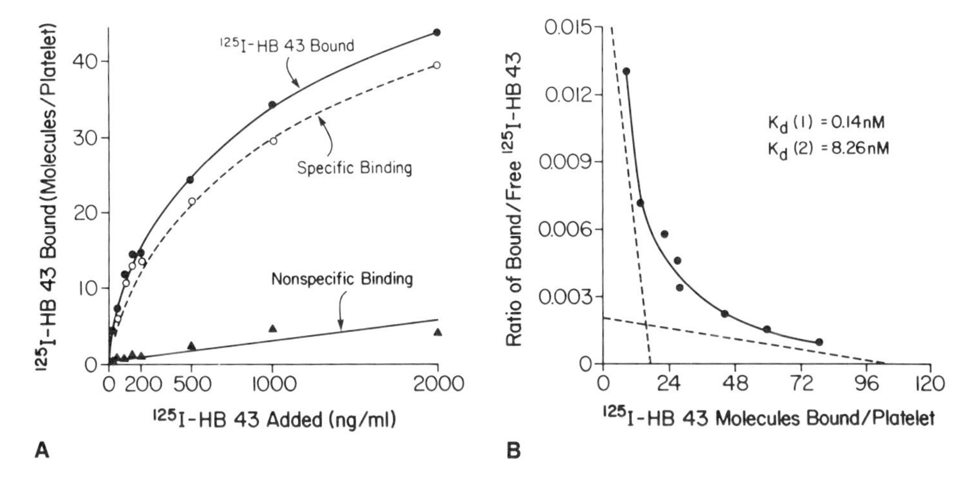

Figure 16-3. Binding of ^{125}I-labeled HB-43 to normal human platelets. Nonspecific binding was measured by adding a 1000-fold concentration of unlabeled HB-43 to the platelets immediately before the addition of ^{125}I-labeled-HB-43. The experimental method is given in Table 16-5. (*A*) presents a direct plot of the binding data. (*B*) presents a Scatchard analysis using the LIGAND program. The K_d and B_{max} values, also shown in Table 16-6, were calculated from the computer-derived (broken) lines.

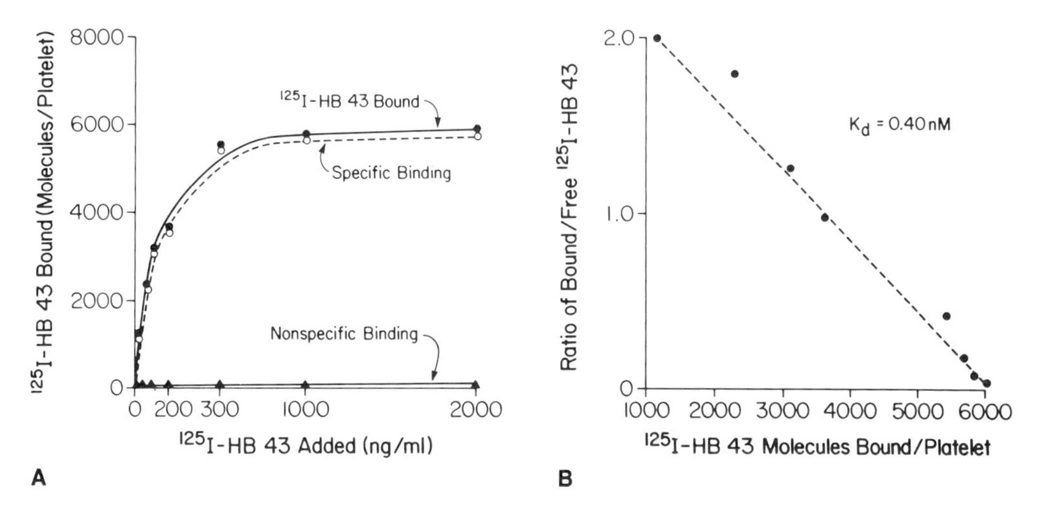

Figure 16-4. Binding of ^{125}I-labeled HB-43 to Pl^{A1}-positive platelets sensitized with anti-Pl^{A1} antibody. Platelets were isolated and fixed as described in Table 16-5, then incubated with a subsaturating concentration of anti-Pl^{A1} antibody, for 30 min at 37°C, conditions that had previously been shown to cause maximal platelet lysis with this antiserum. After this incubation, the platelets were washed four more times before measuring bound ^{125}I-labeled HB-43. Nonspecific binding was determined by addition of a 50-fold excess concentration of unlabeled HB-43 to the platelets immediately before the addition of ^{125}I-labeled HB-43. The experimental method is given in Table 16-5. (*A*) presents the direct plot of the data. (*B*) presents the Scatchard analysis by the LIGAND program. In contrast to ^{125}I-labeled HB-43 binding to untreated normal platelets (*see* Fig. 16-3), only a single class of high-affinity binding sites was present.

Table 16-6
Binding of ^{125}I-labeled HB-43, a Mouse Monoclonal Antibody to Human IgG, to Normal Human Platelets

Experimental Conditions	K_d (nM)	B_{max} (molecules/platelet)
Intact HB-43	0.3	19
$Ca^{++}-Mg^{2+}$ buffer (4)	810.0	2168
HB-43 Fab fragment	4.2	12
$CA^{2+}-Mg^{2+}$ buffer (1)	11,600.0	6048
Intact HB-43	0.1	10
EDTA buffer (3)	16.0	142
HB-43 Fab fragment	3.0	11
EDTA buffer (2)	313.0	129
Thrombin-treated platelets	1.0	81
Intact HB-43	13.2	199
EDTA buffer (2)		

Data are presented for the binding of intact ^{125}I-labeled HB-43 or ^{125}I-labeled HB-43 Fab fragments to normal, fixed, unstimulated platelets or thrombin-treated, fixed platelets. The number of experiments in each group is given in parentheses. In each experiment, the data were analyzed by computer using the LIGAND program,[64] and two independent classes of binding sites were apparent. For each site the dissociation constant (K_d) and maximum antibody molecules bound (B_{max}) are given.
Platelets were isolated from blood anticoagulated with 0.1 volume 3.8% sodium citrate containing PGE_1 (final whole blood concentration, 50 ng/ml) and washed four times in Tyrode's buffer, *p*H 6.5, containing 0.1% glucose, 0.35% BSA, and 50 ng/ml PGE_1. Washed platelets were resuspended in Tyrode's buffer, *p*H 7.4, with the same concentrations of glucose, BSA, and PGE_1 and also containing either 2 mM Ca^{2+} and 1 mM Mg^{2+}, or 4 mM EDTA. After resuspension, platelets were fixed by adding an equal volume of freshly prepared 3% of paraformaldehyde for 5 min at 22°C, then diluted with an equal volume of 0.05 M TRIS, 0.10 M glycine buffer, *p*H 7.4. Thrombin-treated platelets were incubated in a concentraation of 10^8/ml in 4 mM EDTA with 0.5 U/ml thrombin for 10 min at 37°C. The reaction was stopped by adding 2 U/ml hirudin, then the platelets were fixed as described above. Fab fragments of HB-43 were prepared by papain digestion with 10 mM β-mercaptoethanol for 4 hr at 37°C. The reaction was stopped by the addition of iodoacetamide, and Fab fragments isolated by DEAE-cellulose column chromatography. Binding assays were performed in 0.5-ml samples containing 0.5×10^8 platelets and 5-1000 ng of ^{125}I-labeled HB-43 or ^{125}I-labeled HB-43 (Fab). The antibodies were radioiodinated to a specific activity of 1000-3000 cpm/ng.[22] At each antibody concentration, nonspecific binding was determined by the addition of 50- to 1000-fold nonradioactive antibody.

attachment to Fc receptors.[38,78] This orientation may cause HB-43, which is directed against an epitope on the IgG Fc region, to bind less effectively and with a lower affinity.

Although defining the two independent binding sites for HB-43 on the platelet surface is important for a precise understanding of the nature of normal platelet surface IgG, this does not preclude routine clinical measurements of platelet surface IgG. As demonstrated in Figure 16-4, our standard ^{125}I-labeled HB-43 concentration of 2 μg/mg (13.3 nM) used in clinical studies[22] is a concentration 33-fold higher than the K_d of HB-43 binding to platelet surface antibody and is approximately eightfold greater than the concentration required to saturate 6000 molecules of antibody IgG on the platelet surface. The concentrations of HB-43 (0.8-1.0 μg/ml) used by LoBuglio et al.[54] and Court et al.[10,11] (*see* Table 16-4) would also be satisfactory single concentrations for estimation of the total number of high-affinity binding sites. In agreement with Court et al.,[11] the nonspecific binding of HB-43 to Pl^{A1}-sensitized platelets, in our hands, was less than 1% (*see* Fig. 16-4).

Because thrombin-stimulated platelets seemed to bind more HB-43 (*see* Table 16-6) and some secreted α-granule proteins are known to rebind to the platelet surface,[61] and because the platelet α-granule IgG concentration is much greater than the platelet surface IgG concentration, we were concerned that inadvertent platelet activation during blood collection and platelet preparation could significantly affect platelet surface IgG measurements. Also, because platelets are isolated from a plasma milieu that contains a 5000-fold greater concentration of IgG, we were concerned that if platelet activation even minimally enhanced the association of plasma IgG with the platelet surface, the number of surface IgG molecules could be greatly increased. To study this problem, we purposefully activated platelets in whole blood with low concentration of ADP and thrombin, then proceeded with the platelet isolation and ^{125}I-labeled HB-43 binding assay (Table 16-7). The agonist concentrations chosen caused a visible change in the appearance of the platelet pellet and notable difficulty in platelet resuspension during the washing procedure. Nonetheless, single platelets could be obtained. The thrombin concentrations used, 0.1 to 0.4 U/ml or 38 to 152 ng/ml, are capable of causing sizable platelet secretion,[36] and are similar to concentrations present in whole blood during clot formation.[85] These conditions caused no change in the amount of platelet surface IgG. Therefore, secreted IgG must bind minimally, or not at all, to the platelet surface, and platelet activation does not cause an increased association of plasma IgG with the platelet surface. This indicates that assays of platelet surface IgG are not vulnerable to significant artifactual changes if the blood collection of platelet isolation are complicated by the occurrence of platelet activation.

Table 16-7
Effect of Platelet Activation on the Platelet Surface Concentration of IgG

Platelet Sample	Platelet Surface IgG (molecules/platelet)
Control (3)	93 (75–107)
ADP-stimulated	
0.1 μM (1)	112
0.3 μM (2)	78 (76–79)
Thrombin-stimulated	
0.01 U/ml (1)	155
0.02 U/ml (2)	79 (66–92)
0.04 U/ml (1)	89

The data are the mean values for the number of experiments given in parentheses. The range of values is given in the right-hand column.
Blood was anticoagulated with 0.1 volume of 3.8% sodium citrate and 0.001 volume of 50 μg/ml PGE_1. Platelet-rich plasma (PRP) was obtained by centrifugation of 22°C. To aliquots of PRP, ADP or thrombin was added to achieve final concentrations of 0.1–0.3 μM ADP and 0.01–0.04 U/ml thrombin. The PRP was immediately centrifuged at 1500 *g* for 10 min at 22°C, the supernatant plasma was removed, Tyrode's EDTA buffer added, and the platelet pellet incubated for 15 min at 37°C before attempting resuspension. Then the platelets were washed four times and ^{125}I-labeled HB-43 binding measured as described in Table 16-5. Platelet resuspension was more difficult after ADP treatment, but adequate. In the sample treated with 0.04 U/ml thrombin, a plasma clot formed, but some platelets were recovered and resuspended satisfactorily with subsequent washing. No plasma clots were observed with 0.01 and 0.02 U/ml thrombin, although platelet resuspension during washing was noticeably more difficult than normal.

The data in Table 16-4 indicate that normal platelets have only about 100 molecules of IgG on their surface, but considerable variability among published reports is obvious. These differences probably represent variations in laboratory techniques. A critical step appears to be the preparation, storage, and use of ^{125}I-labeled HB-43. We design our radioiodination procedure to achieve a specific activity of 1000 to 3000 cpm/ng with over 98% of the labeled antibody precipitable by 10% tricloroacetic acid (TCA). Labeling to achieve a tenfold greater specific activity causes rapid loss of antibody binding to IgG. We store our labeled antibody at 4°C in 0.1 M glycine, 0.05 M TRIS buffer, pH 8.0, containing 0.35% bovine serum albumin and 0.02% sodium azide. Freezing and thawing or omission of albumin from the storage buffer also causes a loss of antibody activity. Before each use, the ^{125}I-labeled HB-43 is centrifuged in an Eppendorf microfuge at 12,000 *g* for 10 min at 4°C to remove aggregated complexes of IgG. These technical details seem important to avoid unpredictable results: either falsely high apparent binding caused by precipitable ^{125}I-labeled HB-43 complexes or binding of complexes to platelet Fc receptors, or falsely low apparent binding because of deterioration of antibody activity. Platelet preparation is also important. We have used four-times washed platelets because that number of washes appeared to be optimal for removal of trace contamination by plasma IgG (*see* Table 16-2). We fix the platelets with fresh paraformaldehyde, because our previous experience demonstrated unavoidable changes of platelet surface glycoproteins that occurred over a few hours at room temperature.[21] Even though we demonstrated that platelet activation, presumably causing secretion of the preponderant intracellular α-granule IgG, did not result in an increased number of platelet surface IgG molecules (*see* Table 16-7), we assumed that fixation would provide more stable platelets for a more reproducible assay. However, in four experiments, duplicate platelet samples that were assayed with or without paraformaldehyde fixation bound the same amount of ^{125}I-labeled HB-43 (Table 16-8).

"Indirect" Measurement of Platelet Surface Immunoglobulin G: Detection of Antiplatelet Antibodies in Plasma

Analogous to the indirect Coombs test, platelet IgG has also been measured after incubation of test platelets in allogeneic plasma under a variety of conditions. The assumption implicit in these studies was that an increase in platelet IgG after incubation in plasma results from the binding of antiplatelet antibody in the plasma. In some studies, total platelet IgG was actually being measured instead of the stated goal of measuring surface IgG. As an example, Hedge et al.[30] measured platelet IgG by the antiglobulin consumption-complement lysis assay of Dixon et al.[15] (*see* Table 16-1), obtaining a normal value of 4.5 fg (18,000 molecules) per platelet, which they referred to as "surface-bound IgG." Incubation of washed platelets in normal serum for 60 min at 37°C caused no increase in platelet IgG. Although this is not surprising, it is surprising that incubation of normal platelets in serum from 14 of 22 patients with ITP caused an increased platelet IgG, with values ranging up to almost 160,000 molecules per platelet. Kelton et al. used the same basic method of platelet IgG measurement to study sera from normal persons and from patients for "platelet-bindable" IgG, but found different results.[41] For the direct assay of platelet IgG, platelets were isolated from blood anticoagulated with 0.15% EDTA and their IgG content was 3.0 fg (12,000 molecules) per platelet. Although this was referred to as "platelet surface IgG," it represents most of the total platelet IgG. When platelets were isolated from EDTA-anticoagulated blood and then incubated with control serum (obtained by spontaneous clotting, then heat-inactivated; details not given), a value of 25 fg (100,000 molecules) of IgG per platelet was obtained. Although the details of incubation and postincubation washing are not given, higher IgG values for serum-incubated platelets occurred with all conditions tested. Others have reported similar data.

The explanations for these results are not clear, although it seems that under certain conditions of incubation, a significant amount of serum IgG can become associated with the platelets. An increase in total platelet IgG to 225 fg/platelet may still represent contamination by a negligible amount of serum IgG. Assuming an incubation with 10^8 platelets per milliliter[41] and a serum IgG concentration of 11 mg/ml (see Table 16-12), the increase of platelet IgG from 3 to 25 fg/platelet[41] represents a loss of only 2.2 μg of the total 11 mg of serum IgG, or 0.02%, into the platelet pellet. Perhaps the antiglobulin consumption method, which is sensitive not only to platelet IgG but also to all IgG in the incubation system, will detect 0.02% of trapped serum IgG after three washes, and perhaps patients with ITP may have complexes of IgG that are more difficult to separate from platelets by washing.

No analysis of the direct binding of ^{125}I-labeled HB-43 to assess the results of platelets incubated in serum has been published. The only mention of this type of experiment is found in the study of Court et al., who reported that platelets incubated in autologous or allogeneic plasma expressed an average of 447 and 471 molecules of IgG on their surface, respectively.[11] These values are 3.8-fold higher than the surface IgG found in a direct assay of washed platelets.[10] More recent data from the

Table 16-8
Effect of Paraformaldehyde Fixation on the Measurement of Platelet Surface IgG

	Platelet Surface IgG (molecules/platelet)	
Sample	***Unfixed***	***Fixed***
1	99	119
2	108	113
3	126	109
4	99	119
Mean ± SD	108 ± 11	115 ± 4

Blood was anticoagulated either with 5 mM EDTA (sample 1) or 0.38% sodium citrate (samples 2–4) and platelets were isolated and washed four times (*see* Table 16-4) immediately (samples 1–3) or after standing at 22°C for 2 hr (sample 4). Washed platelets were diluted with an equal volume of freshly prepared 3% paraformaldehyde in PBS or with the Tyrode's resuspension buffer, incubated at 22°C for 5 min, then further diluted with the TRIS (0.05M)-glycine (0.1M) buffer for the ^{125}I-labeled HB-43 binding assay, described in Table 16-5.

same laboratory, using unwashed platelets resuspended to 2×10^8/ml in acid, citrate, dextrose (ACD)-anticoagulated blood group AB plasma, incubated at 37°C for 1 hr, then washed three times before assay by ^{125}I-labeled HB-43 binding, demonstrated 657 (SD = 342) molecules of surface IgG per platelet in 32 experiments (range: 108 to 1218). This value is 5.4-fold higher than the number of molecules found in concurrent direct assays.* Similar results are obtained when the indirect assay is performed with a rabbit polyclonal anti-IgG. With EDTA-anticoagulated plasma incubated with allogeneic type O platelets for 45 min at 37°C, the value of platelet surface IgG was found to be 7.5-fold the amount measured in direct assays of washed platelets.† These results indicate that the apparently simple procedure of incubating platelets in normal plasma results in a significant increase in surface IgG.

We have performed preliminary experiments addressing this problem (Table 16-9). Platelets were washed and assayed by our standard direct method (*see* Table 16-5), and then aliquots of the washed platelets were incubated in the assay buffer (Tyrode's buffer containing 0.1% glucose, 0.35% bovine serum albumin, 50 ng/ml PGE_1, and 2 mM EDTA, pH 7.4), or in autologous plasma, or in allogeneic plasma from an ABO-matched individual who had had no risk for developing alloantibodies (no transfusions, no pregnancies). Incubation caused no change in platelet surface IgG. In confirmation of the observations of Court et al.[11] and the communications of Shaw, LoBuglio, and Cines just discussed, incubation in plasma, either autologous or allogeneic, caused more than a twofold increase in platelet surface IgG. The risk of this artifact is increased by simply freezing the plasma before incubation with platelets, which caused a fourfold increase in the amount of surface IgG observed. This must result from the formation of IgG aggregates, as the platelet-reactive IgG can be removed from frozen-thawed plasma by centrifugation at 12,000 for 10 min. Not shown in Table 16-9 are erratic results from earlier experiments conducted before the development of the systematic approach outlined in the legend to that table. We had observed on two separate days 1 month apart, using the same normal donor (JNG) and the method described in Table 16-9, the following results: day 1, direct assay of 72 molecules per platelet and, after incubation in fresh autologous plasma, 274 molecules per platelet; day 2, direct assay of 96 molecules per platelet and, after incubation in fresh autologous plasma, 5248 molecules per platelet! We have other isolated observations of such surprisingly high results.

In summary, assays for antiplatelet antibodies in plasma may be complicated by the reactivity of IgG even from fresh autologous, anticoagulated plasma with washed platelets. Routine procedures, such as the freezing of plasma, can increase the platelet-reactive IgG,

*Shaw, D.R. and LoBuglio, A.F.: Personal communication.

†Cines, D.B.: Personal communication.

Table 16-9
Comparison of the Direct Assay of Platelet Surface IgG to Assays Following Incubation in Buffer, Autologous Plasma, or Allogeneic Plasma

Platelet Sample	Platelet Surface IgG (molecules/platelet)
Direct assay	88 ± 28 (7)
Incubated platelets	
Buffer	101 ± 32 (7)
Fresh autologous plasma	225 ± 86 (4)
Frozen autologous plasma	914 ± 254 (3)
Frozen, spun autologous plasma	260 ± 68 (3)
Fresh allogeneic plasma	233 ± 116 (8)

The data are the mean values ±1 SD for the number of experiments shown in parentheses. Buffer-incubated platelets were not different from the directly assayed platelets. Platelets incubated in plasma all had more surface IgG than control platelets incubated in buffer ($p < 0.05$). Platelets incubated in frozen plasma had more surface IgG than platelets incubated in fresh plasma ($p < 0.01$); and platelets incubated in frozen, spun plasma had less surface IgG than platelets incubated in unspun frozen plasma ($p < 0.005$). Allogeneic plasma was no different than autologous plasma.
Platelet surface IgG was measured by the binding of ^{125}I-labeled HB-43, as described in Table 16-5. In the direct assay, platelets were washed four times and resuspended in Tyrode's buffer containing 4 mM EDTA. For the indirect assays, platelets, 4×10^8/ml, were incubated for 30 min at 37°C with buffer or plasma. Plasma was obtained from blood anticoagulated with 5 mM EDTA, 50 ng/ml PGE_1 (final concentrations) by centrifugation at 1500 *g* for 10 min. Frozen plasmas were stored at −20°C for at least 24 hr. Centrifugation of plasma samples after freezing and thawing was performed at 12,000 *g* for 10 min at 4°C. Allogeneic plsma samples were obtained from ABO-matched donors who had had no opportunity for alloimmunization by transfusion or pregnancy. Following the 30 min incubation, the platelets were washed four more times, fixed, and assayed.

and other unknown variables can cause extreme inconsistency in this type of assay. Therefore, reports of assays aimed at the detection of antiplatelet antibodies in plasma must be interpreted with caution.

THE α-GRANULE LOCATION OF PLATELET IMMUNOGLOBULIN G AND ITS ORIGIN FROM PLASMA

Davy and Lüscher originally observed that platelet IgG was secreted in response to thrombin stimulation and was located in a dense particulate fraction when homogenized platelets were separated in a sucrose density gradient.[12] The particulate fraction enriched in IgG was heterogeneous, containing membrane vesicles, lyzosomes, and α granules.[86] However, as reviewed previously, subsequent data were interpreted to suggest that platelet IgG was located on the cell surface. On the assumption, from the recent literature, that platelet IgG was largely on the cell surface, we developed an assay for total IgG in Lubrol-solubilized platelets with the intention of studying the nature of the platelet surface IgG in normal platelets. Our hypothesis was that this may be an accumulation of naturally occurring antibodies interacting with senescence anti-

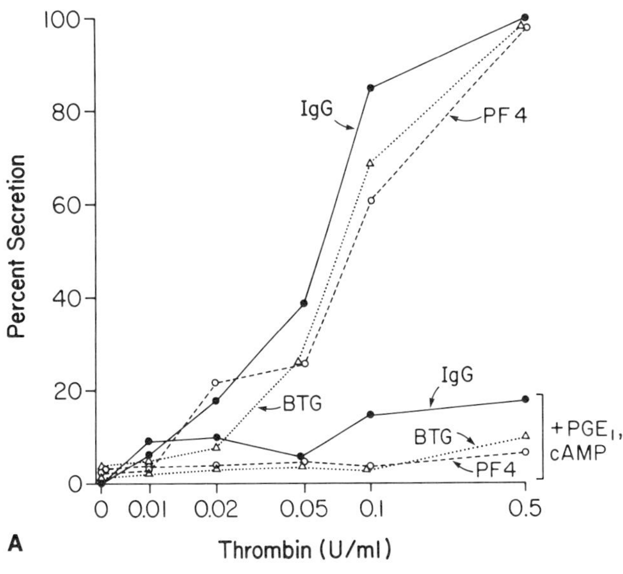

Figure 16-5. Secretion of platelet IgG, platelet factor 4 (PF4), and β-thromboglobulin (βTG). Washed platelets, 10^8/ml, were treated with different concentrations of thrombin (*A*), ionophore (*B*), ADP (*C*), or buffer alone, at 37°C for 10 min. Secretion was measured by comparing supernatant concentrations to whole platelet concentrations of the three proteins. Where indicated, PGE_1 (10 μg/ml) and dibutyryl-cyclic AMP (1 mM) were added before thrombin (George JN, Saucerman S, Levine SP et al: J Clin Invest 76:2020, 1985, with permission).

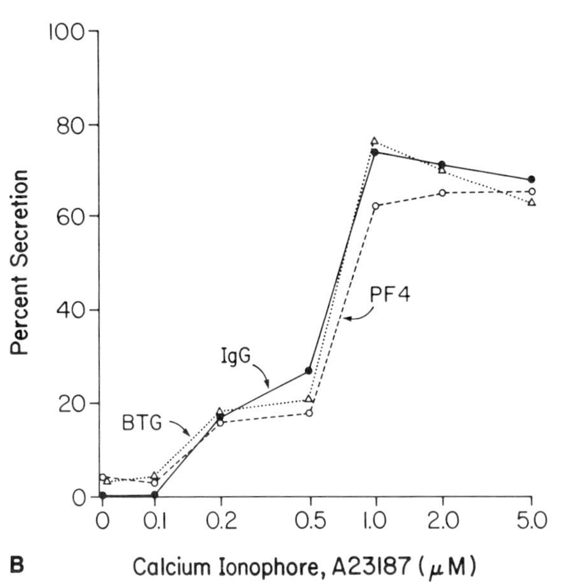

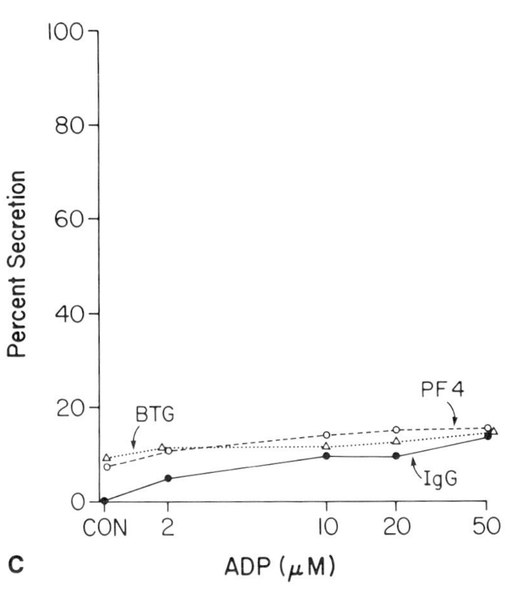

gens.[20] In our initial experiment to determine the subcellular location of platelet IgG, we measured IgG in thrombin-treated platelets, a standard technique in our laboratory used to assess one intracellular protein pool, the α granules. To our surprise, IgG was totally secreted from the thrombin-stimulated platelets! Experiments with Dr. S. Levine demonstrated that the secretion of IgG was parallel and quantitatively identical with the secretion of two known β-granule proteins, platelet factor 4 and β-thromboglobulin, with a variety of agonists: thrombin, thrombin inhibited by PGE_1 and cyclic AMP, calcium ionophore A23187, and ADP (Fig. 16-5). Further studies in collaboration with Dr. D. Bainton demonstrated conclusively the α-granule location of platelet IgG by morphologic analysis (Fig. 16-6). Essentially all

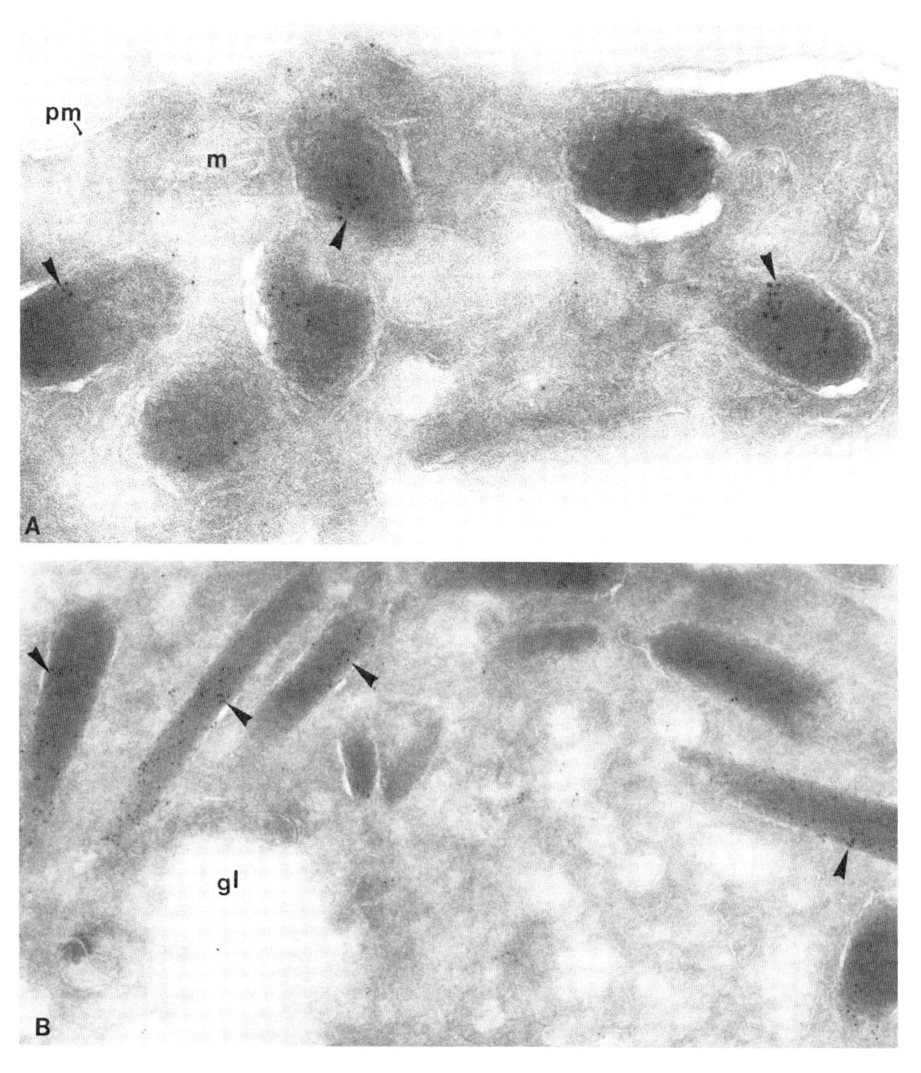

Figure 16-6. Transmission electron micrographs showing the α-granule location of IgG in resting platelets. The frozen thin sections were incubated with anti-IgG and then the immunogold probe, GAR-5 (goat antirabbit IgG linked to 5-nm colloidal gold particles), was applied. Note label (arrows) over many of the α granules. The α granules are heterogeneous in size and shape, and elongated granules, as shown in (*B*), are commonly seen in our preparations of unanticoagulated blood that have been fixed immediately after venipuncture at 37°C. pm, plasma membrane; m, mitochondria. The other intracellular membranes probably represent surface-connected cannicular system. The large extracted area is glycogen (gl). (Original magnifications: *A*, × 100,000; *B*, × 50,000; George JN, Saucerman S, Levine SP et al: J Clin Invest 76:2020, 1985, with permission).

platelet IgG, over 99%, was contained in α granules,[20] thereby confirming the earlier observations of Davy and Lüscher.[12,14]

Not only IgG, but also the major plasma protein, albumin, has been localized to platelet α granules.[87] For this reason, we studied albumin and IgA as examples of other abundant plasma proteins and demonstrated that, like IgG, they were also completely secreted from platelets in response to thrombin and ionophore (Fig. 16-7).

Previous data have suggested an equilibrium between the platelet and plasma pools of plasma proteins. For example, McMillan et al. reported absent platelet IgG in a patient with agammaglobulinemia,[58] and McGrath et al. reported increased platelet IgG concentrations in patients with IgG myeloma and benign hypergammaglobulinemia, but not in patients with IgA myeloma.[57] Previous studies have also demonstrated that platelet IgG has a distribution of heavy-chain subtypes similar to plasma

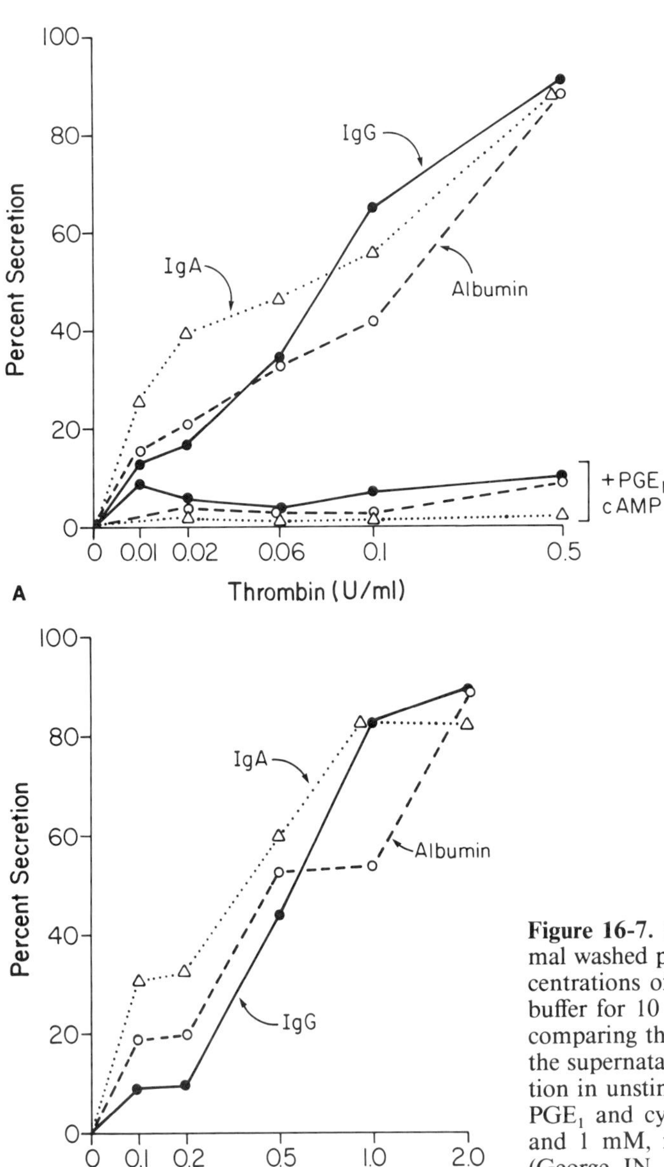

Figure 16-7. Secretion of IgG, IgA, and albumin. Normal washed platelets were incubated with different concentrations of thrombin (*A*) or ionophore (*B*) or with buffer for 10 min at 37°C. Secretion was measured by comparing the concentration IgG, IgA, and albumin in the supernatant fluid with the corresponding concentration in unstimulated control platelets. Where indicated, PGE_1 and cyclic-AMP (final concentrations, 10 μg/ml and 1 mM, respectively) were added before thrombin (George JN, Saucerman S: Blood 72:362, 1988, with permission).

Table 16-10
Comparison of IgG Heavy-Chain Subtypes in Platelets and Plasma

	IgG_1	IgG_2	IgG_3	IgG_4
	(% distribution)			
Normal plasma*	68	21	7	4
Normal platelets†	62	21	5	12
ITP platelets†	56	18	9	17
ITP platelets‡	65	21	9	4

The data are from: *Natvig and Kunkel,[68] who averaged the results from four earlier studies; †Rosse et al.[80] and ‡Hymes et al.[33]

IgG (Table 16-10). We have demonstrated a close correlation between the total platelet and serum concentrations of IgG, IgA, and albumin in normal subjects (Fig. 16-8).[22] These data demonstrate that platelet α granules contain the major plasma proteins, and that their α-granule concentration is proportional to their plasma concentration. It is possible that platelet α granules may contain all plasma proteins, proportional to their plasma concentration.

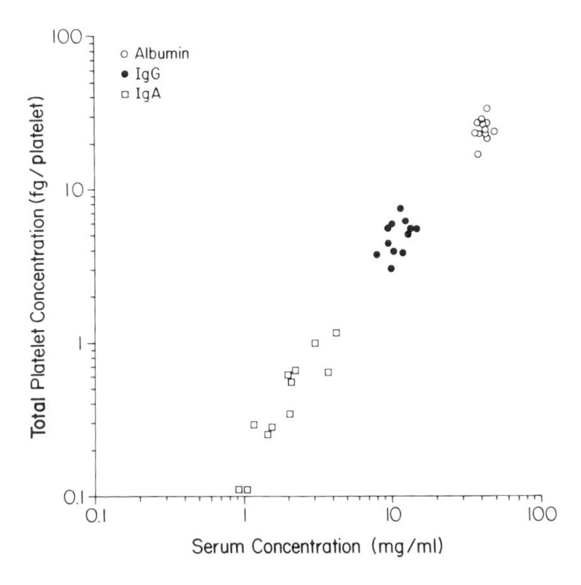

Figure 16-8. Correlation of total platelet and serum concentrations of IgG, IgA, and albumin in normal subjects. The data are presented on a double logarithmic scale for conciseness of illustration. When the data were plotted on a linear scale, they fit a straight line ($y = -1.11 + 0.59x$) with a correlation coefficient (r) of 0.98. IgM was not measurable in normal platelets. For IgG, 1 fg = 4000 molecules (George JN, Saucerman S: Blood 72:362, 1988, with permission).

A recent study by Handagama et al. demonstrated that megakaryocytes can incorporate a circulating protein into developing α granules.[26] Horseradish peroxidase, a protein tracer with a relative molecular mass of 40,000, was injected intravenously into guinea pigs and its uptake into megakaryocyte α granules was rapid and extensive. Figure 16-9 presents electron micrographs of megakaryocytes, demonstrating detectable peroxidase reaction with coated vesicles by 45 min and positive reaction in approximately one-half of the α granules by 75 min. No peroxidase reaction product was seen in the Golgi complex, supporting the hypothesis that the peroxidase was incorporated from the external milieu by endocytosis and not by endogenous synthesis with passage through the Golgi complex. Figure 16-10 illustrates circulating platelets with peroxidase-positive α granules 7 hr after the injection of horseradish peroxidase. When these platelets were stimulated with thrombin, peroxidase was completely secreted (*see* Fig. 16-10). More recent experiments by Handagama et al.[25,27] have demonstrated the same pattern and time course of uptake of intravenously injected human albumin, biotinylated guinea pig albumin, and human IgG by guinea pig megakaryocytes. These studies provide evidence that megakaryocytes possess an endocytic mechanism for uptake and concentration of circulating proteins into secretory granules.

A distinction between the platelet α-granule incorporation of the plasma proteins, IgG and albumin, and endogenously synthesized α-granule proteins is apparent in the gray platelet syndrome. In this rare hereditary disorder, there is a defective formation of α granules and a selective deficiency of α-granule proteins (Table 16-11). However, among the α-granule proteins, IgG and albumin are preserved at

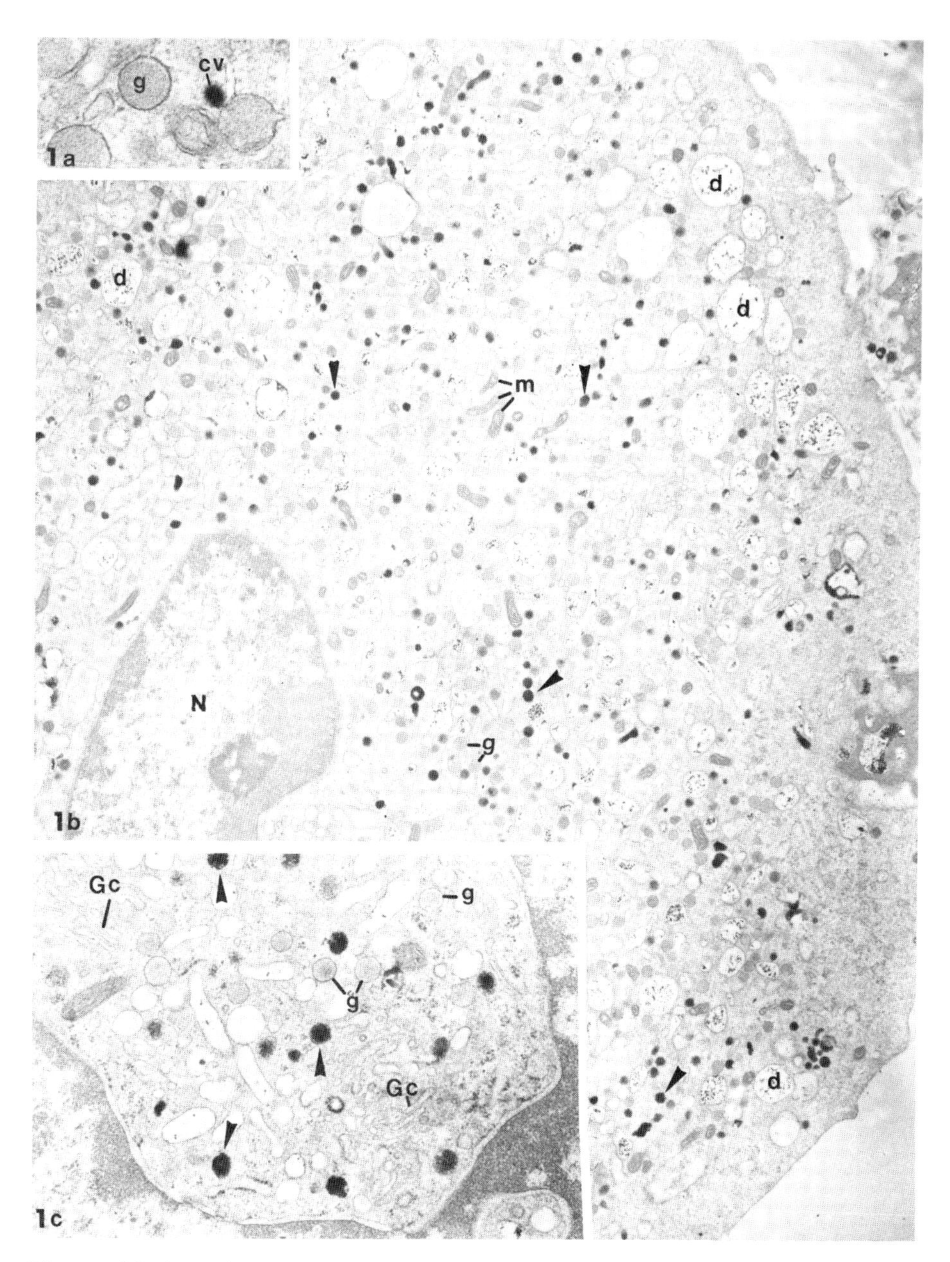

Figure 16-9. Maturing megakaryocytes were isolated at various times after intravenous injection of horseradish peroxidase (HRP) into guinea pigs and assayed for peroxidase activity. (*1a*) At 45 min, coated vesicles (cv) contained dense peroxidase reaction product. The adjacent α granules (g) were peroxidase negative. (*1b*) at 75 min, moderate amounts of enzyme reaction product were present within the demarcation membrane system (d). Many of the granules were peroxidase-positive (arrowheads), although some were peroxidase-negative (g). N, nucleus; m, mitochondrion. This point is better appreciated at higher magnification, as shown in *1c*. The Golgi complex (Gc) was never peroxidase-positive, whereas some of the adjacent granules (arrowheads) contained HRP (original magnifications: *1a*, × 63,400; *1b*, × 12,480; *1c*, × 23,000; Handagama PJ, George JN, Shuman MA et al: Proc Natl Acad Sci USA 84:861, 1987).

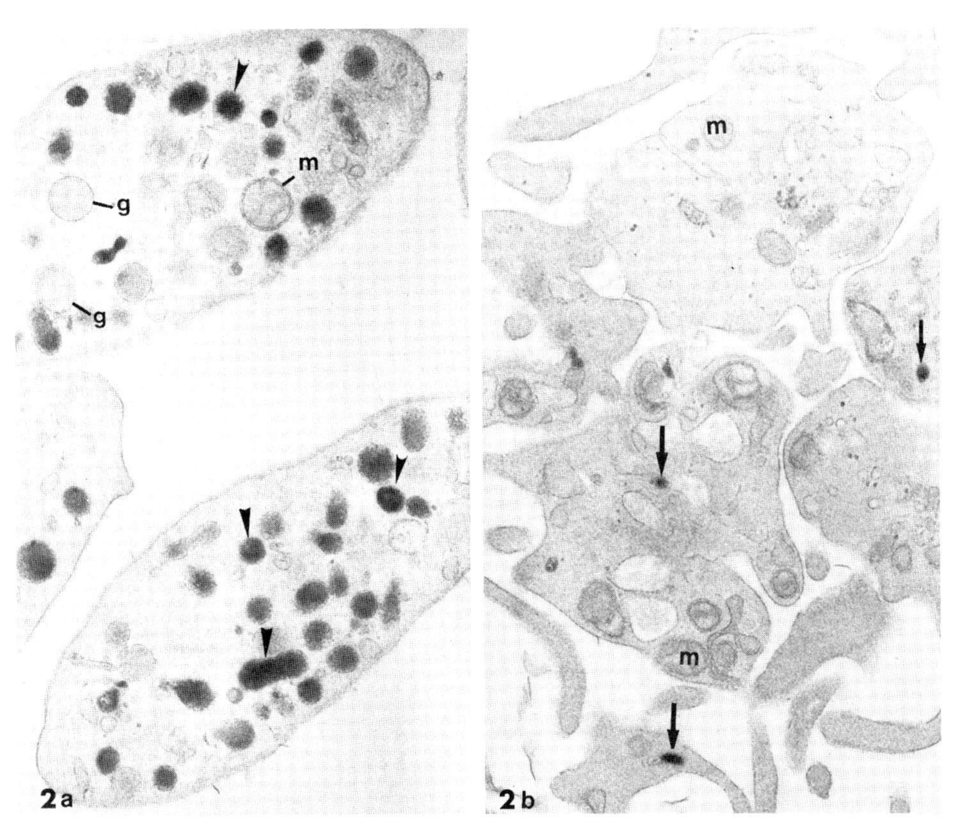

Figure 16-10. Guinea pig platelets from blood collected 7 h after the injection of horseradish peroxidase. (*2a*) Peroxidase reaction product was found exclusively in granules (arrowheads), although some granules (g) were negative. (*2b*) When these platelets were stimulated with thrombin, shape change occurred and almost all the granules were secreted. Only limited amounts of residual enzyme could be observed in some platelets (arrows). M, Mitochondrion (original magnifications: (*2a*, × 32,600; *2b*, × 35,500; Handagama PJ, George JN, Shuman MA et al: Proc Natl Acad Sci USA 84:861, 1987).

Table 16-11
Platelet Concentrations of α-Granule Proteins in the Gray Platelet Syndrome

α-Granule Protein	Platelet Concentration (% or normal)	Data from Refs.
Platelet factor 4	< 5%	2, 19
α-Thromboglobulin	< 5%	2, 19, 53
von Willebrand factor	< 5%	2, 71
Thrombospondin	Absent	2, 19, 71
Fibrinogen	<10%	2, 71
Fibronectin	< 5%	71
Platelet-derived growth factor	Absent	19
IgG	62%	77
Albumin	47%, 46%	71, 77

about half normal concentrations. Rosa et al. have developed a hypothesis that the defect in the gray platelet syndrome may be the absence of a signal molecule that targets newly synthesized secretory proteins to α granules.[77] Without this signal the proteins are constitutively secreted and the α granules remain undeveloped vacuoles. In this hypothesis, plasma proteins, such as IgG and albumin, are normally endocytosed but incompletely incorporated into the defective α granules. However, gray platelets can still effectively secrete their contents of IgG and albumin.[77]

Therefore, our current understanding is that almost all platelet IgG is contained within α granules and is secreted in response to stimulation by physiologic agonists. Megakaryocytes may acquire IgG by endocytosis from the plasma, and this would explain why the α-granule IgG concentration correlates with the plasma IgG level. Other plasma proteins, such as albumin and IgA, may also be endocytosed by megakaryocytes and packaged into α granules, and their platelet concentration would also be expected to correlate with their plasma concentration, as is observed. In this model, only a small fraction of platelet IgG, less than 1%, is on the platelet surface and may potentially represent antibody specific for surface antigens.

PLATELET IMMUNOGLOBULIN G IN DISEASE STATES

The goal of most studies on platelet IgG has been to develop a clinical assay analogous to that used in red cell serology, the Coombs test. The development of a technique to identify weak and "incomplete" Rh agglutinins on red cells by Coombs and coworkers, in 1945,[9] and its prompt application to the identification of autoimmune hemolytic anemia by Boorman and associates, in 1946,[4] were landmark investigations. The Coombs test, the detection of IgG on the red cell surface that could cause agglutination in the presence of heterologous anti-IgG, quickly became a routine laboratory method. In 1951, Harrington et al. dramatically demonstrated that whole blood, or plasma, from ITP patients could cause severe thrombocytopenia when infused into normal volunteers.[29] These investigators concluded that the pathogenesis of ITP and autoimmune hemolytic anemia was similar, and it must have seemed that the serologic evaluation of autoimmune platelet disorders would also soon be established. Now, 36 years later, the significance of platelet IgG assays is still unclear, leading Harrington, himself, to title a recent editorial, *Are platelet antibody tests worthwhile?*[28]

Total Platelet Immunoglobulin G

The values for total IgG in normal platelets in 19 studies from seven laboratories over a 10-year period are very consistent, averaging 5.2 fg/platelet, or 20,800 molecules per platelet (*see* Table 16-1). Even more impressive than the great amount of IgG present in normal platelets are the enormous quantities found in the platelets of patients with ITP. Table 16-1 records ten studies in which the average patient with ITP had a platelet IgG concentration of 57 fg/platelet, equivalent to 228,000 molecules per platelet. In 14 studies, the highest reported values averaged 187 fg/platelet, or 748,000 molecules per platelet. The highest value recorded in Table 16-1 is 750 fg/platelet, or 3 million molecules per platelet. The enormity of this IgG concentrations must be viewed in light of observations that platelets can be rapidly destroyed in vivo by drug-dependent antibodies or alloantibodies at concentrations of 200 to 800 molecules per platelet (0.05–0.2 fg/platelet).[83] One would, thus, suspect that not all of the IgG found in ITP platelets is specific antibody, for these levels exceed, by more than 1000-fold, the amount of antibody that can cause platelet destruction. Because platelet IgG was originally thought to be on the cell surface, common hypotheses incorporated the idea that younger platelets somehow absorbed more plasma IgG. When the platelet content of other plasma proteins was also found to be increased in ITP, [32,44] a more generalized platelet membrane abnormality in ITP was postulated, one that caused trapping of plasma proteins.

A notable frequency of high platelet IgG levels has also been found in apparently nonimmune thrombocytopenia. For example, Barrison et al. reported that platelet IgG was increased in 14 patients with alcoholic liver cirrhosis: their mean platelet IgG was 82 fg/platelet compared with the normal value of 2.8 fg/platelet.[1] Similar observations have been made by Mueller-Eckhardt et al.[63] and Panzer et al.[72] Additional data from this laboratory have further documented that circulating immune complexes have no definite role in the pathogenesis of ITP.[46]

Kelton et al. reported a prospective study, in 1982, on the clinical usefulness of platelet IgG assays. They found that an elevated platelet IgG had a strong association with decreased platelet counts, regardless of the etiology as determined by clinical evaluation. They concluded that measurement of platelet IgG was of limited value in the diagnosis of ITP, but they still considered that platelet IgG was equivalent to antiplatelet antibody and, therefore, suggested "that immune mechanisms mediate many more thrombocytopenic disorders than had been previously thought likely."[43]

The implicit assumption that platelet IgG is antiplatelet antibody severely limited previous interpretations. Now platelet IgG must be considered simply as the α-granule pool of an abundant plasma protein, comparable with albumin, and past data need to be reinterpreted in the light of this knowledge.

We have found a close correlation between the total platelet concentrations of IgG, IgA, IgM, and albumin and their respective serum concentrations in normal subjects, in patients with abnormalities of their plasma proteins, and in patients with ITP.[22] In normal subjects, the total platelet and serum concentrations of IgG, IgA, and albumin had exhibited a near perfect correlation (*see* Fig. 16-7). In patients with abnormal serum protein concentrations, the data were more scattered, but the correlation was still highly significant (Fig. 16-11). For example, patients with IgA myeloma and very high serum concentrations of IgA had comparably high total-platelet IgA. Patients with advanced liver cirrhosis and low serum albumin concentrations had comparably low total-platelet albumin. These data are also presented in Table 16-12. The calculated regression lines for the comparison of total-platelet and serum concentrations of IgG, IgA, and albumin were the same (Fig. 16-12), consistent with an equilibration of these proteins between their platelet and plasma compartments. Platelet IgM was not measurable in normal subjects, indicating a concentration less than 0.1 fg (68 molecules) per platelet, but it was measurable in four patients with macroglobulinemia, again indicating a correlation between plasma and platelet compartments (*see* Fig. 16-11). However, the data for IgM was different from the regression line calculated for IgG, IgA, and albumin, suggesting that IgM had less access to the platelet compartment. This may reflect the more limited extravascular distribution of IgM (24%) compared with IgG, IgA, and albumin (48–55%)[88,89] and, therefore, less incorporation into developing α-granules by marrow megakaryocytes.

The data on patients with ITP were differ-

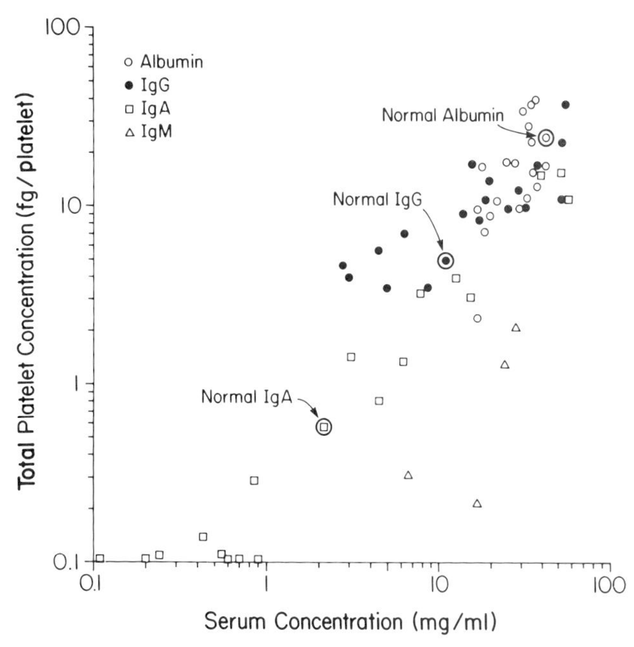

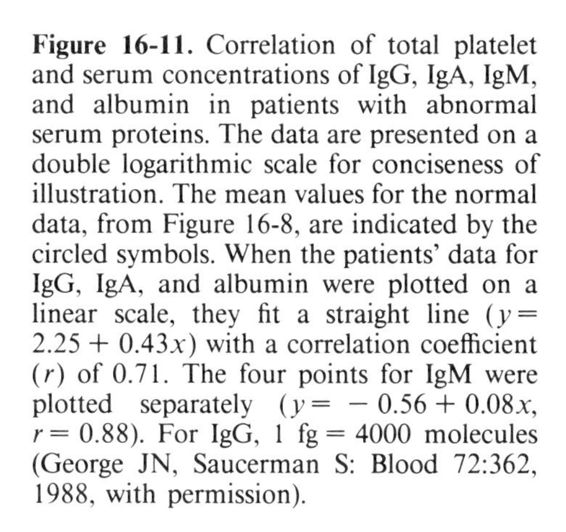
Figure 16-11. Correlation of total platelet and serum concentrations of IgG, IgA, IgM, and albumin in patients with abnormal serum proteins. The data are presented on a double logarithmic scale for conciseness of illustration. The mean values for the normal data, from Figure 16-8, are indicated by the circled symbols. When the patients' data for IgG, IgA, and albumin were plotted on a linear scale, they fit a straight line ($y = 2.25 + 0.43x$) with a correlation coefficient (r) of 0.71. The four points for IgM were plotted separately ($y = -0.56 + 0.08x$, $r = 0.88$). For IgG, 1 fg = 4000 molecules (George JN, Saucerman S: Blood 72:362, 1988, with permission).

Table 16-12
Protein Concentrations of Platelets and Serum from Normal Subjects and Patients*

Subjects	Platelet Count (number/μl)	Platelet Surface IgG (molecules/platelets)	Total Platelet (fg/platelets)†				Serum (mg/ml)			
			IgG	*IgA*	*IgM*	*Albumin*	*IgG*	*IgA*	*IgM*	*Albumin*
Normal (12)	260,160	79 ± 27‡	5.0 ± 1.2	0.5 ± 0.3	<0.1§	24.3–3.5	11.3 ± 1.8	2.2 ± 1.0		42.8 ± 2.9
IgG myeloma (6)	143,500	201 ± 80	18.7 ± 9.5	0.1 ± 0.1		23.4 ± 12.6	41.8 ± 14.0	0.4 ± 0.3		32.0 ± 7.0
IgA myeloma (3)	282,300	73 ± 20	4.8 ± 0.7	13.9 ± 2.0		19.7 ± 2.6	3.5 ± 0.8	50.4 ± 7.3		29.3 ± 4.2
Macroglobulinemia (4)	225,000	207 ± 153	7.9 ± 5.7	0.4 ± 0.6	1.0 ± 0.8	19.2 ± 9.2	9.0 ± 4.1	1.3 ± 1.0	18.8 ± 8.2	37.3 ± 4.3
Liver cirrhosis (5)	113,200	371 ± 185	10.4 ± 2.1	2.5 ± 1.2		13.6 ± 6.0	21.8 ± 6.4	9.5 ± 4.2		18.6 ± 1.9
ITP (10)	71,000	1105 ± 1067	9.7 ± 5.5	1.5 ± 1.4		57.8 ± 37.8	8.9 ± 3.5	3.0 ± 3.8		36.7 ± 4.6
Nonimmune thrombocytopenia (10)	79,000	476 ± 227	8.1 ± 4.8				11.4 ± 4.4			

*Data are the mean ±150 for the number of subjects in parentheses.
†1 femtogram of IgG = 4000 molecules.
‡Data on 20 subjects.
§Data on 5 subjects.

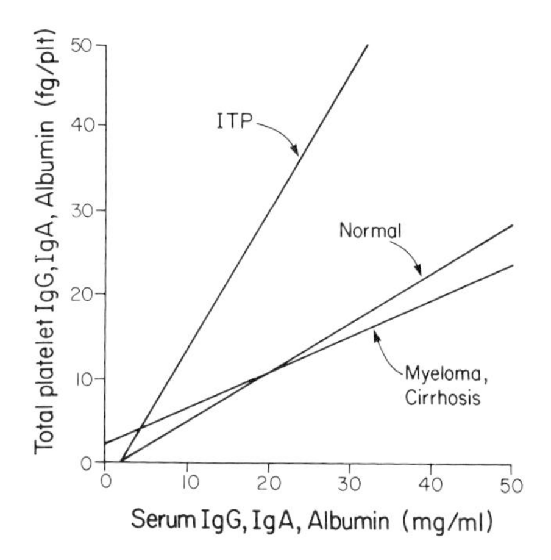

Figure 16-12. Correlation of total platelet and serum concentrations of IgG, IgA, and albumin in normal subjects, in patients with abnormal serum proteins, and in patients with idiopathic thrombocytopenic purpura (ITP). The calculated linear regression lines are shown for data on: (1) normal subjects; (2) patients with IgG or IgA myeloma or with liver cirrhosis; and (3) patients with ITP. The data here represented by the regression lines for groups 1 and 2 are given in Figures 16-8 and 16-11. For the patients with ITP, the data fit a straight line ($y = -3.09 + 1.61x$) with a correlation coefficient (r) of 0.74. The regression analyses for each of the three groups of patients were compared using the P1R algorithm in the BMDP statistical software,[16] taking into account both the slopes and intercepts. The regression equations for normal subjects and the myeloma/cirrhosis patients were not different from each other ($p = 0.19$). However the slope of the line for the ITP patients was significantly greater than for either the normal subjects or the myeloma/cirrhosis patients ($p < 0.001$) (George JN, Saucerman S: Blood 72:362, 1988, with permission).

ent. The total platelet concentrations of IgG, IgA, and albumin were all increased in patients with ITP (*see* Table 16-12) and the platelet concentrations correlated with their respective serum concentrations (*see* Fig. 16-12). However, the regression equation for the platelet–serum relationship was significantly different from those of both normal subjects and patients with abnormal plasma proteins. For any serum concentration of IgG, IgA, or albumin, the platelet concentration was two- to threefold greater (*see* Fig. 16-12). If plasma proteins are incorporated into α granules during megakaryocyte maturation in the marrow, perhaps younger platelets have higher concentrations of these α-granule proteins, and the abnormality in ITP simply reflects the younger mean age of the platelet population. This interpretation is consistent with the observations that ITP patients with lower platelet counts and shorter platelet survival times have higher concentrations of platelet IgG.[15,30,34,39,45,48,55,69] This interpretation is also consistent with the regular observation of an increased total platelet IgG concentration in ITP (*see* Table 16-1), even if the platelet IgG is not antiplatelet antibody.

Platelet Surface Immunoglobulin G

If the increased total platelet concentration of IgG in ITP is an innocent marker for platelet age, the measurement of platelet surface IgG is thought to be a more accurate assessment of antiplatelet antibody. The development of assays specific for the small amount of IgG restricted to the platelet surface was considered, therefore, an important step in the "search for a platelet Coombs test."[65] The first publication on the use of an ^{125}I-labeled monoclonal anti-IgG to clearly measure only platelet surface IgG changed the context of thinking about platelet IgG.[54] As Table 16-4 demonstrates, surface IgG is also increased in almost all patients with ITP, regardless of the method of assay.

In contrast to the results with total-platelet IgG, measurements of platelet surface IgG in patients with ITP have not correlated with the degree of thrombocytopenia.[10,54,82] This is comparable with the experience in autoimmune hemolytic anemia, in which the amount of autoantibody bound to the red cells does not correlate with the degree of shortening of red cell survival.[8] Presumably, qualitative characteristics of both autoantibodies and the autoantigens recognized by them, such as their role in cell membrane integrity or the interaction with macrophages, are more critical determinants of the severity of disease.

Even the accurate measurement of platelet surface IgG has not completely resolved the issue of defining patients with ITP. Here again, the platelet has proved to be a formidably complicated cell. The key issue has been the ability to differentiate patients with ITP from patients with apparently nonimmune thrombocytopenia, who also commonly have high concentrations of platelet surface IgG. In a recent study of 67 patients with a clinical diagnosis of ITP and 55 patients with nonimmune thrombocytopenia, using an ^{125}I-labeled HB-43 binding assay, Court et al. demonstrated a clear difference between these two groups.[10] The platelet surface IgG in ITP patients was 4210 ± 4043 (1 SD) molecules per platelet. In nonimmune ITP, that value was 360 ± 255 molecules per platelet, compared with their normal value of 122 ± 81 molecules per platelet. The widespread and skewed distribution of the values in each group is apparent from the high standard deviations. However, to achieve this distinction, some patient selection was required. Twenty-seven patients with ITP who had been receiving therapy for more than 48 hr were excluded because normal platelet surface IgG concentrations could be found in treated patients with rising platelet counts.[10] Patients with more chronic and treatment-resistant ITP, the group in whom a diagnostic assay may be of more clinical importance, had a lower platelet surface IgG and were grouped separately. Their platelet surface IgG was 2100 ± 3481, with significant overlap into the normal range and the range typical for patients with nonimmune thrombocytopenia. Patients with nonimmune thrombocytopenia were also selected to avoid patients who were severely ill with acute leukemia and were receiving multiple antibiotics. It was stated that these patients could have even higher platelet surface concentrations of IgG than other patients with nonimmune thrombocytopenia.

Our studies of platelet surface IgG measured by ^{125}I-labeled HB-43 binding confirmed the distinction between patients with ITP and normal subjects, even though none of our ten patients were studied before treatment was started.[22] Three of our patients had been treated with prednisone for 3 to 6 days and had rising platelet counts, and seven had had ITP for durations of 6 weeks to 6 years (*see* Table 16-12; Fig. 16-13). Therefore, none of our ITP patients would be among those in the group with the highest platelet surface IgG, as defined by Court et al.[10] However, a variety of patients with presumably nonimmune thrombocytopenia also had high platelet surface IgG concentrations. As a group, platelet surface IgG values for the ten patients with nonimmune thrombocytopenia were higher than those for normal subjects and were no different than those of ITP patients. This was a surprise to us. For example, the platelet surface IgG concentration in a 69-year-old woman with chronic stable myelofibrosis of 8 years duration, enor-

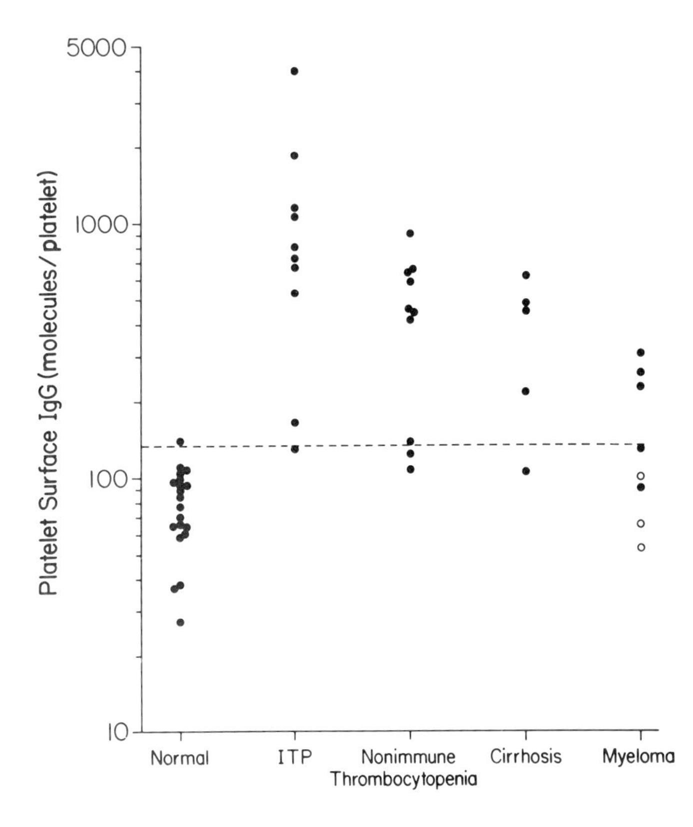

Figure 16-13. Platelet surface IgG in normal subjects and patient groups. Platelet surface IgG was measured by the binding of ^{125}I-labeled HB-43, a murine monoclonal antihuman IgG antibody, as described in Table 16-5. Patients with myeloma had either IgG (●) or IgA (○) paraproteins (George JN, Saucerman S: Blood 72:362, 1988, with permission).

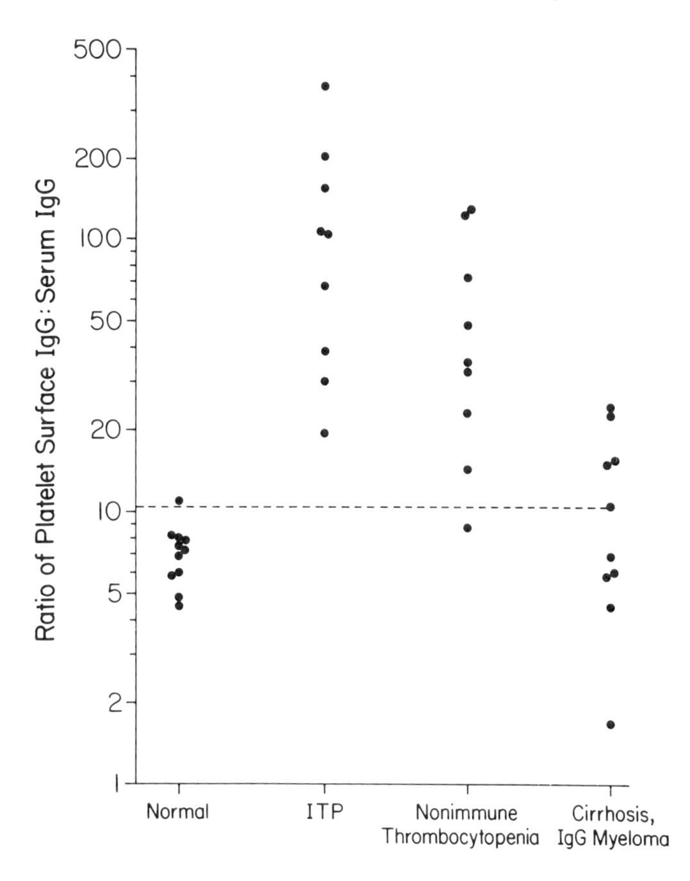

Figure 16-14. Platelet surface IgG in normal subjects and patient groups presented as the ratio of platelet surface IgG concentration (molecules/platelet) to serum IgG (mg/ml). Platelet surface IgG was measured by the binding of ^{125}I-labeled HB-43, a monoclonal antihuman IgG antibody, as described in Table 16-5.

mous splenomegaly, and a constant platelet count of 80,000 to 100,000/μl was 666 molecules per platelet. To check this value, the assay was repeated 2 weeks later, and the result was 618 molecules per platelet. Patients who were studied because their plasma IgG concentrations were high (chronic liver cirrhosis, IgG myeloma) also had high platelet surface IgG concentrations, unrelated to the presence or degree of thrombocytopenia. As a group, the patient with hypergammaglobulinemia could be normalized if their data were expressed as a ratio of platelet surface IgG divided by the serum IgG concentration (Fig. 16-14). However, as individuals there was no correlation between the serum IgG and platelet surface IgG concentrations (Fig. 16-15).

Conditions other than the binding of antiplatelet antibody must be able to cause an increase in platelet surface IgG. The explanation for this observation is unknown. It cannot simply represent equilibrium between plasma and platelet IgG, and it also does not correlate with the degree of thrombocytopenia.[22] Perhaps, as in the in vitro studies of platelet incubation with autologous or allogeneic plasmas, IgG complexes or physically abnormal forms of IgG exist in some patients that allow an increased association with the platelet surface. Altered IgG molecules may bind to the platelet Fc receptor[38,78] in a reaction comparable with the platelet's participation in immunologic responses.[5,37] Perhaps platelet membrane surface alterations that can occur in systemic disease[21] may also expose new antigenic determinants that bind naturally occurring antibodies in plasma.[20] An analogous situation may be the excessive binding of natural anti-α-galactosyl antibodies to sickle erythrocytes.[17] Presumably, red cell membrane alterations occur during the stress of reversible sickling or circulatory trauma, exposing Galα(1-3)Gal on the red cell surface. Antibody to this membrane structure constitute up to 1% of circulating IgG in normal individuals.[17] The platelet membrane may also be vulnerable to similar structural alterations in systemic diseases. Alternatively, alterations in the platelet membrane may expose binding sites for IgG that are unrelated to antigen–antibody interaction. The IgG heavy

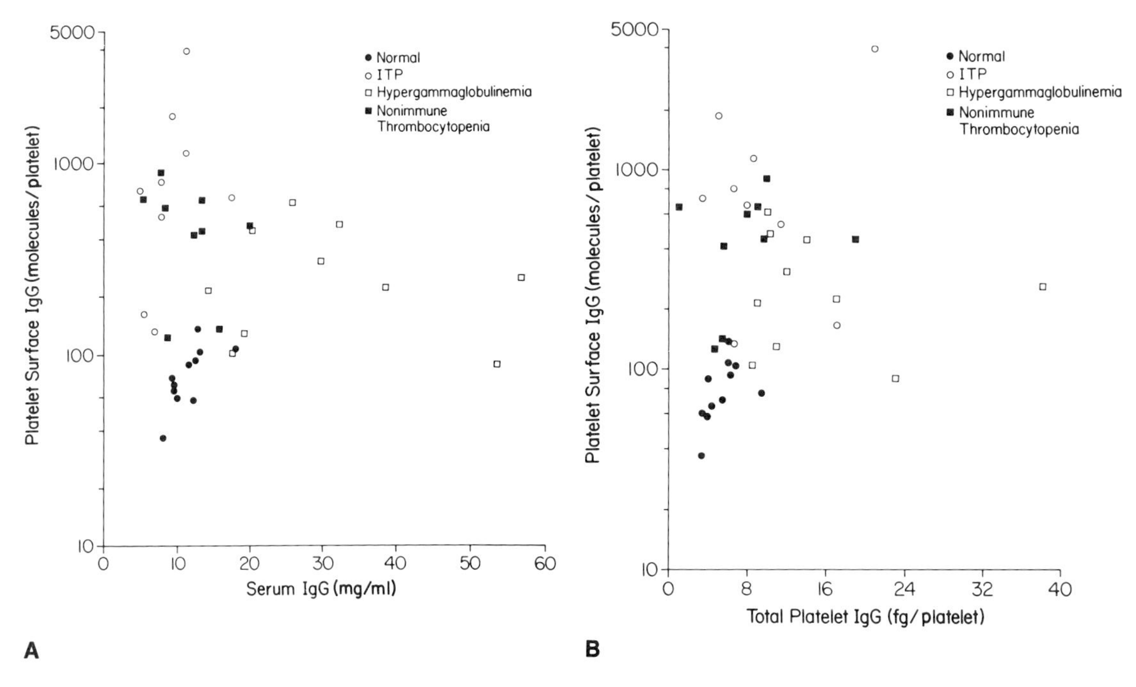

Figure 16-15. Relationship of platelet surface IgG to serum IgG (*A*) and to total platelet IgG (*B*) in normal subjects and in patients with ITP, nonimmune thrombocytopenia, and hypergammaglobulinemia (liver cirrhosis or IgG myeloma). There was some correlation between platelet surface IgG and serum IgG in normal subjects ($r = 0.67$, $p = 0.003$), but there was no correlation in the patient groups (ITP, $r = 0.27$; nonimmune thrombocytopenia, $r = 0.39$; hypergammaglobulinemia, $r = 0.15$). There was no correlation between platelet surface IgG and total platelet IgG in any group (normal subjects, $r = 0.49$; ITP, $r = 0.51$; nonimmune thrombocytopenia, $r = 0.16$; hypergammaglobulinemia, $r = 0.21$) (George JN, Saucerman S: Blood 72:362, 1988, with permission).

chains and κ light chains contain the amino acid sequence of arginine-glycine-aspartic acid-serine (RGDS) that is critical in adhesive proteins (e.g., fibrinogen, fibronectin) for their binding to platelet membrane glycoprotein IIb–IIIa. (These data are on file at the National Biomedical Research Foundation data Bank at Georgetown University, Washington, D.C.)

In summary, the measurement of platelet surface IgG can be used in conjunction with clinical data as an important addition to the definition of ITP. In certain clinical situations, as described on the foregoing, the amount of IgG on the platelet surface may not distinguish between immune thrombocytopenia and thrombocytopenia of obviously nonimmune etiology. However, in untreated patients with acute thrombocytopenia, the platelet surface IgG can be expected to be much higher in ITP than in normal subjects or in patients with nonimmune thrombocytopenia.

CONCLUSION

The bulk of platelet IgG needs to be recognized simply as the platelet pool of an abundant plasma protein. Current evidence suggests that IgG and other plasma proteins, such as albumin and IgA, can be incorporated into megakaryocytes by endocytosis and then packaged into the secretory α granules. Consistent with this hypothesis are the findings that the α granules contain essentially all of the platelet IgG and that the IgG concentration in α granules is directly proportional to the plasma IgG concentration. A function for α-granule IgG is unknown. Perhaps platelets act as messengers in the circulation, carrying packages of plasma proteins to be released at sites of vascular injury. This localized secretion of IgG many be a mechanism of delivering an aliquot of plasma antibodies to a potential site of microbial invasion. This function would be consistent with other observations on the platelet's role in infectious disease.[5,37,67] By transporting plasma albumin, the platelet may also be a vehicle to deliver albumin-bound hormones, enzymes, and metal ions.[18]

The fraction of platelet IgG that may be specific antiplatelet antibody is very small, because surface IgG constitutes less than 1% of total platelet IgG. The role of platelet IgG as antiplatelet antibody has been assumed in most previous investigations, but these studies now need to reinterpreted. In patients with ITP, the high total platelet concentration of IgG may reflect younger cell age and greater α-granule content. The increased platelet surface IgG in ITP probably does represent antiplatelet antibody. Platelet surface IgG can also be increased in nonimmune conditions, and the interactions of plasma IgG with the platelet surface in normal subjects and in patients with nonimmune conditions remain to be more clearly defined. However, if untreated patients with acute thrombocytopenia are studied, the measurement of platelet surface IgG is an important and clinically useful assay to define immune thrombocytopenic purpura.

This work was supported, in part, by the National Heart, Lung, and Blood Institute grant HL 19996.

REFERENCES

1. Barrison IG, Knight ID, Viola L, Boots MA, Murray-Lyon IM, Mitchell TR: Platelet-associated immunoglobulins in chronic liver disease. Br J Haematol 48:348, 1981

2. Berndt MC, Castaldi PA, Gordon S, Halley H, McPherson VJ: Morphological and biochemical confirmation of gray platelet syndrome in two siblings. Aus NZ J Med 13:387, 1983

3. Blumberg N, Masel D, Stoler M: Disparities in estimates of IgG bound to normal platelets. Blood 67:200, 1986

4. Boorman KE, Dodd BE, Loutit JF: Haemolytic icterus (acholuric jaundice) congenital and acquired. Lancet 1:812, 1946

5. Cesbron YJ, Capron A, Vargaftig BB, Lagarde M, Pincemail J, Braquet P, Taelman H, Joseph M: Platelets mediate the action of diethylcarbamazine on microfilariae. Nature 325:533, 1987

6. Cheung NV, McFall P, Schulman I: A microtiter solid-phase radioimmunoassay for platelet-associated immunoglobulin G. J Lab Clin Med 101:393, 1983

7. Cines DB, Schreiber AD: Immune thrombocytopenia. Use of a Coombs antiglobulin test to detect IgG and C3 on platelets. N Engl J Med 300:106, 1979

8. Constantoulakis M, Costra N, Schqartz RS, Dameshek W: Quantitative studies of the effect of red blood cell sensitization on in vivo hemolysis. J Clin Invest 42:1790, 1963

9. Coombs RRA, Bourant AE, Race RR: A new test for the detection of weak and "incomplete" RH agglutinins. Br J Exp Pathol 26:255, 1945

10. Court WS, Bozeman JM, Soong SJ, Saleh MN, Shaw DR, LoBuglio AF: Platelet surface-bound IgG in patients with immune and nonimmune thrombocytopenia. Blood 69:278, 1987

11. Court WS, LoBuglio AF: Measurement of platelet surface-bound IgG by a monoclonal ^{125}I-anti-IgG assay. Vox Sang 30:154, 1986

12. Davey MG, Lüscher EF: Platelet proteins. *In* Kowlaski E, Niewiarowski S (eds): Biochemistry of Blood Platelets, p. 9. New York, Academic Press, 1966

13. Davey MG, Lüscher EF: Actions of thrombin and other coagulant and proteolytic enzymes on blood platelets. Nature 216:857, 1967

14. Davey MG, Lüscher EF: Release reactions of human platelets induced by thrombin and other agents. Biochim Biophys Acta 165:490, 1968

15. Dixon R, Rosse W, Ebbert L: Quantitative determination of antibody in idiopathic thrombocytopenia purpura. N Engl J Med 292:230, 1975

16. Dixon WJ: BMDP Statistical Software. Berkeley, University of California Press, 1981

17. Galili U, Clark MR, Shohet SB: Excessive binding of anti-galactosyl immunoglobulin G to sickle erythrocytes may contribute to extravascular cell destruction. J Clin Invest 77:27, 1986

18. Ganong WF: Review of Medical Physiology, p. 410. Los Alto, CA, Lange Medical Publications, 1979

19. Gerrard JN, Phillips DR, Rao GHR, Plow EF, Walz DA, Ross R, Harker LA, White JG: Biochemical studies of two patients with the gray platelet syndrome. J Clin Invest 66:102, 1980

20. George JN: The role of membane glycoproteins in platelet formation, circulation, and senescence. Review and hypotheses. *In* George JN, Nurden AT, Phillips DR, (eds): Platelet Membrane Glycoproteins, p. 395. New York, Plenum Press, 1985

21. George JN, Pickett EB, Saucerman S, McEver RP, Kunicki TJ, Kieffer N, Newman PJ: Platelet surface glycoproteins. Studies on resting and activated platelet and platelet membrane microparticles in normal subjects, and observations in patients during adult respiratory distress syndrome and cardiac surgery. J Clin Invest 78:340, 1986

22. George JN, Saucerman S: Platelet IgG, IgA, IgM, and albumin: correlation of platelet and plasma concentrations in normal subjects and in patients with ITP or dysproteinemia. Blood 72:362, 1988

23. George JN, Saucerman S, Levine SP, Knieriem LK, Bainton DF: Immunoglobulin G is a platelet alpha granule-secreted protein. J Clin Invest 76:2020, 1985

24. George JN,Thoi LL, Morgan RK: Quantitative analysis of platelet membrane glycoproteins: Effect of platelet washing procedures and isolation of platelet density subpopulations. Thromb Res 23:69, 1981

25. Handagama PJ, Bainton DF: Uptake of intravenously injected human albumin by guinea pig bone marrow megakaryocytes (abstr). Exp Hematol 15:495, 1987

26. Handagama PJ, George JN, Shuman MA, McEver RP, Bainton DF: Incorporation of a circulating protein into megakaryocyte and platelet granules. Proc Natl Acad Sci USA 84:861, 1987

27. Handagama PJ, Shuman MA, Bainton DF: Uptake of circulating albumin IgG, and fibrinogen by guinea pig megakaryocytes in vivo (abstr). Blood 70(Suppl 1):154a, 1987

28. Harrington WJ: Are platelet antibody tests worthwhile? N Engl J Med 316:211, 1987

29. Harrington WJ, Minnich V, Hollingsworth JW, Moore CV: Demonstration of a thrombocytopenic factor in the blood of patients with thrombocytopenic purpura. J Lab Clin Med 38:1, 1951

30. Hegde UM, Gordon-Smith EC, Worlledge S: Platelet antibodies in thrombocytopenic patients. Br J Haematol 35:113, 1977

31. Hegde UM, Powell DK, Bowes A, Gordon-Smith EC: Enzyme-linked immunoassay for the detection of platelet-associated IgG. Br J Haematol 48:39, 1981

32. Hotchkiss AJ, Leissinger CA, Smith ME, Jordan JV, Kautz CA, Shulman NR: Evaluation by quantitative acid elution and radioimmunoassay of multiple classes of immunoglobulins and serum albumin associated with platelets in idiopathic thrombocytopenic purpura. Blood 67:1126, 1986

33. Hymes K, Schur PH, Karpatkin S: Heavy-chain subclass of bound antiplatelet IgG in autoimmune thrombocytopenic purpura. Blood 56:84, 1980

34. Hymes K, Shulman S, Karpatkin S: A solid-phase radioimmunoassay for bound anti-platelet antibody. J Lab Clin Med 94:639, 1979

35. Janson M, McFarland J, Aster RH: Quantitative determination of platelet surface alloantigens using a monoclonal probe. Hum Immunol 15:251, 1986

36. Johnston GI, Pickett EB, McEver RP, George JN: Heterogeneity of platelet secretion in response to thrombin demonstrated by fluorescence flow cytometry. Blood 69:1401, 1987

37. Joseph M. Auriault C, Capron A, Vorng H, Viens P. A new function for platelets: IgE-dependent killing of schistosomes. Nature 30:810, 1983

38. Karas SP, Rosse WF, Kurlander RJ: Characterization of the IgG-Fc receptor on human platelets. Blood 60:1277, 1982

39. Kelton JG, Carter CJ, Rodger C, Bebenek G, Gauldie J, Sheridan D, Kassam YB, Kean WF, Buchanan WW, Rooney PJ: The relationship among platelet-associated IgG, platelet lifespan, and reticuloendothelial cell function. Blood 63:1434, 1984

40. Kelton JG, Denomme G, Lucarelli A, Garvey J, Powers P: Comparison of the measurement of surface or total platelet-associated IgG in the diagnosis of immune thrombocytopenia. Am J Hematol 18:1, 1985

41. Kelton JG, Moore J, Gaudie J, Neame PB, Hirsh J, Tozman E: The development and application of a serum assay for platelet-bindable IgG (S-PBIGg). J Lab Clin Med 98:272, 1981

42. Kelton JG, Neame PB, Bishop J, Ali M, Gauldie J, Hirsh J: The direct assay for platelet-associated IgG: Lack of association between antibody level and platelet size. Blood 53:73, 1979

43. Kelton JG, Powers PJ, Carter CJ: A prospective study of the usefulness of the measurement of platelet associated IgG for the diagnosis of idiopathic thrombocytopenic purpura. Blood 60:1050, 1982

44. Kelton JG, Steeves K: The amount of platelet-bound albumin parallels the amount of IgG on washed platelets from patients with immuno thrombocytopenia. Blood 62:924, 1983

45. Kernoff LM, Blake CH, Shackleton D: Influence of the amount of platelet-bound IgG on platelet survival and site of sequestration in autoimmune thrombocytopenia. Blood 55:730, 1980

46. Kiefel V, Spaeth P, Mueller-Eckhardt C: Immune thrombocytopenic purpura: Autoimmune or immune complex disease? Br J Haematol 64:57, 1986

47. Kieffer N, Boizard B, Didry D, Wautier JL, Nurden AT: Immunochemical characterization of the platelet-specific alloantigen Lek^{a}: A comparative study with the Pl^{A1} alloantigen. Blood 64:1212, 1984

48. Kunicki TJ, Koenig MB, Kristopeit SM, Aster RH: Direct quantitation of platelet-associated IgG by electroimmunoassay. Blood 60:54, 1982

49. Laemmli UK: Cleavage of structural proteins during the assembly of the head of bacteriophage T4. Nature 227:680, 1970

50. Leporrier M, Dighiero G, Auzemery M, Binet JL: Detection and quantification of platelet-bound antibodies with immunoperoxidase. Br J Haematol 42:605, 1979

51. Levine SP, Towell BL, Suarez AM, Knieriem LK, Harris MM, George JN: Platelet activation and secretion associated with emotional stress. Circulation 71:1129, 1985

52. Levine SP, Krentz LS: Development of a radioimmunoassay for human platelet factor 4. Thromb Res 11:673, 1977

53. Levy-Toledano S, Caen JP, Breton-Gorius J, Pendu F, Cywiner-Golenzer C, Dupuy E, Legrand Y, Maclouf J: Gray platelet syndrome: α-Granule deficiency. J Lab Clin Med 98:831, 1981

54. LoBuglio AF, Court WS, Vinocur L, Maglott JG, Shaw FM: Immune thrombocytopenic purpura. Use of a ^{125}I-labeled antihuman IgG monoclonal antibody to quantify platelet-bound IgG. N Engl J Med 309:459, 1983

55. Luiken GA, McMillan R, Lightsey AL, Gordon P, Zevely S, Schulman I, Gribble TJ, Longmire RL: Platelet-associated IgG in immune thrombocytopenic purpura. Blood 50:317, 1977

56. McEver RP, Baenziger NL, Majerus PW: Isolation and quantitation of the platelet membrane glycoprotein deficient in thrombasthenia using a monoclonal hybridoma antibody. J Clin Invest 66:1311, 1980

57. McGrath KM, Stuart JJ, Richards F II: Correlation between serum IgG, platelet membrane IgG and platelet function in hypergammaglobulinemic states. Br J Haematol 42:585, 1979

58. McMillan R, Smith RS, Longmire RL, Yelenosky R, Reid RT, Craddock CG: Immunoglobulins associated with human platelets. Blood 37:316, 1971

59. Morse BS, Giuliani D, Nussbaum M: Quantitation of platelet-associated IgG by radial immunodiffusion. Blood 57:809, 1981

60. Morse BS, Giuliani D, Nussbaum M: A rapid quantitation of platelet-associated IgG by nephelometry. Am J Hematol 12:721, 1982

61. Mosher DF, Presciotta DM, Loftus JC, Albrecht RM: Secreted alpha granule proteins: The race for receptors. *In* George JN, Nurden AT, Phillips DR (eds): Platelet Membrane Glycoproteins. New York, Plenum Press, 1985

62. Mueller-Eckhardt C, Kayser W, Mersch-Baumert K, Mueller-Eckhardt G, Briedenbach M, Kugel HG, Graubner M: The clinical significance of platelet-associated IgG: A study on 298 patients with various disorders. Br J Haematol 46:123, 1980

63. Mueller-Eckhardt C, Mueller-Eckhardt G, Kayser W, Voss RM, Wegner J, Knenzlein E: Platelet-associated IgG, platelet survival, and platelet sequestration in thrombocytopenic states. Br J Haematol 52:49, 1982

64. Munson PJ, Rodbard D: LIGAND: A versatile computerized approach for the characterization of ligand binding systems. Anal Biochem 107:220, 1980

65. Murphy S: In search of a platelet Coombs test. N Engl J Med 309:490, 1983

66. Nachman RL: Platelet proteins. Semin Hematol 5:18, 1968

67. Nachman RL, Weksler BB: The platelet as an inflammatory cell. *In* Weismann G (ed): The Cell Biology of Inflammation, p. 145. Amsterdam, Elsevier/North-Holland, 1980

68. Natvig JB, Kunkel HG: Human immunoglobulins: Classes, subclasses, genetic variants, and idiotypes. Adv Immunol 16:1, 1973

69. Nel JD, Stevens K: A new method for simultaneous quantification of platelet-bound immunoglobulin and complement employing an enzyme-linked immunosorbant assay (ELISA) procedure. Br J Haematol 44:281, 1980

70. Nurden AT, Didry D, Kieffer N, McEver RP: Residual amounts of glycoproteins IIb and IIIa may be present in the platelets of most patients with Glanzmann's thrombasthenia. Blood 65:1021, 1985

71. Nurden AT, Kunicki TJ, Dupuis D, Soria C, Caen JP: Specific protein and glycoprotein deficiencies in platelets isolated from two patients with the gray platelet syndrome. Blood 59:709, 1982

72. Panzer S, Szamait S, Bödeker R-H, Haas OA, Haubenstock A, Mueller-Eckhardt C: Platelet-associated immunoglobulins IgG, IgM, IgA and complement C3 in immune and nonimmune thrombocytopenic disorders. Am J Hematol 23:89, 1986

73. Pfueller SL, Chesterman C, Illes I, Hussein S, Martin JF: Relationship of platelet-associated immunoglobulin G and platelet protein to platelet size and density in normal individuals and patients with thrombocytopenia. J Lab Clin Med 107:299, 1986

74. Pfueller SL, Cosgrove L, Firkin BG, Tew D: Relationship of raised platelet IgG in thrombocytopenia to total platelet protein content. Br J Haematol 49:293, 1981

75. Pfueller SL, Luscher EF: The effects of aggregated immunoglobulins on human blood platelets in relation to their complement-fixing abilities. I. Studies of immunoglobulins of different types. J Immunol 109:517, 1972

76. Rochna E, Hughes-Jones NC: The use of purified ^{125}I-labeled anti-gamma globulin in the determination of the number of D antigen site on red cells of different phenotypes. Vox Sang 10:675, 1965

77. Rosa JP, George JN, Bainton DF, Nurden AT, Caen JP, McEver RP: Gray platelet syndrome:

Demonstration of alpha granule membranes that can fuse with the cell surface. J Clin Invest 80:1138, 1987

78. Rosenfeld SI, Looney RJ, Leddy JP, Phipps DC, Abraham GN, Anderson CL: Human platelet Fc receptor for immunoglobulin G. J Clin Invest 76:2317, 1985

79. Rosse WF, Adams JP, Yount WJ: Subclasses of IgG antibodies in immune thrombocytopenic purpura. Br J Haematol 46:109, 1980

80. Rosse WF, Devine DV, Ware R: Reactions of immunoglobulin G-binding ligands with platelets and platelet-associated immunoglobulin G. J Clin Invest 73:489, 1984

81. Salmon J: Etude immunoelectrophoretique des antigenes plaquettaires humains. Schweiz Med Wochenschr 88;1047, 1958

82. Shaw GM, Axelson J, Maglott JG, LoBuglio AF: Quantification of platelet-bound IgG by ^{125}I-staphylococcal protein A in immune thrombocytopenic purpura and other thrombocytopenic disorders. Blood 63:154, 1984

83. Shulman NR, Jordan JV Jr: Platelet immunology. *In* Colman RW, Hirsh J, Marder VJ, Salzman EW (eds): Hemostasis and Thrombosis, p. 274. Philadelphia, JB Lippencott, 1987

84. Shulman NR, Leissinger CA, Hotchkiss AJ, Kautz CA: The nonspecific nature of platelet-associated IgG. Trans Assoc Am Physicians 95:213, 1982

85. Shuman MA, Levine SP: Relationship between secretion of platelet factor 4 and thrombin generation during in vitro blood clotting. J Clin Invest 65:307, 1980

86. Siegel A, Burri PH, Weibel ER, Bettex-Galland M, Luscher EF: Density gradient centrifugation and electron microscopic characterization of subcellular fractions from human blood platelets. Thromb Diath Haemorrh 25:252, 1971

87. Sixma JJ, van den Berg A, Schiphorst M, Geuze HJ, McDonagh J: Immunocytochemical localization of albumin and factor XIII in thin cryosections of human blood platelets. Thromb Haemostasis 51:388, 1984

88. Sterlin K: The turnover rate of serum albumin in man as measured by ^{131}I-tagged albumin. J Clin Invest 30:1228, 1951

89. Waldmann TA, Johnson JS, Talal N: Hypogammaglobulinemia associated with accelerated catabolism of IgG secondary to its interaction with an IgG-reactive monoclonal IgM. J Clin Invest 50:951, 1971.

90. Waldmann TA, Strober W: Metabolism of immunoglobulins. Prog Allergy 13:1, 1969

91. Woods VL Jr, Wolff LE, Keller DM: Resting platelets contain a substantial centrally located pool of glycoprotein IIb-IIIa complex which may be accessible to some but not other extracellular proteins. J Biol Chem 261:15242, 1986

17

Fc Receptors of Human Platelets

STEPHEN I. ROSENFELD · CLARK L. ANDERSON

The exquisite immunologic specificity of antibody molecules is determined by the structure of the antigen-combining sites contained in the Fab region. However, most of the biologic activity of the immunoglobulin molecules is determined by structures in the Fc portion. Many important biologic activities of immunoglobulin molecules are mediated by interaction of their Fc regions with a variety of cell types. These interactions may occur with monomeric immunoglobulin molecules before the binding of antigen but, for a number of cell types, the interaction occurs only after binding of antibody to antigen and the formation of immunoglobulin aggregates. The structures on cell surfaces responsible for interaction with the Fc region of immunoglobulin molecules are integral membrane glycoproteins termed Fc receptors. In general, these Fc receptors trigger biologic responses after two or more receptors are apposed by interaction with immune complexes. The Fc receptors of most interest react with the immunoglobulins IgG or IgE. The best studied of these receptors in humans are those found on peripheral blood leukocytes and platelets (IgG) and on tissue mast cells and basophils (IgE).

Table 17-1 summarizes the known characteristics and distributions of three receptors for human IgG found on human leukocytes and two receptors for IgE found on leukocytes and other cells. Human platelets have been demonstrated to bear one of the three known types of leukocyte Fc receptors (FcγRII), as well as the low-affinity receptor for IgE (FcϵRII). In addition, other candidate molecules capable of binding IgG Fc regions have been proposed for platelets. The goal of this chapter is to summarize known information about human platelet Fc receptors for IgG and (more briefly) for IgE and to discuss the known and potential biologic importance of these molecules. The emphasis on *human* platelets is important because there are significant species differences in the repertoire of immunologically relevant platelet receptors. This is reflected in the variation among the platelets of different species in their responses to immune complexes. Primate, pig, sheep, goat, and ox platelets bind immune complexes in the absence of complement and are, therefore, presumed to bear Fc receptors, but the platelets of rabbits, dogs, mice, and horses bind immune complexes only if complement components, particularly C3b, are bound to the immune complex.[15] Human platelets do not bear the high-affinity receptor for C3b (CR1) and do not participate in C3b-mediated immune adherence reactions, but other receptors for C3 fragments (gp45–70, CR2, and CR4) have very recently been demonstrated to be present on human platelets. These are discussed and referenced in Chapter 18, "Interaction of Human Platelets with the Complement System."

Table 17-1
Characteristics and Distribution of Human IgG and IgE Receptors on Human Leukocytes and Other Cells

Characteristic	$Fc_{\gamma}RI$	$Fc_{\gamma}RII$	$Fc_{\gamma}RIII$	$Fc_{\epsilon}RI$	$Fc_{\epsilon}RII$
Relative molecular mass (kDa)	72	40	60	$\alpha = 45$	?
Subunits	?	?	?	$\beta = 33$ kDa $2_{\gamma} = 9$ kDa ea	?
Affinity for monomer ligand (K_a, M^{-1})	High ($10^8 - 10^9$)	Low ($<10^6$)	Low ($<10^6$)	High ($>10^9$)	High; low (3×10^7); (8×10^5)
Sites/cell	$1-4 \times 10^4$	[$3-6 \times 10^4$]	[$1 \times 2 \times 10^5$]	3×10^5	10^3 (high, platelet)
Distribution	Macrophages, monocytes	Macrophages, monocytes, PMN, B cells, platelets	Macrophages, PMN, eosinophils, NK cells	Basophils, mast cells	Platelets, eosinophils, monocytes, lymphocytes
hIg specificity	IgG	IgG	IgG	IgE	IgE
hIgG subclass specificity	$1 = 3 > 4$; 2 no	$1 = 3 > 2, 4$	1	NA	NA

Abbreviations: ( ), tentative; NA, not applicable.
(Compiled from: Anderson CL, Looney RJ: Immunol Today 7:264, 1986; Joseph M, Capron A, Amiesen J-C et al: Eur J Immunol 16:306, 1986; Metzger H, Alvarez G, Hohman R et al: Annu Rev Immunol 4:419, 1986)

HISTORICAL BACKGROUND

The classic studies of Humphrey and Jacques[19] were the first to demonstrate that human platelets released serotonin after exposure to antigen-antibody complexes in the absence of complement (C), in contrast to their more extensive studies with rabbit platelets for which C was required. Subsequently, a number of investigators have shown that human platelets can be stimulated to release serotonin or to aggregate by exposure to IgG-containing complexes.[5,13,14,16,21,33,38,39,44] These functional platelet responses were triggered by aggregates of all four subclasses of IgG[16,44] prepared by any of a number of mechanisms, including antigen-antibody complexes, heat aggregation, covalent chemical cross-linking, or aggregation by organic solvents. Coating IgG on solid particles, such as latex, glass, or bacteria, also generates surfaces that stimulate human platelets.[5,14,33,39,42,58] Unaggregated monomers of IgG can inhibit binding of IgG aggregates to platelets, but they do not stimulate the cell. The observations that aggregated Fc fragments, themselves, could stimulate platelet serotonin release, and that unaggregated Fc fragments could inhibit the effect of IgG aggregates on platelets, led Henson and Spiegelberg[16] and Israel et al.[21] independently to propose the existence of an Fc receptor for IgG on the platelet surface. The response of human platelets to soluble IgG aggregates is markedly inhibited in the presence of plasma or high concentrations of monomeric IgG. The inhibitory effect of plasma is accounted for partially by monomeric IgG and partially by C1 in the plasma, which can bind to IgG and, apparently, block its interaction with the platelet Fc receptor, but there may be additional inhibitory effects of plasma that are not fully understood.[45] Insoluble aggregates of immunoglobulin or particles coated with IgG are much more effective than are soluble IgG complexes at stimulating platelets in the presence of plasma. The addition of other ligands, such as fibrinogen or complement, to the complexes can markedly enhance the ability of insoluble IgG aggregates or particle-bound IgG to stimulate platelets in the presence of plasma.[6,12,14,42]

Pfueller and Lüscher[44] and Henson and Speigelberg[16] studied release of serotonin from human platelets triggered by aggregated human IgG myeloma proteins and found that all four subclasses were capable of stimulating platelets, but there was variation in the activity of individual myeloma proteins within subclasses in both studies. The observation that aggregated IgG4 proteins were capable of stimulating platelet release reactions, whereas they are incapable of causing complement fixation, has been taken as evidence that platelet-associated Clq probably does not function as an Fc receptor.

FORMAL LIGAND-BINDING STUDIES OF Fc_γ RECEPTORS ON HUMAN PLATELETS

Although the preceding analyses of the functional responses of platelets to various immune complexes strongly suggested that IgG Fc receptors are present on human platelets, the first formal ligand-binding studies were performed by Karas and associates.[26] These workers reported dose-dependent binding of IgG1 dimers and larger polymers to washed platelets, but the affinity was too low to demonstrate significant specific binding of IgG1 monomers, even at 4°C. The binding of labeled IgG1 dimers to platelets was saturable and yielded a linear Scatchard plot at 4°C. By using both dimers and larger polymers, these workers found approximately 1300 to 1500 binding sites per platelet (assuming one FcR per IgG unit within a polymer.) Unlabeled monomeric IgG1 and IgG3 markedly inhibited the binding of labeled IgG1 dimers to washed platelets, whereas IgG2 and IgG4 monomers were much less inhibitory. Fc, but not Fab, fragments were inhibitory. These workers found that unlabeled IgG1 monomer, in approximately 40-fold molar excess, produced 50% inhibition of binding of labeled IgG1 dimers.

The observation that human platelets bound IgG1 and IgG3 in preference to IgG2 or IgG4 was confirmed by Endressen and Forre[13] using a more qualitative assay than that of Karas et al.[26] This approach involved incubation of platelets with various immunoglobulins and fragments and the subsequent identification with fluorescein-conjugated antibody to human IgG.

POSSIBLE RELATIONSHIP OF Fc RECEPTOR TO GLYCOPROTEIN Ib

The possible association of a platelet IgG Fc receptor with the membrane glycoprotein Ib complex (GPIb) that interacts with von Willebrand factor (VWF) was suggested by the observation of Moore and coworkers that ristocetin-dependent agglutination of human platelets by VWF is inhibited by prior incubation of platelets with aggregated IgG of human or rabbit origin but not by aggregate-free human IgG, Fab fragments, or light chains.[37] These workers also found that the staining of platelets by fluorescein-labeled keyhole limpet hemocyamin (KLH): anti-KLH immune complexes was largely abolished by prior incubation of the platelets with barely agglutinating concentrations of VWF and ristocetin. This relatively high-molecular-mass (M_r) immune complex was found to bind to 80% to 90% of normal platelets, as examined in the fluorescence microscope, but with only one to three small clusters bound per platelet. This staining was interpreted to represent the binding of immune complexes to the platelet Fc receptor, because it was inhibited by Fc fragments. However, the inhibition by VWF and ristocetin was abolished if the platelets were washed once before incubation with the immune complexes. The concept that GPIb may function as an Fc receptor on platelets received a certain degree of support by the observation that quinine- and quinidine-dependent antiplatelet antibodies fail to bind to platelets that lack GPIb, as well as GPIX and GPV, from patients with the Bernard-Soulier syndrome.[29] As the binding of drug-dependent antibodies to platelets had been thought to occur as an immune complex (possibly interacting with a platelet receptor for IgG), this observation was interpreted to support the idea that GPIb functions as an Fc receptor. However, several subsequent observations have failed to support a role for GPIb as a platelet Fc receptor. Pfueller et al. showed that platelets from patients with Bernard-Soulier syndrome could exhibit an IgG-dependent serotonin release reaction upon interaction with latex particles coated with IgG and fibrinogen.[43] Furthermore, these workers showed that the removal of glycocalicin from the GPIb molecule by chymotrypsin digestion abolished the response of normal platelets to ristocetin and VWF but not to heat-aggregated IgG, antigen–antibody complexes, or latex particles bearing IgG or fibrinogen. Spycher et al. confirmed that the removal of glycocalicin with a different enzyme (calpain, the calcium-dependent, neutral protease derived from human blood platelets) also failed to inhibit the stimulation of human blood platelets by chemically aggregated human IgG.[51] These enzyme-treated platelets were no longer capable of reacting with bovine VWF. More recent evidence that the binding of quinine- and quinidine-dependent antibodies to platelets is mediated by the Fab region, rather than the Fc region, of the antibody molecules[10,50] further deemphasizes a role for GPIb as an Fc receptor. Furthermore, Berndt et al.[46] have shown that a mouse monoclonal $F(ab')_2$ directed to GPIX, a component of the GPIb complex, could completely block platelet aggregation induced by (and the binding of) quinidine-dependent antibody, without diminishing the ability of platelets to aggregate in response to acetone-aggregated IgG.

Interest in a relationship between the Bernard-Soulier syndrome and platelet Fc receptors has been resurrected by the recent report of Stricker et al., who showed that a 210-kDa glycoprotein, present on normal platelets but absent from Bernard-Soulier platelets, may have Fc-binding properties.[54] The relationship between this protein (gp210) and GPIb is not completely clear, but these workers found that gp210 is not removed from normal platelets by chymotrypsin treatment sufficient to remove glycocalicin. Although these workers did not study platelet function, they did find that an autoantibody to gp210, found in a patient with "acquired" Bernard-Soulier syndrome, could partially block binding of fluorescein-labeled human Fc fragments to paraformaldehyde-fixed human platelets. They also found that heat-aggregated rabbit or human IgG could bind to a 210-kDa molecule on nitrocellulose immunoblots of sodium dodecylsulfate (SDS)-solubilized human platelet proteins. This appeared to be the same molecule identified by the anti-gp210 autoantibody. Of interest, the anti-gp210 bound to a 40-kDa protein and not to a 210-kDa protein in platelets solubilized with the nonionic detergent NP-40, although the binding of immune complexes to immunoblots derived from NP-40-solubilized platelets was not tested. Because these workers did not perform any functional studies, the relationship of the gp210 molecule to the functional stimulation of platelets by immune complexes or aggregated IgG remains unclear. However, the observation of Pfueller et al.[43] that platelets from patients with the Bernard-Soulier syndrome (which presumably lack gp210) are still capable of a normal functional response to IgG-coated latex particles suggests that gp210 is not absolutely required for platelet responses to IgG-dependent stimuli. Moreover, Kelton et al. have recently shown that platelets from a single patient with the Bernard-Soulier syndrome bind aggregated IgG normally.[26a] Thus, the hypothesis that GPIb or any other components of the GPI complex (GPIX, GPV, or gp210) functions as a Fc_γ receptor of platelets remains to be proved.

AFFINITY ISOLATION OF IMMUNOGLOBULIN G-BINDING PROTEINS FROM HUMAN PLATELETS

The first report of the affinity isolation of an IgG Fc-binding glycoprotein from human platelets[9] used purified Fc fragments of human IgG covalently immobilized to Sepharose 4B by cyanogen bromide. Proteins extracted from whole platelets by the chaotropic agent KBr were applied to this affinity absorbent in low ionic strength buffer containing protease inhibitors. After washing, the column was eluted with 2 M KBr and the effluent was analyzed by sodium dodecyl sulfate–polyacrylamide gel electrophoresis (SDS–PAGE). This revealed a glycoprotein with an apparent M_r of approximately 255,000 unreduced, and 50,000 after reduction. A minor band in the M_r range of 160,000 to 180,000 was also present in both reduced and nonreduced eluates. These authors did not attempt any functional studies with this isolated Fc receptor molecule, but they did show that the isolated radiolabeled Fc fragment-binding protein could associate in vitro with heat-aggregated IgG, as demonstrated by sucrose density gradient ultracentrifugation. They could achieve binding of only approximately 24% of the total radiolabeled protein to aggregated IgG. A similar molecule was also isolated from a platelet membrane preparation, suggesting that the molecule may be a membrane-associated protein.

Our group has more recently approached the problem of the identification of IgG Fc receptor on human platelets by use of techniques and reagents developed in our unit for the study of Fc receptors on human leukocytes.[2,31,32] The most valuable reagent for these studies has been a mouse monoclonal antibody (MAb) to a human Fc receptor produced by immunization with the K562 cell line, designated IV.3 (anti-p40). This IgG2b monoclonal antibody was developed by Dr. R. J. Looney in our unit and has been shown to bind to the 40-kDa Fc receptor ($Fc_{\gamma}RII$) on U937 cells, K562 cells, human peripheral blood monocytes, neutrophils, and eosinophils. By using this monoclonal antibody, we could specifically immunoprecipitate a 40-kDa surface radio-labeled glycoprotein (p40) from NP-40 detergent lysates of washed human platelets.[47] As shown in Figure 17-1, this molecule was very similar to the low-molecular-mass Fc receptor immunoprecipitated by the same monoclonal antibody from the monocytic cell line U937. The p40 glycoprotein showed a slightly higher relative molecular mass on SDS-PAGE gradient gels when reduced (see Fig. 12-1, lanes C and G) than when unreduced (see Fig. 17-1, lane D and H), indicating the presence of intrachain disulfide bonds, but we found no evidence of a higher-molecular-mass precursor in the absence of a reducing agent. All of the unidentified higher-molecular-mass bands were all found in the control (MOPC 141 or myoglobin) immunoprecipitates, as well as the specific (IV.3 or IgG) immunoprecipitates, and presumably represent nonspecific contaminants. The 72 kDa bands in lanes E and F represent $Fc_{\gamma}RI$ from U937 cells, presumably binding to traces of IgG2a contaminating the murine IgG2b preparations. The

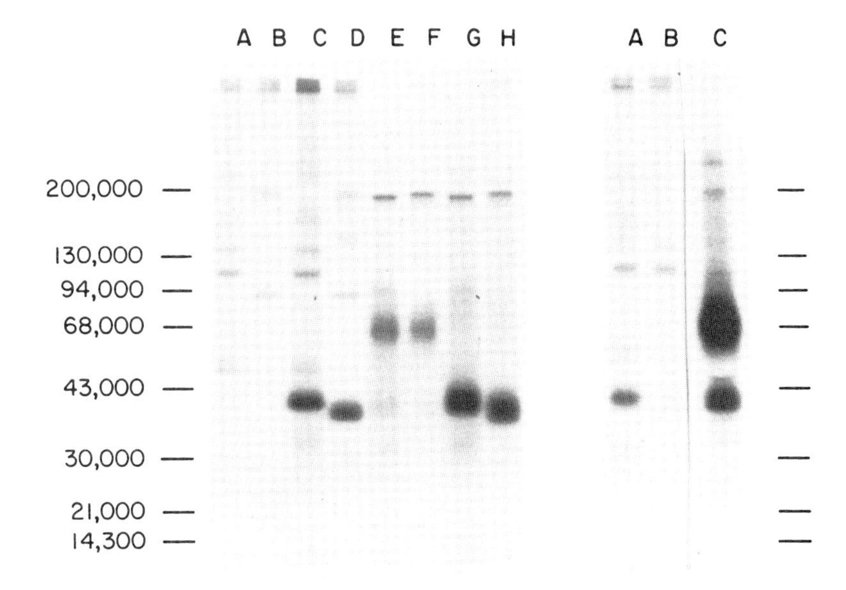

Figure 17-1. Autoradiographs of SDS-PAGE 5% to 15% gradient slab gels. (*left*) Immunoprecipitation from detergent lysates of surface-radiolabeled cells by the anti-p40 (FcR II) murine monoclonal antibody IV.3, or the control murine IgG2b myeloma protein (MOPC 141) followed by Sepharose goat $F(ab')_2$ antimurine Ig; lane A, platelet lysate + MOPC 141 + 20 mM DTT; lane B, same, without DTT; lane C, platelet lysate + anti-p40 (IV.3) + 20 mM DTT; lane D, same, without DTT; lane E, U937 lysate + MOPC 141 + 20mM DTT; lane F, same, without DTT; lane G, U937 lysate + anti-p40 (IV.3) + 20 mM DTT; lane H, same without DTT. (*right*) Eluates from affinity adsorbents as follows; lane A, platelet lysates applied to Sepharose-IgG; lane B, platelet lysates applied to Sepharose-myoglobin; lane C, U937 lysates applied to Sepharose-IgG. All eluates contain 20 mM DTT (Rosenfeld SI, Looney RJ, Leddy JP et al: J Clin Invest 76:2317, 1985, with permission).

right side of Figure 17-1 also demonstrates that a very similar p40 molecule can be isolated from platelets (lane A) and U937 cells (lane C) with a Sepharose IgG immunoadsorbent column. Kelton et al. have also isolated a very similar 40-kDa molecule from surface-labeled human platelets, using human IgG bound to Sepharose.[26a] Here, the binding of the 40-kDa molecule to the immunoadsorbent was inhibited by monomeric IgG and Fc fragments.[26a]

Monoclonal antibody IV.3 could completely inhibit the aggregation of washed platelets by heat aggregated IgG. As seen in Table 17-2, intact MAb IV.3 (43 ng/ml) completely inhibited platelet aggregation by aggregated IgG (500 μg/ml), whereas the control IgG2b murine myeloma protein (MOPC 141) produced little or no inhibition at 1000-fold higher concentrations. The Fab fragments of MAb IV.3 completely inhibited platelet aggregation at concentrations as low as 0.44 μg/ml. We have subsequently repeated this inhibition with MAb IV.3, using a number of other IgG-related platelet stimuli, including tetanus antitetanus immune complexes; zymosan particles coated with human IgG, complement, and fibrinogen; artificial immune complexes composed of IgG molecules chemically cross-linked to a polyacrylic acid backbone; and human erythrocytes heavily coated with mouse antibody to glycophorin (unpublished results). In no instance have we found an IgG-dependent immune complex whose effect on platelets could not be completely inhibited by MAb IV.3. On the other hand, MAb IV.3 has no inhibitory effect on platelet aggregation induced by collagen, ADP plus fibrinogen, or thrombin. In preliminary experiments with ristocetin and platelet-poor plasma as a source of VWF, we have observed no inhibition by MAb IV.3 in two of three experiments, and slight inhibition in one of the three experiments. More recently, we have studied platelet ADP secretion along with aggregation, utilizing a lumiaggregometer, and have found that aggregated IgG-induced secretion and aggregation are inhibited concomitantly by MAb IV.3. Interestingly, MAb IV.3, alone, does not induce

Table 17-2
Inhibition of Aggregated IgG-Induced Platelet Aggregation by $IgG2_b$ Monoclonal Anti-p40 (IV.3) or Control $IgG2_b$ and Their Fragments

Potential Inhibitor	Concentration During Preincubation with Platelets (μg/ml)	Platelet Aggregation by Aggregated IgG max. slope*
None		1.58–1.76†
Intact MOPC 141	0.22	1.35
	2.17	1.49
	10.85	1.32
	21.74	1.12
	43.48	0.88
Intact anti-p40 (IV.3)	0.009	0.98
	0.017	0.35, 0.41
	0.043	0, 0
	0.085	0
Papain digest, anti-p40	0.022	1.76
	0.043	1.61
	0.22	0.41
	0.44	0
Papain digest, MOPC 141	0.22	1.61
	21.74	1.172

*Maximum slope: slope of maximal ascent on aggregometer tracing. Zero slope means no change in light transmission, i.e., a flat tracing.

†Range of four determinations during the experiment. The papain-digested material was used to test the effectiveness of Fab fragments, and continued no detectable intact IgG or Fc fragments. (Rosenfeld SI, Looney RJ, Leddy JP et al: J Clin Invest 76:2317, 1985)

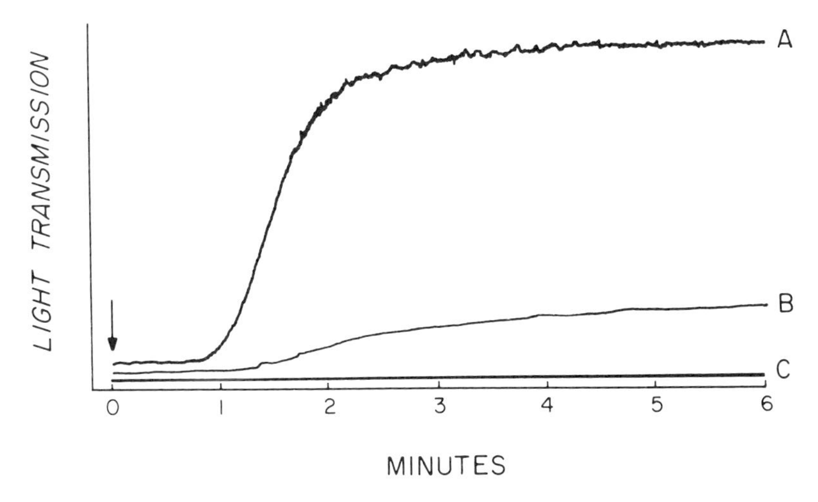

Figure 17-2. Receptor-bridging experiment in which platelet aggregation is induced by monoclonal anti-p40 (IV.3) (43 ng/ml) followed by fluid-phase $F(ab')_2$ goat antimurine Ig (6 μg/ml) (*A*). *B* represents the same reagents in the presence of apyrase (64 μg/ml). *C* is representative of three concurrent controls: anti-p40 (IV.3) (43 ng/ml) alone, and 1/10 UR-1 monoclonal anti-platelet antibody or MOPC 141 (43 ng/ml) followed by $F(ab')_2$ goat antibody alone. (All protein concentrations shown are final concentrations in the reaction mixtures.) The arrow marks the addition of the goat $F(ab')_2$ antibody (Rosenfeld SI, Looney RJ, Leddy JP: J Clin Invest 76:2317, 1985 with permission).

aggregation of washed human platelets when added over a wide concentration range (0.009 to 0.4 μg/ml). However, when platelets are preincubated with MAb IV.3 and then exposed to $F(ab')_2$ goat antimouse immunoglobulin, the platelets aggregate and release ADP. A typical aggregation response is shown in Figure 17-2. The minimal aggregation observed in curve *B* shows that this response is largely inhibitable by apyrase. In other experiments, nearly complete inhibition could be achieved by higher concentrations of apyrase. Tracing *C* represents a response typical of a number of negative controls, including the monoclonal antibody alone, the second cross-linking antibody alone, and an unrelated antiplatelet monoclonal antibody followed by the second cross-linking antibody. These studies, in conjunction with other negative studies using monoclonal antibodies to $Fc_\gamma RI$ and $Fc_\gamma RIII$, strongly suggest that of the Fc receptors known to be present on human blood leukocytes, the only one found on human platelets is $Fc_\gamma RII$.

A different approach to identification of immunoglobulin-binding proteins of human platelets was taken by Steiner and Lüscher.[52] They used a cleavable cross-linking agent to covalently link normal IgG to periodate-labeled platelets and then analyzed the membrane glycoproteins by two-dimensional SDS–PAGE. A glycoprotein with characteristics resembling those of GPIIIa was identified as the major membrane protein cross-linked to IgG. These studies used normal IgG that had not been aggregated. Thus, the membrane protein involved is probably not an Fc receptor. The portion of the IgG molecule (Fc or Fab) that was bound to the glycoprotein resembling GPIIIa was not determined. Nonetheless, the authors concluded that they had identified a possible senescence antigen on human platelets that may contribute to the accumulation of some portion of normally encountered, platelet-bound IgG. It is important to distinguish this type of binding from Fc receptor-mediated binding. The same group, using a different cross-linking agent, has recently claimed that intact monomeric IgG and $F(ab')_2$ fragments bind to GPIIIa, whereas Fc fragments bind to a protein with an M_γ of 200,000 nonreduced and 50,000 reduced.[56] The radioactive protein peaks upon which these claims are based represented trace platelet components, and these data should still be considered preliminary.

FUNCTIONAL RELEVANCE OF IMMUNOGLOBULIN G-BINDING MOLECULES ON PLATELETS

Of the several putative IgG-binding molecules identified by the methods described in the preceding sections, the only molecule that has been subjected to functional analysis is the $Fc_{\gamma}RII$ (p40) which we have studied. As summarized in the foregoing, a monoclonal antibody to this protein is capable of blocking functional responses of platelets to various immune complexes and IgG aggregates, providing strong evidence that this Fc receptor is linked to intracellular mechanisms triggering platelet aggregation and dense-granule release. The actual mechanisms whereby cross-linking of the p40 Fc receptor leads to cellular responses have not yet been elucidated, but they represent an area of ongoing research in our laboratories and those of others. It is of some interest that we, and others, have found that the platelet aggregation response to IgG immune complexes is not dependent upon the presence of extracellular calcium, although we have not ruled out the importance of intracellular calcium fluxes. Because the aggregation response is at least partially (but largely) inhibitable by apyrase, one may presume that secondary responses mediated by the secretion of ADP are involved in the amplification of the initial platelet response to cross-linking of the p40 Fc receptor. Recent experiments by Anderson and Anderson have shown that cross-linking platelet FcR leads to a five-fold increase in inositol phosphate production that is not inhibited by aspirin, but that is, at least partially, inhibited by the guanosine diphosphate (GDP) analogue $GDP_{\beta}S$.[4a] This suggests that signal transduction by the human platelet $Fc_{\gamma}RII$ occurs through G-protein-mediated activation of a phospholipase C.

QUANTITATIVE VARIATION OF PLATELET Fc RECEPTOR EXPRESSION: RELATIONSHIP TO THE PLATELET RESPONSE TO AGGREGATED IMMUNOGLOBULIN G

During the course of our functional studies of washed platelets using aggregated IgG as a stimulus, we became aware of consistent variation among donors in the ability of their platelets to respond to a standardized aggregated IgG stimulus. After preliminary studies suggested that these differences were not related to medication, sex, or menstrual period, we wondered whether these functional differences could be related to quantitative differences in platelet Fc receptor number or expression on the donors' platelets. We therefore studied the same group of donors on multiple occasions over several months, testing both the functional response of their washed platelets to a standardized input (500 μg/ml) of heat-aggregated IgG and (using the same samples) the relative platelet Fc receptor number utilizing a flow cytometer assay that quantitated the binding of either MAb IV.3 or heat aggregated IgG to the platelet surface.[48] The MAb was incubated at saturating concentrations with washed platelets. The platelets were then washed again and the amount of antibody bound was quantitated utilizing a fluorescein-labeled goat anti-mouse immunoglobulin [$F(ab')_2$]. The ability of the same platelets to bind aggregated IgG was tested by incubating the platelets with heat-aggregated IgG, in the presence of EDTA and apyrase. The platelets were then washed, and the amount of aggregated IgG bound was determined by flow cytometry, using a fluorescein-tagged $F(ab')_2$ goat antihuman IgG. These studies were repeated on a group of six normal donors over a 4-month period, and the results of two to four experiments on each donor were combined. These results are summarized in Figure 17-3. Panel *A* shows the main point of these studies, that the slope of the aggregation response to aggregated IgG is highly correlated with the number of p40 platelet receptors as assessed by staining with MAb IV.3. Notice that the platelets of donor c are functionally more active than the number of Fc receptors on his platelets would suggest. This was a consistent observation with this donor and, in subsequent studies, we have identified at least one other donor who has consistently higher functional responses than we would predict from the number of Fc receptors measured via MAb IV.3 binding. This suggests that there must be other factors, besides the number of Fc receptors, that ultimately determine platelet responsiveness to aggregated IgG. The excellent correlation between staining intensity with aggregated IgG and staining intensity with MAb IV.3 (Fig. 16-3, panel *B*) provides additional evidence that these two ligands bind to the same molecule on the surface of the platelets. This conclusion is also reinforced by the

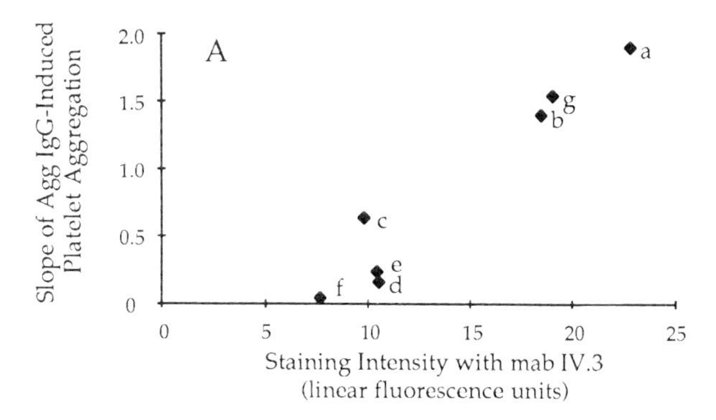

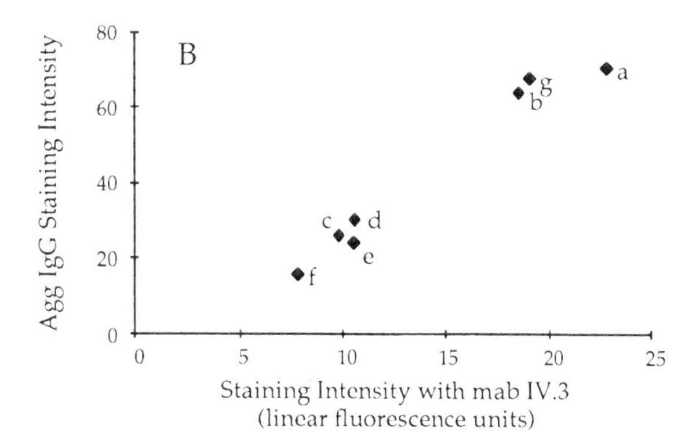

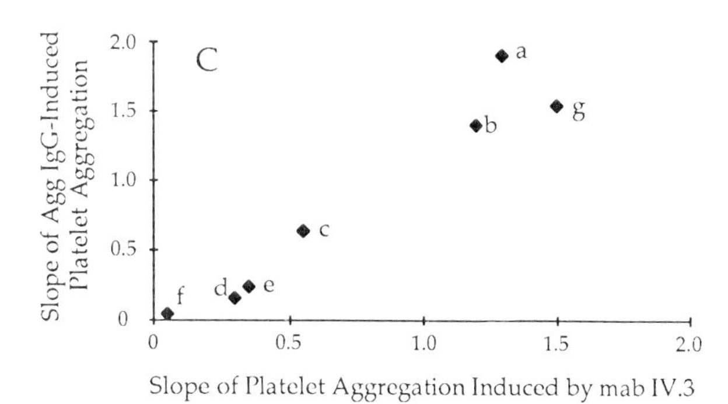

Figure 17-3. Correlation of platelet aggregation and flow cytometric data of various platelet donors. For most points, mean values for each parameter from two to four experiments are shown, but donor g was studied by flow cytometry in only one experiment. (*A*) The binding of MAb IV.3 to platelets by flow cytometry versus functional response of platelets to aggregated IgG. (*B*) The platelet binding of MAb IV.3 versus binding of agg IgG by flow cytometry. (*C*) The platelet aggregation induced by MAb IV.3 plus $F(ab')_2$ goat antimouse Ig versus platelet aggregation by agg IgG. (*D*) The platelet binding of MAb IV.3 versus platelet aggregation response to MAb IV.3 and $F(ab')_2$ goat antimouse Ig (Rosenfeld SI, Ryan DH, Looney RJ: J Immunol 138:2869, 1987).

data in panel *C* which indicate that the slope of platelet aggregation induced by aggregated IgG is highly correlated with the degree of platelet aggregation induced by MAb IV.3 plus a cross-linking $F(ab')_2$ antimouse Ig antibody. Panel *D* shows that the functional response induced by cross-linking p40 correlates with the number of MAb IV.3 molecules bound. In the six donors studied to produce the data in Figure 17-3, the number of Fc receptors or response to aggregated IgG did not correlate with sex, platelet size, platelet count, serum IgG, baseline platelet-associated IgG, or platelet responses to ADP plus fibrinogen or to collagen (Table 17-3). The values for platelet-associated IgG are presented in linear fluorescence units and represent the fluorescence of washed platelets incubated with the fluorescein-tagged $F(ab')_2$ antihuman IgG without prior incubation with aggregated IgG. Values such as these were subtracted from values obtained after incubation of the platelets with aggregated IgG and the fluorescein-tagged anti-IgG to generate the linear fluorescence units of staining intensity shown on the ordinate of panel *B* in Figure 17-3. It can, therefore, be seen that the baseline IgG associated with the washed platelets is much lower than the values obtained after incubation with aggregated IgG, although these baseline values are higher than the control values for staining with the mouse monoclonal antibody, which used a fluorescein tagged antimouse IgG antibody for detection. This latter antibody did not cross-react with human IgG.

The quantitation of Fc receptors using the flow cytometer, of course, can only be relative. To obtain a better estimate of the number of MAb IV.3-binding sites on human platelets we have directly measured the number of radiolabeled MAb IV.3 bound per platelet, in collaboration with Dr. R. J. Looney. We recognize that the use of an intact immunoglobulin molecule could lead to a binding artifact if one molecule of IV.3 is capable of binding to two molecules of p40 (utilizing both antibody-combining sites simultaneously). We intend to perform these studies using Fab fragments of the same antibody, but those data are not yet available. Nevertheless, because we have been unable to induce platelet activation with the intact monoclonal antibody alone over a wide range of concentrations, we believe it is highly

Table 17-3
Variables That Did Not Correlate with Platelet Responsiveness to Aggregated IgG or with Binding of MAb IV.3

						Platelet Aggregation Induced by	
Platelet Donors*	Age/Sex	Mean Platelet Vol.† (μm^3)	Platelet Count† ($\times 10^{-3}$)	Serum IgG‡ (mg/dl)	Platelet-Associated IgG (LFU)§	*ADP Plus Fibrinogen‖ (slope)*	Collagen# *(slope)*
a	25/F	10.5	261	1132	1.25	0.70	2.0
b	29/M	8.8	235	964	1.94	0.67	0.95
c	27/M	9.45	356	1040	1.41	0.5	1.5
d	46/M	8.35	333	876	1.52	0.43	1.4
e	24/F	10.1	291	953	1.72	0.60	1.15
f	25/F	8.9	314	1017	1.31	0.66	1.65

*Letters refer to the same donors used for the data in Figure 17-3.
†Mean platelet volume and platelet counts were measured by electronic impedance on the Coulter S+ analyzer by using EDTA-anticoagulated blood obtained at the time platelets were isolated for two to four of the experiments utilized for Figure 17-3.
‡IgG levels were determined by laser nephelometry on serum obtained at the time of one of the experiments utilized for Figure 17-3.
§LFU, linear fluorescence units, derived from the fluorescence intensity measurements of washed platelets incubated with goat $F(ab')_2$ antihuman IgG. Values represent means from two or three experiments.
‖Human fibrinogen was added to washed platelets to achieve a concentration of 400 mg/ml in the aggregometer cuvette. Values represent means from two or three experiments.
#Concentration of bovine collagen = 1.0 mg/ml in the aggregometer cuvette. Values represent means from two or three experiments.
(Rosenfeld SI, Ryan DH, Looney RJ et al: J Immunol 138:2869, 1987)

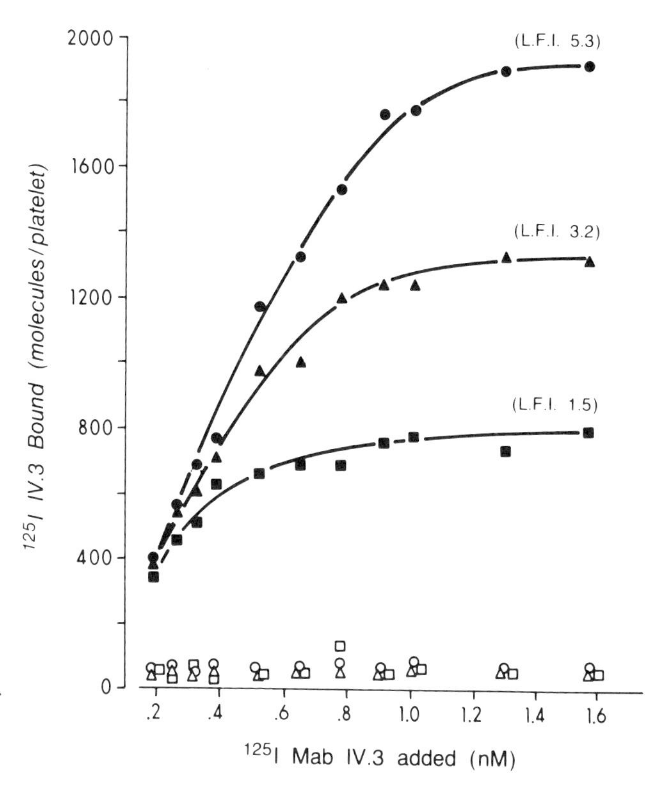

Figure 17-4. Binding of radiolabeled MAb IV.3 to washed platelets from three individual donors (○, ●, △, ▲, □, ■). These donors are not included in Figure 17-3 and Table 17-4. Specific binding is shown by solid symbols; nonspecific binding in the presence of 100-fold excess unlabeled MAb Iv.3 is shown by open symbols. The linear fluorescence index (LFI) was obtained by flow cytometry on the same washed platelet preparations utilizing saturating concentrations of unlabeled MAb IV.3 and fluorescein-labeled $F(ab')_2$ goat antimouse Ig.

unlikely that this monoclonal antibody is capable of binding to two p40 Fc receptors simultaneously.

For the saturation curves shown in Figure 17-4, three different individuals whose platelets displayed high, intermediate, and low reactivity to aggregated IgG were chosen. These donors were not among those used to generate the data for Figure 17-3. Nonspecific binding (shown in the open symbols) was determined by binding of radiolabeled MAb IV.3 in the presence of 100-fold excess of nonlabeled IV.3. Platelets with bound antibody were separated from unbound antibody by centrifugation through phthalate oils. Figure 17-4 shows the saturation binding curves only. Scatchard plots are not shown, but they revealed very similar slopes for all three platelet donors, suggesting that the differences in binding at saturation are not the result of differences in affinity of the monoclonal antibody for the p40 Fc receptor on different donor platelets. These saturation curves yield receptor numbers that are very similar to those obtained from Scatchard plots: approximately 1900 per platelet for the highest donor, 1300 for the middle donor, and 780 for the donor with the lowest number. Values obtained for each of these same platelet preparations by flow cytometry are shown as linear fluorescence index (LFI) values to the right of each curve. These values cannot be directly compared with those in Figure 17-3 because they have not been corrected for day-to-day variation in the calibration of the flow cytometer. It can be seen that the rank order of these values agrees with the values obtained by saturation binding. The number of molecules of MAb IV.3 bound per platelet at saturation agrees very well with the maximum number of binding sites determined for radiolabeled IgG dimers by Karas and colleagues (1350 ± 550),[26] further suggesting that the Fc receptor identified by MAb IV.3 is the same as that identified by ligand-binding studies utilizing IgG oligomers.

In the course of our binding studies with MAb IV.3 and aggregated IgG using platelets from normal human volunteers, we have not found any evidence that a significant fraction of platelets do not bind either of these ligands. Another type of quantitative variability was reported by Moore and Nachman, who used microscopic analysis of fluorescent staining of platelets with fluorescein-conjugated ovalbumin–anti-ovalbumin immune complexes.[36] These workers found that only 3% of the platelets from normal donors exhibited visible staining, whereas an average of 76% of platelets from patients with myeloproliferative diseases demonstrated visible staining. These authors found, by the same technique, that fluorescein-conjugated KLH–anti-KLH complexes stained 80% to 90% of normal platelets. Because the thresholds for detection of binding with the methods used may be very different, we cannot directly compare our results with those of Moore and Nachman,[36] but it is conceivable that their method utilizing ovalbumin–anti-ovalbumin is capable of detecting only those platelets with the highest levels of Fc receptors and that the percentage of such platelets is increased in myeloproliferative diseases. Alternatively, their method may detect a different, lower-affinity Fc receptor not detected on normal platelets by our (or their) methods, which is induced or up-regulated in myeloproliferative diseases. A study of MAb IV.3 binding to platelets of patients with myeloproliferative diseases would obviously be of interest and would probably serve to resolve these discrepancies.

STRUCTURAL POLYMORPHISM OF PLATELET IMMUNOGLOBULIN G Fc RECEPTORS

The 40-kDa Fc receptor for IgG ($Fc_\gamma RII$) on human monocytes is capable of interacting with murine IgG1 anti-T3 monoclonal antibodies to support a human T-lymphocyte proliferative response.[31] This response is supported by the monocytes of approximately 80% of North American Caucasian individuals, whereas $Fc_\gamma RII$ on the monocytes of the remaining individuals fails to support such a response. This ability of an individual's monocyte-bound $Fc_\gamma RII$ to support murine IgG1 anti-T3-mediated lymphocyte proliferation has been correlated with a structural polymorphism of the 40-kDa $Fc_\gamma FII$ as revealed by isoelectric focusing of the receptor isolated by immunoprecipitation with MAb IV.3.[4]

The three distinctive isoelectric focusing patterns of p40 from human monocytes are shown in Figure 17-5. The pattern designated NN has been found only in monocytes from individuals incapable of supporting a murine IgG1 anti-T3 proliferative response. $Fc_\gamma RII$ from individuals capable of supporting such a response have had one of two patterns designated RR or RN. By using similar isoelectric focusing gels to study platelet p40, we have found virtually identical isoelectric focusing patterns from the platelets and monocytes of individuals whose monocytes have already been typed as RR, NN, or RN, except that the banding in the more acidic region tends to be denser in the platelets, whereas the less acidic bands tend to be denser in the monocytes from the same individual.*

In further studies, we have utilized human red blood cells coated with a murine IgG1 monoclonal antibody to stimulate platelets through their p40 Fc receptor. We found that platelets from both of two individuals with the NN isoelectric focusing pattern failed to respond to the mouse IgG1-coated red blood cells, whereas platelets from both of two individuals with the RR pattern gave brisk aggregation and secretion responses to these murine IgG1-coated red blood cells. The platelets from one individual with the RN pattern gave intermediate functional response to the murine IgG1-coated red blood cells. On the other hand, platelets of all of the foregoing individuals tested gave robust and strong responses when stimulated with heat-aggregated human IgG, regardless of isoelectric focusing pattern. Indeed, we found no correlation between the magnitude of response of an individual's platelets to heat aggregated human IgG (which correlates with the number of p40 Fc receptors on their surface) and the individual's isoelectric focusing pattern. Subjects whose platelets gave strong functional responses to human IgG aggregates had isoelectric focusing patterns of any of the three types, as did subjects whose platelets gave poor responses to aggregated IgG. Thus, the ability of the monocyte p40 Fc receptor of specific phenotypes to bind murine IgG1 is shared by the platelet p40 Fc receptor of the same phenotypes.* However, the platelet responsiveness to polyclonal human IgG aggregates is not determined by this structural polymorphism but is more highly correlated with the number of Fc receptors expressed on the platelets. Whether or not this structural polymorphism of the platelet $Fc_\gamma RII$ is corre-

*Looney RJ, Anderson CL, Ryan DH, Rosenfeld SI: J Immunol, in press, 1988.

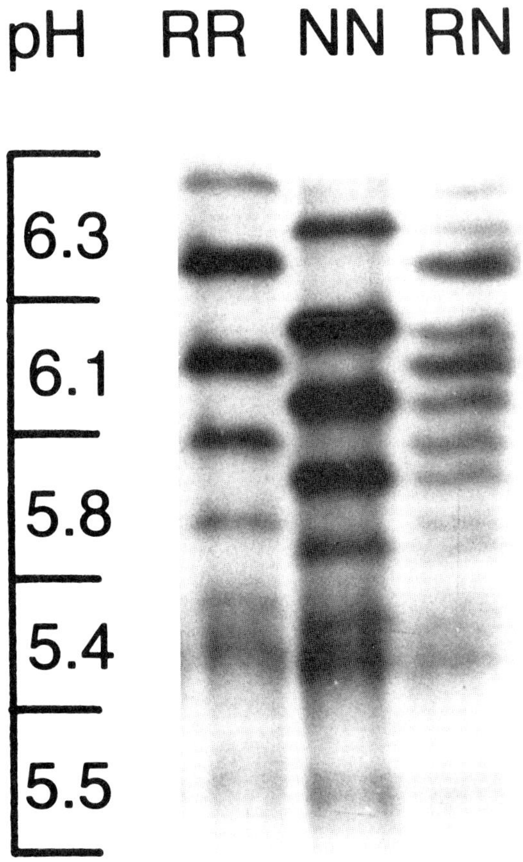

Figure 17-5. Autoradiograph showing the three distinct IEF patterns of the monocyte 40-kDa Fc receptors. Monocytes were purified, surface radioiodinated, and lysed in detergent-containing buffer. The 40-kDa Fc receptor was purified from the monocyte lysate by affinity chromatography by using immobilized MAb IV.3, and was applied to a vertical slab IEF gel. The *p*H gradient, shown on the left of the figure, was obtained by sectioning lateral lanes of the unfixed gel into 1-cm slices and eluting for 24 h with 1 ml of water. The figure shows only the middle third of the vertical dimension of the autoradiograph: The only other significant material on the autoradiograph was a single dense band at the origin of each lane representing about 25% of the total amount of radioactivity seen in each lane (Anderson CL, Ryan DH, Looney RJ, Leary PC: J Immunol 138:2254, 1987).

lated with specificity for human immunoglobulin subclasses is currently under investigation in our laboratories.

RELATIONSHIP OF PLATELET Fc RECEPTORS TO Fc RECEPTORS ON OTHER CELLS

The 40-kDa sialoglycoprotein $Fc_{\gamma}RII$ of human platelets is also found on other cells, according to both molecular size and serologic criteria (*see* Ref. 3 for a brief review). The MAb IV.3 used for characterization of the platelet FcR binds to human macrophages,* monocyte, neutrophils and eosinophils, as well as to the promonocytic cell line U937, the promyelocytic line HL-60, and the erythroblast line K562.[2,3,22,31,32,47,48] A 40-kDa molecule has been isolated from all three of these cell lines and from monocytes and neutrophils by immunoadsorption using immobilized IV.3 or human IgG ligand.[2,31,32,47] Although not recognized by MAb IV.3, a 40-kDa FcR, present on human B cells, cross-reacts immunologically with the 40-kDa FcR of U937 cells.[31] Furthermore, another anti-$Fc_{\gamma}RII$ Mb, KU79, recognizes an epitope common to the 40-kDa FcR of B cells, monocytes, neutrophils, but not the $Fc_{\gamma}FII$ of platelets.[57]

Recently, cDNA for human $Fc_{\gamma}RII$ has been cloned[18,53] by screening U937 cDNA libraries with oligonucleotide probes derived from the murine $Fc_{\gamma}RII$ cDNA.[17,30,46] The sequence of the human cDNA for $Fc_{\gamma}RII$ indicates that the receptor is a 36-kDa transmembrane glycoprotein with leader, extracellular, and transmembrane domains homologous (between 50% and 100%) with the murine $Fc_{\gamma}RII$ receptor and possessing a unique intracellular domain. This unique domain is a surprising finding because the receptors seem to mediate the same functions in both species. Homology with the Ig gene superfamily and with the c-*fms* proto-on-

*Anderson CL et al: Unpublished observations.

cogene and the CSF-1 receptor has also been noted. The $Fc_\gamma RII$ cDNA hybridizes not only with a 1.5-kb mRNA transcript that encodes $Fc_\gamma RII$ but also with a larger 2.5-kb transcript that is a likely candidate for the larger FcRI.[53] Murine L cells transfected with the cDNA bind FcR ligands (e.g., aggregated human IgG) and anti-$Fc_\gamma RII$ MAb IV.3, but not anti-FcRI or anti-$Fc_\gamma RIII$ MAbs. The molecular details of this receptor are expected to differ only slightly from those of the platelet FcR.

THE PLATELET Fc RECEPTOR FOR IMMUNOGLOBULIN E

Platelets have been found to bear specific sites on their surfaces capable of binding IgE and of mediating IgE-dependent killing of parasites such as the schistosomula of *Schistosoma mansoni.*[23,24] Direct-binding studies of human myeloma IgE to human platelets reveal that approximately 20%[11,25] of normal platelets are capable of binding IgE, whereas the percentage of IgE-binding platelets increases to 50% in individuals with asthma or parasite infections.[25] Analysis of binding isotherms by the Scatchard method indicates two binding sites, one relatively sparse (about 1000 binding sites per platelet, assuming that all platelets bind IgE) but with moderately high affinity for ligand ($K_a = 3.3 \times 10^7$ M^{-1}), and another with up to 60,000 sites per cell but of lower affinity ($K^a = 7.8 \times 10^5$ M^{-1}).[25] Further evidence that this binding site is functional comes from studies showing that cross-linking of surface-bound IgE with anti-Ig stimulates the release reaction and platelet aggregation.[11]

The molecular nature of the IgE FcR on platelets is still uncertain. Expression of the GPIIb-IIIa complex is thought to be somehow related to the IgE FcR, based upon the observations that platelets from individuals with Glanzmann's thrombasthenia neither bind IgE nor mediate IgE-dependent schistosomula killing and that monoclonal antibodies directed against the IIb-IIIa complex inhibited IgE binding to platelets.[1,11] A single study in which the receptor was immunoprecipitated from platelet lysates using IgE-affinity chromatography, however, revealed multiple protein bands with relative molecular masses of 97, 45, 43, and 32 kDa. This finding would suggest that the binding site is not actually part of the IIb-IIIa complex[8] or that, in that particular study, significant proteolytic degradation of one or both components of the GPIIb-IIIa complex had occurred during the isolation procedure.

In fact, the platelet FcR for IgE may be a member of a class of low-affinity IgE receptors (distinct from the high-affinity IgE receptor found on basophils and mast cells) common to platelets, monocytes, eosinophils, and lymphocytes. This conclusion is most compellingly suggested by the use of a goat antiserum[35] to abrogate IgE-mediated binding and biologic responses by all of these cells.[8] However, some monoclonal antibodies against this receptor show a more restricted specificity, recognizing epitopes on one or more, but not all, groups of cells bearing a low-affinity IgE FcR.[8,49,55] Given the data obtained with the goat antiserum, it seems likely that the platelet IgE FcR will be similar to the IgE receptor purified from lymphocytes whose amino acid structure has recently been inferred by analysis of cDNA clones.[20,27] This receptor is remarkable on two counts: first, its NH_2-terminus resides inside the cell, whereas its COOH-terminal portion is outside; and second, it has considerable homology to several lectin-binding animal proteins, including the rat asialoglycoprotein receptor, the chicken hepatic lectin, and the rat mannose binding protein.[20,27]

CONCLUSIONS

It is clear from the studies just summarized that human platelets have on their surfaces one or more receptors for the Fc region of IgG, and least one receptor for the Fc region of IgE, and that these receptors are capable of inducing functional responses in the platelets when cross-linked by antibodies or by immune complexes. Whether or not more than one Fc receptor for IgG is present on platelets, as has been documented for mononuclear phagocytes and neutrophils, and whether or not the p40 Fc receptor exists in a complex with other proteins in the platelet membrane, are questions that need to be resolved by further research.

Concerning physiologic and pathologic roles for the platelet Fc receptor, it is most intriguing to speculate that these molecules may be involved in the pathogenesis of thrombocytopenias occurring in patients who have circulating or vessel-deposited immune complexes or in patients with septicemia caused by organisms capable of binding IgG. That thrombocytopenia is by no means universal in these conditions invites further speculation that individuals with larger numbers of Fc receptors on their platelet surfaces may be at greater risk for thrombocytopenia under conditions of marginal immune complex exposure. If the genetic polymorphism of the platelet Fc receptor can be shown to determine specificity for human immunoglobulin subclasses, as it does for murine immunoglobulins, this may be another variable important in determining whether or not thrombocytopenia will be an outcome of immune complex exposure. The potential role of the platelet as an effector cell capable of contributing to the pathogenesis of tissue damage when immune complexes are deposited in vascular walls has thus far received little attention but is intriguing because of the frequent appearance of intravascular thrombosis at sites of immune complex-mediated damage, such as occurs in glomerulonephritis and vasculitis. The participation of platelets in immune-mediated tissue damage could be modulated by platelet properties, such as the number or affinity of Fc receptors, but could also be modulated by important characteristics of the immune reactants deposited, such as the presence or absence of fibrinogen, fibronectin, vitronectin, or complement components, all of which might interact with platelets through receptors independent of the Fc receptor. The potential biologic role of the low-affinity IgE receptors on human platelets, both in immunity to parasite infection and in mediating a possible role for platelets in extrinsic allergic reactions, is very intriguing and may lead to an understanding of new roles for the platelet in host resistance and in allergic diseases.[7]

REFERENCES

1. Ameisen JC, Joseph M, Caen JP, Kusnierz J-P, Capron M, Boizard B, Wautier J-L, Levy-Toledano S, Vorng H, Capron A: A role for glycoprotein IIb–IIIa complex in the binding of IgE to human platelets and platelet IgE-dependent cytotoxic function. Br J Haematol 64:21, 1986

2. Anderson CL, Guyre PM, Whitin JC, Ryan DH, Looney RJ, Fanger MW: Monoclonal antibodies to Fc receptors for IgG on human mononuclear phagocytes: Antibody characterization and induction of superoxide production in a monocyte cell line. J Biol Chem 261:12856, 1986

3. Anderson CL, Looney RJ: Review: Human leukocyte IgG Fc receptors. Immunol Today 7:264, 1986

4. Anderson CL, Ryan DH, Looney RJ, Leary PC: Polymorphism of the human monocyte 40 kD receptor for IgG. J Immunol 138:2254, 1987

4a. Anderson GP, Anderson CL: Signal transduction by the platelet Fc receptor (abst) FASEB J 2: A614, 1988

4b. Berndt MC, Chong BH, Bull HA, Zola H, Castaldi PA: Molecular characterization of quinine/quinidine drug-dependent antibody platelet interactin using monoclonal antibodies. Blood 66:1292, 1985

5. Bettex-Galland M, Luscher ER, Simon G, Vassalli P: Induction of viscous metamorphosis in human blood platelets by means other than thrombin. Nature 200:109, 1963

6. Breckenridge RT, Rosenfeld SI, Graff KS, Leddy JP: Hereditary C5 deficiency in man. III. Studies of hemostasis and platelet responses to zymosan. J Immunol 118:12, 1977

7. Capron A, Ameisen J-C, Joseph M, Auriault C, Fennel AB, Caen J: New functions for platelets and their pathological implications. Int Archs Allergy Appl Immunol 77:107, 1985

8. Capron M, Jourault T, Prin L, Joseph M, Ameisen J-C, Butterworth AE, Papin J-P, Kusnierz J-P, Capron A: Functional study of a monoclonal antibody to IgE Fc receptor (Fc_ER_2) of eosinophils, platelets, and macrophages. J Exp Med 164:72, 1986

9. Cheng CM, Hawiger J: Affinity isolation and characterization of immunoglobulin G Fc fragment-binding glycoprotein from human blood platelets. J Biol Chem 254:2165, 1979

10. Christie DJ, Mullen PC, Aster RH: Fab-mediated binding of drug-dependent antibodies to platelets in quinidine- and quinine-induced thrombocytopenia. J Clin Invest 75:310, 1985

11. Cines DB, Keyl HVD, Levinson AI: In vitro binding of an IgE protein to human platelets. J Immunol 136:3433, 1986

12. Des Prez RM, Steckley S, Stroud RM, Hawiger J: Interaction of *Histoplasma capsulatum* with human platelets. J Infect Dis 142:32, 1980

13. Endresen GK, Forre O: Studies on the binding of immunoglobulins and immune complexes to the surface of human platelets: IgG molecules react with platelet Fc receptors with the CH_3 domain. Int Arch Allergy App Immunol 67:33, 1982

14. Hawiger J, Steckley S, Hammond D, Cheng C, Timmons S, Glick AD, Des Prez RM: Staphylococci-induced human platelet injury mediated by protein A and immunoglobulin G Fc fragment receptor. J Clin Invest 64:931, 1979

15. Henson PM, Ginsberg MH: Immunological reactions of platelets. In Gordon JL (ed): Platelets in Biology and Pathology, p 265. Amsterdam, Elsevier/North-Holland, 1981

16. Henson PM, Spiegelberg HL: Release of serotonin from human platelets induced by aggregated immunoglobulins of different classes and subclasses. J Clin Invest 52:1282, 1981

17. Hibbs ML, Walker ID, Kirszbaum L, Pietersz GA, Deacon NJ, Chambers GW, McKenzie IFC, Hogarth PM: The murine Fc receptor for immunoglobulin: Purification, partial amino acid sequence, and isolation of cDNA clones. Proc Natl Acad Sci USA 83:6980, 1986

18. Hibbs ML, Bonadonna L, Scott BM, McKenzie IFC, Hogarth PM: Molecular cloning of a human IgG Fc receptor. Pro Natl Acad Sci USA 85:2240, 1988

19. Humphrey JH, Jacques RJ: The release of histamine and 5-hydroxytryptamine (serotonin) from platelets by antigen–antibody reactions (in vitro). J Physiol 128:9, 1955

20. Ikuta K, Tahami M, Kim CW, Honjo T, Miyoshi T, Tagaya Y, Kawabe T, Yodoi J: Human lymphocyte Fc receptor for IgE: Sequence homology of its cloned DNA with animal lectins. Proc Natl Acad Sci USA 84:819, 1987

21. Israels ED, Nisli G, Paraskevas F, Israels LG: Platelet Fc receptor as a mechanism for Ag–Ab complex-induced platelet injury. Thromb Diath Haemorrh 29:434, 1973

22. Jones DH, Looney RJ, Anderson CL: Two distinct classes of IgG Fc receptors on a human monocyte line (U937) defined by differences in binding of murine IgG subclasses at low ionic strength. J Immunol 135:3348, 1985

23. Joseph M, Auriault C, Capron A, Ameisen JC, Pancre V, Torpier G, Kusnierz JP, Ovlaque G, Capron A: IgE-dependent platelet cytotoxicity against helminths. Adv Exp Med Biol 184:23, 1985

24. Joseph M, Auriault C, Capron A, Vorng H, Viens P: A new function for platelets: IgE-dependent killing of shistosomes. Nature 303:810, 1983

25. Joseph M, Capron A, Amiesen J-C, Capron M, Vorng H, Pancre V, Kusnierz J-P, Auriault C: The receptor for IgE on blood platelets. Eur J Immunol 16:306, 1986

26. Karas SP, Rosse WF, Kurlander RJ: Characterization of the IgG-Fc receptor on human platelets. Blood 60:1277, 1982

26a. Kelton JG, Smith JW, Santos AV, Murphy WG, Horsewood P: Platelet IgG Fc receptor. Am J Hematol 25:299, 1987

27. Kikutani A, Invi S, Sato R, Barsumian E, Owaki H, Yamasaki K, Kaisho T, Uchebayashi N, Hardy R, Hirano T, Tsunasawa S, Sakyama F, Suemura M, Kishimoto T: Molecular structure of the human lymphocyte receptor for immunoglobulin E. Cell 47:657, 1986

28. Kikutani A, Suemura M, Owaki H, Nahamura H, Sato R, Yamasaki K, Barsumian EL, Hardy RR, Kishimoto T: FcE receptors, a specific differentiation marker transiently expressed on mature B cells prior to isotope switching. J Exp Med 164:1455, 1986

29. Kunicki TJ, Johnson MM, Aster RH: Absence of the platelet receptor for drug-dependent antibodies in the Bernard-Soulier syndrome. J Clin Invest 62:716, 1978

30. Lewis VA, Koch T, Plutner H, Mellman I: A complementary DNA clone for a macrophage–lymphocyte Fc receptor. Nature 324:371, 1986

31. Looney RJ, Abraham GN, Anderson CL: Human monocytes and U937 cells bear two distinct Fc receptors for IgG. J Immunol 136:1641, 1986

32. Looney RJ, Ryan DH, Takahashi K, Fleit HB, Cohen HJ, Abraham GN, Anderson CL: Identification of a second class of IgG Fc receptors on human neutrophils: A 40 kD molecule found also on eosinophils. J Exp Med 163:826, 1986

33. Martin SE, Breckenridge RT, Rosenfeld SI, Leddy JP: Responses of human platelets to immunologic stimuli: Independent roles for complement and IgG in zymosan activation. J Immunol 120:9, 1978

34. Metzger H, Alvarez G, Hohman R, Kinet FP, Pribluda V, Quarto R: The receptor with high affinity for IgE. Annu Rev Immunol 4:419, 1986

35. Milewicz FM, Plummer JM, Spiegelberg HL: Comparison of the Fc receptors for IgE on human lymphocytes and monocytes. J Immunol 129:563, 1982

36. Moore A, Nachman RL: Platelet Fc receptor: Increased expression in myeloproliferative disease. J Clin Invest 67:1064, 1981

37. Moore A, Ross GD, Nachman RL: Interaction of platelet membrane receptors with von Willebrand factor, ristocetin, and the Fc region of immunoglobulin G. J Clin Invest 62:1053, 1978

38. Mueller-Eckhard CL, Lüscher EF: Immune reactions of human blood platelets. I. A comparative study on the effects on platelets of heterologous antiplatelet antiserum, antigen–antibody complexes, aggregated gamma globulins, and thrombin. Thromb Diath Haemorrh 20:155, 1968

39. Mueller-Eckhard CL, Lüscher EF: Immune reactions of human blood platelets. II. The effect of latex particles coated with gamma globulin in relation to complement activation. Thromb Diath Haemorrh 20:168, 1968

40. Nagai T, Adachi M, Noro N, Yodoi J, Uchino H: T and B lymphocytes with immunoglob-

ulin E Fc receptors (Fc_ER) in patients with nonallergic hyperimmunoglobulinemia. Clin Immunol Immunopathol 35:261, 1985

41. Noro N, Yoshioka A, Adachi M, Yasuda K, Masuda T, Yodoi J: Monoclonal antibody inhibiting IgE binding to $Fc_ER(+)$ human lymphocytes. J Immunol 137:1258, 1986

42. Pfueller SL, Cosgrove LJ: Activation of human platelets in PRP via their Fc-receptor by antigen-antibody complexes or immunoglobulin G: Requirement for particle-bound fibrinogen. Thromb Res 20:97, 1980

43. Pfueller SL, Kerlero de Rosbo N, Bilston RA: Platelets deficient in glycoprotein I have normal Fc receptor expression. Br J Haematol 56:607, 1984

44. Pfueller SL, Lüscher EF: The effects of aggregated immunoglobulins on human blood platelets in relation to their complement-fixing abilities. I. Studies of immunoglobulins of different types. J Immunol 109:517, 1972

45. Pfueller SL, Weber S, Lüscher EF: Studies on the mechanism of the human platelet release reaction induced by immunologic stimuli. III. Relationship between the binding of soluble IgG aggregates to the Fc receptor and cell response in the presence and absence of plasma. J Immunol 118:514, 1977

46. Ravetch JV, Luster AD, Weinshank R, Kochan J, Pavlovec A, Portnoy DA, Hulmes J, Pan Y-CE, Unkeless JC: Structural heterogeneity and functional domains of murine immunoglobulin G Fc receptors. Science 234:717, 1986

47. Rosenfeld SI, Looney RJ, Leddy JP, Phipps DC, Abraham GN, Anderson CL: Human platelet Fc receptor for IgG: Identification as a 40 kD membrane protein shared by monocytes. J Clin Invest 76:2317, 1985

48. Rosenfeld SI, Ryan DH, Looney RJ, Anderson CL, Abraham GN, Leddy JP: Human platelet Fc receptors: Quantitative expression correlates with functional responses. J Immunol 138:2869, 1987

49. Sarfati M, Nutman T, Fonteyn C, Delespesse G: Presence of antigenic determinants common to Fc IgE receptors on human macrophages, T and B lymphocytes and IgE-binding factors. Immunology 59:569, 1986

50. Smith ME, Reid DM, Jones CE, Jordan JN, Kantz CA, Shulman MR: Binding of quinine- and quinidine-dependent drug antibodies to platelets is mediated by the Fab domain of the immunoglobulin G and is not Fc dependent. J Clin Invest 79:912, 1987

51. Spycher MO, Nydegger UE, Lüscher EF: The calcium-dependent neutral protease of human blood platelets: A comparison of its effects on the receptors for von Willebrand factor and for the Fc-fragment derived from IgG. Adv Exp Med Biol 167:241, 1984

52. Steiner M, Lüscher EF: Identification of the immunoglobulin G receptor of human platelets. J Biol Chem 261:7230, 1986

53. Stuart SG, Trounstine ML, Vaux DJT, Koch T, Martens CL, Mellman I, Moore KW: Isolation and expression of cDNA clones encoding a human receptor for IgG (Fc_gRII). J Exp Med 166:1668, 1987

54. Stricker RB, Reyes PT, Corash L, Shuman MA: Evidence that a 210,000-molecular-weight glycoprotein (GP210) serves as a platelet Fc receptor. J Clin Invest 79:1589, 1987

55. Suemura M, Kikutani H, Barsumian EL, Hattori Y, Kishimoto S, Sato R, Maeda A, Nakamura H, Owaki H, Hardy R, Kishimoto T: Monoclonal anti-Fc_E-receptor antibodies with different specificities and studies on the expression of Fc_E receptors on human B and T cells. J Immunol 137:1214, 1986

56. Vancura S, Steiner M: Identification of Fc and $F(ab')_2$ IgG receptors on human platelets. Proc Natl Acad Sci USA 84:3575, 1987

57. Vaughn M, Taylor M, Mohanakumar T: Characterization of human IgG Fc receptors. J Immunol 135:4059, 1985

58. Zimmerman TS, Spiegelberg HL: Pneumococcus-induced release froom human platelets. Identification of the participating plasma/serum factor as immunoglobulin. J Clin Invest 56:828, 1975

18

Interaction of Human Platelets with the Complement System

PETER J. SIMS

In addition to accelerating their clearance from the circulation in various disease states, immune reactions affecting blood platelets can lead to platelet aggregation, the secretion of proteolytic enzymes and vasoactive amines from platelet granules, and platelet membrane-catalyzed activation of the coagulation and fibrinolytic pathways. Many of these platelet responses in vivo are suspected to be mediated directly or indirectly through activation of components of the complement system. In this chapter, I will summarize known interactions of human platelets with the various proteins of the complement system and discuss the implications of these interactions in terms of overall platelet function and survival within the vasculature during health and disease.

OVERVIEW OF THE CHEMISTRY AND BIOLOGY OF THE COMPLEMENT SYSTEM

For a comprehensive description of the chemistry and pathobiology of the human complement system, the reader is referred to several excellent recent reviews.[24,130,131] In brief, the complement system includes more than 20 plasma proteins that interact through two interlinked enzymatic reaction pathways to initiate the controlled production of activated species with distinct immunoregulatory, opsonic, or inflammatory activities (Table 18-1 and Fig. 18-1). In addition to these fluid phase reactant and regulatory proteins, the complement system also encompasses a variety of receptor proteins, distributed in the plasma membrane of several cell types, that specifically bind the activated products of this system. As will be briefly described in the following, these complement receptors can serve adherence and regulatory functions, or can serve to mediate stimulus-response transduction across the plasma membrane to initiate cell activation.

Classical Pathway

The classical pathway is initiated through the conformational activation of C1q, one of the components of the $\overline{C1}$* enzyme complex.[21,160] C1 is present in plasma largely as a Ca^{2+}-dependent complex between C1q and the proenzymes C1r and C1s with the stoichiometry $C1q,r_2,s_2$. C1q is a 410-kDa protein formed from six subunits, each comprising three disulfide-bonded chains. Ultrastructurally, the molecule exhibits six globular heads joined by filamentous segments to a helical stemlike core containing the amino-terminus of all 18 polypeptide chains. This helical core is compositionally and structurally similar to collagen, and it can compete for collagen binding to the platelet collagen receptor (discussed later). The

*A bar over a C component indicates that it is in its enzymatically activated form.

Table 18-1
Components and Regulatory Proteins of the Complement System

	Molecular Mass (kDa)	Number of Polypeptide Chains	Approx. Serum Concentration (μ g/ml)	Enzyme or Proenzyme (+) Yes, (−) No	Function in the C-Activation Sequence
Component					
C1q	410	18	70	−	
C1r	83	1	50	+	
C1s	83	1	40	+	Components of classical activation pathway (C1q, C1r, C1s, C4, C2, C3)
C4	200	3	640	−	
C2	117	1	25	+	
C3	185	2	1200	−	
Factor B	93	1	200	+	Components of alternative activation pathway (C3, Factor B, Factor D, Factor P)
Factor D	24	1	1	+	
Factor P	220	4	25	−	
C5	191	2	70		
C6	120	1	65	−	Components of membrane attack complex (C5b–9) (C6, C7, C8, C9)
C7	110	1	55	−	
C8	151	3	55	−	
C9	71	1	60	−	
Regulatory factors					
C1-INH	104	1	240	−	Inactivates $\overline{C1}$ enzyme complex
Carboxypeptidase N	84	1	Trace	+	Inactivates C3a, C4a, C5a
C4b-binding protein	570	5	250	−	Binds C4b; cofactor for factor I
Factor H	150	2	500	−	Binds C3b, C4b; cofactor for factor I
Factor I	88	1	35	+	Cleaves α chains of C3b and C4b (forming iC3b, iC4b)
Vitronectin (S-protein)	83	1	500	−	Blocks C5b67 binding to cell surface
Cell surface components with regulatory function					
CRI	250 (260)	1	NA	−	Cofactor for C3b, C4b, cleavage by factor I
Decay accelerating factor*	70	1	NA	−	Decay dissociates C3/C5-convertases
Homologous restriction factor†		1	NA	−	Blocks C9 activation by membrane C5b–8

*Not present in primate platelets.
†Detected in human erythrocytes; expression by other cells awaits experimental verification.

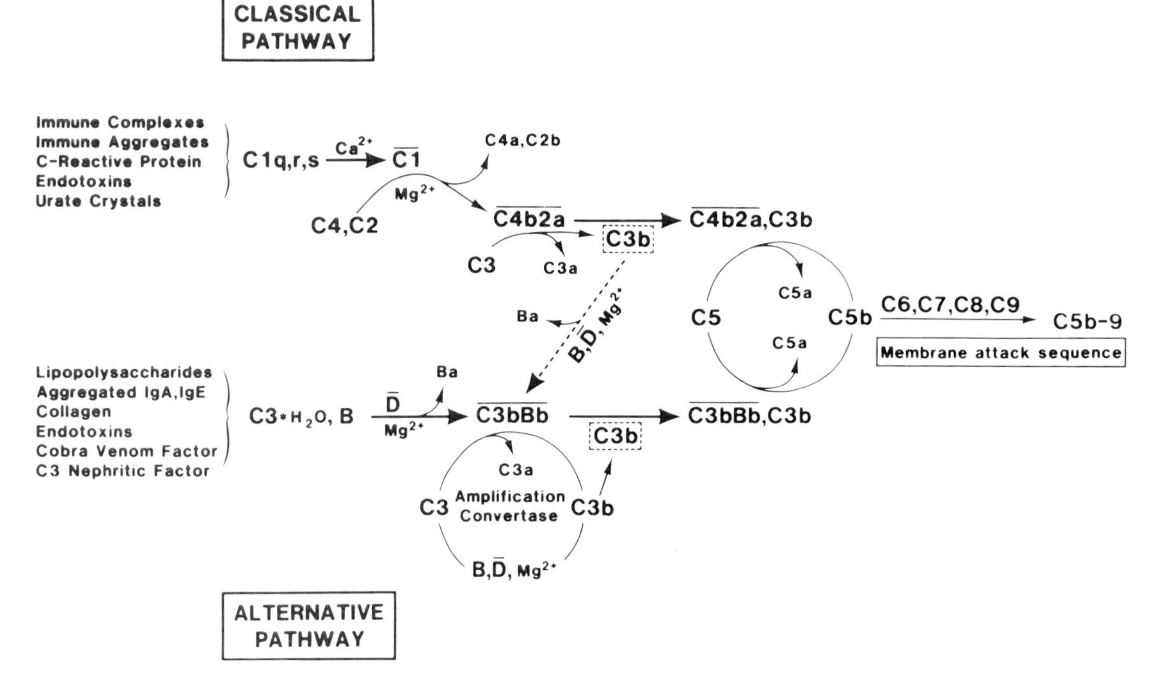

Figure 18-1. The classical and alternative complement activation pathways. A summary of the reaction sequences of the classical and alternative complement activation pathways. Regulatory proteins are not shown (*see* Fig. 18-2). Note the key role of C3b in recruitment of the alternative pathway C3 amplification convertase. Bar over complement component (e.g., $\overline{C1}$) denotes enzyme activity. See text for description.

C1r and C1s dimers bind to the collagenlike tail of C1q, whereas the binding of C1 activators generally occurs through the globular heads of C1q. Activation of C1 requires multipoint attachment of C1q to the Fc domains of immunoglobulin within immune complexes. This can be achieved by simultaneous attachment of two globular heads of C1q to two adjacent IgG molecules or to multiple Fc of a single antigen-complexed molecule of IgM. This requirement for multimeric attachment serves to limit C1 activation by immunoglobulin to those molecules of IgG complexed to antigen at high density on the cell surface or to IgG incorporated into immune complexes. Additionally, attachment through C1q serves to topologically restrict the reactions initiated by the $\overline{C1}$ complex to the close proximity of the antigenic surface. The conformational change in C1q, initiated upon multimeric attachment of the globular heads, is transmitted to the $C1r_2s_2$ subunits, resulting in proteolytic autoactivation of the C1r dimer, which then proteolytically activates C1s. Activated $\overline{C1s}$ possesses the catalytic site for proteolytic activation of C4 and C2. In addition to immune complexes, C1 activation can also be initiated by C-reactive protein, certain viral and bacterial membranes, endotoxin, monosodium urate crystals, cytoskeletal proteins, and heart mitochondrial membranes.

The next reaction step involves proteolytic cleavage of the α chain of C4 by $\overline{C1s}$, generating two fragments C4a and C4b.[108] C4a is a vasoactive peptide of 77 amino acids (removed from the NH_2-terminal end of the α chain). The C4b fragment provides the essential cofactor for assembly of the C3/C5-convertase of the classical pathway. In addition to liberating the C4a peptide, $\overline{C1s}$ cleavage of the α chain of C4 exposes an intrachain thiolester bond within the C4b domain of the molecule, which provides a short-lived and highly reactive carbonyl for covalent attachment of the protein to suitable acceptor residues (primary amines and hydroxyl groups) expressed by the antigen–antibody complex or the cell surface.[139] Once covalently deposited on the cell surface, C4b

Table 18-2
Human Platelet Receptors and Regulatory Proteins That Function in the Complement System

Platelet Component	Location and Function
Clq (collagen) receptor*	Cell surface receptor for Clq and collagen; binds C1q-containing immune complexes; mediates platelet adhesion to vascular collagen, and activates platelet secretion
C1-INH	α-Granule constituent, inhibitor of $\overline{C1}$ enzyme complex
Platelet C3-receptors: (identity tentative)†	
gp45-70	Binds C3b, C4b, iC3b
CR2	Binds C3dg, C3d
CR4	Binds C3dg, iC3b
Factor D	α-Granule constituent; activates factor B of alternative pathway; specific role of platelet factor D unknown
Factor H	α-Granule constituent; regulates platelet-bound C3b restricting $\overline{C3bBb}$ assembly
Decay accelerating factor factor (DAF)	Cell-surface glycoprotein that accelerates decay/dissociation of $\overline{C3bBb}$ complex; absent on affected platelets in PNH
Protein S	Plasma protein present in platelet storage pool; promotes factor Va inactivation by activated protein C at platelet surface; may serve to localize C4b-binding protein to platelet surface, affecting $\overline{C4b2a}$ assembly
GPIIb-IIIa	Binds fibrinogen to mediate platelet aggregation; binds vitronectin (S-protein), potentially affecting C5b-9 assembly at platelet surface
Homologous restriction factor(s)	Expression by human platelets suspected but not confirmed; erythrocyte membrane protein(s) blocks C9 activation by membrane C5b-8

*Molecular identity of Clq receptor to platelet collagen receptor GPIa-IIa awaits experimental verification.
†Functional role of platelet C3 receptors not established.

can bind C2 into a Mg^{2+}-dependent complex. When complexed to C4b, C2 is proteolytically cleaved by $\overline{C1s}$ to liberate the C2b fragment, the C2a domain of the molecule remaining attached to C4b. C2a complexed to C4b provides the catalytic site for subsequent C3 and C5 activation. Covalent attachment of this enzyme complex to immunoglobulin or to the cell surface (through the C4b subunit) topologically restricts activation of C3 and C5 to the vicinity of the target antigen.

In a fashion similar to the activation of C4, peptide cleaveage of the α chain of C3 by the C4b2a enzyme complex liberates the vasoactive peptide C3a from the NH_2-terminus of the molecule and exposes a reactive intrachain thiolester bond within the α chain of the C3b portion of the molecule.[54,139] Multiple C3b are deposited on the cell surface (or within the immune complex) through reaction of this thiolester bond with nearby residues containing primary amines or hydroxyl groups. Those molecules of nascent C3b that fail to immediately react with acceptor residues undergo spontaneous hydrolysis of the internal thiolester bond, thereby losing their capacity for covalent attachment to the target surface (but not their capacity to be recognized by cellular C3b-receptors). In addition to serving as a key ligand for the cellular C3b/C4b-receptor (complement receptor CR1, which mediates immune adherence) C3b functions as a cofactor for the subsequent activation of C5 as well as the cofactor for assembly of the alternative pathway C3/C5-convertase.[34,87,118]

The next step in the classical pathway is the activation of C5, which is also initiated by the C4b2a enzyme complex, through proteolytic cleavage of the α chain of C5. Through a low-affinity binding site for C5, C3b deposited in close proximity to the enzyme complex is thought to facilitate presentation of this substrate (C5) to the active site in C2a, conferring enhanced specificity of the enzyme for C5.[74] Proteolytic cleavage of C5 liberates the potent chemotactic and anaphylactic peptide C5a, leaving the C5b portion of the molecule weakly attached to C3b.[54,74] Interaction of C5b with C6 initiates assembly of the membrane attack complex (C5b-9), which has the potential to insert into lipid-containing structures resulting in plasma membrane damage.[74]

Alternative Pathway

In contrast to the sequentially ordered enzyme cascade of the classical pathway, the alternative pathway entails a positive feedback mechanism, whereby the principal activation product (C3b) serves as the cofactor of the C3-cleaving enzyme complex (C3bBb) that is responsible for its own production (*see* Fig. 18-1).[62,87] This system, therefore, is continuously primed for explosive C3 activation, and the turnover of substrate through this pathway is determined by the stability of the C3bBb enzyme complex. Like the C4b2a complex, C3bBb also serves to activate C5. Activators of this pathway—which include immune complexes, bacterial lipopolysaccharides, yeast cell walls, certain viral membranes, certain viral-infected cell lines, and the autoantibody C3 nephritic factor—share the common property of facilitating stability of the assembled C3bBb enzyme, sequestered away from the regulatory control of fluid-phase inhibitors of the enzyme complex (described later).

Initiation of the alternative pathway involves a spontaneous conformational change of the C3 molecule, which is thought to be closely linked to rupture of the internal thiolester bond within the α chain of the protein.[87,139] One pathway for activation of C3 is by peptide cleavage to C3b (e.g., as initiated by the classical pathway enzyme C4b2a), which exposes the labile thiolester linkage within the C3b portion of the molecule (above). In this manner, C3b formed through the classical pathway can directly initiate assembly of the alternative pathway enzyme complex (see Fig. 18-1). In the absence of classic pathway activation, C3 conversion to an activated state can also occur by spontaneous hydrolysis of the thiolester bond within the intact protein, resulting in a molecule (C3*H_2O) which is conformationally similar to C3b. Slow conversion of C3 to C3*H_2O is believed to proceed continuously under normal plasma conditions. Conversion of C3 to either C3*H_2O or C3b results in expression of a binding site for factor B, the proenzyme of the alternative pathway C3/C5 convertase.

When bound to C3b*H_2O or to C3b, factor B becomes sensitive to proteolytic cleavage by factor D, a trace plasma enzyme normally found in its active state. Cleavage of factor B by factor D liberates a 30-kDa fragment (Ba), leaving the larger Bb fragment (80 kDa) attached to C3*H_2O or to C3b. Through a catalytic site in Bb, the complex of C3*H_2O,Bb can proteolytically convert C3 to C3a and C3b. The nascent C3b generated by this mechanism is capable of binding additional factor B (which is then converted by factor D to active C3bBb), thereby amplifying the reaction. Activation of C5 by the alternative pathway convertase occurs by peptide cleavage identical with that initiated by C4b2a, resulting in formation of C5a and C5b. Again, C3b covalently deposited in the vicinity of the C3bBb complex is believed to be required for proper presentation of C5 to the catalytic site of the enzyme.

Control of the Activation Pathways

The classical and alternative activation pathways are under strict regulatory control designed to limit dissemination of the reactions in plasma as well as to inhibit assembly of the enzyme complexes on exposed blood cell and endothelial surfaces (Fig. 18-2). Inhibitors identified, to date, include several specific binding proteins and enzymes present in plasma, as well as at least two important membrane-anchored glycoproteins.

Control of initiation of the classical pathway is exerted by the plasma glycoprotein C1-inhibitor (C1-INH), which binds irreversibly to C1r and C1s, blocking their enzymatic activity and dissociating their attachment to C1q.[21,160] In the presence of plasma levels of C1-INH, the enzyme activity of C1 decays with a half-life of 13 s. This enzyme inhibitor also plays important roles in the kinin generating, intrinsic coagulation, and fibrinolytic pathways through its interaction with plasmin, kallikrein, and factors XIa and XIIa (reviewed by Sundsmo and Fair[137]). Recently, C1-INH has been identified in platelet α granules.[117]

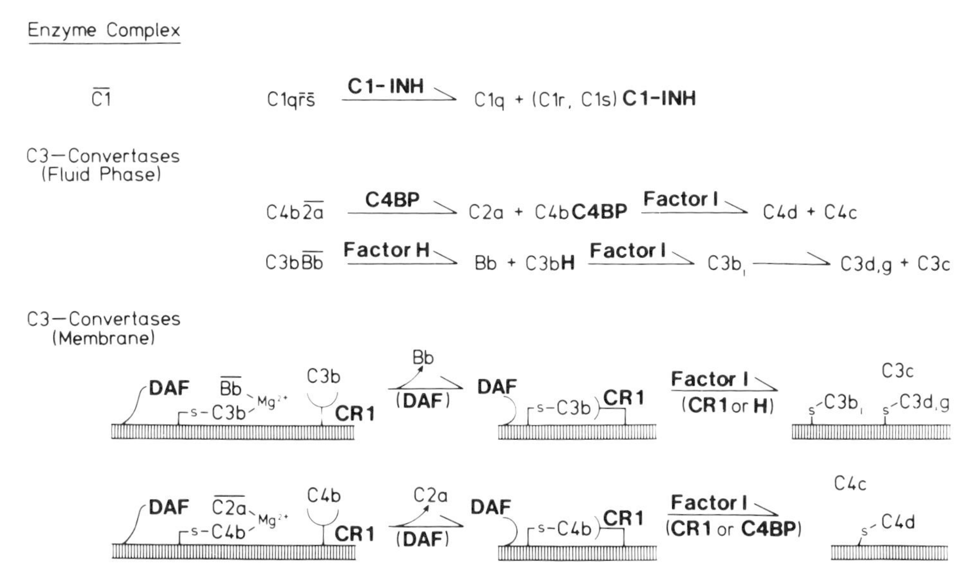

Figure 18-2. Regulation of enzyme complexes of classical and alternative complement activation pathways. Regulatory proteins and their cofactors are depicted in bold type. Bar over complement component (e.g., $\overline{C1}$) denotes active enzyme. Covalent linkage of C3b and C4b to membrane surface through reactive carbonyl of internal α-chain thiolester bond is indicated. Abbreviations: C1-INH, C1-inhibitor; C4BP, C4b-binding protein; H, factor H; DAF, decay accelerating factor; CR1, complement receptor for C3b. CR1 is not present in plasma membrane of primate platelets. See text for explanation.

The classical and alternative pathway C3/C5-convertases are under strict regulatory control by two binding proteins in plasma (C4b-binding protein and factor H) and a proteolytic enzyme (factor I).[62,87] C4b-binding protein is an acute-phase reactant protein that complexes C4b, serving to both block its association with C2 and to accelerate dissociation of the assembled $\overline{C4b2a}$ complex (which in the absence of C4b-binding protein dissociates with a half-life of 3 min). Additionally, C4b-binding protein serves as a cofactor, facilitating proteolytic degradation of C4b by factor I, which splits the larger C4c fragment from the molecule, leaving C4d bound to the original acceptor surface. Approximately 50% of C4b-binding protein normally circulates in plasma as a complex with protein S, a vitamin K-dependent protein having a key regulatory function in the coagulation system.[23]

Through its interaction with C3b, factor H serves to inhibit C3b association with factor B, thereby restricting assembly of the C3bB proenzyme. Factor H will also promote dissociation of the assembled $\overline{C3bBb}$ complex and serve as a cofactor for proteolytic degradation of C3b by factor I.[87] Limited intrachain proteolysis by factor I initially converts C3b to iC3b, which remains covalently bound to its original acceptor surface. Subsequent degradation of the C3b α chain by factor I releases the large C3c fragment (150 kDa), leaving C3dg (41 kDa) still attached to the acceptor surface through the C3d domain of the fragment. The membrane CRl receptor is considerably more efficient than factor H as a cofactor for the factor I mediated conversion of iC3b to C3dg.[69,112] Bound C3dg is normally the final C3b degradation product remaining on circulating cells in vivo. The C3c released into plasma is further degraded by trypsinlike enzymes, liberating the C3e peptide (10 kDa), whereas serine proteases, such as plasmin or elastase, can serve to further degrade C3dg to C3d. In contrast to factor H, which promotes dissociation of $\overline{C3bBb}$, another regulatory protein factor P (properdin) acts to stabilize the alternative pathway enzyme complex.

Regulation of C3/C5-Convertases by Membrane Constituents

It is now recognized that an important aspect of the regulation of the complement activation pathways is also contributed by the cell surface itself.[87] As mentioned earlier, surfaces that activate the alternative pathway are distinguished by their capacity to stabilize the C3bBb complex by inhibiting the binding of factor H, whereas nonactivating surfaces facilitate factor H binding to C3b. Although the exact chemical and physical properties distinguishing activating from nonactivating surfaces remain to be elucidated, it appears that the total content and chemical modification of cell surface sialic acid residues can be a determining factor. Additionally, in blood cells and vascular endothelium, two membrane proteins with specific regulatory functions have been identified: decay-accelerating factor (DAF), which specifically promotes the inactivation of the assembled C3/C5-convertases, and the cellular C3b/C4b receptor (CR1), which binds C3b and C4b and facilitates their degradation by factor I (*see* Fig. 18-2). Additionally, CR1 accelerates decay of the assembled C3/C5 convertases, and inhibits binding of C5 to C3b.[34,36,56,69,81]

Decay-accelerating factor is a 70-kDa single-chain glycoprotein, normally expressed on the surface of red cells, platelets, leukocytes, and endothelium, that serves to accelerate the dissociation of the membrane-assembled C4b2a and C3bBb complexes.[2,81,83,88] Unlike CR1, factor H, or C4b-binding protein, DAF does not function as a cofactor for C4b or C3b inactivation by factor I. Recently, DAF has been shown to belong to an unusual family of membrane proteins (which includes erythrocyte acetylcholinesterase) that are attached to the cell surface by glycosidic linkage to membrane phosphatidylinositol.[25] Decay-accelerating factor has been shown to be missing in the affected blood cells of patients with the acquired stem cell disorder, paroxysmal nocturnal hemoglobinuria (PNH), accounting for the marked capacity of these cells to amplify activation of the C3/C5-convertase.[82,84,88]

CR1, the principal cellular receptor for C3b and C4b, is a membrane glycoprotein of approximately 250 kDa that is distributed on erythrocytes, neutrophils, monocytes, and B-lymphocytes.[34,36,69,112,118] In addition to its important role in the adherence and clearance of C3b-coated cells and immune complexes, this membrane protein also serves as an important cofactor for the proteolytic degradation of both C3b and C4b by factor I. In considering the cellular distribution of CR1 receptors, it is of interest to note that this receptor is conspicuously absent on platelets of humans and other primates.[34,35,118]

Assembly of the Membrane Attack Complex

Membrane damage by the complement system is initiated through the interaction of nascent C5b (generated by either the classical pathway or alternative pathway C3/C5-convertase) with C6, C7, C8, and C9.[7,31,67,74,99] The sequential assembly of each of these proteins into a macromolecular structure is accompanied by major conformational transitions of each protein, which include de novo expression of a binding site for the subsequent component of the complex as well as the unfolding of hydrophobic domains that can insert into the lipid core of biologic membranes (Fig. 18-3). Formation of the C5b–9 complex on permissive cellular membranes can result in marked increases in plasma membrane permeability to aqueous solutes, resulting in the collapse of electrochemical gradients. Under certain conditions, cell lysis can result, either by colloid-osmotic water entry, leading to plasma membrane rupture, or by direct membrane destabilization.

The first step in assembly of the membrane attack complex (MAC) is the formation of a complex between C5b and C6, through a short-lived binding site newly expressed by C5b.[42] Association of C6 with nascent C5b is thought to occur, while C5b remains in contact with membrane-bound C3b.[45,145] The C5b6 complex, which expresses a new binding site for C7, is a stable intermediate that can accumulate in C7-deficient plasma during complement activation.[96] Upon reaction of C7 with the C5b6 complex, a membrane-binding site is transiently expressed (primarily by the C7 subunit), enabling the C5b67 complex to deposit directly onto membrane surfaces.[94] Once bound to a membrane surface, the C5b67 complex expresses a stable binding site for a single molecule of C8. Association of C8 with the complex results in insertion of a portion of the C8 molecule (primarily the α chain) into the hydrophobic core of the membrane, aggregation of C5b–8 complexes on the membrane surface, and expression of a binding site for C9. (This binding site is also within the α chain of C8).[14,132,134] The interaction of C9 with mem-

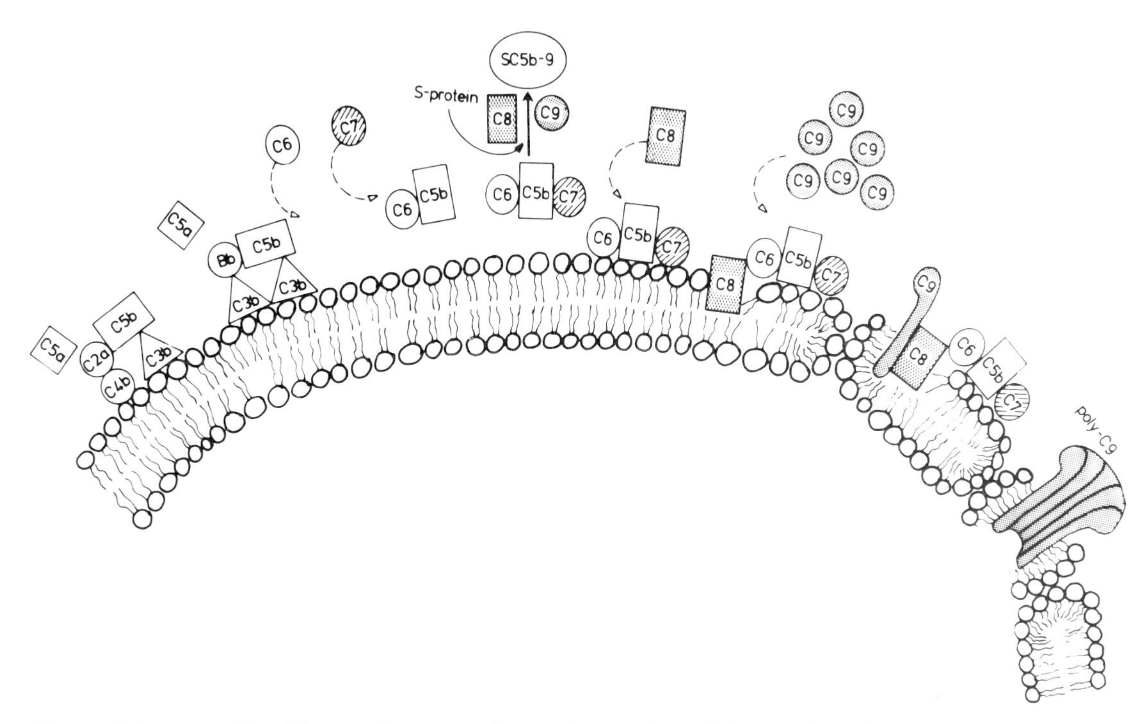

Figure 18-3. Assembly of the membrane attack complex, a schematic illustration of molecular events that initiate the assembly, membrane binding, and membrane insertion of the C5b–9 complex. Both polymerized C9 and nontubular forms of the membrane-inserted C5b–9 complex are depicted. The complement S-protein is identical with vitronectin (also referred to as serum spreading factor). Changes in lipid bilayer structure associated with membrane insertion of the C5b–9 proteins are hypothetical. See text for explanation.

brane-bound C5b–8 initiates a marked conformational transition in C9, resulting in its elongation and insertion into the membrane interior, concomitant with its polymerization into a large, torus-ringed, tubular structure (10 nm id) that can be readily viewed projecting from the membrane surface by electron microscopy.[29,142] This tubular structure forms only if C9 is present at a relatively high concentration, and appears to be composed of 12 to 18 molecules of C9.[98,126,141] Membranes treated with C5b–8, but with only limited amounts of C9, show only aggregated proteins on the surface, with no ringlike lesions. Purified C9 can be induced to spontaneously polymerize into a structure bearing striking ultrastructural identity with the ringlike tubules depicted on the membranes of cells lysed by the C5b–9 complex.[142] One function of the membrane C5b–8 complex is to lower the activation energy required to induce C9 polymerization.[128]

Functional Properties of the Membrane Attack Complex

Insertion of the C5b–9 proteins affects both the structural and functional properties of the plasma membrane. Concomitant with intercalation of hydrophobic domains of C8 and C9, there is a decrease in the anisotropic packing of membrane lipid, suggesting a disordering of bilayer structure.[32,53] Altered packing of membrane lipid can be accompanied by transbilayer migration ("flip-flop") of phospholipid between inner and outer monolayers, leading to exposure of acidic phospholipids on the cell surface.[143] The significance of these physical changes in plasma membrane structure to procoagulant changes accompanying complement-mediated platelet injury will be considered later.

In addition to these alterations in membrane structure, insertion of the C5b–9 proteins can induce significant changes in plasma membrane permeability to aqueous solutes. Although deposition of C5b67 complexes has no measurable effect on membrane permeability, a small dose-dependent increase in membrane permeability to small aqueous solute can be detected in cells treated with C5b–8.[40,107] At very high C5b–8 density, these complexes can initiate the slow lysis of erythrocytes. Addition of C9 to C5b–8-treated membranes greatly increases the permeability of the plasma membrane, resulting in marked changes in membrane potential and cytosolic Na^+, Ca^{2+}, and *p*H.[11,64,154] In the absence of compensatory mechanisms (discussed later), deposition of these proteins at high density on the membrane can lead to complete collapse of electrochemical gradients with cytolytic rupture of the plasma membrane. The actual pore exclusion size of the membrane lesions formed by the C5b–9 proteins has been found to depend on the density and stoichiometry of the bound C5b-9 proteins, as well as the species homology of the target membrane.[9,127]

Control of the Membrane Attack Complex

Initiation of MAC assembly is regulated through control of the C5-convertases, exerted directly by DAF and factor H in conjunction with factor I. The spontaneous decay of the C6-binding site on C5b limits formation of C5b6. Dissemination of the MAC to "innocent" bystander cells is also limited by the very short lifetime of the membrane binding site of the newly formed C5b67 complex.[94] Additionally, the diffusional spread of nascent C5b67 complexes is controlled by the action of plasma vitronectin (also referred to as S-protein), which provides an acceptor surface for C5b67 that competes for the binding of this complex to cell membranes.[97] Upon binding one molecule each of C8 and C9, the vitronectin–C5b–9 complex (SC5b–9) circulates inactively in plasma until cleared (see Fig. 18-3). In addition to this important role in regulating MAC formation, vitronectin can interact with the platelet glycoprotein (GP) IIb–IIIa complex through an Arg-Gly-Asp amino acid sequence in the molecule, as well as bind heparin and antithrombin III, potentially regulating thrombin and factor Xa activity.[95,105,106] In addition to this plasma inhibitor of the C5b67 complex, human erythrocyte membranes (and other blood cells) contain restriction factor(s) that inhibit the cytolytic activity of the C5b–9 complex. These apparently operate by interfering with the interaction of C9 with membrane C5b–8.[109,120] Recently, a membrane glycoprotein (designated homologous restriction factor, HRF) has been isolated from the human erythrocyte and displays the capacity to alter the interaction between membrane-bound C5b–8 and C9, restricting C9 polymerization and inhibiting full expression of the pore-forming and lytic activity of the MAC.[121,159] This protein has been reported to be missing in the abnormal PNH type 3 cell, which would appear to account for the unusual sensitivity of this erythrocyte to lysis by the C5b–9 proteins.[158] This protein is likely to serve a similar function in platelets and other blood cells. The capacity to restrict the interaction between membrane-bound C5b–8 and C9 and to inhibit lytic activity is also shared by high-density lipoproteins and their apolipoproteins.[110]

ACTIVATION OF THE COMPLEMENT SYSTEM ON HUMAN PLATELETS

Despite the well-documented prevalence of thrombocytopenia in association with various intravascular immune reactions and despite the ever-expanding use of immunogenic random donor platelets in transfusion therapy, there is surprisingly little direct information concerning the molecular control of the complement activation pathways at the platelet surface. Accordingly, our understanding of the interaction of the classical and alternative pathway components with blood platelets is derived, for the most part, from results of studies undertaken with red cells (summarized in the previous section). In this section, I will review published data that specifically relate to the assembly and control of the complement system on platelet membranes, with particular emphasis on potential mechanisms whereby these interactions may differ from those observed in erythrocytes. A discussion of the effects of these proteins on platelet function and survival is reserved for a subsequent section.

Initiation of the Classical Pathway at the Platelet Surface

Platelets bind IgG-containing immune complexes by specific interaction with membrane Fc receptors. This surface-expressed immunoglobulin can increase in a variety of circumstances, including during viremia, immune complex disease, immune drug reactions, or the production of antibodies directed specifically against platelet-associated antigens. It would appear, therefore, that platelets potentially provide a favorable surface for binding and activation of C1. Activation of the complement system leading to deposition of complement proteins on the platelet surface has been documented for antibodies directed against histocompatibility (HLA) antigens, platelet-specific antigens, and drugs acting haptenically. Furthermore, platelets isolated from patients with several immune-related disorders have been shown to exhibit eleated levels of surface-bound compelment proteins (platelet-associated complement; PAC). The significance of increased levels of PAC in various disease states is discussed more fully later.

It is noteworthy that normal platelets isolated by gel filtration do not exhibit significant $\overline{C1}$ activity, despite the fact that considerable amounts of C1q are then bound with high affinity to their surface.[52,90,136,147,148] This raises the question of whether or not the $\overline{C1}$ enzyme complex is selectively inhibited at the platelet surface (possibly by mechanisms other than plasma C1-INH). Platelets have been shown to directly bind C1q through a membrane-binding protein that interacts with the collagenlike tail of the molecule.[148] This receptor cross-reacts antigenically with the C1q receptor identified on blood leukocytes.[90] Molecular identity of the platelet C1q receptor to GPIa–IIa (recently identified as the platelet receptor for solid-phase collagen[60a]) awaits experimental verification. C1q binding to its receptor on the platelet can directly alter platelet–collagen interactions, as will be discussed more fully later. As C1r and C1s are known to compete for C1q binding to the C1q receptor from other cells, it is possible that the platelet collagen receptor promotes dissociation of the C1r and C1s subunits from the tail-portion of C1q, thereby constituting a membrane C1 inhibitory function analogous to plasma C1-INH.[140] In this context, it is also interesting that a protein antigenically identical with C1-INH has been detected within platelet α granules, and shown to be secreted upon stimulation of the cells by thrombin or collagen.[117] It is hoped that future study will elucidate the specific role of each of these platelet constituents in the control of C1 activation at the platelet surface.

Inactivation of Platelet-Associated C3b and C4b

As noted previously, primate platelets do not express the C3b/C4b-specific CR1 receptor, a protein present on erythrocytes and virtually all leukocytes. In addition to its role in immune adherence and in the processing of C3b-containing immune complexes, this protein has been shown to act as a membrane cofactor for factor I-mediated inactivation of C3b and C4b deposited on red cells (see Fig. 18-2). This raises the question of how these key subunits of the alternative and classical pathway C3/C5-convertases are normally inactivated on the platelet surface. Although plasma factor H and C4b-binding protein can potentially contribute to the degradation of platelet-bound C3b and C4b by factor I, there are recent data suggesting that the inactivation of these proteins is under regulatory control by additional platelet-associated cofactors. A membrane glycoprotein with affinity for C3b and iC3b (designated gp45-70) has recently been isolated from human platelets and shown, in a solubilized system, to function as a cofactor for factor I inactivation of C3b.[157] Additionally, platelet α granules have been shown to contain factor H, which can potentially provide this cofactor function upon lytic or secretory release.[60] Recent data suggests that this internal pool of factor H is secreted and bound to the platelet surface when C3b deposits on the membrane, providing a mechanism by which these cells may exert feedback inhibitory control of the assembly of C3/C5-convertases on their surface.[26,27] Whether or not the amount of factor H secreted from the α granules is significant against the background of plasma factor H remains to be demonstrated. Finally, recognition that C4b-binding protein (a cofactor for C4b degradation by factor I) circulates in plasma as a complex with protein S of the coagulation system raises the possibility that the inactivation of platelet-bound C4b is regulated through changes in the affinity of protein S for the platelet surface.[23,72] In this context, it is also noteworthy that activation of washed platelets leads to increased expression of cell surface protein S (with increased uptake of C4b-binding protein), reflecting a releasable internal pool of this regulatory protein.

Although data on the stability of the assembled C3/C5-convertases on the platelet surface is limited, these cells are known to contain the

DAF that regulates the $\overline{C4b2a}$ and $\overline{C3bBb}$ complexes on human red cells.[27,83,84] This protein has also been shown to be deficient in affected platelets obtained from patients with PNH, which can exhibit increased sensitivity to complement activation (discussed later). In some (but not all) DAF-deficient platelets, increased C3-convertase activity can be demonstrated, accompanied by increased membrane deposition of C3b.[27] These data suggest that DAF plays an important role in controlling C3-convertase activity on the platelet surface, but that significant control may also be exhibited by other platelet-associated inhibitors.

Participation of Other Proteases in the Deposition of Complement Proteins on the Platelet Surface

Although the complement system is often depicted as an isolated enzyme cascade reacting on the surface of a single cell, it is obvious that, within the vasculature, these proteins interact with a vast collection of plasma and cell-derived constituents. Furthermore, one might expect that this interaction of complement proteins with other components of blood is facilitated when the target cell of complement attack can secrete and specifically bind several enzymes and regulatory proteins, and when it also plays a central role in the organization of other surface-catalyzed proteolytic reactions. In this section, I will briefly review published data relating to the deposition of activated complement proteins on the platelet surface through reaction pathways other than the classical and alternative complement-activation cascades. For a complete discussion of the complex interrelationships between the complement, kinin-generating, coagulation, and fibrinolytic pathways, the reader is referred to several excellent reviews.[8,58,137,138]

A number of plasma enzymes have been shown to exhibit the capacity to activate components of the complement system. These include: activation of C1 by plasmin, Hageman factor fragment, factor XIIa, and kallikrein; of factor B by plasmin and kallikrein; of C3 by plasmin and thrombin; and of C5 by plasmin, thrombin, and kallikrein. In addition to releasing activated complement fragments into plasma (e.g., C3a and C5a) during coagulation, there is considerable evidence that these and potentially other plasma and cell-derived proteases contribute to the deposition of C3b and C5b–9 complexes on the platelet surface.

Polley and Nachman first reported that C5b–9 complexes deposit on the platelet surface during blood coagulation through a mechanism that appeared to require only C3 and thrombin.[103] Zimmerman and Kolb subsequently demonstrated that membrane uptake of C3 and assembly of C5b–9 complexes on the platelet surface also occurs during incubation of platelets in autologous citrated plasma.[162] C5b–9 complex formation was not detected in platelet-poor plasma or when red cells were incubated with autologous plasma under identical conditions. Surprisingly, formation of C5b–9 complexes in platelet–plasma suspensions was not inhibited by EDTA, phenylmethylsulfonylfluoride, or ϵ-aminocaproic acid (EACA), suggesting that this phenomenon occurs independently from known plasma C5-activators. In a plasma-free system, Polley and Nachman demonstrated that incubation of washed platelets with purified C3 and the isolated terminal complement proteins lowers the threshold for thrombin-induced aggregation and granule release (discussed later) and results in membrane deposition of C3 and C5b–9 complexes on the platelet surface.[101,102] Subsequently, it was reported that the assembly of membrane-bound C5b–9 complexes from the purified C5 through C9 proteins also follows stimulation of washed platelets with arachidonic acid, an effect that is blocked by cyclooxygenase inhibitors.[104] Under these conditions, activation of C3 was not observed, and C5 activation (initiating C5b-9 assembly) proceeded in the absence of this protein.

The identity of the protease(s) involved in the platelet-catalyzed assembly of membrane C5b–9 complexes has not been resolved. As previously mentioned, thrombin, plasmin, and kallikrein can each potentially participate in C5 activation. The capacity of stimulated washed platelets to catalyze C5b–9 assembly (presumably in the near-absence of thrombin or other plasma proteins) suggests that C5 activation is initiated either by a surface-bound or by a secreted protease. Of note, Weksler and Coupal described an EACA-sensitive factor in acid-soluble extracts of human platelets that was capable of cleaving C5a from C5.[150] Although EACA and other protease inhibitors were not found to inhibit the uptake of C5b–9 complexes from plasma, it is possible that this enzyme (or other protease) is protected from inactivation when bound to the platelet surface. Finally, leukocyte proteases have also been shown to cleave and activate several components of the complement system, raising the possibility that the apparent participation of platelets in complement activation may be due to leukocytes contaminating platelet suspensions.

THE PLATELET RESPONSE TO ACTIVATED COMPLEMENT COMPONENTS

It has been recognized for many years that immunologic reactions can profoundly alter platelet function and survival within the vasculature.[4,51,66,73,91,92,93,119,163] Some of these effects appear to be mediated directly by immunoglobulin, some entail specific interaction of platelets with components of the complement system, whereas others are mediated through the interaction of platelets with inflammatory mediators released by immune-stimulated leukocytes. In this section, I will focus exclusively upon platelet responses that appear to result from the direct interaction of one or more activated complement proteins with human platelets. A discussion of the significance of these effects mediated directly by activated complement proteins to the overall platelet response to immune or inflammatory insult will be reserved for a subsequent section. Before reviewing these data, a note of caution is warranted: Because of the capacity of activated complement fragments to stimulate a variety of leukocyte responses, including secretion of platelet-activating factor (PAF) and potentially other platelet agonists, the possibility must always be considered that observed complement-induced changes in platelet function are mediated by products released from leukocytes contaminating platelet suspensions.

Expression of Specific Complement Receptors by Human Platelets

In addition to providing a key regulatory function in the complement activation pathways, plasma membrane receptors with specificity for complement components play a central role in the clearance of immune complexes and in mediating cellular responses to complement activation.[34,111,118] In various other blood cells, receptors with specificity for C1q, C3a/C4a, C3b/C4b(CR1), C3dg/C3d (CR2), iC3b (CR3), C3dg/iC3b (CR4), C3e, C5a, and factor H have been identified, and for many, the receptor proteins have been purified. A C3b/C4b/iC3b-binding protein (gp45-70) that is distinct from CR1 has been demonstrated on peripheral blood mononuclear cells.[111] Human platelets have been shown to express receptors for C1q, which are probably identical with the platelet collagen receptors.[90] Recent reports indicate that human platelets also express gp45-70 and potentially two membrane receptors for C3dg (CR2 and CR4), raising the possibility that platelets participate directly in the processing of C3b and in the cellular uptake of C3dg-coated immune complexes.[13,144,157]

Effect of C1q on Platelet–Collagen Interactions

In addition to its role in the activation of the classical pathway, C1q has been shown to modulate collagen-induced platelet aggregation.[12,22,90,136,147] Free C1q inhibits the platelet's collagen response in a competitive fashion, with an apparent dissociation constant of 2–3×10^{-7} M.[90] On the other hand, C1q aggregates initiate platelet aggregation and release reactions, mimicking activation by collagen.[12] The effects of C1q on platelets appear to be directly mediated through the binding of this complement protein to the platelet collagen receptor. Although the interaction between C1q and platelets in vivo remains to be elucidated, one might speculate that C1q (liberated from activated $\overline{C1}$ by the action of C1-INH) can potentially serve to either inhibit platelet adherence to vascular collagen or to function as a platelet activator when clustered by multivalent C1 activators such as immune complexes.[90]

Platelet Activation by C3-Derived Fragments

It is well-established that guinea pig platelets express receptors sensitive to human C3a, which mediate secretory release from dense granules. Nevertheless, experiments with purified C3a (as well as C4a or C5a) have, for the most part, failed to provide conclusive evidence for direct stimulation of human platelets, and it is generally believed that these cells do not express receptors for these peptides.[41,54,70] In a single report, aggregation and dense-granule secretion by human platelets in response to C3a (and to C3a-des-Arg) was described, and evidence for a C3a-specific receptor on these cells was presented.[100] The platelet response to this peptide was observed for gel-filtered, but not washed platelets, and it was not inhibited by aspirin. Platelet secretion was detected at concentrations of the peptide above 10^{-12} M, and the response to C3a exhibited synergy with ADP but not with thrombin. No response to C3b, C3e, or C5a was detected.[100]

In a recent report, Devine and Rosse demonstrate that incubation of washed platelets with purified C3 and a stabilized fluid-phase C3-convertase (cobra venom factor–Bb enzyme complex) results in secretion of factor H from the α granules.[27] α-Granule secretion was blocked by metabolic inhibitors or EDTA. The authors conclude that this release reaction is specifically triggered by membrane-deposited C3b, although the conditions of their experiments do not exclude platelet activation by C3a or alternative pathway proteases. The possibility for direct platelet activation mediated by C3b (or by C3b-derived fragments) is supported by recent evidence for the C3b-related receptors gp45-70, CR2, and CR4 on these cells.[13,144,157]

Platelet Responses to the Membrane Attack Complex

In addition to their well-recognized role in mediating immune cytolysis, there is accumulating evidence that the C5b-9 proteins can also function to nonlytically modulate the permeability properties of the plasma membrane, affecting changes in stimulus–response coupling and cellular function without, causing lytic cell death.[44,57,116,155] The ability of human blood cells to escape cytolytic damage by the complement system resides, in part, with the capacity of their membranes to limit assembly and stability of the C3/C5-convertases as well as by their capacity to restrict the conformational activation of C9 by C5b–8 bound to the cell surface. Recovery from complement-mediated injury is also achieved by compensatory electrochemical changes initiated in the target cell, as well as by removal of functional C5b–9 complexes from the cell surface (discussed later).

Direct participation of the terminal complement proteins in nonlytic platelet activation was first established for the rabbit, in which it was demonstrated that the acceleration of whole blood clotting time or the induction of platelet aggregation and release reactions by various activators of the complement system were abolished in C6-deficient plasma. Addition of purified C6 to this plasma restored the platelet responses.[161] In subsequent studies with human platelets, Breckenridge and associates reported that zymosan-induced platelet aggregation and secretion were abolished when C3-, C5-, C6-, or C7-deficient plasmas were employed as a complement source.[10] The impaired responses in C5-deficient plasma were corrected by addition of C5. Surprisingly, a normal platelet response was observed for C8-deficient plasma, suggesting a requirement only for C5b67 (or, more likely, that the washed platelets employed in these studies carried trace amounts of C8). Similarly, Dixon and Rosse observed that the complement-dependent release of serotonin from normal human platelets treated with anti-I antibodies was virtually abolished in plasma congenitally deficient in C6.[28] By contrast, PNH platelets incubated under similar conditions showed marked serotonin release, suggesting a mechanism mediated through C3 that was independent of the C5b–9 proteins. In experiments using IgG anti-Pl^{A1} antibodies and gel-filtered platelets suspended in heparinized plasma, Cines and Schreiber observed that the release reaction initiated by anti-Pl^{A1} was virtually abolished in plasma deficient in C3, C4, C5, or C6, suggesting requirement of the terminal complement proteins.[17] The cellular mechanism of this nonlytic release reaction was examined by Schreiber et al.[119] They observed that, at low antibody concentration, the complement-dependent release reaction requires metabolic energy and the feedback of ADP, and it could be substantially blocked by either a phosphodiesterase inhibitor (SH869), prostaglandin E_1, or aspirin. At higher antibody concentrations, inhibition by these agents was less complete. The contribution of thrombin (potentially generated in heparinized plasma through activation of the platelet prothrombinase) to the cellular responses observed under the conditions of these experiments was not examined.

In experiments performed with washed human platelets suspended with isolated complement proteins, Polley and Nachman demonstrated that thrombin-mediated platelet aggregation and release reactions were potentiated in the presence of C3 plus the terminal complement components C5–C9.[101,102] Increased secretion in response to low-dose thrombin was inhibited by cyclooxygenase inhibitors and was accompanied by C3 uptake and formation of membrane C5b–9 complexes. Subsequently, it was shown that the secretory response of these cells to exogenous arachidonate was also potentiated by addition of purified C5–C9, by a mechanism totally independent of C3.[104] Potentiation of the platelets' response to arachidonate was accompanied by increased thromboxane production and was inhibited by aspirin. Again, platelet activation was accompanied by deposition of membrane C5b–9 complexes, presumably initiated by a platelet-derived activator of C5 (discussed earlier). Increased thromboxane synthesis by platelets treated with the C5b–9 proteins (in the absence of another agonist) has recently been described by Hansch and coworkers.[47]

These experiments raise two important questions: First, how do platelets forestall cytolytic damage after membrane insertion of the C5b–9 proteins? And second, how are the platelets' normal stimulatory pathways affected by formation of the C5b–9 lesion, resulting in activation or potentiation of the cell's secretory function and accelerated clot formation? To address these questions, we have recently focused our own studies on changes in signal transduction across the plasma membrane arising from insertion of the C5b–9 proteins.[1a,1b,126a,129,151,155] To differentiate responses mediated directly by the C5b–9 proteins from responses to other plasma constituents (including plasma proteases or other complement components), C5b–9 complexes were assembled on gel-filtered platelets, in the absence of plasma, by sequential incubation with purified C5b6 plus C7 (generating approximately 10^3 functional membrane-bound C5b67 complexes per platelet), followed by addition of limiting quantities of purified C8 and C9. The results of these experiments (summarized in Fig. 18-4) indicate:

- Membrane assembly of C5b–9 complexes is accompanied by increased Na^+ conductance across the plasma membrane resulting in rapid depolarization of membrane potential from initial levels of approximately −58 mV (Fig. 18-5). After this initial depolarizing current, the membrane potential re-

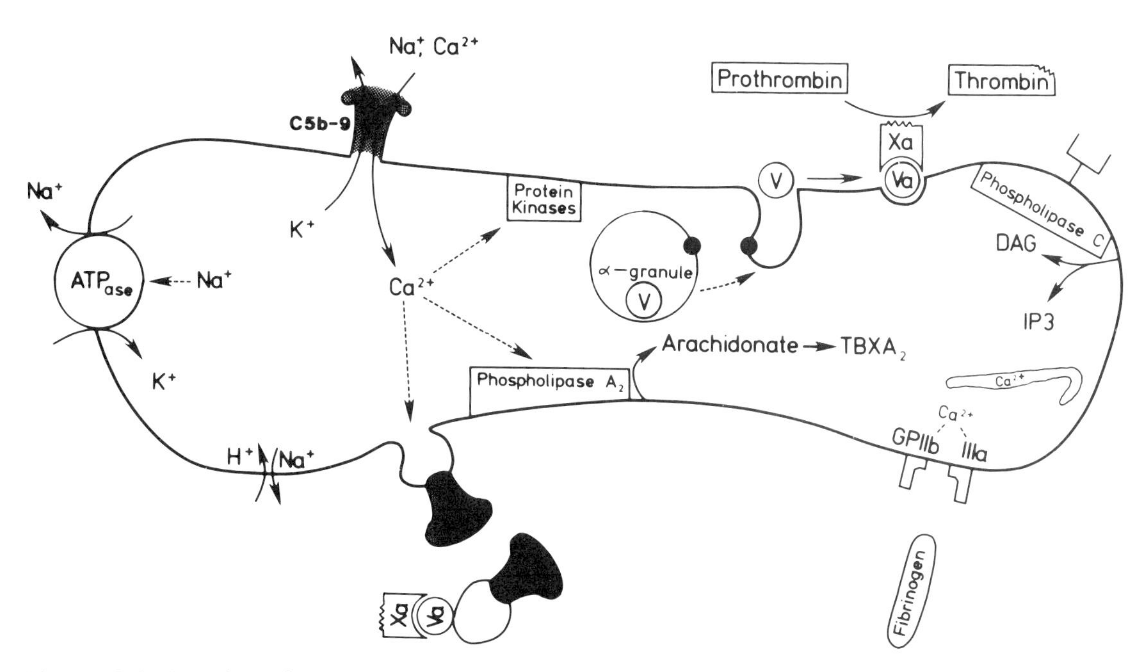

Figure 18-4. Overview of cellular events initiated by C5b–9 insertion into plasma membrane of blood platelets. Elevated intracellular [Ca^{2+}] occurs by diffusional influx across the plasma membrane without release of the ion from internal stores. Activation of phospholipase C to generate diacylglycerol (DAG) and inositol trisphosphate (IP3) requires triggering through cellular receptor pathways and does not occur when C5b–9 binds to the platelet surface in the absence of other plasma proteins. See text for explanation.

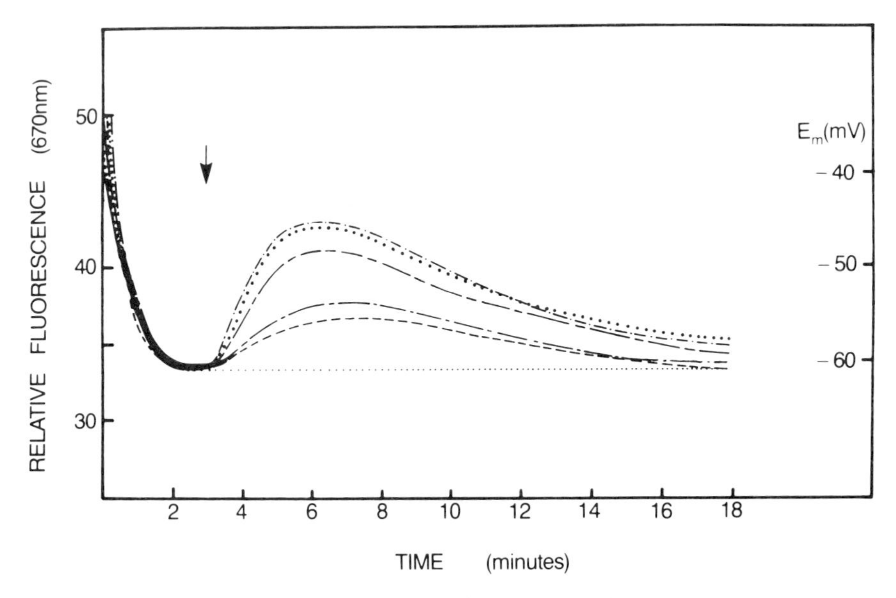

Figure 18-5. Changes in membrane potential accompanying C5b–9 insertion. The fluorescent potentiometric dye indicator diS-C_3-(5) was used to monitor membrane potential (E_m) of human platelets exposed to the purified C5b–9 proteins. Gel-filtered human platelets were exposed to C5b6 (15 μg/1 × 10^8 cells) plus C7 (5 μg/1 × 10^8 cells) to assemble membrane C5b67 complexes. The C5b67 platelets were then suspended (2.5 × 10^7 cells in 2 ml) in a stirred fluorescence cuvet at 37°C, equilibrated with dye, and C8 and C9 added to initiate formation of the C5b–9 complex. Excitation was at 622 nm (8-nm bandwidth) and emission at 670 nm (8-nm bandwidth). At the time indicated by the arrow, all samples received 1.0 μg C9 plus the following amounts of C8: 0 μug (· · · · · · · · ·), 0.07 μg (------), 0.14 μg (— – —), 0.7 μg (- — – —), 1.4 μg (••••••), or 2.8 μg (· - · - · -). Calibration of dye fluorescence (left ordinate) to membrane potential (right ordinate) was performed by reference to the calculated potassium equilibrium potential for platelet suspensions at various external [K^+] in the presence of saturating concentrations of valinomycin (See ref. 155) (Sims PJ, Wiedmer T: J Biol Chem 260:8014, 1985, with permission).

polarizes to near-basal levels, in a process dependent upon active Na^+/K^+ transport, as well as an extracellular Ca^{2+} concentration in the near-millimolar range. Under these conditions (<10^3 C5b–9 complexes per platelet), plasma membrane conductance to monovalent cations returns to near-normal levels, and cell lysis does not occur. With increased input of the C5b–9 proteins, or when active Na^+/K^+ transport is inhibited by metabolic block or exposure to ouabain, repolarization of the membrane potential does not occur, and cell lysis ensues.

- Restoration of the basal conductance of the plasma membrane is associated with vesiculation of the plasma membrane, resulting in selective removal of C5b–9 complexes from the cell surface. Vesiculation of the plasma membrane appears to be triggered by the diffusional influx of Ca^{2+} across the C5b–9 pore, as it is virtually abolished at low external calcium. The capacity of the C5b–9 proteins to trigger plasma membrane vesiculation may account for increased plasma levels of platelet-derived microparticles ("platelet dust") observed after immune injury to platelets in vivo and after thrombin activation of platelets in autologous plasma (conditions known to initiate deposition of C5b–9 complexes on the platelet surface).
- The diffusional influx of Ca^{2+} across the plasma membrane increases the activity of the ion in the cytosol. There is no detectable release of the ion from internal stores (as monitored by the intracellular dye indica-

tors indo-1 or fura-2) and no detectable formation of inositol phosphates, suggesting that the phospholipase C transduction pathway is bypassed during platelet activation by the C5b–9 proteins.

- Assembly of the C5b–9 complex results in activation of protein kinase C as well as myosin light-chain kinase (Fig. 18-6) and results in secretory release from both α granules and dense granules (Fig. 18-7). Prior incubation with sphingosine, a potent protein kinase C inhibitor, completely blocks the secretory response to C5b–9 assembly. C5b–9-induced activation of cellular protein kinases and consequent stimulation of secretion are also completely inhibited by removal of external calcium, suggesting that cell stimulation results directly from the influx of Ca^{2+} across the plasma membrane (Fig. 18-8).
- A small increase in thromboxane A_2 production can be detected, reflecting phospholipase A_2 activation anticipated at elevated cytosolic $[Ca^{2+}]$ or inhibition of arachidonate reacylation.[47] Although this increased prostanoid synthesis is abolished by addition of cyclooxygenase inhibitors, there is no inhibition of the C5b–9-initiated release reaction under these conditions, suggesting that platelet activation is not coupled to feedback by thromboxane.
- No change in platelet function is detected in the presence of the isolated components (C5b6, C7, 8, C9), or in response to mem-

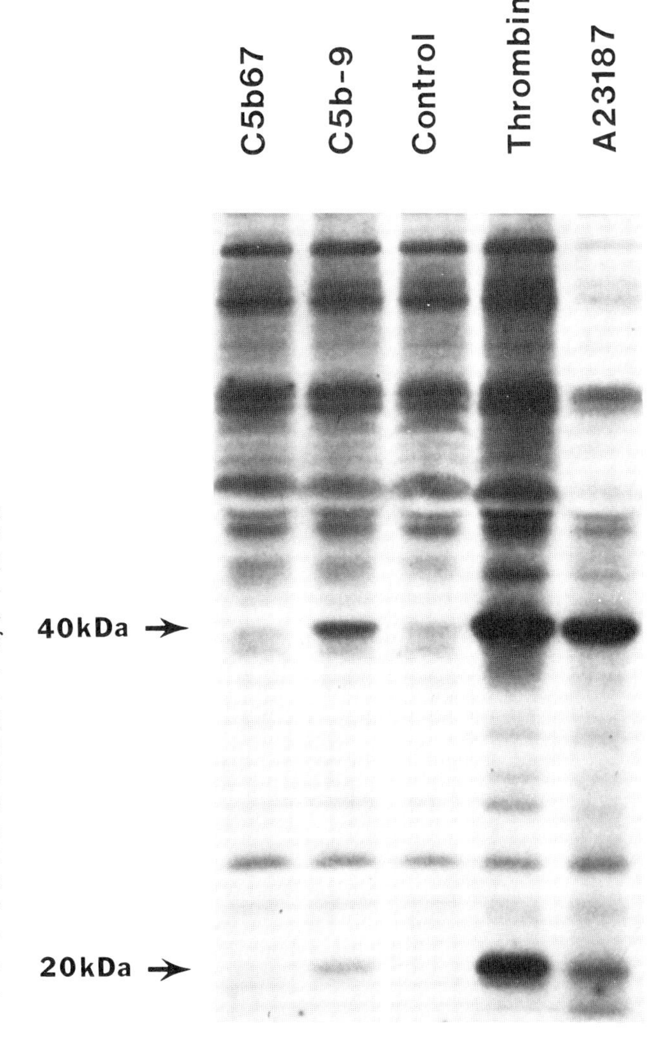

Figure 18-6. Activation of cellular protein kinases by the membrane-inserted C5b–9 proteins. Autoradiograph of ^{32}P-labeled platelets after sodium dodecylsulfate–polyacrylamide gel electrophoresis (SDS–PAGE) demonstrates phosphorylation of 40-kDa and 20-kDa protein bands (substrates of protein kinase C and myosin light-chain kinase, respectively) when gel-filtered platelets are treated with the purified C5b–9 proteins (lane 2). Compare results obtained for platelets treated with thrombin (1 U/ml) or the calcium ionophore A23187 (1 μM; lanes 4 and 5, respectively). Cellular protein kinases were not activated upon membrane deposition of C5b67 complexes (lane 1) or upon exposure of control platelets to purified C8 and C9 proteins (not shown). (Wiedmer T, Ando B, Sims PJ: J Biol Chem 262: 13674, 1987, with permission).

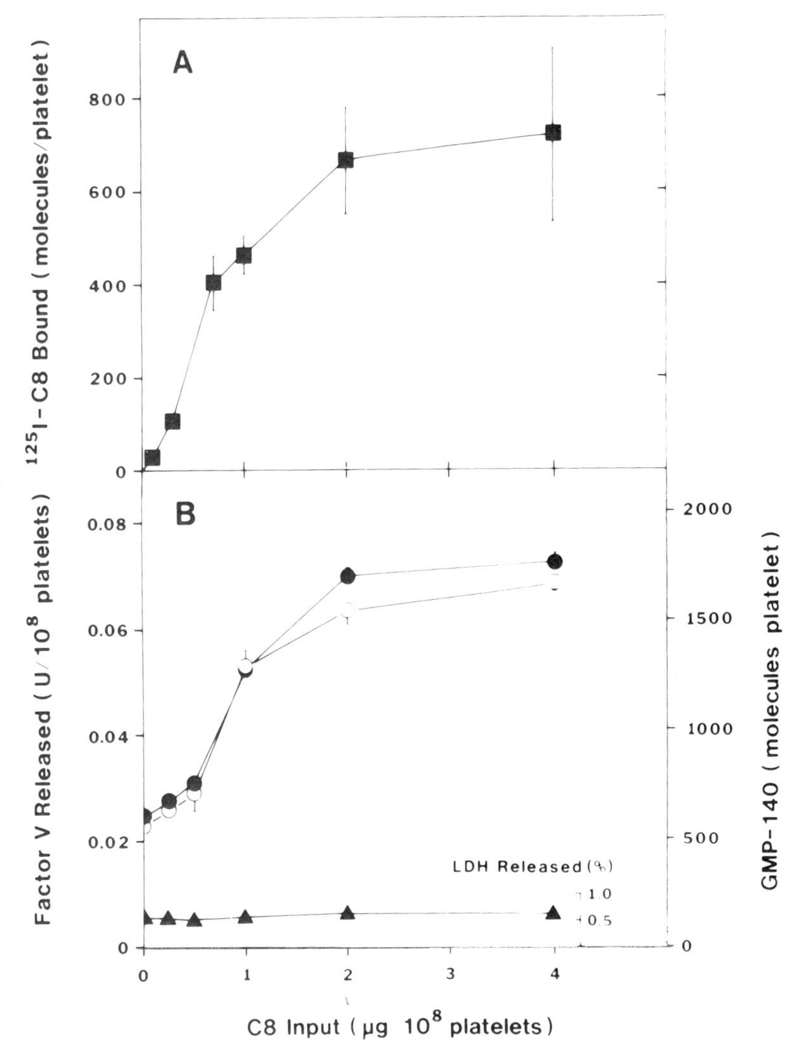

Figure 18-7. Platelet α-granule secretion initiated by membrane C5b–9 complexes. The capacity of the C5b–9 proteins to directly initiate the nonlytic secretion of platelet α-granule contents is demonstrated using gel-filtered human platelets exposed to the purified C5b–9 proteins. In these experiments, gel-filtered platelets were incubated with C5b6 plus C7 (to assemble approximately 800 membrane C5b67 complexes), and C5b–9 complex formation was completed by addition of increasing quantities of C8, in the presence of excess C9. The number of cell-bound C5b–9 complexes under each condition was determined by the specific uptake of ^{125}I-labeled C8 (*A*). As shown by *B* C5b–9 complex formation resulted in a dose-dependent release of factor V from the α granules (closed circles) with concomitant expression of α-granule membrane glycoprotein GMP-140 (open circles) on the platelet surface. This secretory release of factor V from α granules occurred without lytic release of cytoplasmic lactate dehydrogenase (LDH; closed triangles). Under these conditions, a comparable release of [^{14}C]serotonin from platelet dense granules was observed (data not shown) (Wiedmer T, Ando B, Sims PJ: J Biol Chem 262: 13674, 1987).

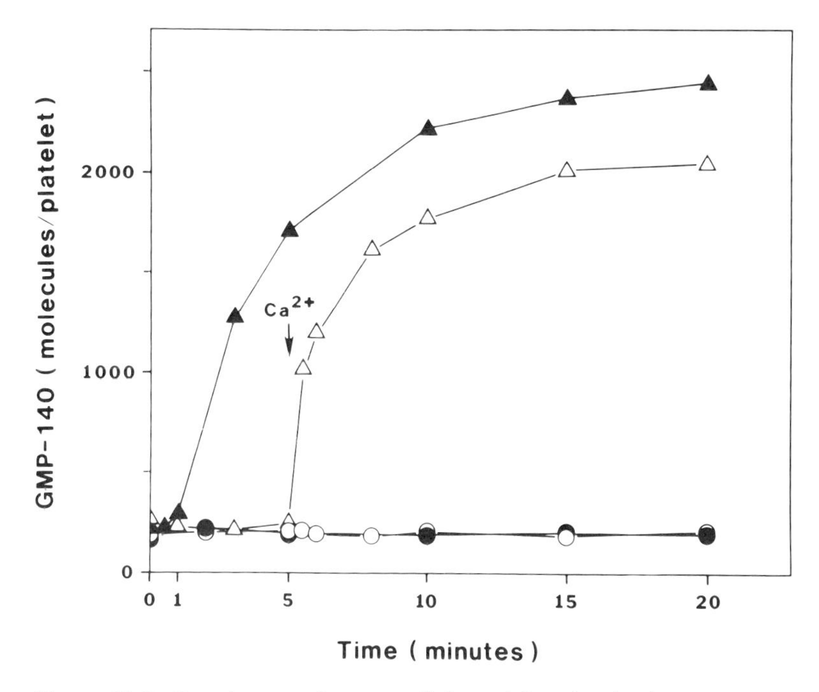

Figure 18-8. Requirement for extracellular calcium in platelet secretory response to the C5b–9 proteins. The relationship of Ca^{2+} influx across the C5b–9-damaged plasma membrane to platelet α-granule secretion is illustrated by the absolute requirement for extracellular Ca^{2+} in the C5b–9-initiated secretory response. Gel-filtered platelets pretreated with C5b6 plus C7 (assembling approximately 1000 C5b67 complexes per cell) were suspended at 37°C in medium containing either 2.5 mM Ca^{2+} (closed triangles) or 0.1 mM EGTA (open triangles).

At time 0, C5b–9 assembly was initiated by the addition of C8 and C9, and α-granule secretion monitored by the expression of α-granule membrane glycoprotein GMP-140 on the platelet surface. In the presence of EGTA (open triangles), the secretory response of the cells to C5b–9 assembly is blocked, but it can be triggered subsequently by the addition of excess Ca^{2+} to the cell suspension (2.5 mM final concentration). Data for control platelets suspended under identical conditions (open and closed circles) are also shown. As 0.1 mM EGTA does not block assembly and functional activation of the C5b–9 pore under these conditions, these data suggest that the platelet secretory response is initiated by the diffusional influx of Ca^{2+} across the plasma membrane. (Wiedmer T, Ando B, Sims PJ: J Biol Chem 262: 13674, 1987, with permission).

brane deposition of C5b67 complexes per se, confirming a requirement for the fully assembled C5b–9 complex. Although a contribution of leukocyte-derived platelet activators cannot be excluded, the C5b–9-mediated responses were unaltered by known inhibitors of platelet-activating factor (PAF), and pretreatment with PAF fails to desensitize platelets to activation by C5b–9.

- By contrast to other known plasma-derived platelet activators, C5b–9-stimulated secretion of platelet storage granules (and, expression of platelet procoagulant activity; see below) occurs without functional activation of the cellular fibrinogen receptors (complexes of plasma membrane glycoproteins GPIIb–IIIa), and aggregation of C5b–9 activated platelets is not observed.[1a,1b] This raises the possibility that C5b–9 deposition in vivo can give rise to activated but nonadherent platelets that persist in the circulation.

Complement Activation of Platelet Procoagulant Response

In addition to providing the initial "hemostatic plug," activated platelets provide an important catalytic surface for assembly and activation of various enzymes of the coagulation system. This catalytic function is thought to be provided by acidic phospholipids (e.g., phosphatidylserine) that become expressed on the platelet surface upon cell activation because of transbilayer exchange of lipid between cytoplasmic and external leaflets.[6] Evidence suggesting participation of specific cell surface receptors in these reactions has also been presented.[71]

Participation of the complement system in expression of platelet procoagulant activity has long been suspected, given the frequent association of vascular thrombosis with complement activation (discussed later). In vitro, zymosan activation of platelet-rich plasma results in deposition of complement proteins on the platelet surface, activation of platelet aggregation and release reactions, and uptake of factor Xa with increased prothrombin activation and accelerated plasma clotting.[86,163,164] This reaction does not occur in plasma deficient in components of the alternative pathway, confirming participation of this complement activation pathway in the procoagulant response.

The exact mechanism by which complement activation initiates thrombin activation and accelerates plasma clotting remains unresolved. With isolated proteins, Fair and colleagues have demonstrated that the properdin-stabilized C3bBb complex can directly activate prothrombin, providing a potential mechanism fcr direct feedback activation of platelet procoagulant responses through thrombin.[33] On the other hand, participation of the terminal complement proteins in thrombin generation is suggested by studies with rabbit platelet-rich plasma, which show a C6-dependent clotting time[161] and by evidence with human platelets that factor Xa-catalyzed plasma clotting is accelerated directly by membrane assembly of the C5b-9 proteins.[153]

The capacity of the C5b-9 proteins to initiate assembly of the platelet prothrombinase (the membrane complex of factors Va and Xa) was recently examined in a plasma-free system with the purified complement and coagulation proteins.[152,153] C5b-9 assembly on gel-filtered human platelets was shown to directly initiate the nonlytic secretion of factor V from the platelet α granules and the slow activation of this protein, resulting in an increase in factor Xa binding to the platelet surface. Factor Xa uptake by the C5b-9-treated cells was accompanied by a concomitant increase in platelet prothrombinase activity (Fig. 18-9). In the presence of exogenous factor Va, factor Xa binding increased to 5500 molecules per cell, approximating the maximum number of potential prothrombinase sites that can be generated under these conditions. Most of these newly-expressed factor Va binding sites are found on small (<0.1 μm) plasma-membrane derived microparticles that are released from the platelet surface upon C5b-9 insertion.[126a] The mechanism for spontaneous activation of secreted factor V (presumably by a platelet-derived protease) and the physical nature of the membrane-associated factor Va binding sites generated under these conditions remain to be elucidated.

PLATELET-ASSOCIATED COMPLEMENT PROTEINS IN DISEASE

Complement-fixing antibodies with specificity for platelet-associated epitopes can lead to deposition of C3b and the C5b-9 proteins on the platelet surface. The binding of these components to the platelet surface has also been demonstrated after fluid-phase activation of the complement system by immune complexes and other soluble complement activators and may also occur by direct C3 or C5 cleavage by other platelet-derived or plasma-generated proteases. Finally, localization of complement-fixing immune complexes to the platelet surface also can potentially be achieved through interaction of immunoglobulin with platelet Fc receptors or through binding of C1q, C3b, iC3b, or C3dg-containing immune complexes with the various complement receptors (C1q, gp45-70, CR2, or CR4) that have recently been reported to be expressed by these cells.

Detection of Platelet-Associated Complement Proteins

By use of an anti-C3 consumption assay (modeled after the antiglobulin consumption assay developed for measurement of platelet-asso-

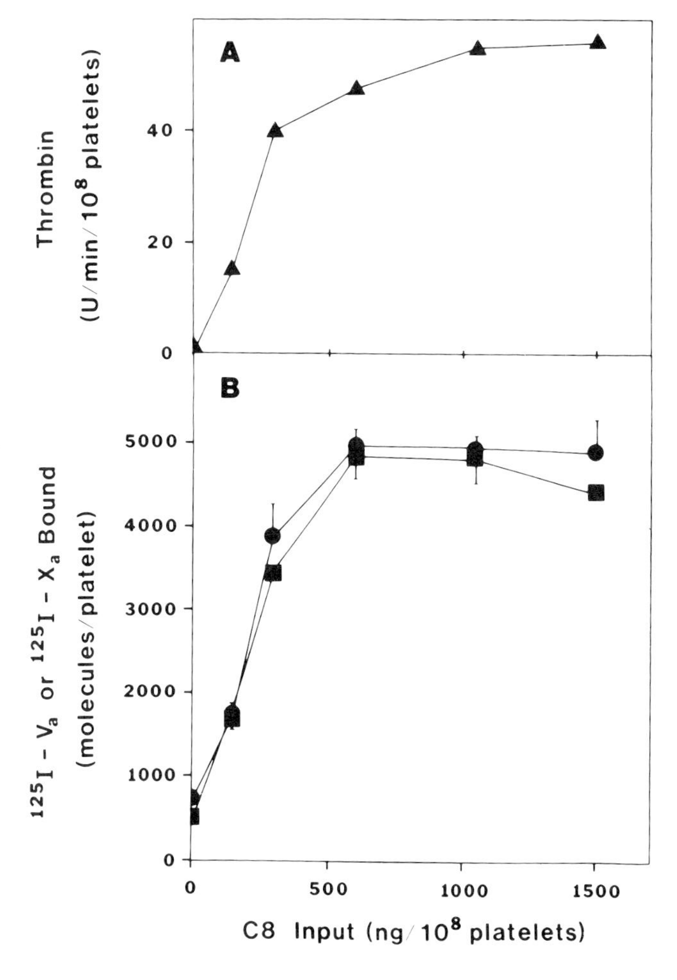

Figure 18-9. Role of the C5b-9 proteins in expression of platelet prothrombinase activity. The capacity of the C5b-9 proteins to initiate assembly and activation of the platelet prothrombinase (the membrane-bound enzyme complex of coagulation factors Va and Xa) was investigated by measuring expression of binding sites for factors Va and Xa by platelets exposed to the purified C5b-9 proteins. Gel-filtered platelets pretreated with C5b6 plus C7 were exposed to increasing amounts of C8 (in the presence of excess C9) and specific uptake of ^{125}I-labeled factors Va and Xa measured in the absence of prothrombin or other plasma proteins. C5b-9 assembly resulted in a coordinate increase in the binding of both factor Va (closed circles) and factor Xa (closed squares) to the platelet surface *B*. The binding of ^{125}I-labeled factor Xa was measured in the presence of 2 μg/ml unlabeled factor Va, and the binding of ^{125}I-labeled factor Va was measured in the presence of 200 ng/ml unlabeled factor Xa. The binding of factors Va and Xa to the C5b-9-treated platelets resulted in a concomitant increase in prothrombinase activity, as measured by the rate of prothrombin conversion to thrombin *A* (Wiedmer T, Esmon CT, Sims PJ: J Biol Chem 261:14587, 1986, with permission).

ciated IgG; PAIgG), Hauch and Rosse first directly demonstrated the presence of C3 antigens on normal washed platelets, and they presented data suggesting that platelet-associated C3 (PAC3) increases in certain cases of ITP, systemic lupus erythematosus (SLE) with thrombocytopenia, and quinidine-induced thrombocytopenias.[49] More recently, direct measurement of platelet-bound C3 (or specific C3b-derived fragments) has also been reported using immunofluorescence, enzyme-linked immunosorbent assays (ELISA), and a variety of radioimmunoassays.[18,19,30,37,50,61,65,68,76,79,89,114,156] Although these reports differ widely in their estimate of the background of C3 antigen on washed, normal platelets, most reported values range from approximately 10^3 to 10^4 molecules per cell. When domain-specific antibodies were employed, bound C3 was often detected as C3dg, indicative of C3b degradation by factor I in vivo.[19,30,50,61,65,89] In addition to C3 (and derived fragments), measurement of platelet-associated C1,[90] C4,[61,115,156] factor H,[26,27,60] factor D,[60] and C9 neoantigen associated with membrane-inserted C5b-9[61] have now been reported.

Platelet-Associated Complement Proteins in Immune Thrombocytopenia

Circulating complement-activating or "fixing" antiplatelet antibodies were first demonstrated by Shulman and coworkers for certain drug-dependent antibodies and alloantibodies to Pl^{A1} or HLA antigens.[122-124] In autoimmune thrombocytopenia (ITP), circulating complement-fixing antibodies are generally not detected, and it was initially assumed that complement activation played no role in this disorder.[125] More recently, complement-fixing antiplatelet antibodies of both IgG and IgM classes have been demonstrated in the plasma or serum of some patients with ITP, and elevated levels of PAC have been detected in this and a variety of other platelet disorders with a known, or suspected, immune cause. Additionally, splenic lymphocytes obtained from patients with ITP have been shown to secrete complement-fixing antibodies that deposit C3 on normal platelets.[68]

The clinical implication of complement activation in thrombocytopenic patients remains unresolved. A relationship between complement activation and in vivo platelet destruction is perhaps best established in cases of alloimmunization to Pl^{A1} and HLA antigens and for certain drug-related thrombocytopenias associated with complement-fixing antibodies against quinidine, heparin, and penicillin.[15-17,38,63,75,124] For these antibodies, complement-dependent platelet-release reactions or evidence of complement-dependent lysis have been reported and, when measured, complement activation and elevated PAC appear to correlate with the severity of thrombocytopenia.

Elevated PAC has also been described in several studies of patients with autoimmune thrombocytopenia, although the implications of this increase remain controversial.[18,19,49,50,59,61,65,76,89,114,156] It is now well established that complement-fixing antibodies do occur in this disorder.[18,49,79] Nevertheless, it is also apparent that severe thrombocytopenia can result from autoantibodies, without evidence of complement activation or of a detectable increase in PAC.[59,76,79,89] Estimates of the frequency with which elevated platelet C3 occurs in patients with ITP vary substantially but, in general, most patients who showed increased PAIg also exhibited elevated C3 on their platelets. In several studies, isolated cases of thrombocytopenia with elevated platelet C3, but normal levels of PAIg, have been documented.[18,59,76,89] In a single study, platelet C3 was shown to positively correlate with the amount of iC3b and C9 antigens on the platelets.[61] No such correlation was found for C4. In individual patients, who were followed over time, the level of PAC3 has been shown to correlate with the severity of thrombocytopenia, with platelet C3 usually returning to normal ranges during remission.[49,76] In comparing different patients with ITP, however, the level of platelet-associated C3 has been found to be either well-correlated or uncorrelated with the platelet count.[49,59,61,76,89] Furthermore, it has been reported that elevated PAC3 can be detected in many cases of thrombocytopenia arising from presumed nonimmunologic causes, contributing to the uncertainty of the diagnostic and prognostic value of this parameter.[59,89] Finally, it should be noted that when interpreting reported values of PAC, consideration must also be given to the potential for nonimmune activation and membrane deposition of complement proteins by platelet-associated proteases generated in autologous platelet-rich plasma suspensions.[162]

Role of Platelet-Associated Complement in Immune Clearance

Despite accumulating data related to quantitative changes in PAC in patients with thrombocytopenia, the actual role of the complement system in altered platelet survival in vivo remains to be established. Data from in vitro study suggests that PAC3b can mediate adherence to monocytes and macrophages which, by analogy to red cells, is likely to accelerate phagocytic clearance by the cells of the reticuloendothelial system (reviewed in Ref. 85). Membrane deposition of large quantities of the C5b–9 proteins can potentially initiate intravascular cytolysis, whereas sublytic amounts of these proteins can evoke a variety of platelet responses affecting function and survival of this cell in the circulation (see above). Although elevations in PAC3 have been correlated with shortened in vivo platelet survival, the relative contribution of cell surface immunoglobulin versus complement in the sequestration and phagocytic removal of these cells from the vasculature has not been defined, nor has it been resolved whether or not the immune-mediated changes in platelet function that can be demonstrated in vitro contribute directly to accelerated clearance of these cells from the circulation. Nevertheless, it is of interest that intracellular storage pool deficiencies, abnormal aggregation, and altered arachidonic acid metabolism have been demonstrated in platelets obtained from patients with chronic ITP, indicative of altered cellular function arising from immune injury in vivo.[135,149]

Paroxysmal Nocturnal Hemoglobinuria

Paroxysmal nocturnal hemoglobinuria (PNH) is an acquired hematopoietic stem cell disorder characterized by anemia and a propensity toward intravascular coagulation. In addition to red cells, platelets and neutrophils can be affected by this disorder. The affected erythrocytes exhibit increased sensitivity to complement-mediated hemolysis, arising from two distinct molecular defects: PNH II erythrocytes exhibit defective regulation of the C3-convertases, resulting from a deficiency of the membrane regulatory protein DAF.[84,88] In addition to lacking DAF, PNH III erythrocytes are defective in their regulation of the MAC because of a deficiency of membrane components that function to restrict C9 activation by membrane C5b–8.[109,120] Recent evidence suggests that this C9-inhibitory factor is a membrane glycoprotein, distinct from DAF, that is missing in the PNH III cell.[121,158,159] In contrast to PNH II and PNH III cells, PNH I cells are biochemically and functionally indistinguishable from normal erythrocytes and are presumed to arise from normal erythroid stem cells. Whereas PNH II erythrocytes are three to five times more sensitive to complement-mediated hemolysis than normal erythrocytes, the combined molecular defects exhibited by PNH III cells render them 15 to 25 times more susceptible to this process.[113] The deficiency in DAF is shared by PNH platelets, monocytes, and granulocytes,[84] although the complete cellular distribution of the unique PNH III defect has not yet been established.

Although platelets from patients with PNH lack DAF (and may also be defective in regulatory control of the MAC), the significance of these molecular defects to the clinical presentation of the disorder has not been completely elucidated. By in vitro assay, PNH platelets show increased sensitivity to complement-mediated lysis initiated by antiplatelet antibodies.[3,28] Increased C3 uptake after fluid-phase activation of the alternative pathway has been observed in some, but not all, studies.[26,28,162] These cells have also been reported to exhibit increased sensitivity to the complement-dependent release reaction resulting from deposition of C3b or the C5b–9 proteins on the plasma membrane.[28] It appears, therefore, that PNH platelets share the membrane defect(s) affecting erythrocytes in this disorder, which gives rise to marked sensitivity to complement activation. Nevertheless, severe thrombocytopenia is not a prominent feature of the clinical presentation of PNH, and many of these patients maintain platelet counts in the normal range.[113] Additionally, in some patients with documented DAF-deficient platelets, autologous ^{111}In-labeled platelet survival is normal.[26]

A possible explanation for why platelet destruction in PNH is less prominent than that observed for erythrocytes is provided by recent data relating to the unique control of the alternative pathway C3-convertase on the platelet surface. Devine and associates measured the activity of this enzyme on platelets obtained from PNH patients who exhibited DAF-negative cells.[27] They report that despite DAF deficiency, normal inhibition of the membrane-bound C3-convertase is observed in more than half of those patients studied, suggesting another mechanism for regulation of this enzyme at the platelet surface. In a subsequent report, they present evidence that suggests that the capacity of DAF-negative platelets to regulate the C3-convertase is directly related to the secretion of factor H from the platelet α granule, which can be triggered by C3b binding to the cell surface.[27]

The increased sensitivity of some PNH platelets to the lytic activity of complement suggests that the C5b-9 inhibitory protein (homologous restriction factor) is expressed on normal platelets and that deficiency of this membrane protein contributes to altered sensitivity of the PNH platelet to the complement system. Finally, it should be noted here that in addition to anemia and thrombocytopenia, patients with PNH exhibit recurrent thrombotic episodes. This property has been variously attributed to increased platelet reactivity or to elevated thromboplastin present in plasma.[80,133] The etiology of these vascular changes remains to be defined. Nevertheless, the C5b–9 proteins have been shown to trigger factor V release and activation, resulting in accelerated thrombin generation through the platelet prothrombinase and to cause release of plasma membrane-derived microvesicles from the cell surface that bind factor Va and express prothrombinase activity, suggesting a direct link between altered regulation of complement activation on the PNH platelet surface and the thrombotic episodes observed in this disorder.[126a,152,153]

Complement–Platelet Interactions in Hemostasis and Thrombosis

It is now widely recognized that vascular hemostasis is regulated through complex and varied interactions among platelets, leukocytes, vascular endothelium and plasma complement, coagulation, kinin, and fibrinolytic systems.[8,58,137,138] One of the implications of this complex interrelationship is that a vascular event initiating recruitment of the mediators of the hemostatic response can potentially activate mediators of the immunoinflammatory response, and vice versa. As discussed previously, there is now considerable evidence from laboratory study that part of this interplay between hemostatic and inflammatory mechanisms is mediated directly through complement–platelet interactions. Additionally, platelet recruitment can potentially be triggered by PAF (and other platelet activators) released by leukocytes exposed to C3a, C5a, and other complement activation products.

The complement system is activated during blood clotting, suggesting participation of these proteins in thrombus formation. Direct participation of the complement system in platelet recruitment for normal hemostasis is best established for the rabbit, for which it has been shown that blood coagulation is retarded in animals deficient in C6.[161] In addition to impaired vascular hemostasis, blood from these animals shows a prolonged whole-blood clotting time and poor prothrombin consumption that is corrected by the addition of C6. Similar results have been documented for the C4-deficient guinea pig.[77]

In humans, a requirement for the complement system in normal hemostasis has not been established. Only a few isolated case studies of coagulation and platelet function in individuals with inherited deficiencies of C3, C5, C6, or C7 have now been reported (reviewed in Refs. 5, 8). The one consistent finding in these individuals has been abnormal platelet release and aggregation in response to zymosan or other activators of the alternative pathway. On the other hand, these individuals do not show impaired hemostasis, and laboratory coagulation and platelet function studies in these individuals have generally been normal. For example, in a C3-deficient patient, normal platelet aggregation responses to ADP, collagen, thrombin, epinephrine, and ristocetin were obtained, and bleeding time was normal.[43] Other investigators have reported similar findings in two individuals deficient in C5, and one deficient in C6.[10] By contrast, Wautier and colleagues have described two individuals deficient in C6 and an individual deficient in C7 who exhibit impaired platelet aggregation in response to thrombin.[1,146] The potential role of the C5b–9 proteins in potentiating the platelet response to subthreshold quantities of thrombin is discussed in the foregoing.

Although normal hemostatic mechanisms in humans do not appear to depend upon complement activation, there is considerable evidence suggesting that complement activation can alter platelet function and contribute to the onset of vascular disease. The potential role of the complement system in the thrombotic episodes associated with PNH has been discussed earlier. Additionally, abnormal platelet function has been noted in patients with immune complex disease and in patients with chronic ITP, suggesting in vivo activation of these cells, either by immune complexes or components of the complement system.[135,149] Although the etiologic significance remains unclear, complement activation has been demonstrated in cases of thrombotic thrombocytopenic purpura, providing a possible mechanism for amplifying platelet activation in this disease.[39,78] Finally, disseminated intravascular coagulation has been shown to follow infusion of endotoxin or other complement activators into experimental animals, and several known activators of the complement system have been implicated in the initiation of these episodes in humans.[20]

CONCLUSIONS

In the past 40 years there has been dramatic progress in defining the immunochemistry of the red cell and the direct translation of this information into diagnostic immunohematology and transfusion practice. Unfortunately, it is now also evident that immunohematologic concepts that derive from studies undertaken with erythrocytes cannot universally be applied to other blood cells that are potential targets of immune attack. The uniqueness of each blood cell's interaction with the body's humoral immunologic defense mechanisms is graphically underscored by considering the interaction of human platelets with the complement system.

In an attempt to rationalize the complex interrelationship that has emerged between the immune–effector function of the complement system, on the one hand, and various reactions underlying platelet-catalyzed hemostasis, on the other, it is useful to recall that the contact–activation systems in both hemolymph and plasma evolved to fulfill two primary functions necessary for maintenance of vascular integrity: a hemostatic and fibrinolytic function required to plug the injured vessel wall while maintaining patency to flow, and an immune recognition and clearance function required to resist colonization by microbial pathogens.

The obvious functional and molecular homologies of those proteins contributing to these humoral effector systems suggests that there has always been an overriding integration of these two ostensibly separate functions of hemostasis and immune defense. One simple example of this integration of function that has apparently been conserved throughout phylogeny is the organization of a clot at the site of bacterial infection, a coagulant response that primarily serves an immune function, restricting dissemination of organisms throughout the vascular bed.

Consideration of this complex interrelationship between the immune and hemostatic effector systems in blood suggests that to completely elucidate the immune mechanisms that affect platelet survival or function in vivo, it will be necessary to take into account the various molecular events associated with expression of this cells' intrinsic hemostatic activity. This will include unraveling the various interactions that occur between immunoglobulin molecules and the complement, coagulation, and fibrinolytic systems when localized within the confines of the unstirred aqueous boundary layer at the platelet surface. Additionally, it will be necessary to delineate the regulatory control of the various contact-activated enzyme complexes that bind to the platelet surface, especially as affected by secretory and other triggered response mechanisms of the platelet itself. And finally, it will be necessary to elucidate the platelet's unique responses to the activated products generated through these various proteolytic reaction cascades as triggered either through ligand binding to specific receptors expressed on the platelet surface, or as a consequence of physical changes produced in the plasma membrane of this cell. Needless to say, there remains much yet to be learned.

This work was supported in part by the National Heart, Lung, and Blood Institute grants HL36946 and HL36061 and an Established Investigatorship Award from the American Heart Association, 85-128.

REFERENCES

1. Alcalay M, Bontoux D, Peltier A, Vial M-C, Vilde J-M, Wautier J-L: C7 deficiency, abnormal platelet aggregation, and rheumatoid arthritis letter. Arthritis Rheum 24:102, 1981

1a. Ando B, Wiedmer T, Hamilton KK, Sims PJ: Complement proteins C5b-9 initiate secretion of platelet storage granules without increased binding of fibrinogen or von Willebrand factor to newly expressed cell surface GPIIb–IIIa. J Biol Chem 263:11907, 1988

1b. Ando B, Wiedmer T, Sims PJ: The secretory release reaction initiated by complement proteins C5b–9 occurs without platelet aggregation through GPIIb–IIIa. Blood (in press), 1989

2. Asch AS, Kinoshita T, Jaffe EA, Nussenzweig V: Decay-accelerating factor is present on cultured human umbilical vein endothelial cells. J Exp Med 163:221, 1986

3. Aster RH, Enright SE: A platelet and granulocyte membrane defect in paroxysmal nocturnal hemoglobinuria. Usefulness for detection of antiplatelet antibodies. J Clin Invest 48:1199, 1969

4. Becker EL, Henson PM: In vitro studies of immunologically induced secretion of mediators from cells and related phenomena. Adv Immunol 17:93, 1973

5. Bennet B, Ogston D: Role of complement, coagulation, fibrinolysis, and kinins in normal hemostasis and disease. In Bloom AL, Thomas DP (eds): Haemostasis and Thrombosis, p 236. New York, Churchill-Livingstone, 1981

6. Bevers EM, Comfurius P, Zwaal RFA: Changes in membrane phospholipid distribution during platelet activation. Biochim Biophys 736:57, 1983

7. Bhakdi S, Tranum-Jensen J: Membrane damage by complement. Biochim Biophys Acta 737:343, 1983

8. Blajchman MA, Ozge-Anwar AH: The role of the complement system in hemostasis. Prog Hematol 14:149, 1986

9. Boyle MDP, Gee AP, Borsos T: Studies on the terminal stages of immune hemolysis. VI. Osmotic blockages of differing Stokes radii detect complement-induced transmembrane channels of differing size. J Immunol 123:77, 1979

10. Breckenridge RT, Rosenfeld SI, Graff KS, Leddy JP: Hereditary C5 deficiency in man. III. Studies of hemostasis and platelet responses to zymosan. J Immunol 118:12, 1977

11. Campbell AK, Daw RA, Hallett MD, Luio JP: Direct measurement of increase in intracellular free calcium ion concentration in response to the action of complement. Biochem J 194:551, 1981

12. Cazenave JP, Assimeh SN, Painter RH, Packham MA, Mustard JF: C1q inhibition of the interaction of collagen with human platelets. J Immunol 116:162, 1976

13. Charriaut-Marlangue C, Nunez D, Barel M, Beneviste J, Frade R: Activation of human platelets by polyclonal or monoclonal antibodies against GP-140, the EBV/C3d receptor (CR2) (abstr). Fed Proc 46:724, 1987

14. Cheng K-H, Wiedmer T, Sims PJ: Fluorescence resonance energy transfer study of the associative state of membrane bound complexes of complement proteins C5b-8. J Immunol 135:459, 1985

15. Chong BH, Grace CS, Rosenberg MC: Heparin-induced thrombocytopenia: Effect of heparin platelet antibody on platelets. Br J Haematol 49:531, 1981

16. Cines DB, Kaywin P, Bina M, Tomaski A, Schreiber AD: Heparin-associated thrombocytopenia. N Engl J Med 303:788, 1980

17. Cines DB, Schreiber AD: Effect of anti-Pl^{A1} antibody on human platelets. I. The role of complement. Blood 53:567, 1979

18. Cines DB, Schreiber AD: Immune thrombocytopenia: Use of Coombs antiglobulin to detect platelet IgG and C3. N Engl J Med 300:106, 1979

19. Cines DB, Wilson SB, Tomaski A, Schreiber AD: Platelet antibodies of the IgM class in immune thrombocytopenic purpura. J Clin Invest 75:1183, 1985

20. Colman RW, Marder VJ: Disseminated intravascular coagulation (DIC). Pathogenesis, pathophysiology, and laboratory abnormalities. In Colman RW, Hirsh J, Marder VJ, Salzman EW (eds): Hemostasis and Thrombosis, p 654. Philadelphia, JB Lippincott, 1982

21. Cooper NR: The classical complement activation pathway: Activation and regulation of the first component. Adv Immunol 37:151, 1985

22. Csako G, Suba EA, Ohanian SH: Interaction of the subcomponent Clq and collagen with isolated platelet membranes in platelet aggregation. Haemostasis 13:288, 1983

23. Dahlback B, Stenflow J: High molecular weight complex in human plasma between vitamin K-dependent protein S and complement component C4b-binding protein. Proc Natl Acad Sci USA 78:2512, 1981

24. Dalmasso AP: Complement in the pathophysiology and diagnosis of human diseases. CRC Crit Rev Clin Lab Sci 24:123, 1986

25. Davitz MA, Low MG, Nussenzweig V: Release of decay-accelerating factor (DAF) from the cell membrane by phosphatidylinositol-specific phosphilipase C (PIPLC). J Exp Med 163:1150, 1986

26. Devine DV, Rosse WF: Regulation of the activity of platelet-bound C3 convertase of the alternative pathway of complement by platelet factor H. Proc Natl Acad Sci USA. 84:5873, 1987

27. Devine DV, Siegel RS, Rosse WF: Interactions of platelets in paroxysmal nocturnal hemoglobinuria with complement. Relationship to defects in the regulation of complement and to platelet survival in vivo. J Clin Invest 79:131, 1987

28. Dixon RH, Rosse WF: Mechanisms of complement-mediated activation of human blood platelets in vitro. J Clin Invest 59:360, 1977

29. Dourmashkin RR: Structural events associated with the attachment of complement components to the cell membranes in reactive lysis. Immunology 35:205, 1978

30. Endresen GKM, Mellbye OJ: Studies on the binding of complement factor C3 to the surface of human blood platelets. Haemostasis 14:269, 1984

31. Esser AF: Interactions between complement proteins and biological and model membranes. In Chapman D (ed): Biological Membranes. New York, Academic Press, 1982

32. Esser AF, Kolb WP, Podack ER, Muller-Eberhard HJ: Reorganization of lipid bilayers by complement: A possible mechanism of membranolysis. Proc Natl Acad Sci USA 76:1410, 1979

33. Fair DS, Sundsmo JS, Schwartz BS, Edgington TS, Muller-Eberhard HJ: Prothrombin activation by factor B (Bb) of the alternative pathway of complement. Thromb Haemostasis 46:301, 1981

34. Fearon DT: The human C3b receptor. Springer Semin Immunopathol 6:159, 1983

35. Fearon DT: Identification of the membrane glycoprotein that is the C3b receptor of the human erythrocyte, polymorphonuclear leukocytes, B lymphocyte, and monocyte. J Exp Med 152:20, 1980

36. Fearon DT: Regulation of the amplification C3 convertase of human complement by an inhibitory protein isolated from human erythrocyte membrane. Proc Natl Acad Sci USA 76:5867, 1979

37. Follea G, Mandrand B, Dechavanne M: Simultaneous enzymoimmunologic assays of platelet associated IgG, IgM, and C3. A useful tool for the assessment of immune thrombocytopenias. Thromb Res 26:249, 1982

38. Gandolfo GM, Afeltra A, Mannella E, Costantini G: Complement-dependence of platelet serotonin release test in polytransfused patients. Br J Haematol 19:355, 1977

39. Garvey MB, Freedman J: Complement in thrombotic thrombocytopenic purpura. Am J Hematol 15:397, 1983

40. Gee AP, Boyle MDP, Borsos T: Distinction between C8-mediated and C8/C9-mediated hemolysis on the basis of independent ^{86}Rb and hemoglobin release. J Immunol 124:1905, 1980

41. Goers JW, Glovsky MM, Hunkapillar MW, Farnsworth V, Richards JH: Studies on $C3a_{hu}$ binding to human eosinophils: Characterization of binding. Int Arch Allergy Appl Immunol 74:147, 1984

42. Goldman JN, Ruddy S, Austen KF: Reaction mechanism of nascent C5,6,7 (reactive lysis). I. Reaction characteristics of production of EC5,6,7 and lysis by C8 and C9. J Immunol 109:353, 1972

43. Gomperts ED, Rabson AR: Coagulation studies in a homozygous C3 deficiency. Br J Haematol 35:165, 1977

44. Hallett MB, Campbell AK: Is intracellular Ca^{2+} the trigger for oxygen radical production by polymorphonuclear leukocytes? Cell Calcium 5:1, 1984

45. Hammer CH, Abramovitz AS, Mayer MM: A new activity of complement component C3: Cell bound C3b potentiates lysis of erythrocytes by C5b,6 and terminal components. J Immunol 117:830, 1976

46. Hansch GM, Gemsa D, Resch K: Induction of prostanoid synthesis in human platelets by the late complement components C5b-9 and channel forming antibiotic nystatin: Inhibition of the reacylation of liberated arachidonic acid. J Immunol 135:1320, 1985

47. Hansch GM, Seitz M, Martinotti G, Betz M, Rauterberg EW, Gemsa D: Macrophages release arachidonic acid, prostaglandin E_2, and thromboxane in response to the late complement components. J Immunol 133:2145, 1984

48. Harrington WJ, Sprague CC, Minnick V, Moore CV, Aulvin RC, Duboch R: Immunologic mechanisms in idiopathic and neonatal thrombocytopenia purpura. Ann Intern Med 38:433, 1952

49. Hauch TW, Rosse WF: Platelet-bound complement (C3) in immune thrombocytopenia. Blood 50:1129, 1977

50. Hedge UM, Bowes A, Roter BLT: Platelet-associated complement components (PAC_{3c} and PAC_{3d}) in patients with autoimmune thrombocytopenia. Br J Haematol 60:49, 1985

51. Henson PM: Role of complement and leukocytes in immunologic release of vasoactive amines from platelets. Fed Proc 28:1721, 1969

52. Henson PM, Ginsberg MH: Immunological reactions of platelets. In Gordon GL (ed): Platelets in Biology and Pathology 2, p 265. New York, Elsevier/North-Holland, 1981

53. Hu VW, Esser AF, Podack ER, Wisnieski BJ: The membrane attack mechanism of complement: Photolabeling reveals insertion of terminal proteins into target membrane. J Immunol 127:380, 1981

54. Hugli TE: Structure and function of the anaphylatoxins. Springer Semin Immunopathol 7:193, 1983

55. Humphrey JH, Jacques R: Release of histamine and 5-hydroxytryptamine (serotonin) from platelets by antigen-antibody reactions (in vitro). J Physiol 128:9, 1955

56. Iida K, Nussenzweig V: Functional properties of membrane-associated complement receptor CR 1. J Immunol 130:1876, 1983

57. Imagawa DK, Osichfin NE, Paznekas WA, Shin ML, Mayer MM: Consequences of cell membrane attack by complement: Release of arachidonate and formation of inflammatory derivatives. Proc Natl Acad Sci USA 80:6647, 1983

58. Kaplan AP, Silverberg M, Dunn JT, Ghebrehiwet B: Interaction of the clotting, kinin-forming, complement, and fibrinolytic pathways in inflammation. Ann NY Acad Sci 389:25, 1982

59. Kayser W, Mueller-Eckhardt C, Bhakdi S, Ebert K: Platelet-associated C3 in thrombocytopenic states. Br J Haematol 54:353, 1983

60. Kenney DM, Davis AE III: Association of alternative complement pathway components with human blood platelets: Secretion and localization of factor D and β1H globulin. Clin Immunol Immunopathol 21:351, 1981

60a. Kunicki TJ, Nugent DJ, Staats SJ, Orchekowski RP, Wayner EA, Carter WG: The human fibroblast class II extracellular matrix receptor mediates platelet adhesion to collagen and is identical to the platelet glycoprotein Ia-IIa complex. J Biol Chem 263:4516, 1988

61. Kurata Y, Curd JG, Tamerius JD, McMillan R: Platelet-associated complement in chronic ITP. Br J Haematol 60:723, 1984

62. Lachmann PJ, Hughes-Jones NC: Initiation of complement activation. Springer Semin Immunopathol 7:143, 1984

63. Lau P, Sholtis CM, Aster RH: Post-transfusion purpura: An enigma of alloimmunization. Am J Hematol 9:331, 1980

64. Lauf PK: Membrane immunology and permeability functions. In Androli TE, Hoffman JF, Fanestil DD (eds): Physiology of Membrane Disorders, p 369. New York, Plenum Press, 1978

65. Lehman HA, Lehman LO, Rustago PK, Plunkett RW, Farolino DL, Conway J, Logue GL: Complement-mediated autoimmune thrombocytopenia (monoclonal IgM antiplatelet antibody associated with lymphoreticular malignant disease). N Engl J Med 316:194, 1987

66. Martin SE, Breckenridge RT, Rosenfeld SI, Leddy JP: Responses of human platelets to immunologic stimuli: Independent roles for complement and IgG in zymosan activation. J Immunol 120:9, 1978

67. Mayer MM: Membrane damage by complement. Johns Hopkins Med J 148:243, 1981

68. McMillan R, Martin M: Fixation of C3 to platelets in vitro by antiplatelet antibody from patients with immune thrombocytopenic purpura. Br J Haematol 47:251, 1981

69. Medof ME, Iida K, Mold C, Nussenzweig V: Unique role of the complement receptor CR1 in the degradation of C3b associated with immune complexes. J Exp Med 156:1739, 1982

70. Meuer S, Hugli TE, Andreatta RH, Hadding U, Bitter-Suermann D: Comparative study on biological activities of various anaphylatoxins (C4a, C3a, C5a). Inflammation 5:263, 1981

71. Miletich JP, Jackson CM, Majerus PM: Properties of the factor Xa binding site on human platelets. J Biol Chem 253:6908, 1978

72. Mitchell CA, Salem HH: Cleavage of protein S by a platelet membrane protease. J Clin Invest 79:374, 1987

73. Mueller-Eckhardt C, Luscher EF: Immune reactions of human blood platelets. I. A comparative study on the effects on platelets of heterologous antiserum, antigen-antibody complexes, aggregated gammaglobulin and thrombin. Thromb Death Haemorrh 20:155, 1968

74. Muller-Eberhard HJ: The membrane attack complex. Springer Semin Immunopathol 7:93, 1984

75. Murphy MF, Riordan T, Minchinton RM, Chapman JF: Demonstration of an immune-mediated mechanism of penicillin-induced neutropenia and thrombocytopenia. Br J Haematol 55:155, 1983

76. Myers TJ, Kim BK, Steiner M, Baldini MG: Platelet-associated complement C3 in immune thrombocytopenic purpura. Blood 59:1023, 1982

77. Nagaki K, Fujikawa K, Inai, S: Studies of the fourth component of complement. II. The fourth component of complement in guinea pig and human platelets. Biken J:129, 1965

78. Neame PB: Immunologic and other factors in thrombotic thrombocytopenic purpura. Semin Thromb Hemostasis 6:416, 1980

79. Nel JD, Stevens K: A new method for the simultaneous quantitation of platelet-bound immunoglobulin (IgG) and complement (C3) employing an enzyme-linked immunosorbant assay (ELISA) procedure. Br J Haematol 44:281, 1980

80. Newcomb TF, Gardner FH: Thrombin generation in PNH. Br J Haematol 9:84, 1963

81. Nicholson-Weller A, Burge J, Fearon DT, Weller PF, Austen KF: Isolation of a human erythrocyte membrane glycoprotein with decay-accelerating activity for C3 convertases of the complement system. J Immunol 129:184, 1982

82. Nicholson-Weller A, March JP, Rosenfeld SI, Austen KF: Affected erythrocytes of patients with paroxysmal nocturnal hemoglobinuria are deficient in the complement regulatory protein, decay-accelerating factor. Proc Natl Acad Sci USA 80:5066, 1983

83. Nicholson-Weller A, March JP, Rosen CE, Spicer DB, Austen KF: Surface membrane expression by human blood leukocytes and platelets of decay-accelerating factor, a regulatory protein of the complement system. Blood 65:1237, 1985

84. Nicholson-Weller A, Spicer DB, and Austen KF: Deficiency of the complement regulatory protein, "decay-accelerating factor," on membranes of granulocytes, monocytes, and platelets in paroxysmal nocturnal hemoglobinuria. N Engl J Med 312:1091, 1985

85. Nydegger UE, Kazatchkine MD: The role of complement in immune clearance of blood cells. Springer Semin Immunopathol 6:373, 1983

86. Ozge-Anwar AH, Freedman JJ, Senyi AF, Cerskus AL, Blajchman MA: Enhanced prothrombin-converting activity and factor Xa binding of platelets activated by the alternative complement pathway. Br J Haematol 57:221, 1984

87. Pangburn MK, Muller-Eberhard HJ: The alternative pathway of complement. Springer Semin Immunopathol 7:163, 1984

88. Pangburn MK, Schreiber RD, Muller-Eberhard HJ: Deficiency of an erythrocyte membrane protein with complement regulatory activity in paroxysmal nocturnal hemoglobinuria. Proc Natl Acad Sci USA 80:5430, 1983

89. Panzer S, Szamait S, Bodeker RH, Haas OA, Haubenstock A, Mueller-Eckert C: Platelet-associated immunoglobulins IgG, IgM, IgA and complement C3 in immune and non-immune thrombocytopenic disorders. Am J Hematol 23:89, 1986

90. Peerschke EIB, Ghebrehiwet B: Human blood platelets possess specific binding sites for C1q. J Immunol 138:1537, 1987

91. Pfueller SL, Lüscher EF: Studies of the mechanisms of the human platelet release reaction induced by immunologic stimuli. I. Complement-dependent and complement-independent reactions. J Immunol 112:1201, 1974

92. Pfueller SL, Lüscher EF: The effects of aggregated immunoglobulins on human blood platelets in relation to their complement-fixing abilities. I. Studies of immunoglobulins of different types. J Immunol 109:517, 1972

93. Pfueller SL, Lüscher EF: The effect of immune complexes on blood platelets and their relationship to complement activation. Immunochemistry 9:1151, 1972

94. Podack ER, Biesecker G, Kolb WP, Muller-Eberhard HJ: The C5b, 6 complex: Reaction with C7, C8, C9. J Immunol 121:484, 1978

95. Podack ER, Dhalback B, Griffin JH: Interaction of S-protein of complement with thrombin and antithrombin III during coagulation. J Biol Chem 261:7387, 1986

96. Podack ER, Kolb WP, Muller-Eberhard HJ. The C5b6 complex: Formation, isolation, and inhibition of its activity by lipoprotein and S-protein of human serum. J Immunol 120:1841, 1978

97. Podack ER, Kolb WP, Muller-Eberhard HJ:

The SC5b–7 complex: Formation, isolation, properties, and subunit composition. J Immunol 119:2024, 1977.

98. Podack ER, Tschopp J, Muller-Eberhard HJ: Molecular organization of C9 within the membrane attack complex of complement: Induction of circular C9 polymerization by the C5b–8 assembly. J Exp Med 156:268, 1982

99. Podack ER, Tschopp J: Membrane attack by complement. Mol Immunol 21:589, 1984

100. Polley MJ, Nachman RL: Human platelet activation by C3a and C3a-des-Arg. J Exp Med 158:603, 1983

101. Polley MJ, Nachman RL: Human complement in thrombin-mediated platelet function: Uptake of the C5b-9 complex. J Exp Med 150:633, 1979

102. Polley MJ, Nachman RL: The human complement system in thrombin-mediated platelet function. J Exp Med 147:1713, 1978

103. Polley MJ, Nachman RL: Ultrastructural lesions on the surface of platelets associated with either blood coagulation or with antibody-mediated immune injury. J Exp Med 141:1261, 1975

104. Polley MJ, Nachman RL, Weksler BB: Human complement in the arachidonic acid transformation pathway in platelets. J Exp Med 153:257, 1981

105. Preissner KT, Wassmuth R, Muller-Berghaus G: Physicochemical characterization of human S-protein and its function in the blood coagulation system. Biochem J 231:349, 1985

106. Pytela R, Pierschbacher MD, Ginsberg MH, Plow EF, Ruoslahti E: Platelet membrane glycoprotein IIb/IIIa: Member of a family of Arg-Gly-Asp-specific adhesion receptors. Science 231:1559, 1986

107. Ramm LE, Whitlow MB, Mayer MM: Size of the transmembrane channel produced by complement proteins C5b-8. J Immunol 129:1143, 1982

108. Reid KBM, Porter RR: The proteolytic activation systems of complement. Annu Rev Biochem 50:433, 1981

109. Rosenfeld SI, Packman CH, Jenkins DE Jr, Countryman JK, Leddy JP: Complement lysis of human erythrocytes. III. Differing effectiveness of human and guinea pig C9 on normal and paroxysmal nocturnal hemoglobinuria cells. J Immunol 125:2063, 1980

110. Rosenfeld SI, Packman CH, Leddy JP: Inhibition of the lytic action of cell-bound terminal complement components by human high density lipoproteins and apoproteins. J Clin Invest 71:795, 1983

111. Ross GD, Atkinson JP: Complement receptor structure and function. Immunol Today 6:115, 1985

112. Ross GD, Lambris JD, Cain JA, Newman SL: Generation of three different fragments of bound C3 with purified factor I or serum. 1. Requirements for factor H vs. CR1 cofactor activity. J Immunol 129:2051, 1982

113. Rosse WF, Parker CJ: Paroxysmal nocturnal hemoglobinuria. Clin Hematol 14:105, 1985

114. Salama M, Mueller-Eckhardt C, Bhakdi S: A two-stage immunoradiometric assay with ^{125}I-staphylococcal protein A for the detection of antibodies and complement on human blood cells. Vox Sang 48:239, 1985

115. Sandvik T, Endresen GKM, Forre O: Studies on the binding of complement factor C4 in human platelets (complement activation by means of cold agglutinins) Int Arch Allergy Appl Immunol 74:152, 1984

116. Schirazi Y, Imagawa DK, Shin ML: Release of leukotrienes B_4 from sublethally-injured oligodendrocytes by terminal complement proteins C5b–9. J Neurochem 48:271, 1987

117. Schmaier AH, Smith PM, Colman RW: Platelet Cl inhibitor: A secreted alpha-granule protein. J Clin Invest 75:242, 1985

118. Schreiber AD: The chemistry and biology of complement receptors. Springer Semin Immunopathol 7:221, 1984

119. Schreiber AD, Cines DB, Zmijewski C, Colman R: Effect of anti-Pl^{A1} antibody on human platelets. II. Mechanism of the complement-dependent release reaction. Blood 53:578, 1979

120. Shin ML, Hansch G, Hu VW, Nicholson-Weller A: Membrane factors responsible for homologous species restriction of complement-mediated lysis: Evidence for a factor other than DAF operating at the stage of C8 and C9. J Immunol 136:1777, 1986

121. Shonermark S, Rauterberg EW, Shin ML, Loke S, Roelcke D, Hansch GM: Homologous species restriction in the lysis of human erythrocytes: A membrane-derived protein with C8-binding capacity functions as an inhibitor. J Immunol 136:1772, 1986

122. Shulman NR: Immunoreactions involving platelets. 1. A steric and kinetic model for formation of a complex from human antibody, quinidine as a haptene, and platelets; and for fixation of complement by the complex. J Exp Med 107:665, 1958

123. Shulman NR, Aster RH, Leitner A, Hiller ML: Immunoreactions involving platelets. V. Post-transfusion purpura due to a complement-fixing antibody against a genetically controlled platelet antigen: A proposed mechanism for thrombocytopenia and its relevance in "auto immunity." J Clin Invest 40:1597, 1961

124. Shulman NR, Marder VJ, Hiller MC, Col-

lier EM: Platelet and leukocyte isoantigens and their antibodies: Serologic, physiologic and clinical studies. Prog Hematol 4:222, 1964

125. Shulman NR, Marder VJ, Weinrach RS: Similarities between known antiplatelet antibodies and the factor responsible for thrombocytopenia in idiopathic purpura. Ann NY Acad Sci 124:499, 1965

126. Sims PJ: Complement protein C9 labeled with fluorescein isothiocyanate can be used to monitor C9 polymerization and formation of the cytolytic membrane lesion. Biochemistry 23:3248, 1984

126a. Sims PJ, Faioni EM, Wiedmer T, Shattil SJ: Complement proteins C5b-9 cause release of membrane vesicles from the platelet surface that are enriched in the membrane receptor for coagulation factor Va and express prothrombinase activity. J Biol Chem (in press), 1989

127. Sims PJ, Lauf PK: Analysis of solute diffusion across the C5b-9 membrane lesion of complement: Evidence that individual C5b-9 complexes do not function as discrete, uniform pores. J Immunol 125:2617, 1980

128. Sims PJ, Wiedmer T: Kinetics of polymerization of a fluoresceinated derivative of complement protein C9 by the membrane-bound complex of complement proteins C5b-8. Biochemistry 23:3260, 1984

129. Sims PJ, Wiedmer T: Repolarization of the membrane potential of blood platelets after complement damage: Evidence for a Ca^{++}-dependent elimination of C5b-9 pores. Blood 68:556, 1986

130. Springer Semin Immunopath 7:92-270, 1984

131. Springer Semin Immunopath 6:117-398, 1983

132. Steckel EW, Welbaum BE, Sodetz JM: Evidence of direct insertion of terminal complement proteins into cell membrane bilayers during cytolysis: Labeling by a photosensitive probe reveals a major role for the eighth and ninth components. J Biol Chem 258:4318, 1983

133. Steinberg D, Carvalho AC, Chesney CM, Colman RW: Platelet hypersensitivity and intravascular coagulation in paroxysmal nocturnal hemoglobinuria. Am J Med 59:845, 1975

134. Stewart JL, Sodetz JM: Analysis of the specific association of the eighth and ninth components of human complement: Identification of a direct role of the α subunit of C8. Biochemistry 24:4598, 1985

135. Stuart MJ, Kelton JG, Allen JB: Abnormal platelet function and arachidonate metabolism in chronic idiopathic thrombocytopenic purpura. Blood 58:326, 1981

136. Suba EA, Csako G: C1q receptor (C1) receptor on human platelets: Inhibition of collagen-induced platelet aggregation by C1q (C1) molecules. J Immunol 117:1, 1976

137. Sundsmo JS, Fair DS: Relationship among the complement, kinin, coagulation, and fibrinolytic systems. Springer Semin Immunopath 6:231, 1983

138. Sundsmo JS, Fair DS: Relationships among the complement, kinin, coagulation, and fibrinolytic systems in the inflammatory reaction. Clin Physiol Biochem 1:225, 1983

139. Tack BF: The β-Cys-γ-Glu thiolester bond in human C3, C4, and α_2-macroglobulin. Springer Semin Immunopathol 6:259, 1983

140. Tenner AJ, Cooper NR: Analysis of receptor-mediated C1q binding to human peripheral blood mononuclear cells. J Immunol 125:1658, 1980

141. Tscopp J, Engel A, Podack ER: Molecular weight of poly C9: 12 to 18 molecules form the transmembrane channel of complement. J Biol Chem 259:1922, 1984

142. Tschopp J, Muller-Eberhard HJ, Podack ER: Formation of transmembrane tubules by spontaneous polymerization of hydrophilic complement protein C9. Nature 298:534, 1982

143. Van derMeer BW, Fugate RF, Tilfod K, Sims PJ: Complement proteins C5b-9 induce transbilayer migration of membrane phospholipid (abstr). Bull Am Phys Soc 32:1423, 1987

144. Vik DP, Fearon DT: Cellular distribution of complement receptor type 4 (CR4): Expression of human platelets. J Immunol 138:254, 1987

145. Vogt W, Schmidt G, van Buttlar B, Dieminger L: A new function of the activated third component of complement: Binding to C5, an essential step for C5 activation. Immunology 34:29, 1978

146. Wautier J-L, Peltier AP, Caen JP: Complement (C6) and platelet activation by thrombin in humans. Thromb Res 15:589, 1979

147. Wautier J-L, Souchon L, Cohen Solal L, Peltier AP, Caen JP: C1 and human platelets. III. Role of C1 subcomponents in platelet aggregation induced by aggregated IgG. Immunology 31:595, 1976

148. Wautier J-L, Souchon H, Reid KBM, Peltier AP, Caen JP: Studies on the mode of reaction of the first component of complement with platelets: Interaction between the collagen-like portion of C1q and platelets. Immunochemistry 14:763, 1977

149. Weiss HJ, Rosove MH, Lages BA, Kaplan KL: Acquired storage pool deficiency with increased platelet-associated IgG. Report of five cases. Am J Med 69:711, 1980

150. Weksler BB, Coupal CE: Platelet-dependent

generation of chemotactic activity in serum. J Exp Med 137:1419, 1973

151. Wiedmer T, Ando B, Sims PJ: Complement C5b-9-stimulated platelet secretion is associated with a Ca^{2+}-initiated activation of cellular protein kinases. J Biol Chem 262:13674, 1987

152. Wiedmer T, Esmon CT, Sims PJ: On the mechanism by which complement proteins C5b-9 increase platelet prothrombinase activity. J Biol Chem 261:14587, 1986

153. Wiedmer T, Esmon CT, Sims PJ: Complement proteins C5b-9 stimulate procoagulant activity through the platelet prothrombinase. Blood 68:875, 1986

154. Wiedmer T, Sims PJ: Cyanine dye fluorescence used to measure membrane potential changes due to assembly of complement proteins C5b-9. J Membr Biol 84:249, 1985

155. Wiedmer T, Sims PJ: Effect of complement proteins C5b-9 on blood platelets: Evidence for reversible depolarization of the membrane potential. J Biol Chem 260:8014, 1985

156. Winiarski J, Holm G: Platelet associated immunoglobulins and complement in idiopathic thrombocytopenic purpura. Clin Exp Immunol 53:201, 1983

157. Yu GH, Holers VM, Seya T, Ballard L, Atkinson JP: Identification of a third component of complement-binding glycoprotein of human platelets. J Clin Invest 78:494, 1986

158. Zalman LS, Wood LW, Frank MM, Muller-Eberhard HJ: Deficiency of the homologous restriction factor in paroxysmal nocturnal hemoglobinuria. J Exp Med 165:572, 1987

159. Zalman LS, Wood LW, Muller-Eberhard HJ: Isolation of a human erythrocyte membrane protein capable of inhibiting expression of homologous complement transmembrane channels. Proc Natl Acad Sci USA 83:6975, 1986

160. Ziccardi RJ: The first component of human complement (C1): Activation and control. Springer Semin Immunopathol 6:213, 1983

161. Zimmerman TS, Arroyave CM, Muller-Eberhard HJ: A blood coagulation abnormality in rabbits deficient in the sixth component of complement (C6) and its correction by purified C6. J Exp Med 134:1591, 1971

162. Zimmerman TS, Kolb WP: Human platelet-initiated formation and uptake of the C5b-9 complex of human complement. J Clin Invest 57:203, 1976

163. Zucker MB, Grant RA: Aggregation and release reaction induced in human blood platelets by zymosan. J Immunol 112:1219, 1974

164. Zucker MB, Grant RA, Alper CA, Goodofsky I, Lepow IH: Requirement for complement components and fibrinogen in the zymosan-induced release reaction of human blood platelets. J Immunol 113:1744, 1974

Part Six ***Clinical Aspects of Platelet Immunology***

19

The Immunologic Thrombocytopenias

RICHARD H. ASTER

Since the 1950s, it has been recognized that platelets can readily be destroyed by immunologic processes. However, progress in understanding the pathogenesis of immunologically mediated thrombocytopenias was delayed by methodologic problems inherent in measuring platelet–immunoglobulin interactions. Laboratory advances of the last decade have led to an explosion of new information about these disorders and to the recognition that platelet destruction can be induced by alloantibodies, drug-dependent alloantibodies, autoantibodies, and probably immune complexes in different conditions. In total, the immune thrombocytopenias constitute a relatively common, diverse, and fascinating group of diseases that affect children and adults.

NEONATAL ALLOIMMUNE THROMBOCYTOPENIA

Etiology

Neonatal alloimmune thrombocytopenic purpura (NATP) is caused by placental transfer of alloantibodies from mother to fetus following sensitization to fetal platelet antigens during pregnancy. The disorder has been recognized for about 30 years.[203,382] The first clear linkage of NATP to maternal alloimmunization against specific platelet antigens was provided by Shulman and his colleagues in 1962.[481] The frequency with which NATP occurs has been estimated to be between 1:2000[62] and 1:5000.[423]

In about one-half of all cases, NATP results from maternal alloimmunization against the antigen Pl^{A1}, a determinant present on platelets of about 98% of the general population. Currently recognized platelet alloantigen systems are shown in Table 19-1. Seven different antigens: Pl^{A1},[481] Pl^{A2},[383] Ko^{a},[192] Pl^{E2},[484] Bak^{a},[541] Pen^{a}/Yuk^{b},[175,475] and Yuk^{a}/Pen^{b},[474] have been implicated in NATP. Sensitization against Pl^{A1} occurs most often in women positive for the histocompatibility (HLA) determinants DR3, DRw52 and, possibly, DR6, DRw52 (relative risk about 10:1).[392,437,438] No association between HLA and sensitization to other platelet-specific antigens has yet been reported.

In about 25% of all cases of NATP, maternal sera contain broadly reactive HLA-specific antibodies and appear to lack antibodies reactive with the platelet-specific alloantigens listed in Table 19-1.[303,482] Experience with such cases has raised the question of whether or not HLA-reactive alloantibodies can cause NATP. HLA-A, HLA-B, and HLA-C antigens are known to be expressed on platelets,[27] but they are also present in other tissues and in plasma. Maternal alloimmunization against these determinants occurs in 25% to 50% of all pregnancies, usually without influencing the fetal platelet count. These facts argue against a causative role for HLA-reactive alloantibodies in

Table 19-1
Platelet-Specific Alloantigens Implicated in Neonatal Alloimmune Thrombocytopenic Purpura (NATP)

Antigen System	Phenotype Frequency	Implicated in NATP	Refs.
$Pl^{A1}(Zw^a)$	0.98	Yes	471
$Pl^{A2}(Zw^b)$	0.25	Yes	383
Ko^a	0.14	Yes	192
Ko^b	0.99	No	
Pl^{E1}	0.99+	No	
Pl^{E2}	0.05	Yes	484
Bak^a	0.91	Yes	541
Bak^b	0.70	No	
$Pen^a(Yuk^b)$	0.99+	Yes	475
$Pen^b(Yuk^a)$	0.01 ?	Yes	474

Adapted from Aster RH, McFarland J: In Bern M (ed): Hematologic Contributions to Fetal Health. New York, Alan R. Liss (in press) 1988

NATP. However, NATP has occurred in association with maternal sensitization against HLA-A2 in a number of instances.[156,423,481] Several of these patients were also amegakaryocytic.[156,423] Sensitization against other HLA determinants has been described in NATP.[26,501] It has been suggested that HLA-reactive antibodies capable of causing NATP may be of unusually high titer or may bind to target antigens with particularly high affinity.[482] The ABO antigens are carried on platelets, but there is, as yet, no published evidence indicating that ABO incompatibility between fetus and mother provokes NATP or protects against it.

Clinical Picture

Neonatal alloimmune thrombocytopenia commonly occurs in a first-born infant, in contrast to erythroblastosis fetalis, the analogous disorder affecting red cells. Subsequent children born to the same mother are also likely to have NATP, especially when Pl^{A1} is the immunizing antigen. Thrombocytopenic infants may be asymptomatic, but often they are born with extensive petechial hemorrhages on the skin and mucosal surfaces. Sometimes these lesions appear in the first few hours after birth. Gastrointestinal and urinary tract bleeding is common. Symptomatic infants usually have platelet levels in the range of 5000 to 25,000/μl.

The most severe complication of NATP is intracranial hemorrhage, which occurred in about 15% of infants reported in the literature. Because publications tend to be biased toward severe cases, the true frequency of intracranial hemorrhage is much lower, perhaps on the order of 1%. Occasionally, intracranial hemorrhage occurs in utero causing porencephalic cysts and severe disability or death.[175,218,487]

Laboratory Findings

By using currently available serologic methods, antibody reactive with paternal platelets can be detected in maternal serum in nearly all cases of NATP.[303,482] Results obtained in 88 cases of suspected NATP studied sequentially are shown in Table 19-2. With the ^{51}Cr-release and indirect immunofluorescent test, positive reactions were obtained in all instances. We have seen a small number of cases in which platelet-reactive antibodies were undetectable at birth but could be measured several weeks later. A method for detection of these presumably low-titer antibodies by absorption and elution from platelets has been described.[385] The HLA-reactive antibodies coexisting with platelet-specific alloantibodies sometimes make the serologic diagnosis of NATP difficult. Newly developed methods in which isolated platelet glycoproteins carrying platelet-specific alloantigens are used as targets should permit this problem to be circumvented in the future (Chap. 20).[117,176] Measurement of platelet-associated IgG on maternal platelets, which is normal in NATP, is sometimes helpful in differentiating NATP

Table 19-2
Serologic Findings in Neonatal Alloimmune Thrombocytopenia

Group No.	*n*	Pl^{A1} Type of Mother	Maternal Antibody Detected Against Paternal Platelets		Number of Maternal Sera with Anti-HLA
			By ^{51}Cr Release	By PSIFT	
1	23	Negative	+	+	10/20
2	18	Negative	−	+	5/15
3	4	Negative	+	−	1/4
4	21	Positive	+	+	14/15
5	20	Positive	−	+	7/16
6	2	Positive	+	−	1/2

Adapted from Kunicki TJ, Aster RH: In McMillan R (ed): Immune Cytopenias. New York, Churchill-Livingston, 1983

from thrombocytopenia associated with maternal autoimmune thrombocytopenic purpura.[266]

The typing of maternal and paternal platelets for platelet-specific alloantigens (*see* Table 19-1) is often helpful in the evaluation of NATP. The finding that the mother is Pl^{A1}-negative, in itself, is strongly suggestive because only 2% of the general population have platelets of this phenotype.

As mentioned, children subsequently born to a woman who gave birth to an infant with NATP, are also likely to be thrombocytopenic. Whether or not serial measurements of maternal antibodies during pregnancy can provide information predictive of NATP has not yet been established.

Treatment and Prognosis

NATP is often so mild that no specific therapy is required. *Corticosteroids* are commonly administered, but it is unclear if their use shortens the duration of thrombocytopenia or reduces the severity of bleeding.[257,367,482] Recovery usually occurs within 1 or 2 weeks, but thrombocytopenia sometimes persists for months.[371] *Platelets* should be transfused to any infant with severe hemorrhage and may be helpful prophylactically in asymptomatic infants with severe thrombocytopenia. Ideally, platelets compatible with the maternal alloantibody should be administered. When it is not possible to confirm the identity of the alloantibody, compatible platelets can be obtained from the mother by plateletpheresis (Fig. 19-1).[11,356] It is essential that they be washed free of maternal plasma containing alloantibody before being transfused. Gamma irradiation can also be considered, although there are no documented cases of graft-vs-host disease being induced by platelet transfusion in NATP. *Intravenous gamma globulin* has been administered to a small number of infants with NATP caused by anti-Pl^{A1} antibody, with apparent beneficial effect,[18,134] and this treatment seems worthy of further trial. *Exchange transfusion* has been utilized in some infants in an attempt to remove maternal alloantibody[179,356] and can be considered in infants with severe symptoms unresponsive to other treatments. There is no basis for *splenectomy* in the treatment of NATP.

Management of subsequent pregnancies poses a number of difficult questions. In utero intracranial hemorrhage can sometimes be diagnosed by ultrasonography, but it is uncertain if early diagnosis by this means can influence the eventual outcome. Transfusion of washed maternal platelets in utero through the umbilical vein was accomplished several hours before delivery by cesarean section in one reported instance,[124] increasing fetal platelets to hemostatic levels. Administration of corticosteroids to the mother for 1 or 2 weeks before delivery is a common practice, but it is uncertain whether or not this influences fetal platelet counts. Infants have been born with severe thrombocytopenia despite such treatment.[367]

Infants at risk to develop NATP are commonly delivered by cesarean section in the belief that this reduces the risk of intracranial hemorrhage,[128,487,490] but it is uncertain whether or not this assumption is valid. Additional experience with prenatal serologic testing may lead to better guidelines for management. It is feasible to sample fetal umbilical vein blood in utero to determine fetal platelet

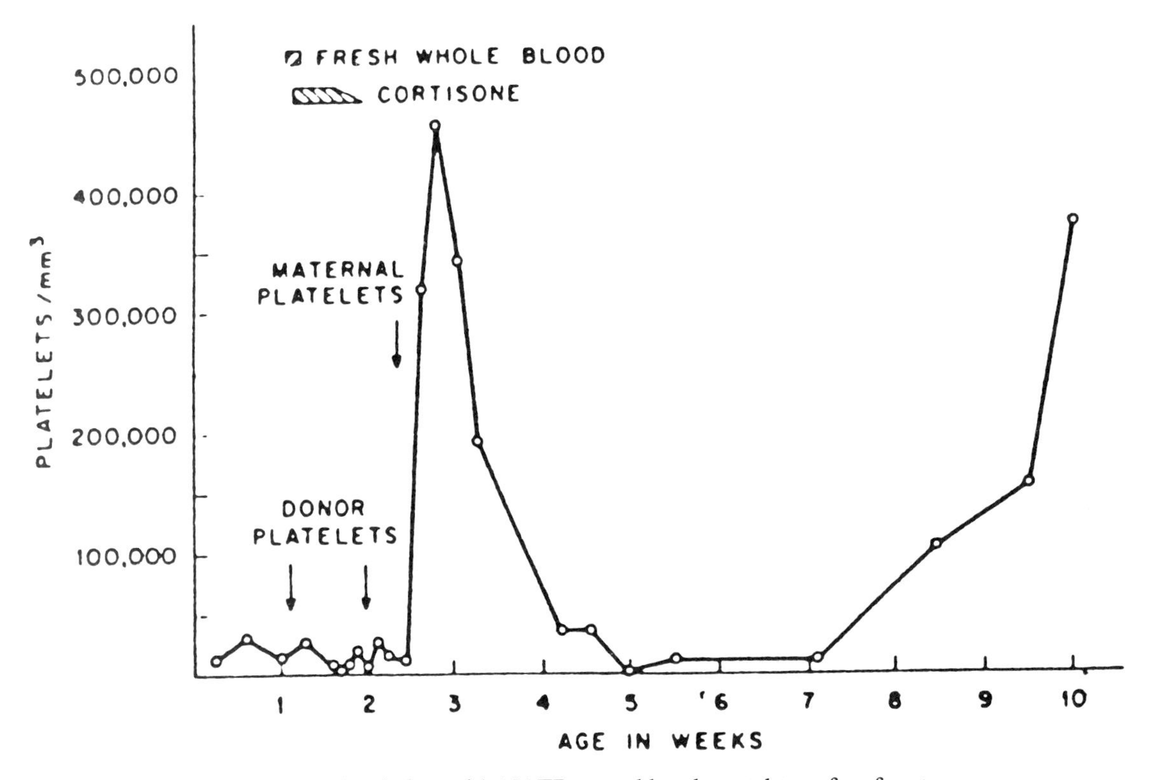

Figure 19-1. Clinical course of an infant with NATP caused by placental transfer of maternal anti-Pl^{A1} antibody. Platelets from random donors were ineffective, but platelets were elevated to normal after transfusion of washed, Pl^{A1}-negative, maternal platelets (McIntosh S, O'Brian RT, Schwartz AD, Pearson HA: J Pediatr 82:1020, 1973).

concentration, and preliminary experience with this approach seems promising.[124] Performance of a platelet count on fetal scalp vein blood obtained early in the course of labor has been advocated as a means of deciding the mode of delivery in infants born to women with idiopathic thrombocytopenic purpura (ITP).[465]

THROMBOCYTOPENIA IN INFANTS BORN TO MOTHERS WITH IDIOPATHIC (AUTOIMMUNE) THROMBOCYTOPENIC PURPURA

Etiology

About half of the infants born to women with active idiopathic (autoimmune) thrombocytopenic purpura (ITP) have low platelet levels at birth because of fetal platelet destruction induced by maternal autoantibody transferred across the placenta.[82,312,416] The syndrome can occur in infants born of women apparently cured of ITP by splenectomy or other means. The incidence of neonatal thrombocytopenia is thought to be highest in infants born of mothers who have severe thrombocytopenia, especially if the mother has been splenectomized.[416,518] However, it is not rare for an infant with a normal platelet count to be born to a woman with severe, active ITP. In one study series, a positive correlation between maternal and fetal platelet counts was observed.[211] This was not found in several other studies.[106,268,466]

Clinical Picture

Spontaneous abortion occurs with increased frequency in ITP.[268,347,416] In the older literature, fetal mortality at term in the range of 10% to 25% was reported. With modern management, mortality is very low.

Findings in full-term infants are essentially the same as in neonatal alloimmune thrombocytopenic purpura. For reasons not yet clear, thrombocytopenia persists longer, on the average, than it does in infants with NATP.

Laboratory Findings

Findings in the mother's blood are essentially the same as those in nonpregnant women with ITP (discussed later). As in NATP, methods to predict whether or not an infant will be born thrombocytopenic have been sought. Two groups found an inverse correlation between platelet counts in the newborn and antiplatelet antibody levels in maternal plasma but not in maternal platelet-associated IgG.[106,353] In a third study that used different methodology, an inverse relationship between maternal platelet-associated IgG and neonatal thrombocytopenia was observed.[268] In another series, the association of maternal antiplatelet antibody with neonatal thrombocytopenia was marginal.[466] In two reported instances, one of a set of twins born to a woman with ITP was thrombocytopenic, but the other was not.[376,466] Thus, there is no consensus at present on the value of serologic testing of the mother in predicting neonatal thrombocytopenia. Rarely, NATP occurs in infants born to mothers with ITP. Serologic studies are helpful in making this distinction.[266]

Treatment and Prognosis

Several recent reviews are available.[211,265,347]

Prenatal Management

Prenatal treatment of ITP in pregnant women is further discussed later under chronic idiopathic (autoimmune) thrombocytopenia (ITP). *Intravenous gamma globulin* is often effective in the mother, appears to be without significant toxicity for mother or fetus, and is now used frequently for women whose disease requires active intervention.[42,317,404,444] Given during the week before delivery, transplacental transfer of gamma globulin may reduce the severity of thrombocytopenia in the neonate,[42,379] but controlled trials will be required to establish if this is true. In a prospective study, prenatal administration of *corticosteroids* was associated with a reduced frequency and severity of thrombocytopenia in neonates.[247,250] In several uncontrolled series, no effect of prenatal steroids on neonatal platelet counts was observed.[268,466] *Cesarean section* has been recommended for women with active ITP, or with a previous history of the disorder, to reduce the chance of intracranial hemorrhage.[82,312,370,518] Unfortunately, there are, as yet, no well established serologic criteria on which to base a decision about the mode of delivery. Measurement of fetal platelet levels in scalp blood obtained early in the course of labor and performance of cesarean section for infants with a platelet count less than 50,000/μl has been advocated.[465]

Postnatal Therapy

Treatment of severely affected infants born to women with ITP is similar to that of infants with NATP, except that platelets "compatible" with the autoantibody are unavailable. *Platelets* from random donors should, nonetheless, be given to infants with severe bleeding. An apparent effect of *prednisone* on platelet levels was described in one study.[247] Prednisolone, which does not require in vivo metabolism may be more effective.[247] Controlled studies of the effect of corticosteroids have not yet been reported. *Exchange transfusion* has been performed with apparent benefit in a few instances.[72] Recently, *intravenous gamma globulin* has been used with rapid and sustained benefit in a number of cases,[93,103,498] and it seems possible that this will become the treatment of choice in the future. There is no definite evidence that *breast feeding* affects the duration or severity of thrombocytopenia in the neonate.[368]

NEONATAL THROMBOCYTOPENIA ASSOCIATED WITH DRUG SENSITIVITY

Drug-induced, immunologic thrombocytopenia is discussed in the following section. If a woman with this disorder ingests the offending drug near term, her infant may be born thrombocytopenic. The best documented examples of this condition have been triggered by quinine.[349] Neonatal thrombocytopenia following treatment with hydralazine[564] may have a similar cause.

DRUG-INDUCED IMMUNOLOGIC THROMBOCYTOPENIA

Etiology

Acute, profound thrombocytopenia following ingestion of certain drugs has been recognized for more than 100 years. In early studies, it was found that this condition is self-limited if the offending drug is discontinued, it can be reinduced by challenge with the drug, and it is mediated by circulating immunoglobulins. These investigations showed that this type of drug-induced thrombocytopenia (DITP) requires the interaction in vivo of the drug, circulating antibody, and platelets.

Drugs studied most intensively relative to the molecular mechanisms responsible for DITP are quinidine, quinine, and allylisopropylacetylurea (Sedormid). Sedormid-induced thrombocytopenia was investigated by Ackroyd in the 1940s, who postulated that, upon being ingested, the drug binds to the membranes of circulating platelets where it acts as a hapten to stimulate antibody production.[8] Arguments against this hypothesis were provided by Shulman in a series of studies done in the 1950s and 1960s.[476,478,479] In this work, it was found that high concentrations of drug fail to inhibit antibody-platelet binding as would be expected if the drug were acting as a hapten. Moreover, binding of drug to the platelet membrane was weak and reversible, whereas haptens must be covalently linked to carrier protein to provoke antibody formation. Moreover, drug-antibody complexes could not be demonstrated in vitro. On the basis of these findings, it was suggested that induction of antibodies by drugs causing DITP occurs without drug-platelet interaction. Once formed, however, these antibodies were thought to combine with ingested drug, producing complexes that bound to platelets with high affinity, causing their destruction.[476]

In the last decade, new information bearing on the molecular mechanisms involved in DITP has been obtained. These observations are described in detail in Chapter 8 and, therefore, will be summarized only briefly here. Several studies have provided convincing evidence that drug-induced antibodies bind to high-affinity platelets by their Fab regions in the presence of drug,[100,492] rather than attaching nonspecifically in the form of immune complexes. Membrane glycoprotein (GP) Ib,[305] the GPIb-GPIX complex,[51] GPV,[506] and the GPIIb-IIIa complex[101] have been identified as targets for this class of antibodies. Together, these observations are consistent with the hypothesis that, in most cases of DITP, the provocative drug combines with one or more constituents of the platelet membrane to induce a reversible, structural modification (neoantigen) that is immunogenic in some patients. Antibodies stimulated by this complex have specificity for both drug and platelet membrane constituent(s) but bind weakly, or not at all, to drug alone or platelets alone. When a drug interacts with platelets to produce the appropriate membrane modification, antibodies bind with high affinity to this target, causing platelet destruction.

In some patients, antibodies appear to be produced that have specificity for the platelet component of the putative drug-platelet complex and are capable of binding to platelets in the absence of drug, causing thrombocytopenia.[319] With some drugs, such as gold salts[539] and α-methyldopa,[344,470] this may be the preferred mechanism. With a few drugs, covalent linkage between the drug and a platelet membrane constituent may allow true hapten-dependent antibodies to be formed. Occasional cases of thrombocytopenia induced by penicillin may represent examples of this phenomenon.[394,453]

Drugs Capable of Causing Immunologically Mediated Thrombocytopenia

Hundreds of drugs have been implicated in DITP (Table 19-3). Quinidine and quinine are the most common offenders. Relevant literature citations can be found in References 28 and 482. Citations are provided in Table 19-3 for recently reported cases involving new drugs. In some instances, the connection between drug ingestion and thrombocytopenia may be coincidental, but cause-and-effect relationships have been convincingly established for quinidine, quinine, sulfonamide antibiotics, and other sulfonamide derivatives. An etiologic role for organic arsenicals, α-methyldopa, *p*-aminosalicylic acid, rifampicin, and other drugs has been demonstrated by reinduction of thrombocytopenia after administration of the drug to sensitive patients in remission. In a small number of patients, immunologic thrombocytopenia appears to have been induced by foods. Claims have been made for the relatively frequent induction of DITP by aspirin,[251,253,407] phenylbutazone,[500] indomethacin,[123] and insecticides,[301] but a causal role for these agents is not fully established. A significant fraction of patients treated with gold salts, thiazide diuretics, and heparin develop thrombocytopenia. These drugs may act by several different mechanisms and are discussed more fully later.

Table 19-3
Drugs and Other Exogenous Substances Implicated in Drug-Induced Immunologic Thrombocytopenic Purpura (DITP)

Analgesics (nonsteroidal, anti-inflammatory)
Acetaminophen, antipyrine, aspirin, clinoril, diclofenac,[299] fenoprofen, indomethacin, oxyphenbutazone, phenylbutazone, piroxicam,[59] sodium salicylate, sulindac,[246] tolmetin[329]
Antibacterials
Ampicillin, cephalexin, cephalothin, cephamandole,[331] gentamicin, lincomycin, methicillin, nitrofurantoin, novobiocin, oxytetracycline, p-*aminosalicylate*, nalidixic acid,[369] *penicillin*,[394,453] pentamidine, *rifampicin*, streptomycin, sulfasalazine,[427] other *sulfonamides*, tobramycin, trimethoprim, vancomycin[547]
Cinchona alkaloids
Quinidine, quinine
Foods
Beans, citrus fruits, others
Sedatives, Hypnotics, Anticonvulsants
Allylisopropylacetylurea, allylisopropylbarbiturate, butabarbitone, *carbamazepine*, centalun, chloridazepoxide, clonazepam, *diazepam*, *diphenylhydantoin*, ethylallylacetylurea, ethylchlorvinyl, ethylphenylhydantoin, imprimine, meprobamate, paramethadione, phenytoin, phthalazinol, primidone, *valproate Na*, *valproic acid*
Sulfonamide derivatives
Acetazolamide, chlorpropamide, chlorthalidone, clopamide, diazoxide, furosemide, glymidine, tolbutamide
Miscellaneous
Allopurinol, *α-methyldopa*, amiodarone,[557] amrinone,[19,293] antazoline, arsenical antiluetics, captopril,[550] chloroquine, *chlorothiazide*, chlorpheniramine, cimetidine,[169,193,340,343,571,575] cyclophosphamide,[383] danazol,[24,433] desimipramine, digitalis, *digitoxin*, *digoxin*, disulfiram, gold salts, *heparin*, heroin, hexopropymate, *hydrochlorothiazide*, hydroxyquinoline, insect bites, insecticides, interferon-α,[1,357] interferon-β[1] iopanoic acid, isoniazide (INH), isoretinoin (vitamin A),[219] levamisole, levodopa, lidocaine, mercurial diuretics, mexiletine,[163] minoxidil, nitroglycerin, nomifensine,[191] oxprenolol, penicillamine, pentagastrin,[23] procainamide, prochlorperazine, propylthiouracil, ranitidine,[178,496] spironolactone, *stibophen*, tetanus toxoid, tetraethylammonium, thioguanine, thiouracil, toluene diisocyanate, turpentine, vinyl chloride

References are provided for drugs recently implicated in DITP. Other literature citations can be found in reviews by Aster[28] and Shulman and Jordan.[482] Drugs in italics have convincingly been shown to cause DITP by in vitro or in vivo criteria.

It should be remembered that antibody-mediated platelet destruction has not been convincingly demonstrated in many of the reported cases of drug-associated thrombocytopenia. There is evidence, for example, that cimetidine may cause thrombocytopenia by a myelotoxic effect,[169,193] especially when given with phenytoin.[575] Drugs such as protamine,[231,529,545] hematin,[400] bleomycin,[533] and ristocetin[233] appear to cause platelet destruction by nonimmunologic mechanisms.

Clinical Picture

Most patients who take the drugs listed in Table 19-3 have no platelet abnormalities. There is, as yet, no way to predict which patients will develop thrombocytopenia, with the possible exception of patients injected with gold salts, who are at greater risk if they are positive for the antigen HLA-DR3.[10] Drug-induced thrombocytopenia has occurred in persons of both sexes and of all ages, including children.

A careful drug history should be taken in all cases of suspected DITP. It is not widely recognized that certain patient medicines, soft drinks, mixers, and aperitifs contain quinine. Quinine used as an adulterant by intravenous drug abusers has also caused DITP.[102] In a few instances, topical medications were thought to provide the immunizing stimulus.[281] Generally, the sensitizing drug will have been ingested within 24 hr of the onset of purpura, with the possible exception of gold salts, which occasionally cause thrombocytopenia months after the last injection.

Commonly, DITP is preceded by flushing and a chill after ingestion of the implicated medication. Purpura, hemorrhagic bullae in the buccal mucosa, and urinary and intestinal bleeding follow 3 to 12 hr later in severe cases. Generally, bleeding symptoms subside over several days as the offending drug is excreted from the body, but I have observed thrombocytopenia of 10 to 14 days duration in patients sensitive to quinidine. As noted, thrombocytopenia induced by gold salts may persist for many months, apparently because the drug is slowly released from tissue depots.

Laboratory Findings

Initial platelet levels are often very low in DITP, ranging from 10,000 to 1000 platelets per microliter. Megakaryocytes are generally normal or increased. Occasionally, there is associated immune destruction of red cells or neutrophils. In such cases, cell destruction appears to be mediated by several drug-dependent antibodies with different tissue specificities.[94,577]

Drug-induced antibodies specific for quinidine and quinine can readily be detected by many different techniques.[27,104,251,270,482] Positive results have been described with many other drugs with use of various assay systems in which patient's serum is mixed with the drug and normal target platelets. However, such antibodies are generally more difficult to detect than those induced by quinidine and quinine. The reasons for this may be several fold: (1) Some drugs implicated in DITP, such as digoxin and furosemide, are relatively insoluble in water, and it may not be possible to achieve a high enough drug concentration in vitro to yield a positive serologic reaction; (2) in some instances, a metabolite of the ingested drug may be the definitive immunogen. This appears to have been demonstrated in cases of DITP induced by acetaminophen,[149] *p*-aminosalicylic acid,[148] and sulfamethoxazole;[286] (3) some drugs may interact with specific platelet alloantigens to facilitate antibody binding.[111] For this, homologous platelets of the appropriate phenotype or autologous platelets would be required to yield a positive test.

Sensitivity to individual drugs can be confirmed by in vivo challenge if it is uncertain which of several drugs necessary for a patient's care caused thrombocytopenia. This should be undertaken with care because 1.3 mg of quinidine was sufficient to produce severe thrombocytopenia in one instance.[477] A dose of Sedormid 1000-fold less caused severe thrombocytopenia in another case.[9] If an in vivo challenge is undertaken, it is wise to begin with a dose less than 1 μg and monitor platelet levels carefully. Failure of a drug to reinduce thrombocytopenia does not exclude it with absolute certainty from a causal role, because time may be required to reinduce antibody.[479] In several reported instances, drugs implicated as the cause of DITP by in vitro testing failed to reinduce either antibody or thrombocytopenia when given at a later date.[330,551]

Treatment and Prognosis

All drugs that are being ingested by a patient suspected of having DITP should be discontinued pending diagnosis. Drugs essential for a patient's welfare should be replaced by others with equivalent pharmacologic actions. Intracerebral hemorrhage is rare, but it has occurred in the acute stage. Fatal pulmonary hemorrhage has been described.[167] Patients with severe thrombocytopenia and significant hemorrhagic symptoms should be hospitalized for at least several days of observation. There is no evidence that glucocorticoids affect the duration of thrombocytopenia, but they are often administered because of their possible effect on capillary integrity. Transfused platelets are often rapidly destroyed, but should be given if there is life-threatening hemorrhage. Platelet levels often return to normal within 2 to 4 days as drug is excreted, but thrombocytopenia occasionally persists for 1 or 2 weeks. Therapeutic plasma exchange appeared to be effective in one patient with persistence of severe thrombocytopenia 3 days after discontinuation of quinidine.[197] In a case of suspected digoxin-induced thrombocytopenia, improvement followed infusion of digoxin-specific antibodies.[220] In most patients, sensitivity to the drug causing DITP is permanent. Therefore, they should be advised to avoid reexposure.

THROMBOCYTOPENIA INDUCED BY THIAZIDE DIURETICS, GOLD SALTS, AND HEPARIN

Thiazide Diuretics

Chlorothiazide and its derivative diuretics cause thrombocytopenia in up to 25% of patients who ingest them.[309] Typically, the drop in platelet levels is less precipitous than in classic DITP and may occur over a period of several weeks or months. Thrombocytopenia is relatively mild; severe hemorrhagic symptoms are distinctly uncommon. In several patients challenged with the drug after recovery, 2 weeks were required for reinduction of thrombocytopenia.[309,409] Associated leukopenia and pancytopenia have been described.[363,443] The appearance of the bone marrow is variable, megakaryocytes being normal[147,413] or decreased[54,443] in different patients. The results of serologic tests have been variable, but evidence for platelet-dependent antibodies has been obtained in a few cases.[147,251,253] In several instances, infants with amegakaryocytic thrombocytopenia were born to women taking thiazides who, themselves, had normal platelet levels.[443] Together, these reports suggest that thiazides may induce thrombocytopenia by suppressing megakaryocytes in the bone marrow of certain sensitive individuals.

Gold Salts

Up to 5% of patients receiving injections of gold salts for treatment of rheumatoid arthritis develop thrombocytopenia.[10] Patients positive for the HLA-DRw3 antigen may be predisposed to develop this complication.[10,546] Fatal hemorrhage has occurred in some instances.[10,258] Generally, thrombocytopenia occurs after 2 to 4 months of treatment, but it can be seen within a few weeks or as late as 6 months after treatment has been discontinued. The onset of thrombocytopenia is usually insidious and is sometimes accompanied by leukopenia or pancytopenia. In patients with isolated thrombocytopenia, megakaryocytes are plentiful in the marrow. Platelet levels usually return to normal over a period of several months after injections are discontinued, but persistence of thrombocytopenia for many years has been described.[216] Tests for gold-dependent antibodies and cellular immune reactions dependent on gold have been inconclusive[133,321] with a few exceptions.[131,270] Evidence that gold-induced thrombocytopenia is mediated by drug-*independent* antibodies, i.e., true autoantibodies, was recently reported.[539]

Gold-induced thrombocytopenia that fails to remit spontaneously often responds to measures effective in idiopathic (autoimmune) thrombocytopenic purpura. Cases managed successfully with glucocorticoids and splenectomy,[115] cyclophosphamide,[298] and vincristine,[38] have been described. In numerous reported cases, recovery appears to have been hastened by promoting excretion of gold with dimercaprol (BAL).[10,115,499]

Heparin

Heparin injected intravenously or subcutaneously is a well-established cause of thrombocytopenia (*see* Chap. 8). The frequency of this complication has ranged from less than 2%[146,190] to as high as 30%[47] in different studies. In 13 prospective studies carried out before 1982, the average incidence was 3.4%.[291] In most cases, there is only a modest reduction in platelet levels (40,000 to 125,000/μl) and, in some instances, platelet levels return to normal despite continued therapy.[264,269,291] In patients with mild thrombocytopenia and no evidence of heparin-dependent antiplatelet activity in their plasma, heparin may act by nonimmunologic mechanisms,[97,462] and the risk of thromboembolism may be minimal. It is not yet certain, however, if heparin can safely be continued under these circumstances.

More striking thrombocytopenia, often associated with arterial and venous thromboembolism, occurs in a few patients who are taking heparin (reviewed in Refs. 20,190,269,264). This development is unrelated to the dose of heparin; it may occur after intravenous or low-dose subcutaneous treatment and even in association with heparin flushes used to maintain patency of IV lines.[210] Low-molecular-weight heparin[120] and a low-molecular-weight heparin analogue, pentosane polysulfate,[171] have been implicated in a few cases. In most recent studies, bovine and porcine heparin caused thrombocytopenia with equal frequency.[20,35,190] Generally, 5 to 7 days of exposure to heparin are required before this complication is seen, but the time interval is sometimes shorter in patients who have received heparin previously. The most common thromboembolic problems are peripheral arterial occlusion, often resulting in gangrene, and pulmonary embolism. Arterial thromboses are more common than venous ones. The arterial clots often consist largely of platelets and fibrin (white thrombi)[520] and may produce a characteristic filling defect on arteriography.[324]

Available evidence indicates that the severe form of heparin-induced thrombocytopenia is mediated by IgG antibodies induced by heparin.[98,105,107,336,473] These antibodies appear to differ from those induced by quinidine and quinine, in that heparin-dependent binding of IgG to platelets has been difficult to demonstrate in vitro. This, however, appears to have been accomplished by one group.[336] The conventional method for detecting heparin-associated antibodies is based on induction of aggregation in normal platelet-rich plasma by added heparin and patient plasma.[98,105] This effect appears to be mediated by thromboxane synthesis[96,98,99] and can be blocked by aspirin.[98,99] Platelet activation induced by this class of antibodies in the presence of pharmacologic quantities of heparin may account for the thromboembolic complications. A recent study raises the interesting possibility that heparin-induced antibodies bind directly to proteoglycans expressed on endothelial cells and induce thromboembolism by damaging vessel walls.[109]

As noted, severe heparin-induced thrombocytopenia complicated by thromboembolism is usually diagnosed by determining if patient plasma induces aggregation of normal platelet-rich plasma at optimal doses of heparin. This test is positive in most, but not all, patients who develop this complication.[273] Greater sensitivity and specificity has been claimed for a test involving release of radiolabeled serotonin from platelets in the presence of patient serum and heparin.[473]

Treatment and Prognosis

Discontinuation of heparin is mandatory in patients with severe heparin-associated thrombocytopenia, especially when in vitro tests for heparin-dependent antibody are positive. It is a common and logical practice to administer inhibitors of platelet activation such as aspirin and dipyridamole, and this may have been effective in some cases (Fig. 19-2). Dextran infusion has also been utilized,[493] but its effectiveness is uncertain. Warfarin (Coumadin) is usually given as an alternative anticoagulant. Surgical intervention is often required for treatment of arterial occlusions but is frequently unsuccessful in preventing loss of an extremity. Patients with demonstrable heparin-dependent antibody who need anticoagulation have been successfully managed with low-molecular-weight heparin,[448,535] the prostacyclin analogue K36374,[244] aspirin,[339] the low-molecular-weight heparinoid ORG 10172,[289,338] and the thrombin inhibitor MD805.[348] One patient tolerated heparin during surgery after an intensive plasma exchange and administration of IV gamma globulin.[531] The value of fibrinolytic therapy in heparin-in-

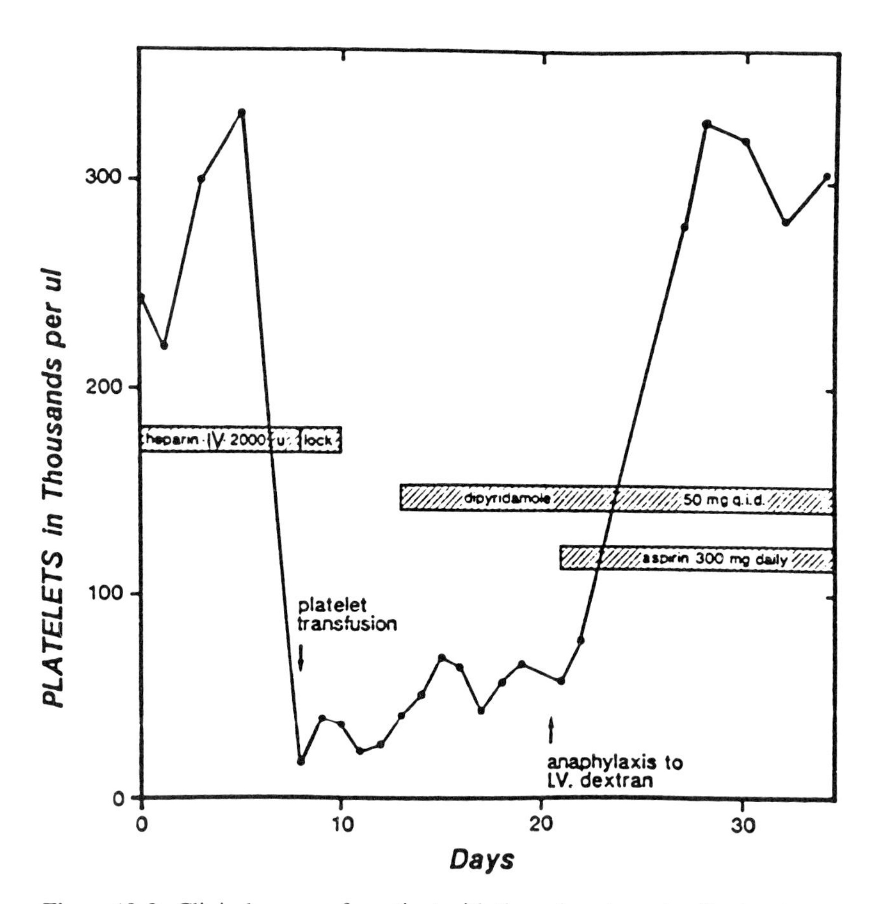

Figure 19-2. Clinical course of a patient with thrombocytopenia after treatment with heparin 2000 U/h IV for 9 days. The apparent response to aspirin may have been coincidental (Green O: Med J Aust 144 (Suppl): H537, 1986).

duced thrombosis has not yet been established. The platelet-aggregating, heparin-dependent immunoglobulin often disappears during convalescence. It has been suggested that such patients can subsequently be treated with heparin for short periods, and this has been demonstrated in a few instances.[414] However, the safety of this approach is not yet fully established.

POSTTRANSFUSION PURPURA

Etiology

Acute thrombocytopenia occurring about 1 week after a blood transfusion and associated with high-titer, platelet-specific alloantibodies was first characterized as a distinct syndrome by Shulman et al. in 1961.[480] The exact frequency of the disorder is not known, but more than 150 cases had been reported by 1986.[384]

Alloantibodies associated with posttransfusion purpura (PTP) have been shown to react with five different platelet-specific alloantigens: Pl^{A1},[480] Pl^{A2},[515] Bak^a/Lek^a,[64,262] Bak^b,[283] and Pen^a/Yuk^b.[488] Anti-Pl^{A2} and anti-Bak^a were present simultaneously in one patient.[89] In more than 90% of cases, the antibodies are directed toward Pl^{A1}. Antigens of the Pl^A (Zw)[302] and Pen (Yuk) systems[176,177] are carried on platelet GPIIIa and those of the Bak/Lek system are carried on GPIIb.[288] Population and gene frequencies of these alloantigens are shown in Table 19-4. Platelets obtained from

Table 19-4
Platelet-Specific Alloantigens Implicated in Posttransfusion Purpura (PTP)

Antigen System	Phenotype Frequency	Implicated in PTP	Refs.
$Pl^{A1}(Zw^a)$	0.98	Yes	480
$Pl^{A2}(Zw^b)$	0.25	Yes	515
Ko^a	0.14	No	
Ko^b	0.99	No	
Pl^{E1}	0.99+	No	
Pl^{E2}	0.05	No	
Bak^a	0.91	Yes	64, 262
Bak^b	0.70	Yes	283
$Pen^a(Yuk^b)$	0.99+	Yes	488
$Pen^b(Yuk^a)$	0.01 ?	No	

[Adapted from Aster RH: In Englfriet CP et al (eds): Baillier's Clinical Immunology and Allergy, p 453. London, WB Saunders 1987.]

Table 19-5
Mechanisms Proposed for the Etiology of Posttransfusion Purpura

Cross-reactive antibodies:	In addition to stimulating an alloantigen-specific antibody, transfused platelets or platelet fragments induce an autoantibody specific for a site on autologous platelets.
Immune complexes:	Alloantigen transfused in the form of platelet fragments or soluble in plasma combines with subsequently formed alloantibody to produce immune complexes that bind with high affinity to autologous platelets.
Acquired antigens:	Alloantigen transfused soluble in plasma or released from platelets after transfusion attaches to autologous platelets, allowing them to be sensitized by subsequently formed alloantibody.

[Adapted from Aster RH: In Englfriet CP et al: Ballier's Clinical Immunology and Allergy. London, WB Saunders (in press) 1987.]

patients with PTP after recovery are invariably found to be negative for the antigen recognized by the alloantibody in their plasma.

How an alloantibody, triggered presumably by platelets contained in a previous blood transfusion, causes destruction of autologous platelets in PTP is as yet unresolved, but several hypotheses have been advanced (Table 19-5). One is that, in addition to alloantibody, a true autoantibody reactive with Pl^{A1}-negative autologous platelets is formed. Support for this proposition was provided by studies in a species of marmoset in which thrombocytopenia followed injection of platelets from another species.[181] Antibodies reactive with intact autologous platelets have not yet been detected unequivocally in acute-phase serum, although an immunoglobulin specific for a 120-kDa protein isolated in gels from detergent-solubilized platelets was identified in one study.[504] A second mechanism suggested for PTP is that alloantibody formed in response to transfusion somehow combines with residual alloantigen to form immune complexes capable of binding with high affinity to autologous platelets and promoting their destruction.[484] The finding that eluates obtained from Pl^{A1}-negative platelets during the acute phase of PTP were capable of sensitizing both autologous platelets obtained after recovery and Pl^{A1} (Zw^{a})-negative platelets from other subjects[424,540] was thought to reflect antibody–antigen complexes, but no direct evidence for platelet destruction by immune complexes in PTP has yet been obtained. A third potential mechanism for PTP is that platelet-specific alloantigen present in the provocative transfusion combines in some way with antigen-negative autologous platelets, rendering them susceptible to destruction by subsequently formed alloantibody. Several observations are consistent with this possibility. Pl^{A1} antigen was detected in polyethylene glycol precipitates prepared from normal Pl^{A1}-positive plasma.[555] However, the possibility that the precipitates contained platelet microparticles[182] was not excluded. In another study, Pl^{A1}-negative platelets acquired Pl^{A1} after being incubated with plasma isolated from Pl^{A1}-positive blood stored at 4°C under blood bank conditions.[284] Together, these reports are consistent with the possibility that, under some circumstances, transfused Pl^{A1} antigen binds to Pl^{A1}-negative platelets of a recipient enabling them to be sensitized by anti-Pl^{A1}. The same mechanism could presumably account for platelet destruction in patients alloimmunized to Pl^{A2}, Bak^{a}, Bak^{b}, and Pen^{a}. Considering that circulating platelets turn over completely in about 8 days, it is hard to envision how the transfused alloantigen could continue to prime platelets for destruction for a month or more, as is seen in some patients with PTP.

The rarity with which PTP occurs despite the fact that most transfusions are mismatched for one or more of the alloantigens listed in Table 19-4 also is unresolved. A partial explanation is provided by the finding that persons positive for the antigen HLA-DRw3[437,438] or possibly the combinations HLA-DR3/DRw52 and DRw6/DR52[136] are much more likely to produce anti-Pl^{A1} than persons lacking these determinants. The relative, but not absolute, requirement for prior exposure to platelet-specific antigens through pregnancy or transfusion for development of PTP is another limiting factor. Whether or not blood from only certain unusual donors can induce the disorder is not yet known.

Clinical Picture

More than 90% of the cases of PTP reported to date have occurred in multiparous women after their first blood transfusion. However, PTP has occurred in nulliparous and previously transfused patients[482] and in a few men.[467] The disorder can be induced by whole blood, packed red cells, or plasma. The onset of severe thrombocytopenia and bleeding typically occurs 6 to 8 days after transfusion. However, cases occurring 2[387] and 10[515] days after the most recent transfusion have been described. Acute PTP resulting from inadvertent passive administration of anti-Pl^{A1} antibody has been reported.[39,408] Extensive petechial hemorrhages in the skin and mucous membranes, together with gross bleeding from the gastrointestinal and urinary tracts, are frequently seen. In about one-third of all cases, the provocative transfusion was accompanied by a febrile reaction.

Laboratory Findings

Thrombocytopenia is usually very severe. Occasionally, platelets are less than 1000/μl. Megakaryocytes are present in normal or increased numbers in the bone marrow. When appropriate serologic studies are performed, a potent, platelet-specific antibody reactive with one of the antigens listed in Table 19-4 can readily be detected by methods such as indirect immunofluorescence,[424] complement fixation,[480] radiolabeled antiglobulin binding,[384] ELISA,[6] and ^{51}Cr release.[303] Sometimes the platelet-specific antibody is obscured by high-titer HLA-reactive antibodies.[262,384]

The Pl^{A1}-reactive antibodies of PTP are nearly always complement-fixing in the acute phase, e.g., capable of causing ^{51}Cr release from labeled, Pl^{A1}-positive target platelets (Table 19-6), in contrast with those found in neonatal alloimmune thrombocytopenia. Some anti-Pl^{A1} antibodies block the response of Pl^{A1}-positive platelets to agonists, such as ADP, apparently by affecting the platelet fibrinogen receptor on the GPIIb–IIIa complex.[7,525] Platelets obtained early in PTP have been shown to carry IgG and IgM[45,424] and, in a few cases, Iga.[540] Anti-Pl^{A1} antibodies are often detected

Table 19-6
Serologic Findings in Posttransfusion Purpura (PTP)

		Number of Sera Positive in			Number of Sera Containing	
Pl^{A1} Type of Patient	*n*	^{51}Cr Release Alone	PSIFT Alone	Both ^{51}Cr Release and PSIFT*	Anti-Pl^{A1} Antibody	Anti-HLA Antibody
Negative	38	0	1	37	35	23/27
Positive	5	0	0	5	0	4/4
Undetermined	13	0	1	12	8	4/7

*PSIFT, platelet suspension immunofluorescent test.
[Adapted from Kunicki TJ, Aster RH: In McMillan R (ed): Immune Cytopenias. New York, Churchill-Livingston, 1983.]

in convalescent plasma, but they are no longer complement-fixing.[313] This may be related to disappearance of alloantibody of the IgG3 subclass present in the acute stage.[514]

Differential Diagnosis

Clinical presentation and laboratory findings of PTP are so distinctive that the diagnosis should readily suggest itself to clinicians aware of this disorder. Many patients with PTP are postoperative and are receiving numerous medications. Therefore, attempts should be made to rule out a drug-induced cause. Disseminated intravascular coagulation, gram-negative sepsis, and other postoperative complications associated with thrombocytopenia should also be considered. It is usually not possible to obtain immediate laboratory confirmation of PTP or drug-induced immunologic thrombocytopenia. Therefore, medications should be discontinued or substitutes given wherever possible.

Treatment and Prognosis

Except when fatal hemorrhage supervenes, even untreated patients recover spontaneously within 1 to 6 weeks. The course of a typical patient treated with only corticosteroids is shown in Figure 19-3. Intracranial hemorrhage, usually fatal, has occurred in about 10% of reported cases.[31,384,482] Therefore, therapeutic intervention should be considered in all cases, particularly those in whom thrombocytopenia is profound and hemorrhagic symptoms are severe. Posttransfusion purpura is invariably treated with *prednisone*, and improvement has been directly attributed to this therapy in a few patients.[491,560] However, prednisone alone usually fails to influence the platelet count. The index case of PTP reported by Shulman and his colleagues[480] was successfully treated by *whole blood exchange transfusions*. In many other instances, recovery has occurred within 1 to 3 days of *plasma exchange* (Fig. 19-4). Despite the lack of controlled studies, the relationship between plasma exchange and recovery from PTP is so striking that it argues strongly for cause and effect. The benefit of plasma exchange cannot be explained by removal of anti-Pl^{A1} antibody alone, because it can persist for at least several years after recovery.[313] Recently, *IV gamma globulin* 0.4 g/kg daily for 5 days has been utilized for treatment.[52,95,185] As reviewed by Mueller-Eckhardt,[384] seven of eight cases treated up to 1986 responded well to this therapy, including two who failed to respond to plasma exchange. If continued experience with IV gamma globulin is favorable, it is likely to become the treatment of choice in this disorder.

Platelet transfusions are generally ineffective in PTP and are often associated with severe fever/chill reactions and sometimes hypotension. If it is necessary to administer platelets because of severe bleeding, reactions should be anticipated. In one instance, Pl^{A1}-negative platelets were ineffective when transfused into a patient with PTP and anti-Pl^{A1}, apparently being destroyed by the same process responsible for destruction of autologous platelets.[183] However, experience with Pl^{A1}-negative platelet transfusion is very limited.

Patients who have recovered from PTP have been transfused at a later date with Pl^{A1}-negative blood without complication.[313] However, recurrence of PTP has been described in several instances.[74,482,494] The suggestion has been

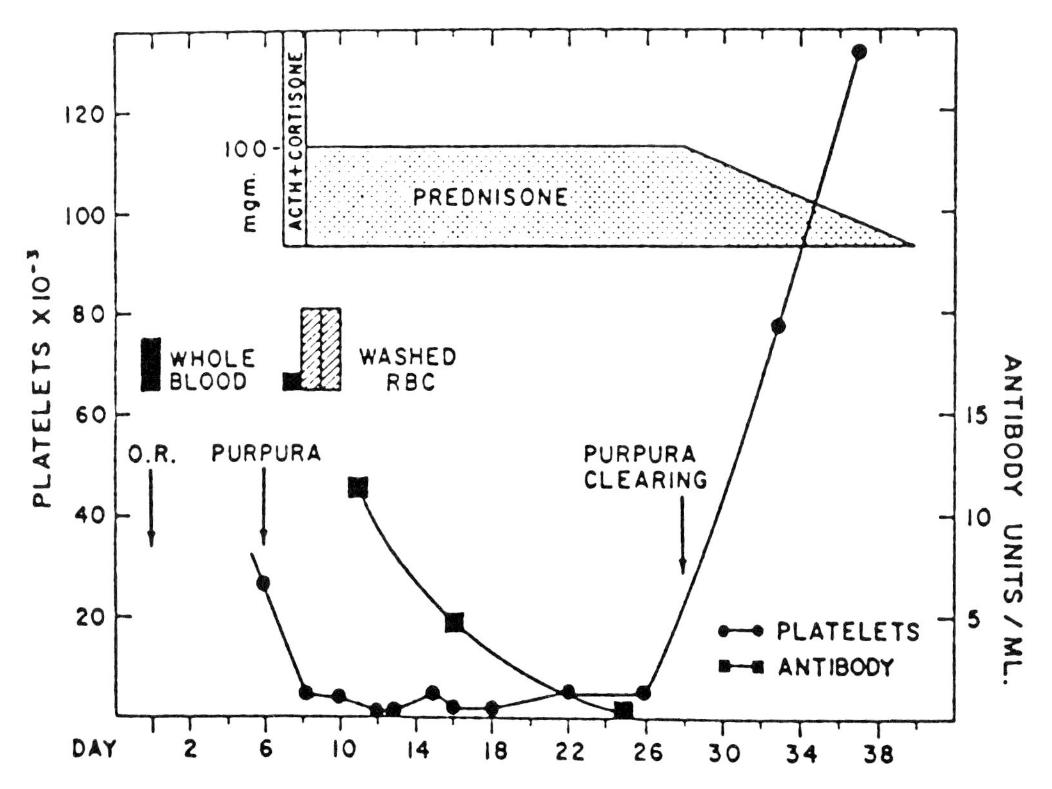

Figure 19-3. Clinical course of a 43-year-old woman who developed PTP 6 days after receiving blood during surgery. Thrombocytopenia lasted for 3 weeks, despite treatment with prednisone. Recovery occurred after disappearance of anti-Pl^{A1} from the patient's plasma (Shulman NR, Aster RH, Leitmer A, Hiller MC: J Clin Invest 40:1597, 1961 with permission).

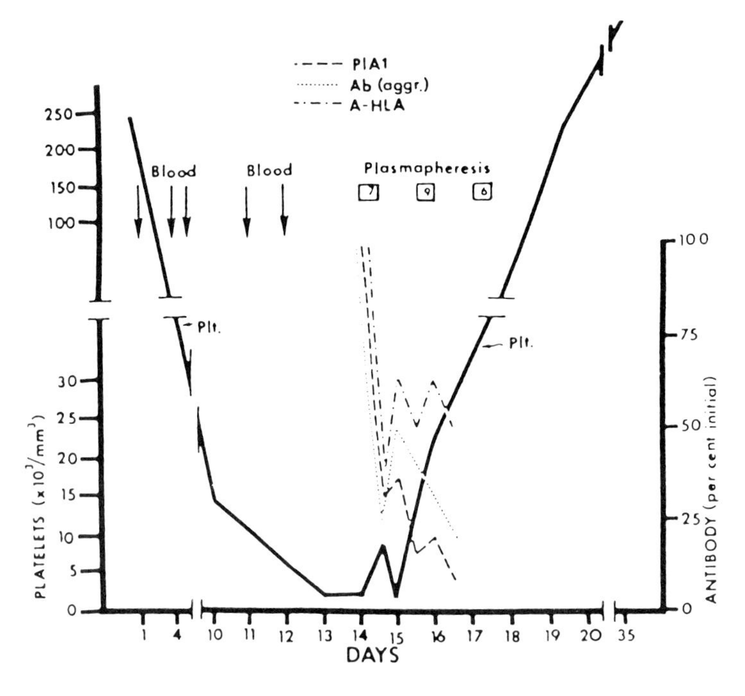

Figure 19-4. Clinical course of a 45-year-old woman with PTP treated by plasma exchange performed 7, 9, and 11 days after the onset of thrombocytopenia (Abramson N, Eisenberg PD, Aster RH: N Engl J Med 291:1163, 1974).

made that recurrent PTP is more likely to occur if many years have elapsed between Pl^{A1}-positive transfusions.[482] In view of the uncertainty about recurrence of PTP, it is reasonable to utilize platelet-poor products, e.g., washed red cells, or Pl^{A1}-negative blood when a patient with a history of PTP required transfusion.

ACUTE IDIOPATHIC (AUTOIMMUNE) THROMBOCYTOPENIC PURPURA

Acute idiopathic thrombocytopenic purpura (ITP) is predominantly a disorder of childhood, characterized by acute, severe thrombocytopenia occurring within 1 or 2 weeks of an infection, usually of viral origin. In about one-third of the children, there is no known antecedent infection. An apparently identical disease occurs rarely in adults of any age. Acute ITP should be distinguished from chronic ITP which, as discussed later, appears to have an entirely different etiology.

Etiology

Despite extensive clinical and laboratory investigations extending over many years, the relationship between infection and the subsequent, sometimes fulminating, destruction of platelets is not yet understood. That platelet destruction occurs at a time when the patient is convalescing from the preceding infection is consistent with the possibility that platelets are somehow injured by the antibody response mounted against the infectious agent. By analogy with posttransfusion purpura, it has been suggested that platelets may be affected by immune complexes whose antigenic component is a constituent of the infecting virus. Platelets are known to express one or more Fc receptors[275,445,505] (*see* Chap. 17) and to be capable of binding immune complexes. In one study, antibodies raised against rubella were found to cause platelet agglutination in the presence of rubella antigen, a property that is not characteristic of postrubella sera of children who did not have thrombocytopenia.[396] However, there is little direct experimental evidence for platelet-binding, circulating immune complexes in acute ITP. An alternative explanation is that a constituent of the infecting organism binds to platelets, priming them for destruction by subsequently produced antibody. In one study, it was found that normal platelets incubated with influenza A virus became susceptible to lysis by autologous serum.[261] This did not appear to be related to the action of viral neuraminidase but, rather, to adhesion of viral hemagglutinin to the cell membrane and subsequent attack by antihemagglutinin antibody. Although influenza A viral infection does not typically provide acute ITP, further studies of this phenomenon with other viruses seem warranted. A third possible basis for acute ITP is inappropriate production of platelet-reactive autoantibodies in association with the immune response against the primary infection. Although elevated levels of platelet-associated immunoglobulin are demonstrable in most patients,[85,91,249,322,326] studies to identify platelet-reactive antibodies in serum have often yielded negative, or inconsistent results.[44,526,573] Positive results have been achieved more consistently in recent studies (*see* Chap. 7). The similarities between etiologies suggested for drug-induced immunologic thrombocytopenia, posttransfusion purpura, and acute ITP offer the hope that elucidation of the cause or causes of one of these conditions will shed light on the others. The antigens HLA-Aw32[157] and HLA-Bw56[189] were marginally increased among patients with acute ITP in two studies. However the rarity with which acute ITP occurs in families argues against a hereditary basis for the disorder.

Clinical Picture

Acute ITP is most common among children 1 to 10 years of age (Fig. 19-5). But a similar

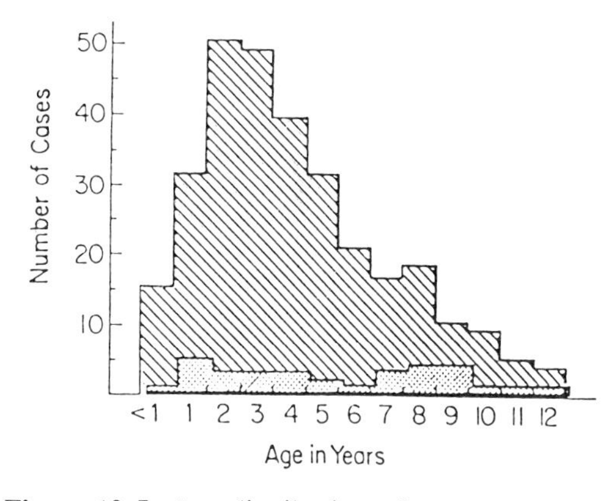

Figure 19-5. Age distribution of acute ITP in 305 children. Cross-hatching indicates age at onset in 32 children with the chronic form of ITP (Lüsher JM, Iyer R: Semin Thromb Hemost 3:175, 1977).

disorder can occur in older children or adults. Males and females are affected with equal frequency. Typically, the onset of petechiae, purpura, and bleeding from the gums, gastrointestinal, and urinary tracts begins abruptly. Pronounced hemorrhagic symptoms usually persist for only a few days, even when platelet levels remain depressed for longer periods. Infections that trigger acute ITP are usually viral and include rubella, rubeola, and varicella, but nonspecific respiratory infections are more common.[335,354] The disorder can also be induced by immunization with live vaccines given prophylactically for measles, chickenpox, mumps, and smallpox.[84,354] Injection of BCG, given for the treatment of cancer in adults, has also been implicated.[410] Acute ITP occurs most often during the winter and spring when the prevalence of viral infections is highest. Physical examination generally reveals consequences of hemorrhage in the skin and gastrointestinal tract, especially in areas exposed to trauma. Hemorrhagic bullae in the oral mucosa are common. Mild hepatosplenomegaly and lymphadenopathy are often found, probably reflecting the preceding viral infection.

Laboratory Findings

The initial thrombocytopenia is usually severe, with platelet levels commonly less than 10,000/μl. Anemia, if present, is secondary to blood loss. Megakaryocytes are almost invariably normal or increased in number in the bone marrow. Immature forms, reflecting megakaryocyte proliferation, are often present.

Platelet-associated immunoglobulins are generally elevated. In several studies, platelet-associated IgG was higher in children with acute ITP than in adults[322,332] or in children with chronic ITP.[552] Studies of platelet-associated immunoglobulins performed, to date, in acute ITP are difficult to interpret because of methodologic problems inherent in these assays (see discussion under chronic ITP). There is now no reliable way to distinguish between platelet-associated autoantibodies and immune complexes.

Differential Diagnosis

The history, physical, and laboratory findings of acute ITP generally suggest the correct diagnosis immediately. It is important, however, to rule out bacterial sepsis, especially meningococcemia, in which purpura and thrombocytopenia are sometimes present. Other conditions associated with thrombocytopenia in childhood, such as leukemia, thrombotic thrombocytopenic purpura, and the hemolytic uremic syndrome, can easily be excluded by appropriate laboratory studies. Thrombocytopenia secondary to a cavernous hemangioma occasionally causes diagnostic difficulties. Fragmented red blood cells (schistocytes) found in the latter condition are helpful in diagnosis. Drug-induced immunologic thrombocytopenia should be considered in patients who have been taking medications.

Treatment and Prognosis

Despite the early, striking hemorrhagic manifestations, more than 80% of patients eventually recover regardless of the treatment regimen.[116,335,354,366,489] The course of a typical patient is shown in Figure 19-6. In about two-thirds of patients, platelet levels return to normal in less than 6 weeks; 80% to 90% recover within 6 months. Most patients remain permanently well, but a few experience recurrences in later years. In some instances, these appear to have been triggered by infection[125,335] or vaccination.[84]

The most important complication of acute ITP is intracranial hemorrhage, which occurs in less than 1% of the cases.[334,354,489,570] The risk of intracranial hemorrhage is greatest in the first 1 or 2 weeks, and most often it occurs within a few days of the onset of symptoms. Patients should restrict physical activity and avoid trauma. Those with striking hemorrhagic symptoms should be hospitalized for observation. It is important that aspirin and other drugs capable of inhibiting platelet function be avoided.

Beyond these routine measures, opinion is divided about whether acute ITP should be treated by observation only, with corticosteroids, or with intravenous gamma globulin.[235] In one series of 469 consecutive cases, untreated children required 3 weeks, on the average, for recovery, a slightly shorter period than children given prednisone.[334] In some studies, the outcome appeared to be unaffected by use or nonuse of medication.[335,354] In contrast, other groups have found that platelet levels rise more rapidly in children given prednisone, 2–3 mg/kg body weight a day.[366,457,461,489] A particularly rapid increase was observed in nine

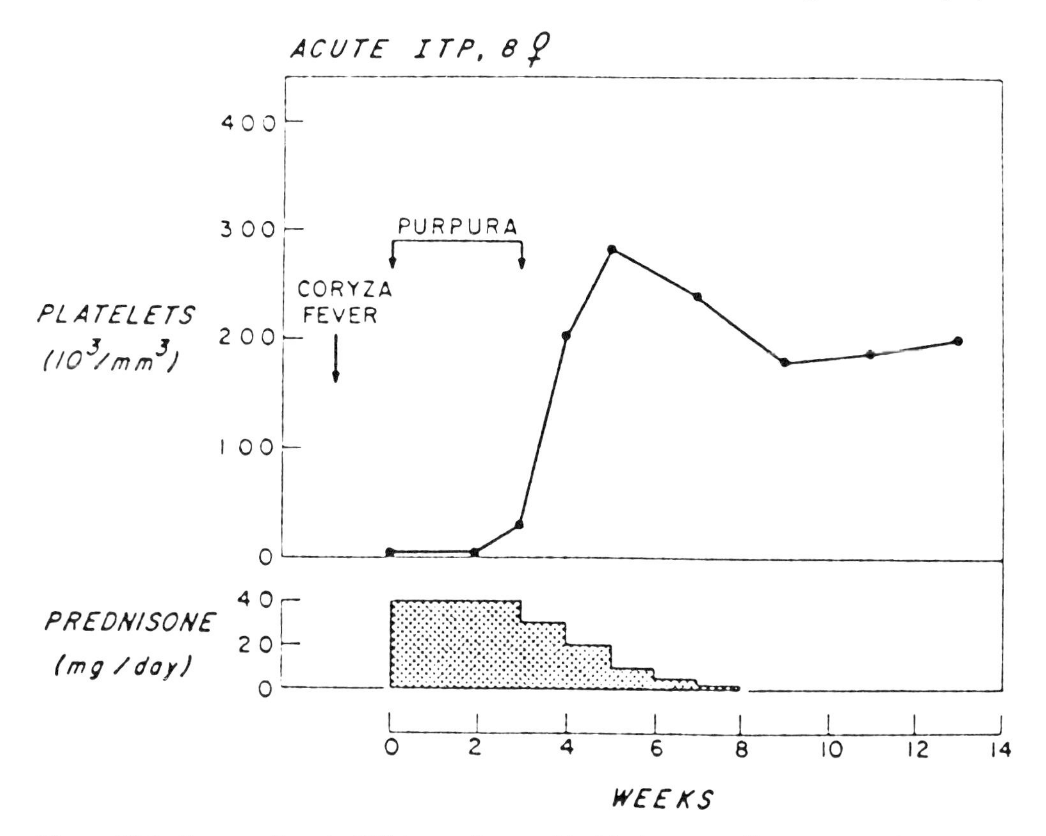

Figure 19-6. Course of acute ITP in an 8-year-old girl. A nonspecific upper respiratory infection occurred 1 week before the onset of symptoms (Aster RH: In Beutler E, Erslev AJ (eds): Hematology; p 1298. New York, McGraw-Hill, 1983).

patients given prednisone at the high dose of 6 to 8 mg/kg per day.[509] Arguments for[143] and against[73] the use of prednisone have recently been summarized.

Interest in the use of intravenous gamma globulin in acute ITP was stimulated by the demonstration of its effectiveness by Imbach and coworkers in 1981.[239] In most series, 50% to 75% of children given IV gamma globulin at a dose of 400 mg/kg per day experienced a rise in platelet count within 1 week, often to normal levels.[79] This treatment is relatively nontoxic, but it is expensive. More than two-thirds of a group of patients given a single injection of IV gamma globulin at a dose of 1 g/kg, achieved platelet levels greater than 50,000/μl within 24 hr and did not require further treatment. It was suggested that this approach might lower costs by reducing the number of injections required.[238]

Whether therapeutic intervention should be attempted in children with acute ITP hinges on the answers to two questions: Can the incidence of intracranial hemorrhage be reduced, and will the frequency with which a permanent remission is achieved be increased? Intracranial hemorrhage in acute ITP of childhood is extremely rare; it was not observed in a recent series of 465 consecutive cases.[334] The number of children that would have to be studied in controlled trials to confirm an effect of any therapeutic intervention on intracranial hemorrhage would be about 14,000.[300] Thus, such a study is unlikely to be undertaken.

Platelet transfusions should not be given routinely in acute ITP because transfused platelets are rapidly destroyed, but they are indicated in patients with severe hemorrhage, especially intracranial.[323,411] In children with intracranial hemorrhage, high-dose glucocorticoids should be administered, and emergency splenectomy should be performed when possible before neurosurgery is attempted.[570,576] Plasma exchange appears to have been helpful in several severe cases.[323,411]

In about 10% of children with acute ITP,

permanent remission is not achieved. After 6 months, the condition is designated "chronic," although in rare instances, remission has occurred more than 1 year after onset.[354] These children appear to have autoimmune thrombocytopenia similar to that seen in adults with chronic ITP.

Children with chronic ITP, like adults, respond transiently to corticosteroid therapy, but they almost invariably relapse when the drug is discontinued. Long-term administration of corticosteroids in developing children may cause retardation of growth and other complications.[327] Gamma globulin may be helpful in long-term management of some cases.[553] The alternative therapy for children with chronic thrombocytopenia who require maintenance steroid therapy is splenectomy. Because of the small, but significant, risk of serious infection after splenectomy,[335] surgery should be deferred until the child is at least 4 to 5 years of age, whenever possible. In most series, 80% to 90% of children have recovered completely after removal of the spleen. Immunosuppressive therapy has occasionally been used in children with chronic ITP. Regimens that have been used include azathioprine with glucocorticoids[310,327,354,436] and vincristine.[342,468] Improvement has been observed in about one-third of children so treated. Because of the uncertainty about long-term side effects of such treatment, it should be reserved for the most severe cases.

CHRONIC IDIOPATHIC (AUTOIMMUNE) THROMBOCYTOPENIC PURPURA

Chronic ITP differs from the acute disorder in being primarily a disease of adults that rarely resolves spontaneously. It is considerably more common than the analogous disorder, autoimmune hemolytic anemia. As will be noted, convincing evidence now indicates that chronic ITP is a true autoimmune condition in which platelets are targeted for destruction by humoral, and possibly cellular, immune mechanisms. As better methods of laboratory diagnosis are developed, the name "autoimmune thrombocytopenic purpura" is likely to be adopted. For purposes of this discussion, the abbreviation ITP will be used.

Etiology

Early studies demonstrated that platelets transfused for therapeutic purposes to patients with ITP were rapidly destroyed in nearly all instances.[252,359] Similar observations were later made with radiolabeled autologous and isologous platelets.[30,67,201,440] Plasma from about half of patients with ITP was shown to cause thrombocytopenia when transfused to normal subjects.[202,554] The active substance was found to be an IgG immunoglobulin that could be absorbed by human platelets and was incapable of causing thrombocytopenia in animals.[485]

As evidence implicating autoantibodies in the pathogenesis of ITP accumulated in the 1950s and 1960s, a multitude of assays were applied to its laboratory diagnosis. For the most part, these were nonspecific, insensitive, and difficult to reproduce. In the mid-1970s, two groups described direct immunochemical assays for platelet-associated IgG,[139,332] stimulating many subsequent studies of platelet-associated immunoglobulins and complement in ITP. The methods used in these initial studies and problems encountered in their interpretation are discussed in Chapter 16.

Platelet-Associated IgG, IgM, and IgA

Elevations in platelet-associated IgG (PAIgG) or platelet-associated IgM, or both, are found (PAIgM) is in more than 90% of patients with ITP when studies are performed on platelets isolated from anticoagulated blood and washed in buffer.[108,110,172,212,304,395,401,420,422,523] In about two-thirds of patients, both classes of immunoglobulin are elevated; in the remainder, PAIgG is more often increased than PAIgM. Platelet-associated IgG consists of all four IgG subclasses, comparable with their distribution in plasma.[447,538] Platelet-associated IgA elevations have been found in some patients.[420,538,568] Measurements of PAIgG, PAIgM, and PAIgA in ITP reported up to 1984 have recently been summarized.[537] In many series, values ranging from 10 fg to 100 fg/platelet have been obtained. For IgG, this is equivalent to 40,000 to 400,000 molecules of IgG per platelet, two orders of magnitude higher than values usually obtained in studies of red cells in autoimmune hemolytic anemia. Issues relating to the specificity of such measurements are discussed in detail in Chapter 16. Only brief comment will be provided here.

Platelet-Associated Complement

Platelet-associated complement (PAC) 3 and C3 breakdown products are increased on the platelet surface in 30% to 70% of patients.[108,172,209,214,259,306,395,420,568] Elevations in PAC4 have also been described.[568] In general, increased PAC3 correlates with increased PAIgM,[110,214] but many exceptions have been observed.

Specificity of Platelet-Associated IgG and Platelet-Associated Measurements

Although elevated levels of platelet-associated immunoglobulins and complement are regularly found in ITP, the specificity of these determinations has been questioned. Mueller-Eckhardt,[386] using radiolabeled antiglobulin, Kelton et al.,[272] using a radiolabeled anti-IgG consumption assay, Panzer et al.,[420] using radiolabeled staphylococcal protein A binding, and von dem Borne et al.,[542] using the indirect immunofluorescence test, found that 30% to 88% of patients with thrombocytopenia of apparently nonimmune etiology had elevated levels of PAIgG. In contrast, Sugiura et al,[510] using quantitative fluorescein-labeled antiglobulin binding, Cines and Schreiber,[108] using radiolabeled antiimmunoglobulin binding, Shaw et al.,[472] using radiolabeled staphylococcal protein A binding, and LoBuglio et al.,[328] using radiolabeled monoclonal anti-IgG binding, regularly obtained values for PAIgG in nonimmune throbocytopenia that were less than those found in selected patients with ITP. No fully satisfactory explanation for these apparent discrepancies is yet available.

The surprisingly high values for PAIgs obtained in some studies of immune thrombocytopenia also raise questions about the specificity of such measurements. Several groups have found that platelet-associated albumin increases in proportion to PAIgG in ITP.[232,276] Winiarski[566] observed the platelets incubated in plasma with heat-aggregated IgG take up IgM, IgA, and albumin in proportion to IgG and that this effect was independent of platelet aggregation. Shulman and his colleagues[483] induced thrombocytopenia in dogs with rabbit antidog platelet antibody and found that the resulting increase in PAIgG was almost entirely of dog origin. Together, these findings suggest that antibody-induced damage to circulating platelets somehow promotes nonspecific uptake of plasma proteins, perhaps related to trapping of plasma in the platelet interstices or encapsulation of plasma in microvesicles derived from platelets.[232] Arguments against the latter possibility have been advanced by Kelton et al.[274]

An alternative explanation for high levels of platelet-associated plasma proteins in ITP is that plasma may be incorporated preferentially into young (newly formed) platelets typical of ITP. Platelets may also be capable of internalizing antibodies, aggregated IgG, and immune complexes with which they interact.[46,456,497] This represents another way in which large quantities of IgG might be accumulated by platelets before they are cleared from the circulation. This internal IgG would be measured in assays that involve platelet disruption or allow platelet secretion, intentionally or unintentionally (*see* Chap. 16). A report that increased levels of internal platelet IgG persist after steroid-induced remission in ITP is of interest in this connection.[161]

For reasons not fully clear, some assays appear to detect only platelet-bound autoantibody, and are insensitive to the relatively large quantities of IgG sequestered in platelet granules in normal and in pathologic states (*see* Chap. 16). One technique that appears to detect only surface IgG is based on the binding of radiolableled, monoclonal antihuman IgG.[122,328] With this approach, almost complete discrimination between autoimmune thrombocytopenia, thrombocytopenia of nonimmune etiology, and the normal state was described in a recent report (Fig. 19-7). This distinction may have been aided by studying only untreated patients with severe ITP and by excluding patients with nonimmune thrombocytopenia who were acutely ill. It is of interest that this assay yields values for surface-associated IgG in the range of 50 to 200 molecules per platelet in normals and 400 to 2000 molecules platelet in most patients with ITP, a range comparable with that seen in autoimmune hemolytic anemia. Exclusion of cell fragments by centrifugation of platelets through a Percoll solution may be an advantage of this method.[188]

Serum Autoantibodies

Numerous assays have been employed to detect platelet-reactive antibodies in ITP. In general, positive reactions have been obtained less

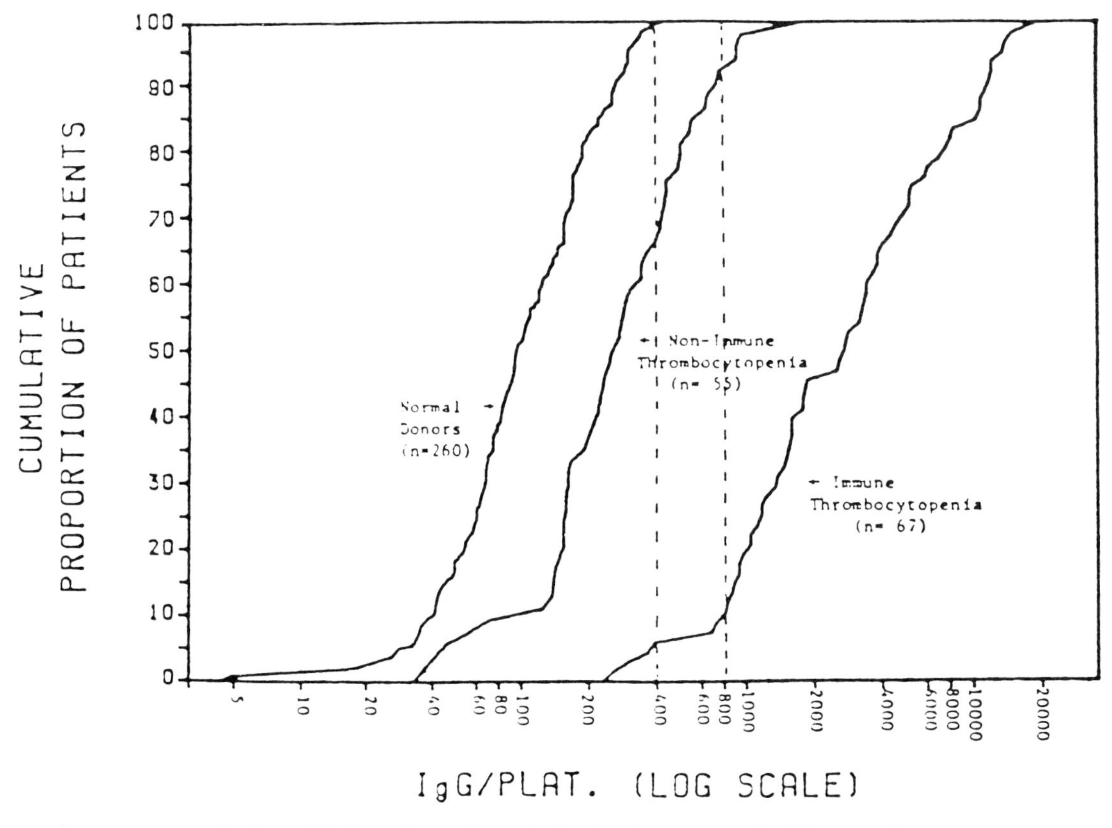

Figure 19-7. Quantitation of IgG on the surface of platelets from normal subjects, patients with thrombocytopenia presumed to be due to nonimmune causes, and platelets from patients with apparent ITP. Expression of IgG on the platelet surface was determined with a radiolabeled monoclonal, Fc-specific, anti-IgG probe (Court WS, Bozeman JM, Soong S-J et al: Blood 69:278, 1987).

often with indirect assays than with direct assays for PAIgG and PAIgM. In many studies of serum and plasma, no special precautions were taken to discriminate among autoreactive antibodies, alloantibodies, circulating immune complexes, and aggregates of normal IgG present in stored sera. Thus, reported values may be higher than the true incidence of circulating autoantibody. In various studies, reactions considered to be positive were obtained in 81% to 95% of cases by the antiglobulin consumption test,[139,271] 33% to 88% by the ^{125}I-antiglobulin test,[178,389,556] 35% to 69% by the indirect immunofluorescence test,[510,528,538] 26% to 37% by the ^{125}I-labeled staphylococcal protein A-binding test,[119,162] 46% to 90% by the ELISA test,[142,160,213,234,567] 27% to 60% by the platelet factor 3-release test,[250,390] and 27% to 60% by the [^{14}C] serotonin-release assay.[225,390]

Circulating Immune Complexes

Circulating immune complexes (CIC) have been detected in 30% to 70% of patients with ITP in some studies,[81,307,432,523] but not in others,[287] and their role promoting platelet destruction in ITP is uncertain. The possible role of CIC in thrombocytopenia associated with human immunodeficiency virus (HIV) will be discussed separately.

Target Antigens

Several studies have provided evidence that epitopes on GPIIb or GPIIIa are recognized by autoantibodies in ITP.[362,526,573] Epitopes on

GPIb[362,513,572] have also been implicated. Target antigens in ITP are fully discussed in Chapter 7.

Cellular Immunity

Apparent cell-mediated antiplatelet activity has been demonstrated in a small number of patients with ITP.[113,380] Studies of T-lymphocyte subsets have demonstrated increased T-suppressor cells,[314,521] decreased helper/suppressor (T4/T8) ratios,[397,426] normal T4/T8 ratios,[315,464] increased numbers of T4+, T8+ lymphocytes,[374,464] in increased numbers of Ia+ T cells.[375] The possible relationship of corticosteroid and other therapies to these seemingly inconsistent results is unclear. Abnormal autologous mixed lymphocyte reactions[578] and leukocyte migration inhibition in lymphocyte–platelet mixtures[65] have also been described.

Genetic Influences

Expression of HLA-A,B,C, and DR markers on lymphocytes of patients with ITP has been studied extensively. An increased prevalence of HLA-B8 and HLA-B12,[186] HLA-DRw2,[254] and HLA-A28[151] has been found in selected groups of patients. In other series, no association between ITP and HLA was observed.[189,350,362,391] In one group of patients, PAIgM was higher in patients with the haplotype HLA-B8/DRw3.[430] Familial occurrence of ITP is distinctly unusual,[63,255] but immunologic abnormalities detected in first-degree relatives of patients with chronic ITP may reflect a hereditary predisposition to develop the disorder.[118,508]

Platelet Production and Destruction

Platelet life span, determined by direct counting of transfused platelets or with radioactive labels, is almost invariably shortened in ITP,[30,40,67,201,221,252,285,359,419,442] and was inversely related to PAIgG in some studies.[278,419] Platelet levels may be influenced by defective reticuloendothelial clearance in some patients.[267] A small subgroup of patients with normal platelet life spans appear to have a different disorder not yet fully characterized.[141,201] Platelet production, calculated indirectly from measurements of platelet turnover, was found to be about five times normal in early studies,[67,201] consistent with the increased numbers of megakaryocytes found in the marrow. In recent investigations that used autologous platelets, normal or decreased rates of platelet production have been observed in patients with both mild and severe disease.[40,194,221,502] A possible explanation for these discrepant findings is that radiolabeled homologous platelets (generally used in early studies) are destroyed more rapidly than autologous platelets.[40,221] Thus, use of homologous cells could lead to a higher estimate of platelet turnover and platelet production. The suggestion that platelet production is inappropriately low in ITP is consistent with reports that autoantibodies bind to megakaryocytes[36,356] and can inhibit megakaryocyte colony formation in vitro.[226,524] However, the number of megakaryocyte colon ly-forming units in ITP marrow appears to be normal[40] or increased.[511]

Evidence cited in the foregoing is consistent with the possibility that inhibition of platelet production contributes to thrombocytopenia in ITP. However, conclusions based on the kinetics of radiolabeled *autologous* platelets are not necessarily authoritative because of the striking heterogeneity of surface marker expression in human platelets[144,241] creating the possibility that platelets available for radiolabeling in the circulation of patients with ITP constitute a subpopulation resistant to autoantibody-mediated destruction. If this is true, *homologous* platelet survival could provide the most accurate index of autologous platelet destruction. Calculations of platelet turnover based on kinetics of radiolabeled autologous platelets remain suspect until this question is resolved.

Body surface scanning after transfusion of radiolabeled platelets has shown that platelet destruction occurs primarily in the spleen in most patients.[30,40,442,482] Hepatic platelet clearance has been observed in patients with the most severe thrombocytopenia and rapid rates of platelet destruction.[29,30,278,486] Scanning results have been interpreted to indicate diffuse destruction of platelets throughout the reticuloendothelial system in some patients.[223] In addition to being the major site in which platelets are destroyed, the spleen appears to be an important site of autoantibody synthesis in ITP.[256,360] Destruction of platelets in the organ may, therefore, be promoted by a high local concentration of autoantibody.[359]

Hormonal Influences

The high frequency with which ITP occurs in postpubertal, premenopausal women, and the rclapses that sometimes occur during pregnancy, are consistent with the possibility that estrogens or other hormones are important in the pathogenesis of ITP, but no clear link has been established. The connection between high expression of Fc receptors on female platelets and the tendency of the disease to occur in women[377] is uncertain.

Platelet Dysfunction

A variety of functional defects have been described in platelets of patients with ITP.[113,222,252] Binding of autoantibodies to functional membrane glycoproteins such as GPIIb-IIIa,[37] GPIb,[135] and perhaps others[512] may explain variability in the severity of bleeding in individual patients.

Association with Other Conditions

Thrombocytopenia apparently indistinguishable from ITP occurs more often than would be expected by chance in patients with other disorders. Often, this is designated *secondary* ITP. Associated conditions thought to be predisposing to ITP were found in about one-half of a series of 508 patients.[215] The PAIgM was elevated more often in uncomplicated ITP and PAIgG more often in the secondary form. The association of ITP with lymphoma (Hodgkin's disease, chronic lymphocytic leukemia, non-Hodgkin's lymphoma),[50,243,294,544] systemic lupus erythematosus,[76,137,204] infectious mononucleosis,[86,87,150,245,351] and thyrotoxicosis[208,217,236,308] is well established. Thrombocytopenia in human immunodeficiency virus (HIV) infection and hemophilia will be discussed separately. An association of ITP with scleroderma,[403] disseminated carcinoma without splenic enlargement or marrow infiltration,[48,290,463] extragonadal germ cell cancer,[180] tuberculosis,[92] brucellosis,[155] histoplasmosis,[21] Hashimoto's thyroiditis,[236] Gaucher's disease,[320] Crohn's disease,[297] sarcoidosis,[71,165,295] ulcerative colitis,[196] and myasthenia gravis[527] has been described. Transient and chronic thrombocytopenia following bone marrow transplantation may have an autoimmune basis.[55,168,372,495] The chronic form is associated with severe graft-vs-host disease and poor prognosis.[168] Idiopathic thrombocytopenia following remission induction therapy for acute leukemia has been described.[90] The underlying abnormality in many of the conditions mentioned may be a defect in immunoregulation, leading to inappropriate production of platelet-reactive autoantibodies.

The simultaneous occurrence of chronic ITP and autoimmune hemolytic anemia (Evans's syndrome) is well recognized.[80,425,431] Paraproteins associated with lymphoma[318] and multiple myeloma[138] sometimes react with platelets and provoke thrombocytopenia. Autoantibodies simultaneously affecting platelets and coagulation factors,[519] or neutrophils,[325,565] have been described in a few instances.

Idiopathic thrombocytopenia commonly occurs during pregnancy.[82,224,248,249,280,312,416] As the disorder chiefly affects women of child-bearing age, this relationship may be coincidental. However, it is not uncommon for platelet levels to return to normal after delivery.[370] Twenty-four percent of 116 pregnant women developed mild thrombocytopenia and increased platelet-associated IgG during gestation in one series.[207] These abnormalities did not persist after delivery and were felt not to reflect typical ITP.

Clinical Picture

Chronic ITP most often affects persons between the ages of 20 and 55 years but can occur at any age. Women are affected three to four times as often as men. A history of preceding infection is distinctly unusual. The condition appears to be rare among black children[335] and adults.[137]

Typically, the onset of the disorder is insidious. For weeks, patients may note occasional petechiae and other minor bleeding symptoms, including menorrhagia. Rarely, these signs are present for months or years before diagnosis. Bleeding manifestations may be present anywhere on the skin or mucosal surfaces, especially the distal upper and lower extremities. In patients with profound thrombocytopenia, hemorrhagic bullae are often present in the buccal mucosa. Bleeding into joints or into the retina is rare.[137] Intracranial hemorrhage is uncommon but is a potential complication in every patient. Slight splenomegaly is seen occasionally. Gross splenomegaly provides evidence against ITP as the primary diagnosis.

Laboratory Findings

Platelet levels are usually in the range from 5000 to 100,000/μl. Fragmented and giant platelets are commonly seen in the peripheral blood smear.[282] Patients with significant blood loss or concomitant autoimmune hemolytic anemia (Evans's syndrome) may be anemic. In patients with markedly increased rates of platelet turnover, plasma acid phosphatase is sometimes increased.[417] Rosetting of platelets about granulocytes has been described in a small number of cases.[563] One or two percent of patients with chronic ITP exhibit positive serologic tests for lupus erythematosus and are suffering from that disorder.[76,137]Anticardiolipin antibodies were found in about one-third of 96 patients by using a sensitive immunoassay.[205] An association between the lupus anticoagulant and thrombocytopenia was found in one series.[33]

Active bleeding in some patients with platelet levels sufficiently high to expect normal hemostasis may reflect inhibition of platelet function by certain autoantibodies.[37,113,135,236,512] Platelet dysfunction secondary to autoantibodies has also been described in patients with normal platelet levels.[236,406,562]

As noted previously, PAIgG or PAIgm levels are elevated in more than 90% of patients. Platelet-associated C3 is increased in a somewhat lower percentage. Platelet-reactive antibodies were detected in serum of 20% to 90% of patients in different studies. In many studies, a rough, inverse relationship between PAIgG and the platelet count has been found.

Megakaryocytes are present in normal or increased numbers in the bone marrow, but are sometimes less granular and smoother in contour than those of normal marrow. As noted earlier, whether or not these abnormalities reflect subnormal platelet production is not fully established.

The surgically removed spleen exhibits increased numbers of lymphatic nodules, with reactive germinal centers in the white pulp, and plasma cells peripheral to small vessels in the marginal zone, suggesting active immunoglobulin synthesis.[517] On electron microscopy, platelets can be demonstrated in various stages of degradation in macrophages.[333,517] Lipid-loaded macrophages containing cholesterol, phospholipid, and ceroid, probably derived from platelets, are often identified.[292,455,516] These "foam cells" appear to be especially prominent in patients treated for prolonged periods with prednisone.[292] Possibly, this phenomenon reflects inhibition of lipoprotein metabolism by platelet secretory products.[428] "Relative sphingomyelinase deficiency" has been suggested as a cause of the splenic histiocytosis.[228]

Treatment and Prognosis

Several reviews on this subject have recently been published.[252,364,482] Spontaneous recovery occurs in a small fraction, perhaps 10% to 15% of adults with ITP. These individuals may have the acute form of ITP more commonly seen in children. Alternatively, they may have unsuspected sensitivity to drugs or other exogenous agents. There is as yet no way to determine which patients will achieve spontaneous remission.

Platelet Transfusions

Platelets should not be given routinely to patients with ITP because they are rapidly destroyed by the same mechanisms responsible for clearance of autologous platelets. Moreover, platelets present in the circulation, although few, are newly formed and may have superior hemostatic function. There should be no hesitation about transfusing platelets to patients with apparent life-threatening hemorrhage, however, because reasonable posttransfusion increments can be transiently achieved in a significant percentage of cases.[3,85] The life span of transfused platelets can be prolonged by prior injection of IV gamma globulin.[43]

Corticosteroids

Glucocorticoids appear to benefit patients with ITP primarily by suppressing the phagocytic activity of the monocyte–macrophage system, especially in the spleen,[199,355,482] thus prolonging the life span of antibody-coated platelets.[30,67] Evidence for inhibition of antibody synthesis by corticosteroids is less convincing. Recent kinetic studies provide evidence that effective production of platelets increases with corticosteroid administration.[87] Improved capillary fragility and normalization of the bleeding time are sometimes seen before platelet levels increase; the mechanism of this effect is uncertain.

The usual initial dose of prednisone is 1.0 mg/kg. Platelet levels sometimes increase within a few days of treatment, but several weeks are often required. The response of a typical patient is shown in Figure 19-8. Platelet-associated immunoglobulin levels do not appear to correlate with prednisone responsiveness.[122,279] When sufficiently large doses are administered, nearly all patients will respond with a rise in platelet levels.[561] If there is no improvement within 2 to 3 weeks, or if massive doses of steroids are required to maintain hemostatic platelet levels, splenectomy should be performed in patients who are operative candidates.[132] In patients who respond, dosage should be reduced gradually for several weeks to a point at which platelet levels can be maintained at about 50,000/μl. Patients who remain steroid-dependent for 2 to 4 months should also be considered for splenectomy.[68,70,132,166,252,337]

Splenectomy

It seems clear that the beneficial effect of splenectomy in ITP results largely from removal of the primary site in which platelets are destroyed and a major site of platelet autoantibody production.[359] An effect of splenectomy on platelet production, independent of these actions, has been suggested.[40] Where possible, platelets should be raised to hemostatic levels by administering prednisone preoperatively. Where this is not possible, platelets can sometimes be elevated by transfusions given after a single dose of intravenous gamma globulin, 400 mg/kg[43] or immediately after clamping the splenic artery. Many thrombocytopenic patients do well without platelet transfusions, however. During surgery, a search should be made for accessory spleens. Usually, these are found near the base of the splenic pedicle.[137]

Between 70% and 95% of patients improve after splenectomy. Platelet levels are restored

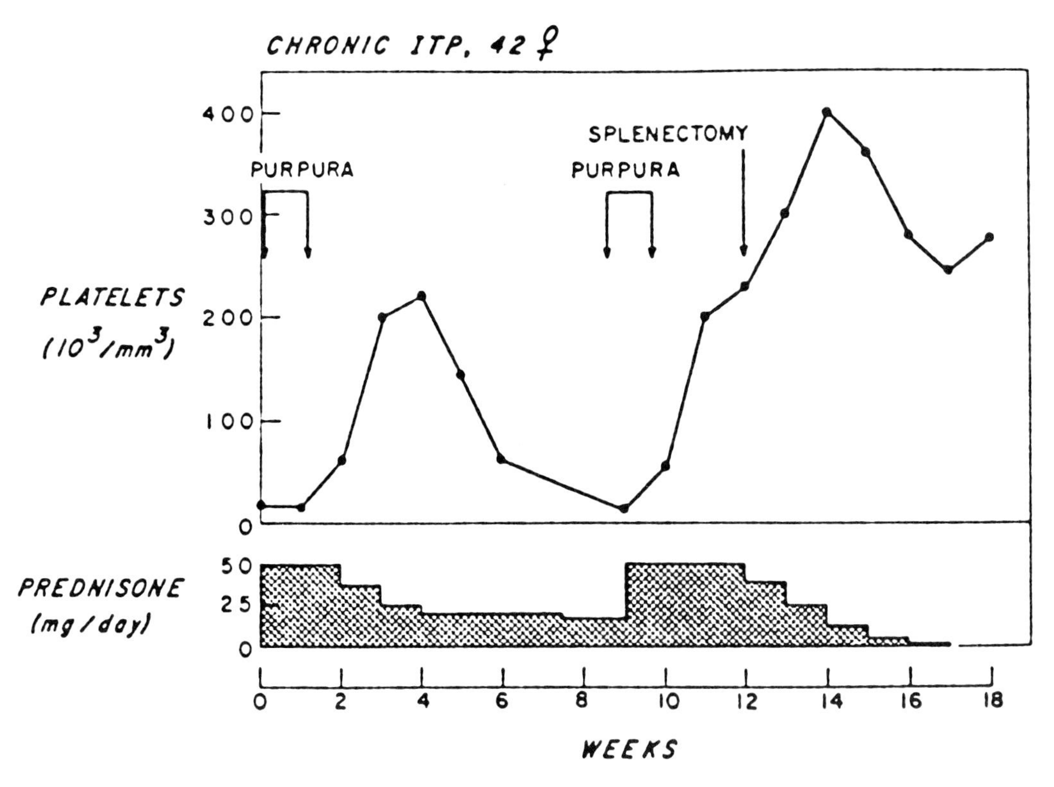

Figure 19-8. Course of chronic ITP in a 42-year-old woman. Platelet levels rose to normal after 3 weeks of prednisone therapy, but thrombocytopenia recurred after the dose was tapered. A sustained remission was achieved after splenectomy [Aster RH: In Williams W, Butler E, Erslev (eds): Hematology, p 1298. New York McGraw-Hill, 1983).

permanently to normal in about two-thirds of these.[70,132,137,166,252,337,429] A rise in platelet levels is usually apparent within 1 or 2 days of surgery, but occasionally patients require 1 or 2 weeks to respond. Nonresponders can often be managed, thereafter, on lower dosages of corticosteroids.

In patients responding to splenectomy, plasma- and platelet-associated immunoglobulins generally return to normal. However, persistent elevation of PAIgG was found in 30% to 40% of the patients in several studies.[172,237,322,332]

There is, as yet, no reliable means of predicting which patients will respond to splenectomy. In one series,[260] but not in another,[279] patients with lowest values of PAIgG did somewhat better. In one small series, patients with detectable autoantibodies in plasma had responded poorly to splenectomy.[358] Patients over the age of 50 years are less likely to achieve complete remission than are younger patients.[137] Those who develop marked thrombocytosis after splenectomy are more likely to sustain remission than those in whom platelets rise only to normal levels.[137,337] Patients splenectomized early in their course did better than those in whom splenectomy was delayed in one series.[83]

The demonstration by body surface scanning that platelets labeled with ^{51}Cr or ^{111}In are destroyed in the spleen is thought by some to offer a way to select candidates for surgery.[77,195,398,534] However, the prevailing view is that studies of the sites of platelet clearance are not useful in predicting a surgical outcome.[30,439,440]

Occasionally, systemic lupus erythematosus becomes clinically apparent following splenectomy for ITP, but the operation, itself, appears not to be a causative factor.[53,229] In one series, patients with combined lupus and ITP responded poorly to splenectomy.[198] This has not been the experience of others.[229,240]

After splenectomy, corticosteroid dosage can be reduced over a period of 2 to 4 weeks and discontinued indefinitely if platelet levels remain elevated. Relapses of ITP sometimes occur many years later. In one series, this was most likely to happen in patients with spleens weighing less than 125 g.[66] In patients who relapse, a search should be made for an accessory spleen by using appropriate imaging techniques.[127] Surgical removal of accessory splenic tissue leads to restoration of normal platelet levels in more than half of these patients.[127,137,200,536] After a splenectomy, appropriate precautions should be taken to reduce the risk of catastrophic infection associated with the asplenic state.

Intravenous Gamma Globulin

Reports in 1981 that patients with ITP sometimes respond to infusion of large doses of intravenous gamma globulin[239,460] stimulated a flurry of interest in this approach to treatment. More than 50 publications have appeared since that time documenting the effectiveness of this treatment. Numerous IV gamma globulin preparations, some containing intact and others chemically modified monomeric IgG, are now on the market. The recommended therapeutic dose is 400 mg/kg body weight per day for 5 days. Clinical trials intended to establish a firm basis for the use of intravenous IgG are still in progress, but results published to date allow some general comments to be made about its therapeutic effectiveness. Overall, about two-thirds of patients with severe ITP respond to high-dose intravenous IgG.[80,173,405,459,543] Patients older than 50 years of age are less likely to respond than are younger persons.[412] Pretreatment levels of platelet-associated immunoglobulins and complement appear not to correlate well with responsiveness.[405] A recent extensive literature review[80] concluded that: unmodified IgG preparations may be superior to those that have been chemically modified; patients with ITP of long duration do less well than those treated early; the initial platelet level is not predictive of responsiveness; and the higher the initial rise in platelet levels after infusion, the longer the duration of the response. In responding patients, platelet levels rise within 1 to 7 days of treatment, often to normal. Concomitant with the rise in platelets, platelet-associated immunoglobulin and complement levels are partially or totally corrected toward normal.[173,415,459,569] In more than 90% of cases, however, platelets return to preinfusion levels within 1 to 4 weeks.[2,80,296,405,415,543] A small percentage of patients are permanently benefited; in some of these, the platelet count becomes normal.

Few dose-response studies have been performed to determine optimum doses of IV gamma globulin. In a recent study, 6 of 10 patients receiving 400 mg/kg for 5 days responded, whereas only 3 of 11 receiving 165 mg/kg did so.[153] Two patients treated initially with standard doses of IV gamma globulin followed by intermittent booster treatments of 1 g/kg for 100 to 150 days eventually achieved sustained remission.[56]

Despite extensive clinical application, the mechanism(s) by which IV gamma globulin treatment results in elevation of platelet levels in ITP is not fully understood. One mode of action appears to be reticuloendothelial blockade lasting up to 30 days.[164,378] No inhibition of the interaction of macrophages with antibody-coated platelets by high doses of IV gamma globulin was detected in an in vitro study[454] and, in another study, inhibition of reticuloendothelial function in vivo by IV gamma globulin infusion was achieved only in patients who were not receiving prednisone.[75] Yet, IgG is often effective in patients taking corticosteroids. The suggestion has been made that aggregates of IgG contaminating gamma globulin preparations may be primarily responsible for their therapeutic effects.[32] A report that pepsin-generated F(ab')^2 fragments, given at the low dose of 0.03 mg/kg, produced lasting responses in five patients refractory to conventional treatment requires confirmation.[152] Other studies performed in vitro and in vivo provide evidence that IV gamma globulin may act to regulate autoantibody production[69,78,126,129,522] or to inhibit autoantibody–platelet binding.[569] An effect on natural killer cells has also been described.[154]

A course of treatment with IV gamma globulin costs several thousand dollars for an adult. Despite its efficacy and low toxicity, this treatment should, therefore, be reserved for patients refractory to conventional therapy.

Anti-Rh$_0$ Immunoglobulin

One group, who argued that the action of intravenous gamma globulin in ITP may in part result from sensitization of recipient red cells, resulting in low-grade hemolysis and reticuloendothelial blockade,[452] treated a series of patients with ITP with low doses (200–1000 μg) of IgG-anti-**Rh**$_0$(D) intravenously for 1 to 5 days.[450,451] Significant elevations of platelet levels occurred in 13 of 15 Rh-positive, but not in either of two Rh-negative patients.[450] Benefits were transient in most patients but were sustained for many months in five instances. Only minor side effects were observed. Similar results were obtained in two other small studies,[399,418] but benefits were less striking. Further evaluation of this relatively inexpensive treatment seems warranted.

Immunosuppression

Immunosuppressive therapy is effective in a variable proportion of patients with ITP. Azathioprine in combination with prednisone resulted in good or excellent responses in 25% of 92 patients described before 1981.[359] Three to nine months was required for improvement in most cases. About half of 61 patients given cyclophosphamide and prednisone achieved good responses in 1 to 2 months.[166,359,532] A higher frequency of more rapid responses has been described in patients given vincristine 1–2 mg weekly.[15,311,359,441] Slow intravenous infusion over 4 hr or longer is thought to be more effective than bolus injection by some groups.[14,341] However, responses to vinca alkaloids have been minor and transient in many studies.[34,137,184,359] Cyclosporine appeared to be effective in several recently reported cases.[263,530] In a recent retrospective study, response to an immunosuppressive regimen was distinctly unusual in patients failing to respond to corticosteroids and splenectomy.[132]

It is reasonable to consider a trial of immunosuppression in patients who fail to achieve a sustained response to the aforementioned therapies or in those who are not candidates for splenectomy. The risks of immunosuppressive therapy, such as infection and predisposition to malignancy, should be carefully considered before utilizing this approach.

Vinca Alkaloid-Loaded Platelets

Transfusion of platelets "loaded" with vinblastine sometimes results in an elevation in platelet levels and, occasionally, sustained remission.[17] Serious side effects have occurred in some patients[277] and, because vinblastine dissociates rapidly from platelets in vivo, this treatment is likely to be effective only in patients with extremely short platelet survival times.[277] In a small number of patients, response rates exceeding 50%, and rates of sustained remission ranging from 33% to 75% were achieved with platelets loaded in vitro with vincristine,[12,13] which appears to bind to platelets more tightly than vinblastine.[12] Despite its inconvenience, this approach seems warranted in selected patients refractory to other treatments.

Colchicine

Three of 14 patients refractory to splenectomy and corticosteroids achieved normal platelet levels when treated with colchicine, 1.2 mg daily for at least 2 weeks.[507] Inhibition of microtubule-dependent events in macrophages was suggested as the mechanism of action. This benign therapy seems worthy of trial in selected patients.

Danazol

Treatment with danazol, an attenuated androgen, in dosages ranging from 400 to 800 mg/day was followed by improvement in platelet levels in 15 of 22 patients, most of whom were refractory to conventional treatment, in the first reported series.[16] Eleven of these patients achieved sustained normalization of platelet counts. Each of three patients with thrombocytopenia associated with lupus erythematosus were benefited in another study, but treatment was limited by the occurrence of hypersensitivity dermatitis in two patients.[346] In two other series, only 1 of 20 patients showed sustained improvement in platelet levels when taking danazol.[352,365] Hepatosplenic peliosis,[402] drug-induced thrombocytopenia,[24,433] and other apparent side effects[352] have been described. The mechanism of action of danazol in some patients with ITP, and the variable response rates observed in different series, are currently unexplained.

Plasma Exchange

Intensive plasma exchange totaling 3 to 5 plasma volumes over a period of several days was followed by a significant rise in platelet levels in eight of ten patients with chronic ITP;[61] however, this improvement was only transient. Sustained remission after plasma exchange in acute ITP is not uncommon.[61,345] Whether or not this reflects a cause-and-effect relationship is difficult to establish in this self-limited disorder. In view of its high cost and marginal benefit in chronic ITP, plasma exchange should be reserved for patients with life-threatening hemorrhage.[230,559]

Anti-Fc Gamma-Receptor Antibody

Infusion of a murine monoclonal antibody reactive with an Fc receptor shared by neutrophils and macrophages to a patient with severe refractory ITP was followed by a dramatic rise in platelet levels lasting about 10 days, but a second infusion given 1 month later was ineffective.[114] The value of this approach to treatment remains to be established.

IDIOPATHIC THROMBOCYTOPENIC PURPURA IN PREGNANCY

The natural history of ITP does not appear to be influenced by pregnancy,[82,224,242,280,312,416] and treatment should be essentially as in nonpregnant women, except for precautions appropriate to protection of the fetus. Intravenous gamma globulin has been used effectively in women with ITP at various stages of gestation.[42,317,404,444] Whether or not this treatment will reduce the severity of thrombocytopenia in the newborn is not yet established. Splenectomy has been performed successfully in the second and third trimester,[170,312] but it is associated with increased fetal mortality and should be postponed until after delivery whenever possible.

Prenatal and postnatal management of infants born to women with ITP was discussed earlier.

THROMBOCYTOPENIA ASSOCIATED WITH HUMAN IMMUNODEFICIENCY VIRUS INFECTION

Reports of apparent autoimmune thrombocytopenia in otherwise healthy homosexual men first appeared in 1982.[381] Later, similar findings were made in homosexual men, drug addicts, and others with acquired immunodeficiency syndrome (AIDS) or AIDS-related complex (ARC).[5,121,187,227,446,548,549]

Etiology

The human immunodeficiency virus (HIV) may be capable of infecting bone marrow stem cells and can produce various marrow abnormalities.[140,579] Selective ablation of megakaryocytes was found in one child with this syndrome.[558] In patients with HIV-associated thrombocytopenia, however, the bone marrow is usually hypercellular, with normal or increased numbers of megakaryocytes.[471,579] Moreover, platelet transfusions are only transiently effective, and platelet-associated immunoglobulins and complement are almost universally elevated.[5,49,381,458,503,549] Together, these findings are indicative of immunologically mediatcd platelet destruction.

In one study, eluates prepared from platelets of patients with HIV-associated thrombocytopenia failed to react with normal target platelets, in contrast with eluates prepared from platelets in ITP.[549] Platelet-associated immunoglobulin levels were increased in proportion to circulating immune complexes (CIC) detected by polyethylene glycol precipitation.[549] These findings implied that CIC, present in a high proportion of patients with HIV infection, might bind to platelets and promote their destruction. Subsequently, evidence was obtained that the CIC consist of anti-F(ab')$_2$ antibodies complexed with the F(ab')$_2$ portion of normal IgG.[574] Some antibodies appeared to have limited specificity, possibly for certain IgG idiotypes. It was suggested that these antibodies might be provoked by prolonged exposure to exogenous antigens or be a result of disordered immunoregulation.[574]

Somewhat different findings were made by another group, who detected an IgG antibody reactive with a 25-kDa protein located in normal platelets and in herpes virus-infected green monkey kidney cell lines but not in other blood cells in 29 of 30 homosexual men with apparent autoimmune thrombocytopenia.[503] This antibody disappeared in one patient after splenectomy-induced remission and reappeared after relapse. No direct laboratory evidence showing that the antibody binds to intact platelets was presented, however. In another small group of patients, platelet-reactive autoantibodies were demonstrated in the absence of detectable CIC.[393] Together, these observations support the possibility that platelet destruction in HIV-associated thrombocytopenia is immunologically mediated by mechanisms that differ from those responsible for classic ITP.

Clinical Presentation

An HIV-associated thrombocytopenia has been described in infants,[471,558] children,[449] and adults of all ages infected with HIV. It can occur in asymptomatic carriers of HIV, but in one large series, it was limited to patients with ARC or AIDS.[393] In several studies, it was found that thrombocytopenic patients had the same probability of developing ARC and full-blown AIDS as HIV-infected persons with normal platelet levels.[227,446] In patients without stigmata of ARC or AIDS, clinical presentation is indistinguishable from classic ITP.

Laboratory Findings

Platelet levels range from profoundly thrombocytopenic to slightly subnormal. Lymphopenia and reversed T-helper/T-suppressor cell ratios are found in the same frequency as in nonthrombocytopenic patients infected with HIV.[4,579] An increased frequency of the antigen HLA-DR5 was found in one group of patients.[434] Serologic tests for anti-HIV antibody are positive. The bone marrow generally contains normal or increased numbers of megakaryocytes.[88,471,579] Lymphoid infiltration, plasmacytosis, and dysplasia typical of HIV infection are often present.[579] Platelet-associated immunoglobulins and complement are elevated.[4,5,386,458,503,549] Positive indirect tests for antiplatelet antibodies are often obtained.[121,393,549] Circulating immune complexes can be detected in more than 75% of patients.[5,49,503,549]

Treatment and Prognosis

In some patients, platelet levels return to normal spontaneously.[4,548] Sixty to ninety percent of patients respond to corticosteroid therapy or splenectomy.[4,458,548] The potential risk of administering corticosteroids to patients with HIV infection has been stressed.[449,469] However, conventional doses of corticosteroids were tolerated in one series of 24 patients, 19 of whom achieved an increase in platelet levels.[4] A retrospective analysis suggested that full-blown AIDS is more likely to develop after splenectomy.[41] In several studies, satisfactory but transient responses to intravenous gamma globulin were obtained in adults[130,316] and children.[449] Failure to respond to gamma globulin has also been observed.[58,449] Elevations in platelet levels were seen after treatment of three patients with Kaposi's sarcoma with vincristine,[373] but the hazard of using this drug in HIV-infected patients has not been defined. Several patients achieved transient elevations in platelet counts following treatment with anti-**Rh**$_o$(D) immunoglobulin given to induce low-grade hemolysis and reticuloendothelial blockade.[57,145] Antibodies specific for the **Rh** c antigen was effective in one **Rh**$_o$(D)-negative patient.[57]

THROMBOCYTOPENIA IN PATIENTS WITH HEMOPHILIA

A condition clinically similar to ITP occurs in children and adults with hemophilia treated with commercially produced antihemophilic factor.[421,435] Except for concomitant hemophilia, clinical presentation is identical with that of chronic ITP. Concomitant autoimmune hemolytic anemia has been reported.[206] Megakaryocytes are increased in the bone marrow,[435] platelet life span is shortened,[421] and platelet immunoglobulins are elevated.[421,435] Lymphopenia and subnormal helper/suppressor cell ratios are commonly found,[158,159,421,435] as they are in HIV-associated thrombocytopenia. These observations favor an immune etiology for hemophilia-associated thrombocytopenia. In view of the high incidence of anti-HIV antibodies in this group of patients, a connection with HIV infection has been suggested. However, a significant association between hemophilia A and thrombocytopenia was observed in a retrospective study of 1551 patients on whom information was available from the period 1975 to 1979.[159] It was argued that low platelet levels in these patients could not have been a complication of HIV, which was not prevalent during that time interval.[159] In some patients, reduced platelet levels appeared to be associated with chronic viral hepatitis. Nonetheless, a significant association between thrombocytopenia and eventual development of AIDS was found in a recent study of 84 patients.[158] This is in contrast with the pattern in homosexual males.

The similarities between the thrombocytopenia/hemophilia and the thrombocytopenia/HIV syndromes are apparent, and it seems possible that the etiologies of the two conditions are the same. However, epidemiologic studies confirming this connection unequivocally have not yet been performed.

Hemophiliacs with immune-mediated thrombocytopenia respond well to corticosteroids and splenectomy.[421,435] Intravenous gamma globulin is also effective.[130,316]

REFERENCES

1. Abdi EA, Brien W, Venner PM: Auto-immune thrombocytopenia related to interferon therapy. Scand J Haematol 36:515, 1986

2. Abe T, Matsuda J, Kawasugi K, Yoshimura Y, Kinoshita T, Kazama M: Clinical effect of intravenous immunoglobulin on chronic idiopathic thrombocytopenic purpura. Blut 47:69, 1983

3. Abraham J, Ellman L: Platelet transfusion in immune thrombocytopenic purpura. J Am Med Assoc 236:1847, 1976

4. Abrams DI, Kiprov DD, Goedert JJ, Sarngadharan MG, Gallo RC, Volberding PA: Antibodies to human T-lymphotropic virus type III and development of the acquired immunodeficiency syndrome in homosexual men presenting with immune thrombocytopenia. Ann Intern Med 104:47, 1986

5. Abrams DI, Kiprov DD, Volberding PA: Isolated thrombocytopenia in homosexual men—longitudinal follow-up. Adv Exp Med Biol 187:117, 1985

6. Abramson M, Pfueller S, Sheridan W: Post-transfusion purpura. Aust NZ J Med 15:763, 1986

7. Abramson N, Eisenberg PD, Aster RH: Post-transfusion purpura: Immunologic aspects and therapy. N Engl J Med 291:1163, 1974

8. Ackroyd JF: Allergic purpura, including purpura due to food, drugs and infections. Am J Med 14:605, 1953

9. Ackroyd JF: The pathogenesis of thrombocytopenic purpura due to hypersensitivity to Sedormid. Clin Sci 7:249, 1949

10. Adachi JD, Bensen WG, Kassam Y, Powers PJ, Bianchi FA, Cividino A, Kean WF, Rooney PJ, Craig GL, Buchanan WW, Tugwell PX, Gordon DA, Lucarelli A, Singal DP: Gold induced thrombocytopenia: 12 cases and a review of the literature. Semin Arthritis Rheum 16:287, 1987

11. Adner MM, Fisch GR, Starobin SG, Aster RH: Use of "compatible" platelet transfusions in treatment of congenital isoimmune thrombocytopenic purpura. N Engl J Med 280:244, 1969

12. Agnelli G, De Cunto M, Gresele P, Nenci GG: Vinca-loaded platelets (letter). N Engl J Med 311:599, 1984

13. Ahn YS, Byrnes JJ, Harrington WJ, Pall LM: Vinca-loaded platelets (letter). N Engl J Med 311:600, 1984

14. Ahn YS, Harrington WJ, Mylvaganam R, Allen LM, Pall LM: Slow infusion of vinca alkaloids in the treatment of idiopathic thrombocytopenic purpura Ann Intern Med 100:192, 1984

15. Ahn YS, Harrington WJ, Seelman RC, Eytel CS: Vincristine therapy of idiopathic and secondary thrombocytopenias. N Engl J Med 291:376, 1974

16. Ahn YS, Harrington WJ, Simon SR, Mylvaganam R, Pall LM, So AG: Danazol for the treatment of idiopathic thrombocytopenic purpura. N Engl J Med 308:1396, 1983

17. Ahn YS, Byrnes JJ, Harrington WJ, Cayer

ML, Smith DS, Brunskill DE, Pall LM: The treatment of idiopathic thrombocytopenia with vinblastine-loaded platelets. N Engl J Med 298:1101, 1978

18. Amran D, Schved JF, Contal M, Lesbros D: Traitement par immunoglobulines intraveineuses d'une thrombopenie neonatale par allo-immunisation plaquettaire: Ann Pediatr 34:143, 1987

19. Ansell J, Tiarks C, McCue J, Parrilla N, Benotti JR: Amrinone-induced thrombocytopenia. Arch Intern Med 144:949, 1984

20. Ansell JE, Price JM, Shah S, Beckner RR: Heparin-induced thrombocytopenia. What is its real frequency? Chest 88:878, 1985

21. Armitage JO, Sheets RF: Idiopathic thrombocytopenic purpura in patients with histoplasmosis. J Am Med Assoc 21:2323, 1977

22. Arnott J, Horsewood P, Kelton JG: Measurement of platelet-associated IgG in animal models of immune and nonimmune thrombocytopenia. Blood 69:1294, 1987

23. Arnved J, Skov PS, Winter K: Pentagastrin-induced thrombocytopenia (letter). Lancet 2:1068, 1985

24. Arrowsmith JB, Dreis M: Thrombocytopenia after treatment with danazol (letter). N Engl J Med 315:585, 1986

25. Aster RH: Post-transfusion purpura. In Engelfriet CP et al (eds): Bailliere's Clinical Immunology and Allergy, p 453. London, WB Saunders, 1987

26. Aster RH: Clinical significance of platelet-specific antigens and antibodies. In McCullough J, Sandler S (eds): Advances in Immunobiology and Bone Marrow Transplantation. New York, Alan R Liss, 1984

27. Aster RH: Platelet antigen systems. In Engelfriet C, van Loghem JJ, von dem Borne AEG Kr (eds): Immunohematology. Amsterdam, Elsevier Science Publishers, 1984

28. Aster RH: Thrombocytopenia due to enhanced platelet destruction. In Williams W, Beutler E, Erslev AJ (eds): Hematology, p 1298. New York, McGraw-Hill, 1983.

29. Aster RH, Jandl JH: Platelet sequestration in man. II. Immunological and clinical studies. J Clin Invest 43:856, 1964

30. Aster RH, Keene WR: Sites of platelet destruction in idiopathic thrombocytopenic purpura. Br J Haematol 16:61, 1969

31. Aster RH, McFarland J: Neonatal alloimmune thrombocytopenia. In Bern M (ed): Hematologic Contributions to Fetal Health. New York, Alan R Liss, 1987 (in press)

32. Augener W, Friedmann B, Brittinger G: Are aggregates of IgG the effective part of high-dose immunoglobulin therapy in adult idiopathic thrombocytopenic purpura (ITP)? (letter) Blut 50:249, 1985

33. Averbuch M, Koifman B, Levo Y: Lupus anticoagulant, thrombosis and thrombocytopenia in systemic lupus erythematosus. Am J Med Sci 293:1, 1987

34. Awida AS, El-Khateeb MS, Abu Khalaf MM, Tarawneh MS, Shannak MS: A controlled trial of steroids and splenectomy versus bolus intravenous vincristine in the treatment of adult idiopathic thrombocytopenic purpura. Curr Ther Res 40:809, 1986

35. Bailey RT, Ursick JA, Heim KL, Hilleman DE, Reich JW: Heparin-associated thrombocytopenia: A prospective comparison of bovine lung heparin, manufactured by a new process, and porcine intestinal heparin. Drug Intell Clin Pharm 20:374, 1986

36. Baldini MG: Platelet production and destruction in idiopathic thrombocytopenic purpura: A controversial issue. J Am Med Assoc 239:2477, 1978

37. Balduini CL, Grignani G, Sinigaglia F, Bisio A, Pacchiarini L, Scalabrini DR, Balduini C, Mauri C, Ascari E: Severe platelet dysfunction in a patient with autoantibodies against membrane glycoproteins IIb–IIIa. Haemostasis 7:98, 1987

38. Ball GV: Gold-induced thrombocytopenia: Response to vincristine? (letter) Arthritis Rheum 20:1288, 1977

39. Ballem PJ, Buskard NA, Decary F, Doubroff P: Post-transfusion purpura secondary to passive transfer of anti-Pl^{A1} by blood transfusion. Br J Haematol 66:113, 1987

40. Ballem PJ, Segal GM, Stratton JR, Gernsheimer T, Adamson JW, Slichter SJ: Mechanisms of thrombocytopenia in chronic autoimmune thrombocytopenic purpura. Evidence of both impaired platelet production and increased platelet clearance. J Clin Invest 80:33, 1987

41. Barbui T, Cortelazzo S, Minetti B, Galli M, Buelli M: Does splenectomy enhance risk of AIDS in HIV-positive patients with chronic thrombocytopenia? (letter) Lancet 2:342, 1987

42. Barton JC, Saleh MN, Stedman CM, LoBuglio AF: Case report: Immune thrombocytopenia: Effects of maternal gamma globulin infusion on maternal and fetal serum, platelet, and monocyte IgG. Am J Med Sci 293:112, 1987

43. Baumann MA, Menitove JE, Aster RH, Anderson T: Urgent treatment of idiopathic thrombocytopenic purpura with single-dose gammaglobulin infusion followed by platelet transfusion. Ann Intern Med 104:808, 1986

44. Beardsley DS, Spiegel JE, Jacobs MM, Handin RI, Lux SE IV: Platelet membrane glycoprotein IIIa contains target antigens that bind anti-platelet

antibodies in immune throbocytopenias. J Clin Invest 74:1701, 1984

45. Becker T, Panzer S, Maas D, Kiefel V, Sprenger R, Kirschbaum M, Mueller-Eckhardt C: High-dose intravenous immunoglobulin for post-transfusion purpura. Br J Haematol 61:149, 1985

46. Behnke O: Surface membrane clearing of receptor–ligand complexes in human blood platelets. J Cell Sci 87:465, 1987

47. Bell WR, Royall RM: Heparin-associated thrombocytopenia: A comparison of three heparin preparations. N Engl J Med 303:902, 1980

48. Bellone JD, Kunicki JK, Aster RH: Immune thrombocytopenia associated with carcinoma. Ann Intern Med 99:470, 1983

49. Bender BS, Quinn TC, Spivak JL: Homosexual men with thrombocytopenia have impaired reticuloendothelial system Fc receptor-specific clearance. Blood 70:392, 1987

50. Berkman AW, Kickler T, Braine H: Platelet-associated IgG in patients with lymphoma. Blood 63:944, 1984

51. Berndt MC, Chong BH, Bull HA, Zola H, Castaldi PA: Molecular characterization of quinine/quinidine drug-dependent antibody platelet interaction using monoclonal antibodies. Blood 66:1292, 1985

52. Berney SI, Metcalfe P, Wathen NC, Waters AH: Post-transfusion purpura responding to high-dose intravenous IgG: Further observations on pathogenesis. Br J Haematol 61:627, 1985

53. Best WR, Darling DR: A critical look at the splenectomy-SLE controversy. Med Clin N Am 46:19, 1962

54. Bettman JW Jr: Drug hypersensitivity purpuras. Arch Intern Med 112:840, 1963

55. Bierling P, Cordonnier C, Fromont P, Rodet M, Tanzer J, Vernant J-P, Bracq C, Duedari N: Acquired autoimmune thrombocytopenia after allogeneic bone marrow transplantation. Br J Haematol 59:643, 1985

56. Bierling P, Divine M, Farcet J-P, Wallet P, Duedari N: Persistent remission of adult chronic autoimmune thrombocytopenic purpura after treatment with high-dose intravenous immunoglobulin. Am J Hematol 25:271, 1987

57. Bierling P, Karianakis G, Duedari N, Desaint C, Oksenhendler E, Habibi B, Brossard Y: Anti-rhesus antibodies, immune thrombocytopenia, and human immunodeficiency virus infection (letter). Ann Intern Med 106:773, 1987

58. Biniek R, Malessa R, Brockmeyer NH, Luboldt: Anti-Rh(D) immunoglobulin for AIDS-related thrombocytopenia (letter). Lancet 2:627, 1986

59. Bjornstad H, Vik O: Thrombocytopenic purpura associated with piroxicam. Br J Clin Pharmacol 40:42, 1986

60. Blanchette V, Hogan V, Esseltine D, Hsu E, Luke B, Rock G: Evaluation of a simple immunodiffusion technique for quantitation of platelet-associated immunoglobulin G in childhood immune thrombocytopenias. Am J Pediatr Hematol Oncol 7:125, 1985

61. Blanchette VS, Hogan VA, McCombie NE, Drouin J, Bormanis JD, Taylor R, Rock GA: Intensive plasma exchange therapy in ten patients with idiopathic thrombocytopenic purpura. Transfusion 24:388, 1984

62. Blanchette VS, Peters MA, Pegg-Feige K: Alloimmune thrombocytopenia. Review from a neonatal intensive care unit. In Decary F, Rock GA (eds): Platelet Serology. Research Progress and Clinical Implications. Basel, S. Karger, 1986

63. Bogart L, Wittels EG: Idiopathic thrombocytopenic purpura in two elderly siblings. Arch Intern Med 145:2259, 1985

64. Boizard B, Wautier JL: Lek[a], a new platelet antigen absent in Glanzmann's thrombasthenia. Vox Sang 46:47, 1984

65. Borkowski W, Karpatkin S: Leukocyte migration inhibition of buffy coats from patients with autoimmune thrombocytopenic purpura when exposed to normal platelets: Modulation by transfer factor. Blood 63:83, 1984

66. Boughton BJ, Smith P, Fielding J, Hawker R, Wilson I, Chandler S, Howie A: Size of spleen rather than amount of platelet sequestration may determine long term responses to splenectomy in adult idiopathic thrombocytopenic purpura. J Clin Pathol 38:1172, 1985

67. Branehog I, Kutti J, Weinfeld A: Platelet survival and platelet production in idiopathic thrombocytopenic purpura (ITP). Br J Haematol 27:127, 1974

68. Branehog I: Platelet kinetics in idiopathic thrombocytopenic purpura (ITP) before and at different times after splenectomy. Br J Haematol 29:413, 1975

69. Brearley RL, Rowbotham B, Collins RJ: Changes in T-lymphocytes and response to high-dose γ-globulin therapy in idiopathic thrombocytopenic purpura. Scand J Haematol 33:482, 1984

70. Brennan MF, Rappeport JM, Maloney WC, Wilson RE: Correlation between response to corticosteroids and splenectomy for adult idiopathic thrombocytopenic purpura. Am J Surg 129:490, 1975

71. Brent LH: Sarcoidosis with thrombocytopenia. Del Med J 51:341, 1979

72. Bridges JM, Carre IJ: Congenital thrombocy-

topenic purpura during pregnancy. Obstet Gynecol 28:532, 1966

73. Buchanan GR: The nontreatment of childhood idiopathic thrombocytopenic purpura. Eur J Pediatr 146:107, 1987

74. Budd JL, Wiegers SE, O'Hara JM: Relapsing post-transfusion purpura. A preventable disease. Am J Med 78:361, 1985

75. Budde U, Auch D, Niese D, Schäfer G, Reske SN, Schmidt RE: Reticuloendothelial system Fc-receptor function in patients with immune thrombocytopenia after treatment with high dose intravenous immunoglobulin. Scand J Haematol 37:125, 1986

76. Budman DR, Steinberg AD: Hematologic aspects of systemic lupus erythematosus: Current concepts: Ann Intern Med 86:220, 1977

77. Burger T, Schmelczer M, Kett K, Kutas J: Immune thrombocytolytic purpura (ITP): Diagnosis and therapeutic survey of 86 cases with regard to the results of splenectomy and conservative therapy. Acta Med Acad Sci Hung 35:213, 1978

78. Bussel J, Pahwa S, Porges A, Cunningham-Rundles S, Koziner B, Morell A, Barandun S: Correlation of in vitro antibody synthesis with the outcome of intravenous γ-globulin treatment of chronic idiopathic thrombocytopenic purpura. J Clin Immunol 6:50, 1986

79. Bussel JB, Goldman A, Imbach P, Schulman I, Hilgartner MW: Treatment of acute idiopathic thrombocytopenia of childhood with intravenous infusions of gamma globulin. J Pediatr 106:886, 1985

80. Bussel JB, Pham LC: Intravenous treatment with gammaglobulin in adults with immune thrombocytopenic purpura: Review of the literature. Vox Sang 52:206, 1987

81. Campana D, Bergui L, Camussi G, Miniero R, Morgando MP, Sardi A, Novarino A, Cappio FC: Immune-complexes and antiplatelet antibodies in idiopathic thrombocytopenic purpura. Haematologica 68:157, 1983

82. Carloss HW, McMillan R, Crosby WH: Management of pregnancy in women with immune thrombocytopenic purpura. J Am Med Assoc 224:2756, 1980

83. Carpenter AF, Wintrobe MM, Fuller EA, Haut A, Cartwright GE: Treatment of idiopathic thrombocytopenic purpura. J Am Med Assoc 171:1911, 1959

84. Carpentieri U, Haggard ME: Thrombocytopenia and viral diseases. Tex Med 71:81, 1975

85. Carr JM, Kruskall MS, Kaye JA, Robinson SH: Efficacy of platelet transfusions in immune thrombocytopenia. Am J Med 80:1051, 1986

86. Carter RL: Platelet levels in infectious mononucleosis. Blood 24:817, 1965

87. Casey TP, Matthews JRD: Thrombocytopenic purpura in infectious mononucleosis. NZ Med J 77:318, 1973

88. Castella A, Croxson TS, Mildvan D, Witt DH, Zalusky R: The bone marrow in AIDS. A histologic, hematologic, and microbiologic study. Am J Clin Pathol 84:425, 1985

89. Chapman JF, Murphy MF, Berney SI, Ord J, Metcalfe P, Amess JAL, Waters AH: Post-transfusion purpura associated with anti-Bak[a] and anti-Pl[A2] platelet antibodies and delayed haemolytic transfusion reaction. Vox Sang 52:313, 1987

90. Chapman JF, Murphy MF, Minchinton RM, Metcalfe P, Lister TA, Waters AH: Autoimmune thrombocytopenia and neutropenia after remission induction therapy for acute leukaemia. Br J Haematol 63:693, 1986

91. Cheung N-KV, Hilgartner MW, Schulman I, McFall P, Glader BE: Platelet-associated immunoglobulin G in childhood idiopathic thrombocytopenic purpura. J Pediatr 102:366, 1983

92. Chia YC, Machin SJ: Tuberculosis and severe thrombocytopenia. Br J Clin Pract 33:55, 1979

93. Chirico G, Duse M, Ugazio AG, Rondini G: High-dose intravenous gammaglobulin therapy for passive immune thrombocytopenia in the neonate. J Pediatr 103:654, 1983

94. Chong BH, Berndt MC, Koutts J, Castaldi PA: Quinidine-induced thrombocytopenia and leukopenia: Demonstration and characterization of distinct antiplatelet and antileukocyte antibodies. Blood 62:1218, 1983

95. Chong BH, Cade J, Smith JA, Tatoulis J: An unusual case of post-transfusion purpura: Good transient response to high-dose immunoglobulin. Vox Sang 51:182, 1986

96. Chong BH, Castaldi PA: Heparin-induced thrombocytopenia: Further studies of the effects of heparin-dependent antibodies on platelets. Br J Haematol 64:347, 1986

97. Chong BH, Castaldi PA: Platelet proaggregating effect of heparin: Possible mechanism for non-immune heparin-associated thrombocytopenia. Aust NZ J Med 16:715, 1986

98. Chong BH, Grace CS, Rozenberg MC: heparin-induced thrombocytopenia: Effect of heparin platelet antibody on platelets. Br J Haematol 49:531, 1981

99. Chong BH, Pitney WR, Castaldi PA: Heparin-induced thrombocytopenia: Association of thrombotic complications with heparin-dependent IgG antibody that induced thromboxane synthesis and platelet aggregation. Lancet 2:1246, 1982

100. Christie DJ, Mullen PC, Aster RH: Fab-mediated binding of drug-dependent antibodies to platelets in quinidine- and quinine-induced thrombocytopenia. J Clin Invest 75:310, 1985

101. Christie DJ, Mullen PC, Aster RH: Quinine- and quinidine-induced platelet antibodies can react with GPIIb/GPIIIa. Br J Haematol 67:213, 1987

102. Christie DJ, Walker RH, Kolins MD, Wilner FM, Aster RH: Quinine-induced thrombocytopenia following intravenous use of heroin. Arch Intern Med 143:1174, 1983

103. Ciccimarra F, De Curtis M, Paludetto R, Romano G, Troncone R: Treatment of neonatal passive immune thrombocytopenia (letter). J Pediatr 105:677, 1984

104. Cimo P, Pisciotta AV, Desai RG, Pino JL, Aster RH: Detection of drug-dependent antibodies by the ^{51}Cr platelet lysis test: Documentation of immune thrombocytopenia induced by diphenylhydantoin, diazepam and sulfisoxazole. Am J Hematol 2:65, 1977

105. Cimo PL, Moabe JL, Weinger RS, Ben-Menachem Y, Khalil KG: Heparin-induced thrombocytopenia: Association with a platelet aggregating factor and arterial thrombosis. Am J Hematol 6:125, 1979

106. Cines DB, Dusak B, Tomaski A, Mennuti M, Schreiber AD: Immune thrombocytopenic purpura and pregnancy. N Engl J Med 306:826, 1982

107. Cines DB, Kaywin P, Bina M, Tomaski A, Schreiber AD: Heparin-associated thrombocytopenia. N Engl J Med 303:788, 1980

108. Cines DB, Schreiber AD: Immune thrombocytopenia. Use of a Coombs antiglobulin test to detect IgG and C3 on platelets. N Engl J Med 300:106, 1979

109. Cines DB, Tomaski A, Tannenbaum S: Immune endothelial-cell injury in heparin-associated thrombocytopenia. N Engl J Med 316:581, 1987

110. Cines DB, Wilson SB, Tomaski A, Schreiber AD: Platelet antibodies of the IgM class in immune thrombocytopenic purpura. J Clin Invest 75:1183, 1985

111. Claas FHJ, van Rood JJ: The interaction of drugs and endogeneous substances with HLA class I antigens. Prog Allergy 36:135, 1985

112. Clancy R: Cellular immunity to autologous platelets and serum-blocking factors in idiopathic thrombocytopenic purpura. Lancet 1:6, 1972

113. Clancy R, Jenkins E, Firkin B: Qualitative platelet abnormalities in idiopathic thrombocytopenic purpura. N Engl J Med 286:622, 1972

114. Clarkson SB, Bussel JB, Kimberly RP, Valinsky JE, Nachman RL, Unkeless JC: Treatment of refractory immune thrombocytopenic purpura with an anti-Fc γ-receptor antibody. N Engl J Med 314:1236, 1986

115. Coblyn JS, Weinblatt M, Holdsworth D, Glass D: Gold-induced thrombocytopenia: A clinical and immunogenetic study of twenty-three patients. Ann Intern Med 95:178, 1981

116. Cohn J: Thrombocytopenia in childhood: An evaluation of 433 patients. Scand J Haematol 16:226, 1976

117. Collins J, Aster RH: Use of immobilized platelet glycoproteins for detection of platelet-specific alloantibodies in ELISA. Vox Sang, 53:157, 1987

118. Conley CL: Idiopathic thrombocytopenic purpura (letter). Arch Intern Med 146:1244, 1986

119. Connellan JM, Quinn M, Wiley JS: The use of ^{125}I-labelled staphylococcal protein A in the diagnosis of autoimmune thrombocytopenic purpura and other immune mediated thrombocytopenias. pathology 18:111, 1986

120. Copplestone A, Oscier DG: Heparin-induced thrombocytopenia in pregnancy (letter). Br J Haematol 65:248, 1987

121. Costello C, Treacy M, Lai L: Treatment of immune thrombocytopenic purpura in homosexual men. Scand J Haematol 36:507, 1986

122. Court WS, Bozeman JM, Soong S-J, Saleh MN, Shaw DR, LoBuglio AF: Platelet surface-bound IgG in patients with immune and nonimmune thrombocytopenia. Blood 69:278, 1987

123. Cuthbert MD: Adverse reactions to non-steroidal antirheumatic drugs. Curr Med Res Opin 2:600, 1974

124. Daffos F, Forestier F, Muller JY, Reznikoff-Etievant MJ, Habibi B, Capella-Pavlovsky M, Maigret M, Kaplan C: Prenatal treatment of alloimmune thrombocytopenia. Lancet 2:632, 1984

125. Dameshek W, Ebbe S, Greenberg L, Baldini M: Recurrent idiopathic thrombocytopenic purpura. N Engl J Med 269:647, 1963

126. Dammacco F, Iodice G, Campobasso N: Treatment of adult patients with idiopathic thrombocytopenic purpura with intravenous immunoglobulin: Effects on circulating T cell subsets and PWM-induced antibody synthesis in vitro. Br J Haematol 62:125, 1986

127. Davis HH II, Varki A, Andrew Heaton A, Siegel BA: Detection of accessory spleens with indium^{111}-labeled autologous platelets. Am J Hematol 8:81, 1980

128. Deaver JE, Leppert PC, Zaroulis CG: Neonatal alloimmune thrombocytopenic purpura. Am J Perinatol 3:127, 1986

129. Delfraissy JF, Tchernia G, Laurian Y, Wallon C, Galanaud P, Dormont J: Suppressor cell function after intravenous gammaglobulin treatment in adult chronic idiopathic thrombocytopenic purpura. Br J Haematol 60:315, 1985

130. Delfraissy JF, Tertian G, Dreyfus M, Tchernia G: Intravenous gammaglobulin, thrombocyto-

penia, and the acquired immunodeficiency syndrome. Ann Intern Med 103:478, 1985

131. Denman EJ, Denman AM: The lymphocyte transformation test and gold hypersensitivity. Ann Rheum Dis 27:582, 1968

132. den Ottolander GJ, Gratama JW, de Koning J, Brand A: Long-term follow-up study of 168 patients with immune thrombocytopenia. Implications for therapy. Scand J Haematol 32:101, 1984

133. Deren B, Masi R, Weksler M, Nachman RL: Gold-associated thrombocytopenia. Arch Intern Med 134:1012, 1974

134. Derycke M, Dreyfus M, Ropert JC, Tchernia G: Intravenous immunoglobulin for neonatal isoimmune thrombocytopenia. Arch Dis Child 60:667, 1985

135. Devine DV, Currie MS, Rosse WF, Greenberg CS: Pseudo-Bernard-Soulier syndrome: Thrombocytopenia caused by autoantibody to platelet glycoprotein Ib. Blood 70:428, 1987

136. DeWaal LP, van Dalen CM, Engelfriet CP, von dem Borne AEG Kr: Alloimmunization against the platelet-specific Zw^a antigen resulting in neonatal alloimmune thrombocytopenic purpura or posttransfusion purpura is associated with the supertypic DRw52 antigen including DR3 and DRw6. Hum Immunol 17:45, 1986

137. DiFino SM, Lachant NA, Kirshner JJ, Gottleib AJ: Adult idiopathic thrombocytopenic purpura. Clinical findings and response to therapy. Am J Med 69:430, 1980

138. DiMinno G, Coraggio F, Cerbone AM, Capitanio AM, Manzo C, Spina M, Scarpato P, Dattoli GMR, Mattioli PL, Mancini M: A myeloma paraprotein with specificity for platelet glycoprotein IIIa in a patient with a fatal bleeding disorder. J Clin Invest 77:157, 1986

139. Dixon R, Rosse W, Ebbert L: Quantitative determination of antibody in idiopathic thrombocytopenic purpura. N Engl J Med 292:230, 1975

140. Donahue RE, Johnson MM, Zon LI, Clark SC, Groopman JE: Suppression of in vitro haematopoiesis following human immunodeficiency virus infection. Nature 326:200, 1987

141. Donaldson GWK, Parker AC, McArthur M, Richmond J: Thrombocytopenic purpura with normal platelet survival time. J Clin Pathol 24:621, 1971

142. Doughty R, James V, Magee J: An enzyme linked immunosorbent assay for leucocyte and platelet antibodies. J Immunol Methods 47:161, 1981

143. Dunn NL, Maurer HM: Prednisone treatment of acute idiopathic thrombocytopenic purpura of childhood. Am J Pediatr Hematol Oncol 6:159, 1984

144. Dunstan RA, Simpson MB: Heterogeneous distribution of antigens on human platelets demonstrated by fluorescence flow cytometry. Br J Haematol 61:603, 1985

145. Durand JM, Harle JR, Verdot JJ, Weiller PJ, Mongin M: Anti-**Rh**(D) immunoglobulin for immune thrombocytopenic purpura (letter). Lancet 2:49, 1986

146. Eika C, Godal HC, Laake K, Hamborg T: Low incidence of thrombocytopenia during treatment with hog mucosa and beef lung heparin. Scand J Haematol 25:19, 1980

147. Eisner EV, Crowell EB: Hydrochlorothiazide-dependent thrombocytopenia due to IgM antibody. J Am Med Assoc 215:480, 1971

148. Eisner EV, Kasper K: Immune thrombocytopenia due to a metabolite of para-aminosalicylic acid. Am J Med 53:709, 1972

149. Eisner EV, Shaidi NT: Immune thrombocytopenia due to a drug metabolite. N Engl J Med 287:376, 1972

150. Ellman L, Carvallo A, Jacobson BM, Colman RW: Platelet autoantibody in a case of infectious mononucleosis presenting as thrombocytopenic purpura. Am J Med 55:723, 1973

151. El-Khateeb MS, Awidi AS, Tarawneh MS, Abu-Khalaf M: HLA antigens, blood groups and immunoglobulin levels in idiopathic thrombocytopenic purpura. Acta Haematol 76:110, 1986

152. Emilia G, Sacchi S, Torelli G, Selleri L, Torelli U: Low-dose intravenous pepsin-treated gamma-globulin for idiopathic thrombocytopenic purpura in adults (letter). Br J Haematol 58:761, 1984

153. Emmerich B, Hiller E, Woitinas F, Maubach PA, Riess H, Nerl C, Geursen RG. Dose-response relationship in the treatment of idiopathic thrombocytopenic purpura with intravenous immunoglobulin. Klin Wochenschr 65:369, 1987

154. Engelhard D, Waner JL, Kapoor N, Good RA: Effect of intravenous immune globulin on natural killer cell activity: Possible association with autoimmune neutropenia and idiopathic thrombocytopenia. J Pediatr 108:77, 1986

155. Erb BD: Thrombocytopenic purpura accompanying brucellosis: A case report with demonstration of a granuloma in the bone marrow. J Tenn Med Assoc 59:876, 1966

156. Evans DIK: Immune amegakaryocytic thrombocytopenia of the newborn: Association with anti-HLA-A2. J Clin Pathol 40:258, 1987

157. Evers K-G, Thouet R, Haase W, Kruger J: HLA frequencies and haplotypes in children with idiopathic thrombocytopenic purpura (ITP). Eur J Pediatr 129:267, 1978

158. Eyster ME, Gail MH, Ballard JO, Al-Mondhiry H, Goedert JJ: Natural history of human immunodeficiency virus infections in hemophiliacs: Effects of T-cell subsets, platelet counts, and age. Ann Intern Med 107:1, 1987

159. Eyster ME, Whitehurst DA, Catalano PM, McMillan CW, Goodnight SH, Kasper CK, Gill JC, Aledort LM, Hilgartner MW, Levine PH, Edson JR, Hathaway WE, Lusher JM, Gill FM, Poole WK, Shapiro SS: Long-term follow-up of hemophiliacs with lymphocytopenia or thrombocytopenia. Blood 66:1317, 1985

160. Fabris F, Casonato A, Crociani E, Zanchetta R, Busolo F, Girolami A: A new ELISA method for the detection of serum bindable anti-platelet antibodies (SPBIG). Clin Chim Acta 146:223, 1985

161. Fabris F, Casonato A, Randi ML, Luzzatto G, Girolami A: Clinical significance of surface and internal pools of platelet-associated immunoglobulins in immune thrombocytopenia. Scand J Haematol 37:215, 1986

162. Faig D, Karpatkin S: Cumulative experience with a simplified solid-phase radioimmunoassay for the detection of bound antiplatelet IgG, serum auto-, allo-, and drug-dependent antibodies. Blood 60:807, 1982

163. Fasola GP, Dosualdo F, Depanghe V, Barducci E: Thrombocytopenia and mexiletine (letter). Ann Intern Med 100:162, 1984

164. Fehr J, Hofmann V, Kappeler U: Transiet reversal of thrombocytopenia in idiopathic thrombocytopenic purpura by high-dose intravenous gamma globulin. N Engl J Med 306:1254, 1982

165. Field SK, Poon M-C: Sarcoidosis presenting as chronic thrombocytopenia. West J Med 156:481, 1987

166. Finch SC, Castro O, Cooper M, Covery W, Erickson R, McPhedran P: Immunosuppressive therapy of chronic idiopathic thrombocytopenic purpura. Am J Med 56:4, 1974

167. Fireman Z, Yust I, Abramov AL: Lethal occult pulmonary hemorrhage in drug-induced thrombocytopenia (Technical Note). Chest 79:358, 1981

168. First LR, Smith BR, Lipton J, Nathan DG, Parkman R, Rappeport JM: isolated thrombocytopenia after allogeneic bone marrow transplantation: Existence of transient and chronic thrombocytopenic syndromes. Blood 65:368, 1985

169. Fitchen JH, Koeffler HP: Cimetidine and granulopoiesis: Bone marrow culture studies in normal man and patients with cimetidine-associated neutropenia. Br J Haematol 46:361, 1980

170. Fitzgerald G, McCarthy D, O'Connell LG, McCann SR: Hyperimmune thrombocytopenia and pregnancy treated by splenectomy. Acta Haematol 59:315, 1978

171. Follea G, Hamandjian I, Trzeciak M-C, Nedey C, Streichenberger R, Dechavanne M: Pentosane polysulphate associated thrombocytopenia. Thromb Res 42:413, 1986

172. Follea G, Mandrand B, Dechavanne M: Simultaneous enzymo-immunologic assays of platelet associated IgG, IgM and C_3. A useful tool in assessment of immune thrombocytopenias. Thromb Res 26:249, 1982

173. Follea G, Souillet G, Clerc M, Philippe N, Bordet JC, Dechavanne M: Intravenous plasmin-treated gammaglobulin therapy in idiopathic thrombocytopenic purpura. Nouv Rev Fr Hematol 27:5, 1985

174. Freedman J, Cheong T, Garvey MB: Use of the indirect platelet radioactive antiglobulin test with anti-IgG and anti-C3 in immune and nonimmune thrombocytopenias. Am J Hematol 18:297, 1985

175. Friedman JM, Aster RH: Neonatal alloimmune thrombocytopenic purpura with congenital porencephaly in two siblings associated with a "new" maternal antiplatelet antibody. Blood 65:1412, 1985

176. Furihata K, Nugent DJ, Aster RH, Kunicki TJ: Anti-Pen^a binds specifically to an epitope on platelet glycoprotein IIIa. Blood 68(Suppl 1):107a, 1986

177. Furihata K, Nugent D, Bissonette A, Aster RH, Kunicki TJ: On the association of the platelet-specific alloantigen, Pen^a, with glycoprotein IIIa. J Clin Invest 80:1624, 1987

178. Gafter U, Komlos L, Weinstein T, Zevin D, Levi J: Thrombocytopenia, eosinophilia, and ranitidine (letter). Ann Intern Med 106:477, 1987

179. Galea P, Patrick MJ, Goel KM: Isoimmune neonatal thrombocytopenic purpura. Arch Dis Child 56:112, 1981

180. Garnick MB, Griffin JD: Idiopathic thrombocytopenia in association with extragonadal germ cell cancer. Ann Intern Med 98:926, 1983

181. Gengozian N, McLaughlin CL: IgG^+ platelets in the marmoset: Their induction, maintenance, and survival. Blood 55:885, 1980

182. George JN, Thoi LL, McManus LM, Reimann TA: Isolation of human platelet membrane microparticles from plasma and serum. Blood 60:834, 1982

183. Gerstner JB, Smith MJ, Davis KD, Cimo PL, Aster RH: Post-transfusion purpura: Therapeutic failure of Pl^{A1}-negative platelet transfusion. Am J Hematol 6:71, 1979

184. Ghosh MI: Long-term effect of vincristine in chronic idiopathic thrombocytopenic purpura (ITP). J Ir Med Assoc 69:167, 1976

185. Glud TK, Rosthøj S, Jensen MK et al:

High-dose intravenous immunoglobulin for post-transfusion purpura. Scand J Haematol 31:495, 1983

186. Goebel KM, Hahn E, Havemann K: HLA matching in autoimmune thrombocytopenic purpura. Br J Haematol 35:341, 1977

187. Goldsweig HG, Grossman R, William D: Thrombocytopenia in homosexual men. Am J Hematol 21:243, 1986

188. Gottschall, JL, Collins J, Kunicki TJ, Nash R, Aster RH: Effect of hemolysis on apparent values of platelet-associated IgG. Am J Clin Pathol 87:218, 1987

188. Gratama JW, D'Amaro J, de Koning J, den Ottolander GJ: The HLA-system in immune thrombocytopenic purpura: Its relation to the outcome of therapy. Br J Haematol 56:287, 1984

189. Gratama JW, D'Amaro J, de Koning J, den Ottolander GJ: The HLA-system in immune thrombocytopenic purpura: Its relation to the outcome of therapy. Br J Haematol 56:287, 1984

190. Green D: Heparin-induced thrombocytopenia. Med J Aust 144(Suppl):HS37, 1986

191. Green PJ, Nagrosea SM: Nomifensine and thrombocytopenia (Technical Note). Br Med J 288:830, 1984

192. Grenet P, Dausset J, Dugas M, Petit D, Badoual J, Tangun Y: Purpura thrombopenique neonatal avec isoimmunisation foeto-maternelle anti-Ko[a]. Arch Fr Pediatr 22:1165, 1965

193. Gross S, Worthington-White DA: Cimetidine suppression of CFU-C in males. Am J Hematol 17:279, 1984

194. Grossi A, Vannucchi AM, Casprini P, Guidi S, Rafanelli D, Pecchioli MG, Ferrini PR: Different patterns of platelet turnover in chronic idiopathic thrombocytopenic purpura. Scand J Haematol 31:206, 1983

195. Gugliotta L, Isacchi G, Guarini A, Ciccone F, Motta MR, Lattarini C, Bachetti G, Mazzucconi MG, Baccarani M, Mandelli F, Tura S: Chronic idiopathic thrombocytopenic purpura (ITP): Site of platelet sequestration and results of splenectomy. A study of 197 patients. Scand J Haematol 26:407, 1981

196. Gupta S, Saverymuttu SH, Marsh JCW, Hodgson HJF, Chadwick VS: Immune thrombocytopenic purpura, neutropenia and sclerosing cholangitis associated with ulcerative colitis in an adult. Clin Lab Haematol 8:67, 1986

197. Guthrie TH, Pallas CW, Squires JE: Quinidine-induced thrombocytopenia successfully treated with plasma exchange. Plasma Ther Transfusion Technol 5:361, 1984

198. Hall S, McCormick JL, Greipp PR, Michet CJ, McKenna CH: Splenectomy does not cure the thrombocytopenia of systemic lupus erythematosus. Ann Intern Med 102:325, 1985

199. Handin RI, Stossel TP: Effect of corticosteroid therapy on the phagocytosis of antibody-coated platelets by human leukocytes. Blood 51:771, 1978

200. Hansen S, Järhult J: Accessory spleen imaging. Radionuclide, ultrasound and CT investigations in a patient with thrombocytopenia 25 yr after splenectomy for ITP. Scand J Haematol 37:74, 1986

201. Harker LA: Thrombokinetics in idiopathic thrombocytopenic purpura. Br J Haematol 19:95, 1970

202. Harrington WJ, Minnich V, Hollingsworth JW, Moore CV: Demonstration of a thrombocytopenic factor in the blood of patients with thrombocytopenic purpura. J Lab Clin Med 38:1, 1951

203. Harrington WJ, Sprague CC, Minnich V, Moore CV, Aulvin RC, Dubach R: Immunologic mechanisms in idiopathic and neonatal thrombocytopenic purpura. Ann Intern Med 38:433, 1953

204. Harris EN, Asherson RA, Gharavi AE, Morgan SH, Derue G, Hughes GRV: Thrombocytopenia in SLE and related autoimmune disorders: Association with anticardiolipin antibody. Br J Haematol 59:227, 1985

205. Harris EN, Gharavi AE, Hegde U, Derue G, Morgan SH, Englert H, Chan JKH, Asherson RA, Hughes GRV: Anticardiolipin antibodies in autoimmune thrombocytopenic purpura. Br J Haematol 59:231, 1985

206. Harris PJ, Kessler CM, Lessin LS: Acquired hemolytic anemia and thrombocytopenia (Evans' syndrome) in hemophilia (letter). N Engl J Med 309:50, 1983

207. Hart D, Dunetz C, Nardi M, Porges RF, Weiss A, Karpatkin M: An epidemic of maternal thrombocytopenia associated with elevated antiplatelet antibody. Am J Obstet Gynecol 154:878, 1986

208. Haubenstock A, Zalusky R: Autoimmune hyperthyroidism and thrombocytopenia developing in a patient with chronic lymphocytic leukemia. Am J Hematol 19:281, 1985

209. Hauch TW, Rosse WF: Platelet-bound complement (C3) in immune thrombocytopenia. Blood 50:1129, 1977

210. Heeger PS, Backstrom JT: Heparin flushes and thrombocytopenia (letter). Ann Intern Med 105:143, 1986

211. Hegde UM: Immune thrombocytopenia in pregnancy and the newborn (letter). Br J Obstet Gynaecol 92:657, 1985

212. Hegde UM, Ball S, Zuiable A, Roter BLT: Platelet associated immunoglobulins (PAIgG and PAIgM) in autoimmune thrombocytopenia. Br J Haematol 59:221, 1985

213. Hegde UM, Bowes A, Powell DK, Joyner MV: Detection of platelet-bound and serum antibodies in autoimmune thrombocytopenia by enzyme-linked assay. Vox Sang 41:306, 1981

214. Hegde UM, Bowes A, Roter BLT: Platelet associated complement components (PAC_{3c} and PAC_{3d}) in patients with autoimmune thrombocytopenia. Br J Haematol 60:49, 1985

215. Hegde UM, Zuiable A, Ball S, Roter BLT: The relative incidence of idiopathic and secondary autoimmune thrombocytopenia: A clinical and serological evaluation in 508 patients. Clin Lab Haematol 7:7, 1985

216. Herbst KD, Store WH, Flannery EP: Chronic thrombocytopenia following gold therapy. Arch Intern Med 135:1622, 1975

217. Herman J, Resnitzky P, Fink A: Association between thyroxicosis and thrombocytopenia. Isr J Med Sci 14:469, 1978

218. Herman JH, Jumbelic MI, Ancona RJ, Kickler TS: In utero cerebral hemorrhage in alloimmune thrombocytopenia. Am J Pediatr Hematol Oncol 8:312, 1986

219. Hesdorffer CS, Weltman MD, Raftopoulos H, Mendelow B, Bezwoda WR: Thrombocytopenia caused by isotretinoin (letter). S Afr Med J 70:705, 1986

220. Hess T, Riesen W, Scholtysik G, Stucki P: Digitoxin intoxication with severe thrombocytopenia: Reversal by digoxin-specific antibodies. Eur J Clin Invest 13:159, 1983

221. Heyns A DuP, Fraser J, Retief FP: Platelet aggregation in chronic idiopathic thrombocytopenic purpura. J Clin Pathol 31:1239, 1978

222. Heyns A DuP, Badenhorst PN, Lötter MG, Pieters H, Wessels P, Kotzé HF: Platelet turnover and kinetics in immune thrombocytopenic purpura: Results with autologous ^{111}In-labeled platelets and homologous ^{51}Cr-labeled platelets differ. Blood 67:86, 1986

223. Heyns A duP, Lötter MG, Badenhorst PN, de Kock F, Pieters H, Herbst C, van Reenen OR, Kotze H, Minnaar PC: Kinetics and sites of destruction of ^{111}indium-oxine-labeled platelets in idiopathic thrombocytopenic purpura: A quantitative study. Am J Hematol 12:167, 1982

224. Heys RF: Child bearing and idiopathic thrombocytopenic purpura. J Obstet Gynaecol Br Commonw 73:205, 1966

225. Hirschman RJ, Shulman NR: The use of platelet serotonin release as a sensitive method for detecting anti-platelet antibodies and a plasma anti-platelet factor in patients with idiopathic thrombocytopenic purpura. Br J Haematol 24:793, 1973

226. Hoffman R, Zaknoen S, Yang HH, Bruno E, LoBuglio AF, Arrowsmith JB, Prchal JT: An antibody cytotoxic to megakaryocyte progenitor cells in a patient with immune thrombocytopenic purpura. N Engl J Med 312:1170, 1985

227. Holzman RS, Walsh CM, Karpatkin S: Risk for the acquired immunodeficiency syndrome among thrombocytopenic and nonthrombocytopenic homosexual men seropositive for the human immunodeficiency virus. Ann Intern Med 106:383, 1987

228. Hom BL Belles Q, Oishi N: Splenic histiocytosis in idiopathic thrombocytopenic purpura: A relative sphingomyelinase deficiency? Hum Pathol 16:1175, 1985

229. Homan WP, Dineen P: The role of splenectomy in the treatment of thrombocytopenic purpura due to systemic lupus erythematosus. Ann Surg 187:52, 1978

230. Hoots WK, Huntington D, Devine D, Schmidt C, Bracey A: Aggressive combination therapy in the successful management of life-threatening intracranial hemorrhage in a patient with idiopathic thrombocytopenic purpura. Am J Pediatr Hematol Oncol 8:225, 1986

231. Horrow JC: Clinical Report. Thrombocytopenia accompanying a reaction to protamine sulfate. Can Anaesth Soc J 32:49, 1985

232. Hotchkiss AJ, Leissinger CA, Smith ME, Jordan JV, Kautz CA, Shulman NR: Evaluation by quantitative acid elution and radioimmunoassay of multiple classes of immunoglobulins and serum albumin associated with platelets in idiopathic thrombocytopenic purpura. Blood 67:1126, 1986

233. Howard M, Firkin BG: The effect of ristocetin on platelet-rich plasma. J Aust Soc Med Res 2:195, 1968

234. Howe SE, Lynch DM, Lynch JM: An enzyme-linked immunosorbent assay for the quantification of serum platelet-bindable IgG. Transfusion 24:348, 1984

235. Humbert JR, Sills R: Controversies in treatment of idiopathic thrombocytopenic purpura in children. Am J Pediatr Hematol Oncol 6:147, 1984

236. Hymes K, Blum M, Lackner H, Karpatkin S: Easy bruising, thrombocytopenia, and elevated platelet immunoglobulin G in Graves' disease and Hashimoto's thyroiditis. Ann Intern Med 94:27, 1981

237. Hymes K, Shulman S, Karpatkin S: A solid-phase radioimmunoassay for bound anti-platelet antibody. Studies on 45 patients with autoimmune platelet disorders. J Lab Clin Med 94:639, 1979

238. Imbach P, Berchtold W, Hirt A, Mueller-Eckhardt C, Rossi E, Wagner HP, Gaedicke G, Joller P, Müller B, Barandun S: Intravenous immunoglobulin versus oral corticosteroids in acute immune thrombocytopenic purpura in childhood. Lancet 2:464, 1985

239. Imbach P, D'Apuzzo V, Hirt A, Rossi E, Vest M, Barandun S, Baumgartner C, Morell A, Schöni M, Wagner HP: High-dose intravenous gamma-globulin for idiopathic thrombocytopenic purpura in childhood. Lancet 1:1228, 1981

240. Jacobs P, Wood L, Dent DM: Splenectomy and the thrombocytopenia of systemic lupus erythematosus. Ann Intern Med 105:97, 1986

241. Jennings LK, Ashmun RA, Wang WC, Dockter ME: Analysis of human platelet glycoproteins IIb–IIIa and Glanzmann's thrombasthenia in whole blood by flow cytometry. Blood 68:173, 1986

242. Jones RW, Innes Asher M, Rutherford CJ, Munro HM: Autoimmune (idiopathic) thrombocytopenic purpura in pregnancy and the newborn. Br J Obstet Gynaecol 84:679, 1977

243. Kaden BR, Rosse WF, Hauch TW: Immune thrombocytopenia in lymphoproliferative diseases. Blood 53:545, 1979

244. Kappa JR, Cottrell ED, Berkowitz HD, Fisher CA, Sobel M, Ellison N, Addonizio VP: Carotid endarterectomy in patients with heparin-induced platelet activation: Comparative efficacy of aspirin and iloprost (ZK36374). J Vasc Surg 5:693, 1987

245. Kappers-Klunne MC, van Vliet HHDM: IgM and IgG platelet antibodies in a case of infectious mononucleosis and severe thrombocytopenia. Scand J Haematol 32:145, 1984

246. Karachalios GN, Parigorakis JG: Thrombocytopenia and sulindac (letter). Ann Intern Med 104:128, 1986

247. Karpatkin M: Clinical and laboratory observations. Corticosteroid therapy in thrombocytopenic infants of women with autoimmune thrombocytopenia. J Pediatr 105:623, 1984

248. Karpatkin M, Forges RF, Karpatkin S: Platelet counts in infants of women with autoimmune thrombocytopenia: Effect of steroid administration to the mother. N Engl J Med 305:936, 1981

249. Karpatkin M, Karpatkin S: Immune thrombocytopenia in children. Am J Pediatr Hematol Oncol 3:213, 1981

250. Karpatkin M, Porges RF, Karpatkin S: Platelet counts in infants of women with autoimmune thrombocytopenia. Effect of steroid administration to the mother. N Engl J Med 305:936, 1981

251. Karpatkin M, Siskind GW, Karpatkin S: The platelet factor 3 immunoinjury technique reevaluated: Development of a rapid test for antiplatelet antibody: Detection in various clinical disorders, including immunologic drug-induced and neonatal thrombocytopenias. J Lab Clin Med 82:400, 1977

252. Karpatkin S: Autoimmune thrombocytopenic purpura. Semin Hematol 22:260, 1985

253. Karpatkin S: Drug-induced thrombocytopenia. Am J Med Sci 262:68, 1971

254. Karpatkin S, Fotino M, Gibofsky A, Winchester RJ: Association of HLA-DRw2 with autoimmune thrombocytopenic purpura. J Clin Invest 63:1085, 1979

255. Karpatkin S, Fotino M, Winchester R: Hereditary autoimmune thrombocytopenic purpura: An immunologic and genetic study. Ann Intern Med 94:781, 1981

256. Karpatkin S, Struck N, Siskind GW: Detection of splenic anti-platelet antibody synthesis idiopathic autoimmune thrombocytopenic purpura (ATP). Br J Haematol 23:167, 1972

257. Katz J, Hodder FS, Aster RS, Bennetts GA, Cairo MS: Neonatal isoimmune thrombocytopenia. Clin Pediatr 23:159, 1984

258. Kay A: Depression of bone marrow and thrombocytopenia associated with chrysotherapy. Ann Rheum Dis 32:277, 1973

259. Kayser W, Mueller-Eckhardt C, Bhakdi S, Ebert K: Platelet-associated complement C3 in thrombocytopenic states. Br J Haematol 54:353, 1983

260. Kayser W, Mueller-Eckhardt C, Mueller-Eckhardt G: The value of platelet-associated IgG in predicting the efficacy of splenectomy in autoimmune thrombocytopenia. Scand J Haematol 30:30, 1983

261. Kazatchkine MD, Lambré CR, Kieffer N, Maillet F, Nurden AT: Membrane-bound hemagglutinin mediates antibody and complement-dependent lysis of influenza virus-treated human platelets in autologous serum. J Clin Invest 74:976, 1984

262. Keimowitz RM, Collins J, Davis K, Aster RH: Posttransfusion purpura associated with alloimmunization against the platelet-specific antigen, Bak[a]. Am J Hematol 21:79, 1986

263. Kelsey PR, Schofield KP, Geary CG: Refractory idiopathic thrombocytopenic purpura (ITP) treated with cyclosporine (letter). Br J Haematol 60:197, 1985

264. Kelton JG: Heparin-induced thrombocytopenia. Haemostasis 16:173, 1986

265. Kelton JG: Management of the pregnant patient with idiopathic thrombocytopenic purpura. Ann Intern Med 99:796, 1983

266. Kelton JG, Blanchette VS, Wilson WE, Powers P, Mohan Pai KR, Effer SB, Barr RD: Neonatal thrombocytopenia due to passive immunization. N Engl J Med 302:1401, 1980

267. Kelton JG, Carter CJ, Rodger C, Bebenek G, Gauldie J, Sheridan D, Kassam YB, Kean WF, Buchanan WW, Rooney PJ, Bianchi F, Denburg J: The relationship among platelet-associated IgG platelet lifespan, and reticuloendothelial cell function. Blood 63:1434, 1984

268. Kelton JG, Inwood MJ, Barr RM, Effer SB, Hunter D, Wilson WE, Ginsburg DA, Powers PJ:

The prenatal prediction of thrombocytopenia in infants of mothers with clinically diagnosed immune thrombocytopenia. Am J Obstet Gynecol 144:449, 1982

269. Kelton JG, Levine MN: Heparin-induced thrombocytopenia. Semin Thromb Hemostas 12:59, 1986

270. Kelton JG, Meltzer D, Moore J, Giles AR, Wilson WE, Barr R, Hirsch, Neame PB, Powers PJ, Walker I, Bianchi F, Carter CJ: Drug-induced thrombocytopenia is associated with increased binding of IgG to platelets both in vivo and in vitro. Blood 58:524, 1981

271. Kelton JG, Moore J, Gauldie J, Neame PB, Hirsh J, Tozman E: The development and application of a serum assay for platelet-bindable IgG (S-PBIgG). J Lab Clin Med 98:272, 1981

272. Kelton JG, Powers PJ, Carter CJ: A prospective study of the usefulness of the measurement of platelet-associated IgG for the diagnosis of idiopathic thrombocytopenic purpura. Blood 60:1050, 1982

273. Kelton JG, Sheridan D, Brain H, Powers PJ, Turpie AG, Carter CJ: Clinical usefulness of testing for a heparin-dependent platelet-aggregating factor in patients with suspected heparin-associated thrombocytopenia. J Lab Clin Med 103:606, 1984

274. Kelton JG, Sheridan D, Neame PB, Simon GT: Platelet fragments do not contribute to elevated levels of platelet associated IgG. Br J Haematol 61:707, 1985

275. Kelton JG, Smith JW, Santos AV, Murphy WG, Horsewood P: Platelet IgG Fc receptor. Am J Hematol 25:299, 1987

276. Kelton JG, Steeves K: The amount of platelet-bound albumin parallels the amount of IgG on washed platelets from patients with immune thrombocytopenia. Blood 62:924, 1983

277. Kelton JG, McDonald JWD, Barr RM, Walker I, Nicholson W, Neame PB, Hamid C, Wong TY, Hirsh J: The reversible binding of vinblastine to platelets: Implications for therapy. Blood 57:431, 1981

278. Kernoff LM, Blake CH, Shackleton D: Influence of the amount of platelet-bound IgG on platelet survival and site of sequestration in autoimmune thrombocytopenia. Blood 55:730, 1980

279. Kernoff LM, Malan E: Platelet antibody levels do not correlate with response to therapy in idiopathic thrombocytopenic purpura. Br J Haematol 53:559, 1983

280. Kernoff LM, Malan E, Gunston K: Neonatal thrombocytopenia complicating autoimmune thrombocytopenia in pregnancy. Ann Intern Med 90:56, 1979

281. Khaleeli AA: Quinaband-induced thrombocytopenia purpura in a patient with myxoedema coma. Br Med J 2:562, 1976

282. Khan I, Zucker-Franklin D, Karpatkin S: Microthrombocytosis and platelet fragmentation associated with idiopathic/autoimmune thrombocytopenic purpura. Br J Haematol 31:449, 1975

283. Kickler TS, Furihata K, Kunicki TJ, Herman JH, Aster RH: A new platelet alloantigen allelic to Bak[a] and its association with post-transfusion purpura (abstr). Blood 68(Suppl 1):111a, 1986

284. Kickler TS, Ness PM, Herman JH, Bell WR: Studies on the pathophysiology of post-transfusion purpura. Blood 68:347, 1986

285. Kiefel V, Becker TH, Mueller-Eckhardt G, Grebe S, Mueller-Eckhardt C: Platelet survival determined with ^{51}Cr versus ^{111}In. Klin Wochenschr 63:84, 1985

286. Kiefel V, Santoso S, Schmidt S, Salama A, Mueller-Eckhardt C: Metabolite-specific (IgG) and drug-specific antibodies (IgG, IgM) in two cases of trimethoprim-sulfamethoxazol-induced immune thrombocytopenia. Transfusion 27:262, 1987

287. Kiefel V, Spaeth P, Mueller-Eckhardt C: Immune thrombocytopenic purpura: Autoimmune or immune complex disease? Br J Haematol 64:57, 1986

288. Kieffer N, Boizard B, Didry D, Wautier JL, Nurden AT: Immunochemical characterization of the platelet-specific alloantigen Lek[a] a comparative study with the Pl[A1] alloantigen. Blood 64:1212, 1984

289. Kiers L, Grigg LE, Cade JF, Street PR, Chong BH: Use of ORG 10172 in the treatment of heparin-induced thrombocytopenia and thrombosis (letter). Aust NZ J Med 16:719, 1986

290. Kim HD, Boggs DR: A syndrome resembling idiopathic thrombocytopenic purpura in 10 patients with diverse forms of cancer. Am J Med 67:371, 1979

291. King DJ, Kelton JG: Heparin-associated thrombocytopenia. Ann Intern Med 100:535, 1984

292. King FM, Harsock RJ: Histochemical identification of lipid in spleens of patients with idiopathic thrombocytopenic purpura. Am J Clin Pathol 49:250, 1968

293. Kinney EL, Ballard JO, Carlin B, Zelis R: Amrinone-mediated thrombocytopenia. Scand J Haematol 31:376, 1983

294. Kirshner JJ, Zamkoff KW, Gottleib AJ: Idiopathic thrombocytopenic purpura and Hodgkin's disease: Report of two cases and a review of the literature. Am J Med Sci 280:21, 1980

295. Knodel AR, Beekman JF: Severe thrombocytopenia and sarcoidosis. J Am Med Assoc 243:258, 1980

296. Korninger C, Panzer S, Graninger W, Neumann E, Niessner H, Lechner K, Deutsch E: Treatment of severe chronic idiopathic thrombocyto-

penic purpura in adults with high-dose intravenous gamma-globulin. Scand J Haematol 34:128, 1985

297. Kosmo MA, Bordin G, Tani P, McMillan R: Immune thrombocytopenia and Crohn's disease (letter). Ann Intern Med 104:136, 1986

298. Kozloff M, Votaw M, Penner JA: Gold-induced thrombocytopenia responsive to cyclophosphamide. South Med J 72:1490, 1979

299. Kramer MR, Levene C, Hershko C: Severe reversible autoimmune haemolytic anaemia and thrombocytopenia associated with diclofenac therapy. Case Report. Scand J Haematol 36:118, 1986

300. Krivit W, Tate D, White JG, Robinson LL: Idiopathic thrombocytopenic purpura and intracranial hemorrhage. Pediatrics 67:570, 1981

301. Kulis JC: Chemically induced selective thrombocytopenic purpura. Arch Intern Med 116:559, 1965

302. Kunicki TJ, Aster RH: Isolation and immunologic characterization of the human platelet alloantigen, Pl^{A1}. Mol Immunol 16:353, 1979

303. Kunicki TJ, Aster RH: Qualitative and quantitative tests for platelet alloantibodies and drug-dependent antibodies. In McMillan R (ed): Immune Cytopenias. New York, Churchill-Livingston, 1983

304. Kunicki TJ, Koenig MB, Kristopeit SM, Aster RH: Direct quantitation of platelet-associated IgG by electroimmunoassay. Blood 60:54, 1982

305. Kunicki TJ, Russell N, Nurden AT, Aster RH, Caen JP: Further studies of the human platelet receptor for quinine- and quinidine-dependent antibodies. J Immunol 126:398, 1981

306. Kurata Y, Curd JG, Tamerius JD, McMillan R: Platelet-associated complement in chronic ITP. Br J Haematol 60:723, 1985

307. Kurata Y, Hayashi S, Aochi H, Nagamine K, Oshida M, Mizutani H, Tomiyama Y, Tsubakio T, Yonezawa T, Tarui S: Analysis of antigen involved in circulating immune complexes in patients with idiopathic thrombocytopenic purpura. Clin Exp Immunol 67:293, 1987

308. Kurata Y, Nishioed Y, Tsubakio T, Kitani T: thrombocytopenia in Graves' disease: Effect of T3 on platelet kinetics. Acta Haematol 63:185, 1980

309. Kutti J, Weinfeld A: The frequency of thrombocytopenia in patients with heart disease treated with oral diuretics. Acta Med Scand 183:245, 1968

310. Kuzemo JA, Keidan SE: Treatment of chronic idiopathic thrombocytopenic purpura and azathioprine and prednisilone: A clinical trial with three children. Clan Pediatr (Bologna) 7:216, 1968

311. Lacey JV, Penner JA: Management of idiopathic thrombocytopenic purpura in the adult. Semin Thromb Hemostas 3:160, 1977

312. Laros RK Jr, Sweet RL: Management of idiopathic thrombocytopenic purpura during pregnancy. Am J Obstet Gynecol 122:182, 1975

313. Lau P, Sholtis CM, Aster RH: Post-transfusion purpura: An enigma of alloimmunization. Am J Hematol 9:331, 1980

314. Lauria F, Mantovani V, Catovsky D, Gaurini A, Gobbi M, Gugliotta L, Mirone E, Tura S: T gamma cell deficiency in idiopathic thrombocytopenic purpura (ITP). Scand J Haematol 26:156, 1981

315. Lauria F, Raspadori D, Gobbi M, Guarini A, Gugliotta L, Aieta M, Tura S: T-cell subsets defined by monoclonal antibodies in autoimmune thrombocytopenic purpura (ATP). Haematologica 68:600, 1983

316. Laurian Y, Le Bras P, Ellrodt A, Alvin P: Immune thrombocytopenia gammaglobulin, and seropositivity to the human T-lymphotrophic virus type III. Ann Intern Med 105:145, 1986

317. Lavery JP, Koontz WL, Liu YK, Howell R: Immunologic thrombocytopenia in pregnancy; use of antenatal immunoglobulin therapy: Case report and review. Obstet Gynecol 66:41S, 1985

318. Lehman HA, Lehman LO, Rustagi PK, Rustgi RN, Plunkett RW, Farolino DL, Conway J, Logue GL: Complement-mediated autoimmune thrombocytopenia. Monoclonal IgM antiplatelet antibody associated with lymphoreticular malignant disease. N Engl J Med 316:194, 1987

319. Lerner W, Caruso R, Faig D, Karpatkin S: Drug-dependent and non-drug-dependent antiplatelet antibody in drug-induced immunologic thrombocytopenic purpura. Blood 66:306, 1985

320. Lester TJ, Grabowski GA, Goldblatt J, Leiderman IZ, Zaroulis CG: Immune thrombocytopenia and Gaucher's disease. Am J Med 77:569, 1984

321. Levin HA, McMillan R, Tavassoli M, Longmire RL, Yelonsky R, Sacks PV: Thrombocytopenia associated with gold therapy: Observations on the mechanism of platelet destruction. Am J Med 59:274, 1975

322. Lightsey AL, Koenig HM, McMillan R: Platelet-associated immunoglobulin G in childhood idiopathic thrombocytopenic purpura. J Pediatr 94:201, 1979

323. Lightsey AL, McMillan R, Koenig HM: Childhood idiopathic thrombocytopenic purpura: Aggressive management of life-threatening complications. J Am Med Assoc 232:734, 1975

324. Lindsey SM, Maddison FE, Towne JB: Heparin-induced thromboembolism: Angiographic features. Radiology 131:771, 1979

325. Linker CA, Newcom SR, Nilsson CM, Wolf JL, Shuman MA: Combined idiopathic neutropenia

and thrombocytopenia: Evidence for an immune basis for the syndrome. Ann Intern Med 93:704, 1980

326. Ljung R, Nilsson IM, Frohm, Holmberg L: Platelet-associated IgG in childhood idiopathic thrombocytopenic purpura: Measurements on intact and solubilized platelets and after gammaglobulin treatment. Scand J Haematol 36:402, 1986

327. Lo SS, Hitzig WH, Sigg P: Management of chronic ITP in children with particular reference to immunosuppressive therapy. Acta Haematol 41:1, 1969

328. LoBuglio AF, Court WS, Vinocur L, Maglott G, Shaw GM: Immune thrombocytopenic purpura. Use of a ^{125}I-labeled antihuman IgG monoclonal antibody to quantify platelet-bound IgG. N Engl J Med 309:459, 1983

329. Lockhart JM: Tolmetin-induced thrombocytopenia (letter). Arthritis Rheum 25:1144, 1982

330. Loiseau P: Sodium valproate, platelet dysfunction and bleeding. Epilepsia 22:141, 1981

331. Lown J, Barr A: Immune thrombocytopenia induced by cephalosporins specific for thiomethyltetrazole side chain (letter). J Clin Pathol 40:700, 1987

332. Luiken GA, McMillan R, Lightsey AL, Gordon P, Zevely S, Schulman I, Gribble TJ, Longmire RL: Platelet-associated IgG in immune thrombocytopenic purpura. Blood 50:317, 1977

333. Luk SC, Musclow E, Simon GT: Platelet phagocytosis in the spleen of patients with idiopathic thrombocytopenic purpura (ITP). Histopathology 4:127, 1980

334. Lüsher JM, Emami A, Ravindranath Y, Warrier AI: Idiopathic thrombocytopenic purpura in children. The case for management without corticosteroids. Am J Pediatr Hematol Oncol 6:149, 1984

335. Lüsher JM, Iyer R: Idiopathic thrombocytopenic purpura in children. Semin Thromb Hemost 3:175, 1977

336. Lynch DM, Howe SE: Heparin-associated thrombocytopenia: Antibody binding specificity to platelet antigens. Blood 66:1176, 1985

337. MacPherson AIS, Richmond J: Planned splenectomy in ITP. Br Med J 1:64, 1975

338. Makhoul RG, Greenberg CS, McCann RL: Heparin-associated thrombocytopenia and thrombosis: A serious clinical problem and potential solution. J Vasc Surg 4:522, 1986

339. Makhoul RG, McCann RL, Austin EH, Greenberg CS, Lowe JE: Management of patients with heparin-associated thrombocytopenia and thrombosis requiring cardiac surgery. Ann Thorac Surg 43:617, 1987

340. Mann HJ, Schneider JR, Miller JB, Delaney JP: Cimetidine-associated thrombocytopenia. Drug Intell Clin Pharm 17:126, 1983

341. Manoharan A: Slow infusion of vincristine in the treatment of idiopathic thrombocytopenic purpura. Am J Hematol 21:135, 1986

342. Manoharan A: Vincristine by infusion for childhood acute immune thrombocytopenia (letter). Lancet 1:317, 1986

343. Mar DD, Brandstetter RD, Miskovitz PF, Fotino M: Cimetidine-induced, immune-mediated leukopenia and thrombocytopenia. South Med J 75:1283, 1982

344. Marcus GJ, Stevenson M, Brown T: Alphamethyldopa-induced immune thrombocytopenia: Report of a case. Am J Clin Pathol 64:113, 1975

345. Marder VJ, Nusbacher J, Anderson FW: One-year follow-up of plasma exchange therapy in 14 patients with idiopathic thrombocytopenic purpura. Transfusion 21:291, 1981

346. Marino C: Danazol for lupus thrombocytopenia. Arch Intern Med 145:2251, 1985

347. Martin JN, Morrison JC, Files JC: Autoimmune thrombocytopenic purpura: Current concepts and recommended practices. Am J Obstet Gynecol 150:86, 1984

348. Matsuo T, Nakao K, Yamada T, Matsuo O: A new thrombin inhibitor MD805 and thrombocytopenia encountered with heparin hemodialysis. Thromb Res 44:247, 1986

349. Mauer AM, DeVaux LO, Lahey MD: Neonatal and maternal thrombocytopenic purpura due to quinine. Pediatrics 19:84, 1957

350. Mayr WR, Mueller-Eckhardt G, Kruger M, Mueller-Eckhardt C, Lechner K, Niessner H: HLA-DR in chronic idiopathic thrombocytopenic purpura (ITP). Tissue Antigens 18:56, 1981

351. Mazza J, Magin GE: Severe thrombocytopenia in infectious mononucleosis. Wis Med J 74:124, 1975

352. Mazzucconi MG, Francesconi M, Falcione E, Ferrari A, Gandolfo GM, Ghirardini A, Tirindelli MC: Danazol therapy in refractory chronic immune thrombocytopenic purpura. Acta Haematol 77:45, 1987

353. Mazzucconi MG, Francesconi M, Fidani P, Conti L, Martelli MC, Paesano R, Pachi A, Purpura M, Gandolfo GM: Pregnancy, delivery and detection of antiplatelet antibodies in women with idiopathic thrombocytopenic purpura. Haematologica 70:506, 1985

354. McClure PD: Idiopathic thrombocytopenic purpura in children: Diagnosis and management. Pediatrics 55:68, 1975

355. McElfresh AE: Idiopathic thrombocytopenic purpura: To treat or not to treat. J Pediatr 87:160, 1975

356. McIntosh S, O'Brien RT, Schwartz AD, Pearson HA: Neonatal isoimmune purpura: Response to platelet infusions. J Pediatr 82:1020, 1973

357. McLaughlin P, Talpaz M, Quesada JR, Saleem A, Barlogie B, Gutterman JU: Immune thrombocytopenia following α-interferon therapy in patients with cancer. J Am Med Assoc 254:1353, 1985

358. McMillan R: Annotation. Platelet autoantigens in chronic ITP. Br J Haematol 57:1, 1984

359. McMillan R: Chronic idiopathic thrombocytopenic purpura. N Engl J Med 304:1135, 1981

360. McMillan R, Longmire RL, Xelenosky R, Donnel RL, Armstrong S: Quantitation of platelet-binding IgG produced in vitro by spleens from patients with idiopathic thrombocytopenic purpura. N Engl J Med 291:812, 1974

361. McMillan R, Luiken GA, Levy R, Yelenosky R, Longmire RL: Antibody against megakaryocytes in idiopathic thrombocytopenic purpura. J Am Med Assoc 239:2460, 1978

362. McMillan R, Pellegrino MA, Ferrone S: Letter to the Editor. Blood 55:709, 1980

363. McMurdo R: Thrombocytopenic purpura due to chlorothiazide. Practitioner 192:403, 1964

364. McVerry BA: Clinical Annotation. Management of idiopathic thrombocytopenic purpura in adults. Br J Haematol 59:203, 1985

365. McVerry BA, Auger M, Bellingham AJ: The use of danazol in the management of chronic immune thrombocytopenic purpura. Br J Haematol 61:145, 1985

366. McWilliams NB, Mauer HM: Acute idiopathic thrombocytopenic purpura in children. Am J Hematol 7:87, 1979

367. Mennuti M, Schwarz RH, Gill F: Obstetric management of isoimmune thrombocytopenia. Am J Obstet Gynecol 118:565, 1974

368. Meschengieser S, Lazzari MA: Breast-feeding in thrombocytopenic neonates secondary to maternal autoimmune thrombocytopenic purpura (letter). Am J Obstet Gynecol 154:1166, 1986

369. Meyboom RHB: Thrombocytopenia induced by nalidixic acid. Br Med J 289:962, 1984

370. Michlewitz H, Kawada CY, Kennison R: Cesarean delivery and severe idiopathic thrombocytopenic purpura. A case report. J Reprod Med 30:781, 1985

371. Miller DT, Etzel RA, McFarland JG, Aster RH, White JG: Prolonged neonatal alloimmune thrombocytopenic purpura associated with anti-Bak^a. Two cases in siblings. Am J Perinatol 4:55, 1987

372. Minchinton RM, Waters AH, Malpas JS, Starke I, Kendra JR, Barrett AJ: Platelet- and granulocyte-specific antibodies after allogeneic and autologous bone marrow grafts. Vox Sang 46:125, 1984

373. Mintzer DM, Real FX, Jovino L, Krown SE: Treatment of Kaposi's sarcoma and thrombocytopenia with vincristine in patients with the acquired immunodeficiency syndrome. Ann Intern Med 102:200, 1985

374. Mizutani H, Katagiri S, Uejima K, Ohnishi M, Tamaki T, Kanayama Y, Tsubakio T, Kurata Y, Yonezawa T, Tarui S: T-cell abnormalities in patients with idiopathic thrombocytopenic purpura: The presence of OKT4+8+ cells. Scand J Haematol 35:233, 1985

375. Mizutani H, Tsubakio T, Tomiyama Y, Katagiri S, Tamaki T, Kurata Y, Yonezawa T, Tarui S: Increased circulating Ia-positive T cells in patients with idiopathic thrombocytopenic purpura. Clin Exp Immunol 67:191, 1987

376. Moise KJ, Cotton DB: Discordant fetal platelet counts in a twin gestation complicated by idiopathic thrombocytopenic purpura. Am J Obstet Gynecol 156:1141, 1987

377. Moore A, Weksler BB, Nachman RL: Platelet Fc IgG receptor: Increased expression in female patients. Thromb Res 21:469, 1981

378. Morfini M, Vannucchi AM, Grossi A, Cinotti S, Rafanelli D, Ferrini PR: Direct evidence that high dose intravenous gammaglobulin blocks splenic and hepatic sequestration of ^{51}Cr-labeled platelets in ITP. Thromb Haemostasis 54:554, 1985

379. Morgenstern GR, Measday B: Autoimmune thrombocytopenia in pregnancy: New approach to management. Br Med J 287:584, 1983

380. Morimoto C, Abe T, Hara M, Homma M: Cell-mediated immune response in idiopathic thrombocytopenic purpura. Clin Immunol Immunopathol 8:181, 1977

381. Morris L, Distenfeld A, Amorosi E, Karpatkin S: Autoimmune thrombocytopenic purpura in homosexual men. Ann Intern Med 96:714, 1982

382. Moulinier J: Iso-immunization maternelle anti-plaquettaire et purpura neo-natal. Le systeme de groupe plaquettaire "Duzo." Trans Sixth Congress of European Society of Haematology, 1957, Part II, p. S817. Basel, S Karger, 1958

383. Mueller-Eckhardt C, Becker T, Weisheit M, Witz C, Santoso S: Neonatal alloimmune thrombocytopenia due to fetomaternal Zw^b incompatibility. Vox Sang 50:94, 1986

384. Mueller-Eckhardt C: Post-transfusion purpura. Br J Haematol 64:419, 1986

385. Mueller-Eckhardt C, Kayser W, Forster C, Mueller-Eckhardt G, Ringenberg C: Improved assay for detection of platelet-specific Pl^{A1} antibodies in neonatal alloimmune thrombocytopenia. Vox Sang 43:76, 1982

386. Mueller-Eckhardt C, Kayser W, Mersch-Baumert K, Mueller-Eckhardt G, Breidenbach M, Kugel H-G, Graubner M: The clinical significance

of platelet-associated IgG: A study on 298 patients with various disorders. Br J Haematol 46:123, 1980

387. Mueller-Eckhardt C, Kiefel V, Mueller-Eckhardt G, Bambauer R, Baur J, Behringhoff B, Deuss U, Heinrich D, Klein HO, Lechner K, Maas D, Panzer S, Sprenger R, Stählin, Vahrson H: Posttransfusion purpura. A survey of 13 cases. Klin Wochenschr 64:1198, 1986

388. Mueller-Eckhardt C, Küenzlen E, Kiefel V, Vahrson H, Graubner M: Cyclophosphamide-induced immune thrombocytopenia in a patient with ovarian carcinoma successfully treated with intravenous gamma globulin. Blut 46:165, 1983

389. Mueller-Eckhardt C, Mahn I, Schulz G, Mueller-Eckhardt G: Detection of platelet autoantibodies by a radioactive anti-immunoglobulin test. Vox Sang 35:357, 1978

390. Mueller-Eckhardt C, Mersch-Baumert K: The problem of platelet autoantibodies. I. Evaluation of the platelet factor 3 availability test for their detection. Vox Sang 33:221, 1977

391. Mueller-Eckhardt C, Myr W, Lechner K, Muller-Eckhardt G, Niessner H, Pralle H: HLA antigens in immunologic thrombocytopenic purpura. Scand J Haematol 23:348, 1979

392. Mueller-Eckhardt G, Mueller-Eckhardt C: Alloimmunization against the platelet specific Zw[a] antigen associated with HLA-DRw52 and/or DRw6? Hum Immunol 18:181, 1987

393. Murphy MF, Metcalfe P, Waters AH, Carne CA, Weller VD, Linch DC, Smith A: Incidence and mechanism of neutropenia and thrombocytopenia in patients with human immunodeficiency virus infection. Br J Haematol 66:337, 1987

394. Murphy MF, Riordan T, Minchinton RM, Chapman JF, Amess JAL, Shaw EJ, Waters AH: Demonstration of an immune-mediated mechanism of penicillin-induced neutropenia and thrombocytopenia. Br J Haematol 55:155, 1983

395. Myers TJ, Kim BK, Steiner M, Baldini MG: Platelet-associated complement C3 in immune thrombocytopenic purpura. Blood 59:1023, 1982

396. Myllyla G, Vaheri A, Vesikari T, Penttinen K: Interaction between human blood platelets, viruses, and antibodies. IV. Post-rubella thrombocytopenic purpura and platelet aggregation by rubella antigen–antibody interaction. Clin Exp Imunol 4:323, 1969

397. Mylvaganam R, Ahn YS, Harrington WJ, Kim CI, Gratzner HG: Differences in T cell subsets between men and women with idiopathic thrombocytopenic purpura. Blood 66:967, 1985

398. Najean Y, Ardaillou N: The sequestration site of platelets in idiopathic thrombocytopenic purpura: Its correlation with the results of splenectomy. Br J Haematol 21:153, 1971

399. Nakamura S, Yoshida T, Ohtake S, Matsuda T: Hemolysis due to high-dose intravenous gamma-globulin treatment for patients with idiopathic thrombocytopenic purpura. Acta Haematol 76:115, 1986

400. Neely SM, Gardner DV, Reynolds N, Green D, Ts'Ao C-H: Mechanism and characteristics of platelet activation by haematin. Br J Haematol 58:305, 1984

401. Nel JD, Stevens K, Mouton A, Pretorius FJ: Platelet-bound IgM in autoimmune thrombocytopenia. Blood 61:119, 1983

402. Nesher G, Dollberg L, Zimran A, Hershko C: Hepatosplenic peliosis after danazol and glucocorticoids for ITP. N Engl J Med 312:242, 1985

403. Neucks SH, Moore TL, Lichtenstein JR, Baldassare R, Weiss TD, Zuckner J: Localized scleroderma and idiopathic thrombocytopenia. J Rheumatol 7:741, 1980

404. Newland AC, Boots MA, Patterson KG: Intravenous IgG for autoimmune thrombocytopenia in pregnancy (letter). N Engl J Med 310:261, 1984

405. Newland AC, Treleaven JG, Minchinton RM, Waters AH: High-dose intravenous IgG in adults with autoimmune thrombocytopenia. Lancet 1:84, 1983

406. Niessner H, Clemetson KJ, Panzer S, Mueller-Eckhardt C, Santoso S, Bettelheim P: Acquired thrombasthenia due to GPIIb/IIIa-specific platelet autoantibodies. Blood 68:571, 1986

407. Niewig HO, Bouma HG, DeVries K, Jansz A: Haematologic side effects of some anti-rheumatic drugs. Ann Rheum Dis 22:240, 1963

408. Nijjar TS, Bonacosa IA, Israels LG: Severe acute thrombocytopenia following infusion of plasma containing anti-Pl[A1]. Am J Hematol 25:219, 1987

409. Nordquist P, Cramer G, Bjorntorp P: Thrombocytopenia during chlorothiazide treatment. Lancet 1:271, 1959

410. Norton JA, Shulman NR, Corash L, Smith RL, Au F, Rosenberg SA: Severe thrombocytopenia following intralesional BCG therapy. Cancer 41:820, 1977

411. Novak R, Wilimas J: Plasmapheresis in catastrophic complications of idiopathic thrombocytopenic purpura. J Pediatr 92:434, 1978

412. Ogier C, Ballerini G: Age-related effect of high-dose IgG infusion in autoimmune thrombocytopenia (ATP). Analysis of 87 treated patients reported in 13 studies. Acta Haematol 72:67, 1984

413. Okafor KC, Griffin C, Ngole PM: Hydrochlorothiazide-induced thrombocytopenic purpura. Drug Intell Clin Pharm 20:60, 1986

414. Olinger GN, Hussey CV, Olive JA, Malik MI: Cardiopulmonary bypass for patients with pre-

viously documented heparin-induced platelet aggregation. J Thorac Cardiovasc Surg 87:673, 1984

415. Oral A, Nusbacher J, Hill JB, Lewis JH: Intravenous gamma globulin in the treatment of chronic idiopathic thrombocytopenic purpura in adults. Am J Med 76:187, 1984

416. O'Reilly RA, Taber B-Z: Immunologic thrombocytopenic purpura and pregnancy. Obstet Gynecol 51:509, 1978

417. Oski FA, Naiman JL, Diamond LK: Use of the plasma acid phosphatase volume in the differentiation of thrombocytopenic states. N Engl J Med 273:845, 1965

418. Panzer S, Grümayer ER, Haas OA, Niessner H, Graninger W: Efficacy of Rhesus antibodies (anti-**Rh**$_0$(D)) in autoimmune thrombocytopenia: Correlation with response to high dose IgG and the degree of haemolysis. Blut 52:117, 1986

419. Panzer S, Niessner H, Lechner K, Dudczak, Jäger U, Mayr WR: Platelet-associated immunoglobulins IgG, IgM, IgA and complement C3c in chronic idiopathic autoimmune thrombocytopenia: Relation to the sequestration pattern of ^{111}indium labelled platelets. Scand J Haematol 37:97, 1986

420. Panzer S, Szamait S, Bödeker R-H, Haas OA, Haubenstock A, Mueller-Eckhardt C: Platelet-associated immunoglobulins IgG, IgM, IgA and complement C3 in immune and nonimmune thrombocytopenic disorders. Am J Hematol 23:89, 1986

421. Panzer S, Zeitelhuber U, Hach V, Brackmann HH, Niessner H, Mueller-Eckhardt C: Immune thrombocytopenia in severe hemophilia A treated with high-dose intravenous immunoglobulin. Transfusion 26:69, 1986

422. Pawha J, Giuliani D, Morse BS: Platelet-associated IgM levels in thrombocytopenia. Vox Sang 45:97, 1983

423. Pearson HA, Shulman NR, Marder VJ, Cone TE: Isoimmune neonatal thrombocytopenic purpura. Clinical and therapeutic considerations. Blood 23:154, 1964

424. Pegels JG, Bruynes ECE, Engelfriet CP, von dem Borne AEG Kr: Post-transfusion purpura: A serological and immunochemical study. Br J Haematol 49:521, 1981

425. Pegels JG, Helmerhost FM, van Leeuwen EF, Engelfriet CP, von dem Borne AEGKr: The Evans syndrome: Characterization of the responsible autoantibodies. Br J Haematol 51:445, 1982

426. Peller S, Kaufman S, Shaked U: Immunoregulatory defect in patients with autoimmune thrombocytopenic purpura (ATP). Thymus 8:361, 1986

427. Pena JM, Gonzalez JJ, Garciaal J, Barbado FJ, Vazquez JJ: Thrombocytopenia and sulfasalazine (letter). Ann Intern Med 102:277, 1985

428. Phillips DR, Arnold K, Innerarity TL: Platelet secretory products inhibit lipoprotein metabolism in macrophages. Nature 316:746, 1985

429. Pizzuto J, Ambriz R: Therapeutic experience on 934 adults with idiopathic thrombocytopenic purpura: Multicentric trial of the cooperative Latin American group on hemostasis and thrombosis. Blood 64:1179, 1984

430. Porges A, Bussel J, Kimberly R, Schulman I, Pollack M, Pandey J, Barandun S, Hilgartner M: Elevation of platelet associated antibody levels in patients with chronic idiopathic thrombocytopenic purpura expressing the B8 and/or DR3 allotypes. Tissue Antigens 26:132, 1985

431. Pui CH, Wilimas J, Wang W: Evans syndrome in childhood. J Pediatr 97:754, 1980

432. Puram V, Giuliani D, Morse BS: Circulating immune complexes and platelet IgG in various diseases. Clin Exp Immunol 58:672, 1984

433. Rabinowe SN, Miller KB: Danazol-induced thrombocytopenia (letter). Br J Haematol 65:383, 1987

434. Raffoux C, David V, Couderc LD, Rabian C, Clauvel JKP, Seligmann M, Colombani J: HLA-A, B and DR antigen frequencies in patients with AIDS-related persistent generalized lymphadenopathy (PGL) and thrombocytopenia. Tissue Antigens 29:60, 1987

435. Ratnoff OD, Menitove JE, Aster RH, Lederman MM: Coincident classic hemophilia and "idiopathic" thrombocytopenic purpura in patients under treatment with concentrates of antihemophiliac factor (factor VIII). N Engl J Med 308:439, 1983

436. Reiquam CW, Prosper JC: Chronic idiopathic thrombocytopenia: Treatment with prednisone, 6-mercaptopurine, vincristine, and fresh plasma transfusions. J Pediatr 68:885, 1966

437. Reznikoff-Etievant MF, Muller JY, Julien F, Patereau C: An immune response gene linked to MHC in man. Tissue Antigens, 22:312, 1983

438. Reznikoff-Etievant MF, Muller JY, Kaplan C, Patereau C, Clemenceau S: L'Immunisation contre l'antigene plaquettaire Zw^a (Pl^{A1}): Groupe à risque, prevention des complications. Pathol Biol 34:783–787, 1986

439. Richards JDM, Thompson DS: Assessment of thrombocytopenic patients for splenectomy. J Clin Pathol 32:1248, 1979

440. Ries CA: Platelet kinetics of autoimmune thrombocytopenia: Relationship between splenic platelet sequestration and response to splenectomy. Ann Intern Med 86:194, 1977

441. Ries CA: Vincristine for treatment of refractory autoimmune thrombocytopenia. N Engl J Med 295:1136, 1976

442. Ries CA, Price DC: Platelet kinetics in thrombocytopenia: Correlation between splenic se-

questration of platelets and response to splenectomy. Ann Intern Med 80:702, 1974

443. Rodriguez SU, Leikin SL, Hiller MC: Neonatal thrombocytopenia associated with ante-partum administration of thiazide drugs. N Engl J Med 270:881, 1964

444. Rose VL, Gordon LI: Idiopathic thrombocytopenic purpura in pregnancy. Successful management with immunoglobulin infusion. J Am Med Assoc 254:2626, 1985

445. Rosenfeld SI, Looney RJ, Leddy JP, Phipps DC, Abraham GN, Anderson CL: Human platelet Fc receptor for immunoglobulin G. Identification as a 40,000-molecular-weight membrane protein shared by monocytes. J Clin Invest 76:2317, 1985

446. Rosenfelt FP, Rosenbloom BE, Weinstein IM: Thrombocytopenia in homosexual men. Ann Intern Med 106:911, 1987

447. Rosse WF, Adams JP, Yount WJ: Subclasses of IgG antibodies in immune thrombocytopenic purpura (ITP). Br J Haematol 46:109, 1980

448. Roussi JH, Houbouyan LL, Goguel AF: Use of low-molecular-weight heparin in heparin-induced thrombocytopenia with thrombotic complications. Lancet 1:1183, 1984

449. Rubinstein A: Pediatric AIDS. Curr Probl Pediatr 16:365, 1986

450. Salama A, Kiefel V, Amberg R, Mueller-Eckhardt C: Treatment of autoimmune thrombocytopenic purpura with rhesus antibodies (anti-$\mathbf{Rh}_0$ (D)). Blut 49:29, 1984

451. Salama A, Kiefel V, Mueller-Eckhardt C: Effect of IgG anti-$\mathbf{Rh}_0$ (D) in adult patients with chronic autoimmune thrombocytopenia. Am J Hematol 22:241, 1986

452. Salama A, Mueller-Eckhardt C, Kiefel V: Effect of intravenous immunoglobulin in immune thrombocytopenia. Competitive inhibition of reticuloendothelial system function by sequestration of autologous red blood cells? Lancet 2:193, 1983

453. Salamon DJ, Nusbacher J, Stroupe T, Wilson JH, Hanrahan JB: Red cell and platelet-bound IgG penicillin antibodies in a patient with thrombocytopenia. Transfusion 24:395, 1984

454. Saleh MN, Court WS, LoBuglio AF: In vitro effects of gammaglobulin (IgG) on human monocyte Fc receptor function. I. Effect on monocyte membrane-associated IgG and Fc receptor-dependent binding of antibody-coated platelets. Am J Hematol 23:197, 1986

455. Salzstein SL: Phospholipid accumulation in histiocytes of splenic pulp associated with thrombocytopenic purpura. Blood 18:73, 1961

456. Santoso S, Zimmermann U, Neppert J, Mueller-Eckhardt C: Receptor patching and capping of platelet membranes induced by monoclonal antibodies. Blood 67:343, 1986

457. Sartorius JA: Steroid treatment of idiopathic thrombocytopenic purpura in children. Preliminary results of a randomized cooperative study. Am J Pediatr Hematol Oncol 6:165, 1984

458. Saulsbury FT, Boyle RJ, Wykoff RF, Howard TH: Thrombocytopenia as the presenting manifestation of human T-lymphotropic virus type III infection in infants. J Pediatr 109:30, 1986

459. Schmidt RE, Budde U, Bröschen-Zywietz C, Schäfer G, Mueller-Eckhardt C: High dose gammaglobulin therapy in adults with idiopathic thrombocytopenic purpura (ITP) clinical effects. Blut 48:19, 1984

460. Schmidt RE, Budde U, Schäfer G, Stroehmann I: High-dose intravenous gammaglobulin for idiopathic thrombocytopenic purpura. Lancet 2:475, 1981

461. Schulman I: Diagnosis and treatment: Management of idiopathic thrombocytopenic purpura. Pediatrics 33:979, 1964

462. Schwartz KA, Royer G, Kaufman DB, Pennar JA: Complications of heparin administration in normal individuals. Am J Hematol 19:355, 1985

463. Schwartz KA, Slichter SJ, Harker LA: Immune-mediated platelet destruction and thrombocytopenia in patients with solid tumours. Br J Haematol 51:17, 1982

464. Scott CS, Wheeler R, Ford P, Bynoe AG, Roberts BE: T lymphocyte subpopulations in idiopathic thrombocytopenic purpura (ITP). Scand J Haematol 40:401, 1983

465. Scott JR, Cruikshank DP, Kochenour NK, Pitkin RM, Warenski JC: Fetal platelet counts in the obstetric management of immunologic thrombocytopenic purpura. Am J Obstet Gynecol 136:495, 1980

466. Scott JR, Rote NS, Cruikshank DP: Antiplatelet antibodies and platelet counts in pregnancies complicated by autoimmune thrombocytopenic purpura. Am J Obstet Gynecol 145:932, 1983

467. Seidenfeld AM, Owen J, Glynn MFX: Post-transfusion purpura cured by steroid therapy in a man. Can Med Assoc J 118:1285, 1978

468. Seip M: Vincristine in the treatment of postinfectious and neonatal thrombocytopenia (letter). Acta Paediatr Scand 69:253, 1980

469. Shafer RW, Offit K, Macris NT, Horbar BM, Ancona L, Hoffman IR: Possible risk of steroid administration in patients at risk for AIDS (letter). Lancet 1:934, 1985

470. Shalev O, Brezis M: Methyldopa-induced thrombocytopenia in chronic lymphocytic-leukemia (letter). N Engl J Med 297:1471, 1977

471. Shannon KM, Ammann AJ: Acquired immune deficiency syndrome in childhood. J Pediatr 106:332, 1985

472. Shaw GM, Axelson J, Maglott JG, LoBuglio AF: Quantification of platelet-bound IgG by ^{125}I-staphylococcal protein A in immune thrombocytopenic purpura and other thrombocytopenic disorders. Blood 63:154, 1984

473. Sheridan D, Carter C, Kelton JG: A diagnostic test for heparin-induced thrombocytopenia. Blood 67:27, 1986

474. Shibata Y, Matsuda I, Miyaji T, Ichikawa Y: Yuk^a, a new platelet antigen involved in two cases of neonatal alloimmune thrombocytopenia. Vox Sang 50:177, 1986

475. Shibata Y, Miyaji T, Ichikawa Y, Matsuda I: A new platelet antigen system, Yuk^a/Yuk^b. Vox Sang 51:334, 1986

476. Shulman NR: A mechanism of cell destruction in individuals sensitized to foreign antigens and its implications in autoimmunity. Ann Intern Med 60:506, 1964

477. Shulman NR: Immunologic reactions to drugs. N Engl J Med 287:408, 1972

478. Shulman NR: Immunoreactions involving platelets. III. Quantitative aspects of platelet agglutination, inhibition of clot retraction, and other reactions caused by the antibody of quinidine purpura. J Exp Med 107:697, 1958

479. Shulman NR: Immunoreactions involving platelets. IV. Studies on the pathogenesis of thrombocytopenia in drug purpura using test doses of quinidine in sensitized individuals. Their implications in idiopathic thrombocytopenic purpura. J Exp Med 107:711, 1958

480. Shulman NR, Aster RH, Leitner A, Hiller MC: Immunoreactions involving platelets. V. Post-transfusion purpura due to a complement-fixing antibody against a genetically controlled platelet antigen. A proposed mechanism for thrombocytopenia and its relevance in 'autoimmunity.' J Clin Invest 40:1597, 1961

481. Shulman NR, Aster RH, Pearson HA, Hiller MC: Immunoreactions involving platelets. VI. Reactions of maternal isoantibodies responsible for neonatal purpura. Differentiation of a second platelet antigen system. J Clin Invest 41:1059, 1962

482. Shulman NR, Jordan JV Jr: Platelet immunology. In Colman RW, Harsh J, Marder VJ, Salzman EW (eds): Hemostasis and Thrombosis, pp 452–529. Philadelphia, JB Lippincott, 1987

483. Shulman NR, Leissinger CA, Hotchkiss AJ, Kautz CA: The nonspecific nature of platelet-associated IgG. Trans Assoc Amer Physicians 95:213, 1982

484. Shulman NR, Marder VJ, Hiller MC, Collier EM: Platelet and leukocyte isoantigens and their antibodies: Serologic, physiologic and clinical studies. Prog Hematol 4:222, 1964

485. Shulman NR, Marder VJ, Weinrach RS: Similarities between known antiplatelet antibodies and the factor responsible for thrombocytopenia in idiopathic purpura: Physiologic, serologic and isotopic studies. Ann NY Acad Sci 124:499, 1965

486. Shulman NR, Weinrach RS, Libre EP, Andrews HL: The role of the reticuloendothelial system in the pathogenesis of idiopathic thrombocytopenic purpura. Trans Assoc Am Physicians 78:374, 1965

487. Sia CG, Amigo NC, Harper RG, Kochen GF: Failure of caesarian section to prevent intracranial hemorrhage in siblings with isoimmune neonatal thrombocytopenia. Am J Obstet Gynecol 153:79, 1985

488. Simon T, Collins J, Kunicki T, Furihata K, Smith K, Aster R: Post-transfusion purpura with antiplatelet antibody specific for the platelet antigen Pen^a (abstr). Blood 68:117a, 1986

489. Simons SM, Main CA, Yaish HM, Rutzky J: Idiopathic thrombocytopenic purpura in children. J Pediatr 87:16, 1975

490. Sitarz AL, Driscoll JM, Wolff JA: Management of isoimmune neonatal thrombocytopenia. Am J Obstet Gynecol 124:39, 1976

491. Slichter SJ: Post-transfusion purpura: Response to steroids and association with red blood cell and lymphocytotoxic antibodies. Br J Haematol 50:599, 1982

492. Smith ME, Reid DM, Jones CE, Jordan JV, Kautz CA, Shulman NR: Binding of quinine- and quinidine-dependent drug antibodies to platelets is mediated by the Fab domain of the immunoglobulin G and is not Fc dependent. J Clin Invest 79:912, 1987

493. Sobel M, Adelman B, Greenfield LJ: Dextran 40 reduces heparin-mediated platelet aggregation. J Surg Res 40:382, 1986

494. Soulier JP, Pattereau C, Gobert N, Achach P, Muller JY: Post-transfusional immunologic thrombocytopenia. A case report. Vox Sang 37:21, 1979

495. Spruce W, Forman S, McMillan R, Farbstein M, Turner M, Blume K: Idiopathic thrombocytopenic purpura following bone marrow transplantation. Acta Haematol 69:47, 1983

496. Spychal RT, Wickham NWR: Thrombocytopenia associated with ranitidine (letter). Br Med J 291:1687, 1985

497. Spycher MO, Nydegger UE: Part of the activating cross-linked immunoglobulin G is internalized by human platelets to sites not accessible for enzymatic digestion. Blood 67:12, 1986

498. Stabile A, Pesaresi MA, Sopo SM, Segni G: Effective high-dose intravenous gammaglobulin

therapy for passive immune thrombocytopenia in the neonate. Eur J Pediatr 146:90, 1987

499. Stafford BT, Crosby WH: Late onset of gold-induced thrombocytopenia with a practical note on injections of dimercaprol. (Technical Note) J Am Med Assoc 239:50, 1978

500. Stephens CAL, Yoeman EE, Holbrook WP, Hill DF, Goodin WL: Benefits and toxicity of phenylbutazone (Butazolidin) in rheumatic arthritis. J Am Med Assoc 150:1084, 1952

501. Sternbach MS, Malette M, Nadon F, Guevin RM: Severe alloimmune neonatal thrombocytopenia due to specific HLA antibodies. In Decary F, Rock GA (eds): Platelet Serology. Research Progress and Clinical Implications. Basel, S Karger, 1986

502. Stoll D, Cines DB, Aster RH, Murphy S: Platelet kinetics in patients with idiopathic thrombocytopenic purpura and moderate thrombocytopenia. Blood 65:584, 1985

503. Stricker RB, Abrams DI, Corash L, Shuman MA: Target platelet antigen in homosexual men with immune thrombocytopenia. N Engl J Med 313:1375, 1985

504. Stricker RB, Lewis BH, Corash L, Shuman MA: posttransfusion purpura associated with an autoantibody directed against a previously undefined platelet antigen. Blood 69:1458, 1987

505. Stricker RB, Reyes PT, Corash L, Shuman MA: Evidence that a 210,000-molecular-weight glycoprotein (gp210) serves as a platelet Fc receptor. J Clin Invest 79:1589, 1987

506. Stricker RB, Shuman MA: Quinidine purpura: Evidence that glycoprotein V is a target platelet antigen. Blood 67:1377, 1986

507. Strother SV, Zuckerman KS, LoBuglio AF: Colchicine therapy for refractory idiopathic thrombocytopenic purpura. Arch Intern Med 144:2198, 1984

508. Stuart MJ, Tomar RH, Miller ML, Davey FR: Chronic idiopathic thrombocytopenic purpura: A familial immunodeficiency syndrome? J Am Med Assoc 239:939, 1978

509. Suarez CR, Rademaker D, Hasson A, Mangogna L: High-dose steroids in childhood acute idiopathic thrombocytopenia purpura. Am J Pediatr Hematol Oncol 8:111, 1986

510. Sugiura K, Steiner M, Baldini MG: Platelet antibody in idiopathic thrombocytopenic purpura and other thrombocytopenias. A quantitative, sensitive, and rapid assay. J Lab Clin Med 96:640, 1980

511. Sugiyama H, Yagita M, Takahashi T, Nakamura K, Iho S, Hoshino T, Imura H: Megakaryocytopoiesis in idiopathic thrombocytopenic purpura. Acta Haematol Jpn 50:119, 1987

512. Sugiyama T, Okuma M, Ushikubi F, Sensaki S, Kanaji K, Uchino H: A novel platelet aggregating factor found in a patient with defective collagen-induced platelet aggregation and autoimmune thrombocytopenia. Blood 69:1712, 1987

513. Szatkowski NS, Kunicki TJ, Aster RH: Identification of glycoprotein Ib as a target for autoantibody in idiopathic (autoimmune) thrombocytopenic purpura. Blood 67:310, 1986

514. Taaning E, Killmann S-A, Morling N, Ovesen H, Svejgaard A: Post-transfusion purpura (PTP) due to anti-Zw^{b} ($-Pl^{A2}$): The significance of IgG3 antibodies in PTP. Br J Haematol 64:217, 1986

515. Taaning E, Morling N, Ovesen H, Svejgaard A: Post-transfusion purpura and anti-Zw^{b} ($-Pl^{A2}$). Tissue Antigens 26:143, 1985

516. Takahashi K, Hakozaki H, Terashima K, Kojima M: Two distinctive types of lipid histiocytes appearing in the spleen of idiopathic thrombocytopenic purpura: Sea-blue histiocyte and foam cell. Acta Pathol Jpn 27:447, 1977

517. Tavassoli M, McMillan R: Structure of the spleen in idiopathic thrombocytopenic purpura. Am J Clin Pathol 64:180, 1975

518. Territo M, Finkelstein J, Oh H, Habel C, Kattlove H: Management of autoimmune thrombocytopenia in pregnancy and in the neonate. Obstet Gynecol 41:579, 1973

519. Torres A, Lucia JF, Oliveros A, Vazquez C: Anti-factor IX circulating anticoagulant and immune thrombocytopenia in a case of Takayasu's arteritis. Acta Haematol 64:338, 1980

520. Towne JB, Bernhard VM, Hussey C, Garancis JC: White clot syndrome. Arch Surg 114:372, 1979

521. Trent R, Adams E, Erhardt C, Basten A: Alterations in T-gamma-cells in patients with chronic idiopathic thrombocytopenic purpura. J Immunol 127:621, 1981

522. Tsubakio T, Kurata Y, Katagiri S, Kanakura Y, Tamaki T, Kuyama J, Kanayama Y, Yonezawa T, Tarui S: Alteration of T cell subsets and immunoglobulin synthesis in vitro during high dose γ-globulin therapy in patients with idiopathic thrombocytopenic purpura. Clin Exp Immunol 53:697, 1983

523. Uike N: Pathophysiological significance of platelet-associated IgG in idiopathic thrombocytopenic purpura. Acta Haematol Jpn 48:1459, 1985

524. Usuki Y, Kohsaki M, Nagai K, Ohe Y, Hara H: Complement-dependent cytotoxic factor to megakaryocyte progenitors in sera from patients with idiopathic thrombocytopenic purpura. Int J Cell Cloning 4:447, 1986

525. van Leeuwen EF, Leeksma OC, van Mourik JA, Engelfriet CP, von dem Borne AEG Kr: Effect of the binding of anti-Zw^{a} antibodies on platelet function. Vox Sang 47:280, 1984

526. van Leeuwen EF, van der Ven JTHM, Engelfriet CP, von dem Borne AEG Kr: Specificity of autoantibodies in autoimmune thrombocytopenia. Blood 59:23, 1982

527. Veenhoven WA, Oosterhuis HJ, van der Schans GS: Myasthenia gravis and Werlhof's disease. Acta Med Scand 206:131, 1979

528. Veenhoven WA, van der Schans GS, Nieweg HO: Platelet antibodies in idiopathic thrombocytopenic purpura. Clin Exp Immunol 39:645, 1980

529. Velders AJ, Wildevuur CHRH: Platelet damage by protamine and the protective effect of prostacyclin: An experimental study in dogs. Ann Thorac Surg 42:168, 1986

530. Velu TJ, Debusscher L, Stryckmans PA: Cyclosporine for the treatment of refractory idiopathic thrombocytopenic purpura (letter). Eur J Haematol 38:95, 1987

531. Vender JS, Matthew EB, Silverman IM, Konowitz H, Dau PC: Heparin-associated thrombocytopenia: Alternative managements. Anesth Analg 65:520, 1986

532. Verlin M, Laros Jr RK, Penner JA: Treatment of refractory thrombocytopenic purpura with cyclophosphamide. Am J Hematol 1:97, 1976

533. Verwey J, Breed WPM, Hillen HFP: Bleomycin-induced early-onset transient decrease in platelet counts. Neth J Med 27:202, 1984

534. Viala JJ, Dechevanne M, Ville D: Les Epreuves radioisotopiques sont les meilleures indications de la splenectomie au cours de purpura thrombopenie idiopathiques chroniques? A propos de 50 observations. Lyon Med 234:419, 1975

535. Vitoux J-F, Mathieu J-F, Roncato M, Fiessinger J-N, Aiach M: Heparin-associated thrombocytopenia treatment with low molecular weight heparin. Thromb Haemostasis 55:37, 1986

536. Voet D, Afschrift M, Nachtegaele P, Delbeke MJ, Schelstraete K, Benoit Y: Sonographic diagnosis of an accessory spleen in recurrent idiopathic thrombocytopenic purpura. Pediatr Radiol 13:39, 1983

537. von dem Borne AEG Kr: Autoimmune thrombocytopenias. In Engelfriet CP et al (eds): Immunohematology, p 222. Amsterdam, Elsevier Science Publishers, 1984

538. von dem Borne AEG Kr, Helmerhorst FM, van Leeuwen EF, Pegels JG, von Riesz E, Engelfriet CP: Autoimmune thrombocytopenia: Detection of platelet autoantibodies with the suspension immunofluorescence test. Br J Haematol 45:319, 1980

539. von dem Borne AEG Kr, Pegels JG, van der Stadt RJ, van der Plas-van Dalen CM, Helmerhorst FM: Thrombocytopenia associated with gold therapy: A drug-induced autoimmune disease? Br J Haematol 63:509, 1986

540. von dem Borne AEG Kr, van der Plas-van Dalen CM: Further observation on post-transfusion purpura (PTP). Br J Haematol 61:374, 1985

541. von dem Borne AEG Kr, von Riesz E, Verheugt FWA, ten Cate JW, Koppe JG, Engelfriet CP, Nijenhuis LE: Bak[a], a new platelet-specific antigen involved in neonatal alloimmune thrombocytopenia. Vox Sang 39:113, 1980

542. von dem Borne AEG Kr, Vos JJE, van der Lelie J, Bossers B, van Dalen CM: Clinical significance of positive platelet immunofluorescence test in thrombocytopenia. Br J Haematol 64:767, 1986

543. Vos JJE, van Aken WG, Engelfriet CP, von dem Borne AEG Kr: Intravenous gammaglobulin therapy in idiopathic thrombocytopenic purpura. Vox Sang 49:92, 1985

544. Waddell CC, Cimo PL: Idiopathic thrombocytopenic purpura occurring in Hodgkin's disease after splenectomy: Report of two cases and review of the literature. Am J Hematol 7:381, 1979

545. Wakefield TW, Bouffard JA, Spauldin SA, Petry NA, Gross MD, Lindblad B, Stanley JC: Sequestration of platelets in the pulmonary circulation as a consequence of protamine reversal of the anticoagulant effects of heparin. J Vasc Surg 5:187, 1987

546. Walker DJ, Saunders P, Griffiths ID: Gold induced thrombocytopenia. J Rheumatol 13:225, 1986

547. Walker RW, Heaton A: Thrombocytopenia due to vancomycin (letter). Lancet 1:932, 1985

548. Walsh C, Krigel R, Lennette E, Karpatkin S: Thrombocytopenia in homosexual patients. Prognosis, response to therapy, and prevalence of antibody to the retrovirus associated with the acquired immunodeficiency syndrome. Ann Intern Med 103:542, 1985

549. Walsh CM, Nardi MA, Karpatkin S: On the mechanism of thrombocytopenic purpura in sexually active homosexual men. N Engl J Med 311:635, 1984

550. Walsh KP, Branagan JP, Walsh MJ: Reversible severe thrombocytopenia associated with captopril therapy. Ir Med J 79:43, 1986

551. Wanamaker WM, Wanamaker SJ, Celesia GG, Koeller AA: Thrombocytopenia associated with long-term levodopa therapy. J Am Med Assoc 235:2217, 1976

552. Ware R, Kinney TR, Friedman HS, Falletta JM, Rosse WF: Prognostic implications for direct platelet-associated IgG in childhood idiopathic thrombocytopenic purpura. Am J Pediatr Hematol Oncol 8:32, 1986

553. Warrier IA, Lusher JM: Intravenous gammaglobulin (Gamimune) for treatment of chronic idiopathic thrombocytopenic purpura (ITP): A two-year follow-up. Am J Hematol 23:323, 1986

554. Watkins SP Jr, Cowan DH, Shulman NR: Differentiation of immunologic from non-immunologic forms of idiopathic thrombocytopenic purpura. J Clin Invest 46:1129, 1967

555. Wautier JL, Boizard B, Doan R, Caen JP, Hartmann L: Identification of the platelet alloantigen (Pl^{A1}) in circulating immune complexes of normal human serum. Can Immunol Immunother 13:44, 1982

556. Wautier JL, Boizard B, Patereau C, Muller JY: Studies of platelet antibodies in patients with thrombocytopenic purpura by two different techniques. Haemostasis 11:170, 1982

557. Weinberger I, Rotenberg Z, Fuchs J, Ben-Sasson E, Agmon J: Amiodarone-induced thrombocytopenia. Arch Intern Med 147:735, 1987

558. Weinblatt ME, Scimeca PG, James-Herry AG, Pahwa S: Thrombocytopenia in an infant with AIDS (letter). Am J Dis Child 141:15, 1987

559. Weir AB, Poon MC, McGowan EI: Plasma-exchange in idiopathic thrombocytopenic purpura. (Technical Note) Arch Intern Med 140:1101, 1980

560. Weisberg LJ, Linker CA: Prednisone therapy of post-transfusion purpura. Ann Intern Med 100:76, 1984

561. Weisberger AS, Suhrland LG: Massive corticosteroid therapy in the management of resistant thrombocytopenic purpura. Am J Med Sci 236:425, 1958

562. Weiss HJ, Rosove MH, Lages BA, Kaplan KL: Acquired storage pool deficiency with increased platelet-associated IgG: Report of five cases. Am J Med 69:711, 1980

563. White LA Jr, Brubaker LH, Aster RH, Henry PH, Adelstein EH: Platelet satellitism and phagocytosis by neutrophils: Association with antiplatelet antibodies and lymphoma. Am J Hematol 4:313, 1978

564. Widerlov E, Karlman I, Storsater J: Hydralazine-induced neonatal thrombocytopenia (letter). N Engl J Med 303:1235, 1980

565. Wiesneth M, Pflieger H, Frickhofen N, Heimpel H: Idiopathic combined immunocytopenia. Br J Haematol 61:339, 1985

566. Winiarski J: Immunoglobulin binding to platelets. The effect of aggregated IgG. Blut 51:259, 1985

567. Winiarski J, Ekelund E: Antibody binding to platelet antigens in acute and chronic idiopathic thrombocytopenic purpura: A platelet membrane ELISA for the detection of antiplatelet antibodies in serum. Clin Exp Immunol 63:459, 1986

568. Winiarski J, Holm G: Platelet associated immunoglobulins and complement in idiopathic thrombocytopenic purpura. Clin Exp Immunol 53:201, 1983

569. Winiarski J, Kreuger A, Ejderhamn J, Holm G: High dose intravenous IgG reduces platelet associated immunoglobulins and complement in idiopathic thrombocytopenic purpura. Scand J Haematol 31:342, 1983

570. Woerner SJ, Abildgaard CF, French BN: Intracranial hemorrhage in children with idiopathic thrombocytopenic purpura. Pediatrics 67:453, 1981

571. Wong YY, Lichtor T, Brown FD: Severe thrombocytopenia associated with phenytoin and cimetidine therapy. Surg Neurol 23:169, 1985

572. Woods VL, Kurata Y, Montgomery RR, Tani P, Mason D, Oh EH, McMillan R: Autoantibodies against platelet glycoprotein Ib in patients with chronic immune thrombocytopenic purpura. Blood 64:156, 1984

573. Woods VL, Oh EH, Mason D, McMillan R: Autoantibodies against the platelet glycoprotein IIb/IIIa complex in patients with chronic ITP. Blood 63:368, 1984

574. Yu J-R, Lennette ET, Karpatkin S: Anti-$F(ab')_2$ antibodies in thrombocytopenic patients at risk for acquired immunodeficiency syndrome. J Clin Invest 77:1756, 1986

575. Yue CP, Mann KS, Chan KH: Severe thrombocytopenia due to combined cimetidine and phenytoin therapy. Neurosurgery 20:963, 1987

576. Zarella JT, Martin LW, Lampkin BC: Emergency splenectomy for idiopathic thrombocytopenic purpura in children. J Pediatr Surg 13:243, 1978

577. Ziegler Z, Shadduck RK, Winkelstein A, Stroupe TK: Immune hemolytic anemia and thrombocytopenia secondary to quinidine: In vitro studies of the quinidine-dependent red cell and platelet antibodies. Blood 53:396, 1979

578. Zinberg M, Francus T, Weksler ME, Siskind GW, Karpatkin S: Abnormal autologous mixed lymphocyte reaction in autoimmune thrombocytopenic purpura. Blood 59:148, 1982

579. Zon LI, Arkin C, Groopman JE: Haematologic manifestations of the human immune deficiency virus (HIV). Br J Haematol 66:251, 1987

20

Laboratory Methods for the Detection of Platelet Antibodies and Identification of Antigens

CHRISTIAN MUELLER-ECKHARDT · VOLKER KIEFEL

Ever since the famous in vivo demonstration by Harrington et al.,[24,25] in the early 1950s, that certain forms of idiopathic and neonatal thrombocytopenic purpura are due to an immunologic mechanism, the need to correlate laboratory findings with clinical diagnoses and the outcome of patient management has stimulated the development of an endless list of new antibody assays. Thus, the history of platelet immunology reflects the history of these methods, each with its inherent peculiarities. Platelets, fragile tiny blood elements, are the cellular components of the blood coagulation system. Their inherent functions, namely adhesion to surfaces and mutual aggregation elicited by a large number of agonists (thrombin, ADP, collagen, immune complexes, and many others), are the reasons why serologic handling of them has been so difficult. Therefore, advances in correctly diagnosing the manyfold disease conditions in which platelet antibodies are implicated, e.g., neonatal alloimmune thrombocytopenic purpura (NATP), posttransfusion purpura (PTP), refractoriness to platelet transfusion, drug-induced thrombocytopenia, and thrombocytopenic or thrombocytopathic autoimmune disorders, have been relatively slow. Nevertheless, considerable progress in clinical platelet immunology has been made in the last decade, thanks to the introduction of sophisticated modern technology.

It is not the purpose of this chapter to give an extensive description of the literally hundreds of assays and their modifications that have been published over the years. For older work, the reader is referred to comprehensive reviews.[46,63,88,93,101] In this contribution we shall outline the principles of those methods that are still of importance in the clinically oriented laboratory and give an account of their diagnostic value based on our personal, knowledgeable (but possibly biased) experience as one of the larger reference laboratories.

METHODS AND THEIR PRINCIPLES

Methods of antibody detection may be classified by whether they are employed for detection of free serum antibodies (indirect assays) or in vivo platelet-associated immunoproteins, such as antibodies or complement components (direct assays). Other classifications subdivide serologic platelet assays into qualitative and quantitative tests. Assays that use ligands for determination of platelet-associated immunoproteins may employ xenogeneic secondary antibodies of polyclonal or monoclonal origin or ligands that are not antibodies such as staphylococcal protein A (SPA) or lectins. Ligands in turn may be used either unlabeled (which necessitates their detection by a tertiary reaction) or labeled with radioactive isotopes (e.g., ^{125}I or ^{3}H), fluorescent dyes (e.g., fluorescein or rhodamine), or enzymes (e.g., peroxidase or alkaline phosphatase). Finally, platelet-bound antibody may be detected by functional assays in which the presence of antibody on the platelet surface either enhances or inhibits an inherent function of platelets (e.g., aggregation or release of granule contents). None of these classifications is entirely satisfactory, and modern technology makes increasing use of various combinations of the aforementioned approaches. The classification presented is oriented toward the viewpoint of the practical immunohematology laboratory.

Platelet Agglutination

Platelet agglutination is the oldest technique used in platelet serology. The physiologic tendency of platelets to aggregate and, thereby, invalidate serologic results has been overcome by using heat-inactivated, thrombin-depleted serum in the presence of EDTA and native or phenol-treated platelets, with constant rotation. The simplified agglutination technique introduced in 1954 by Dausset and Malinvaud[14] is still the basis of all modifications. It is insensitive, but gives unequivocally reproducible results with strong platelet agglutinins that arise, albeit rarely, in multiply transfused patients. A platelet agglutination assay was used to establish the first two diallelic platelet-specific alloantigen systems (Zw^a Zw^b, identical with Pl^{A1} Pl^{A2}, and Ko^a Ko^b; for a review *see* Ref. 101).

Platelet Complement Fixation

Quantitative platelet complement fixation (PCF) was introduced to platelet serology in the early 1960s by Shulman et al.[88] In this type of assay, platelets are incubated with the serum to be investigated and a fixed amount of complement before the indicator cells (sheep red blood cells sensitized with rabbit antisheep red blood cell antibodies) are added. In a famous series of studies, Shulman and associates used this technique to define the Pl^{A1} antigen ($=Zw^a$), the diallelic platelet-specific alloantigen system Pl^{E1}/Pl^{E2}, and a number of alloantigens shared by platelets, lymphocytes, and other cells, that were later found to represent HLA antigens. These authors were also the first to associate platelet-specific antibodies (anti-Pl^{A1}) with the syndrome of posttransfusion purpura (PTP); the first to demonstrate platelet-specific, incomplete "blocking" antibodies responsible for neonatal alloimmune thrombocytopenic purpura (NATP); and they provided insights into the functional abnormalities responsible for immune blood cell destruction which, in many respects, remain valid today. Quantitative PCF, in their hands, proved more sensitive and yielded more reliable results than platelet agglutination.

A considerable advantage of PCF is that platelet suspensions can be stored refrigerated for months, thereby facilitating the construction of large platelet panels. A semiquantitative PCF modification was described by Svejgaard[93] and was used for the determination of HLA antigens and cross-reactive HLA antibodies. In 1971, a micromodification of PCF was adopted as the international standard technique.[10] It is still widely used, requires very small amounts of material, has a high degree of reproducibility, and can easily be modified for quantitative applications. The overall sensitivity, however, is rather low by modern standards, and its use is restricted to the detection of complement-activating antibodies.

Complement-Dependent ^{51}Cr or ^{111}In Release

The ^{51}Cr-release assay, introduced and extensively employed by Aster and coworkers (for references and a detailed description of the method *see* Ref. 47), used platelets that are first tagged with ^{51}Cr and then sensitized with complement-fixing antibodies. After addition of complement, the lytic activity of platelet antibodies can be quantitated by the percentage of ^{51}Cr released. By using enzyme- or 2-aminoethylisothiouronium bromide (AET)-treated platelets or platelets of patients with paroxysmal nocturnal hemoglobinuria, the sensitivity of the procedure can be considerably enhanced[7,47] because the cells become more prone to complement-dependent lysis. The ^{51}C-release assay is sensitive and has a high degree of reproducibility. It has been useful for the analysis of a variety of clinically relevant antibodies, particularly drug-dependent antibodies (for a review, see Chap. 8).

A platelet microcytotoxicity assay that uses ^{111}In-labeled platelets and antithymocyte globulin was described by Hawker and Hawker.[26]

Antiglobulin Consumption Assays

Early attempts to measure consumption of an antiglobulin reagent by titration with sensitized red blood cells were unreliable and insensitive (for references *see* Ref. 63). The quantitative complement lysis inhibition assay described by

Dixon et al.[16] was a major development in that it allowed one to determine platelet-associated immunoglobulins with considerable precision. In this assay the degree of platelet sensitization, i.e., the amount of immunoglobulins bound by platelets, is quantitated by the consumption of a fixed amount of hemolytically active antihuman IgG, as monitored by the degree of inhibition of complement-dependent lysis of human red blood cells added subsequently. Although the applicability of this assay for the determination of platelet-associated IgG has been confirmed in many subsequent studies, it has been replaced in most laboratories by antiglobulin-binding tests. It is not recommended for the detection of free serum antibodies because the background is usually high, and it is, therefore, less suitable than assays employing labeled antiglobulin ligands.[30]

Assays Using Labeled Antiglobulin Reagents

The assays that use labeled antiglobulins are the most versatile and sensitive tests for routine purposes. To target the antiglobulin reagent, fluorescent dyes, radioactive tracers, or enzymes are employed (Table 20-1). Platelets are used in suspension, fixed to surfaces, or after detergent lysis. Platelet-bound antibodies can be measured directly on autologous platelets (i.e., after in vivo sensitization) or indirectly after incubation of serum with allogeneic platelets in vitro. Separation of bound and unbound antibodies is usually achieved by several washing steps, but centrifugation through Percoll, oil, or sucrose solutions of appropriate density has also been employed. A detailed description of the various techniques is beyond the scope of this chapter. For clinical applications, two types of assays have gained general acceptance: The immunofluorescent test and the enzyme-linked immunosorbent assay (ELISA). These will, therefore, be considered in greater detail here.

Immunofluorescent Tests

Previous attempts to analyze platelets in suspension by immunofluorescence were hampered by a high level of nonspecific fluorescence (for references *see* Ref. 63). Von dem Borne et al.[106] described a platelet suspension immunofluorescent test (PSIFT) in which nonspecific staining was prevented by fixation of cells with paraformaldehyde (PFA). The PSIFT is now being used in many laboratories as the standard test for the demonstration of free serum antibodies. Its disadvantages are the necessity to use fresh (or freshly frozen and thawed) platelets and PFA fixation, which requires numerous wash steps and leads to considerable loss of platelets. In patients with chronic renal failure, false-positive results have been obtained with PFA-fixed platelets caused by anti-N-like antibodies.[55] These antibodies are probably linked to the use of dialysis equipment sterilized with PFA and are stimulated by the in vivo presence in these patients of aldehydes that alter the antigenicity of the patient's cells.[55] This results in the production of an autoantibody reacting only with PFA-treated platelets.[55]

A very useful micromodification of the immunofluorescent test was reported in 1981 by Schneider and Schnaidt[83] and designated platelet adhesion immunofluorescent test (PAIFT). It is performed on Hamax glass slides with 60 rings, originally manufactured for the two-color fluorescent test used to determine HLA-DR antigens on B-lymphocytes. A drop of freshly washed platelets in 0.5% EDTA in saline is pipetted into each ring, whereupon the platelets sediment and attach firmly to the glass slides. All subsequent steps are performed on the slides including sensitization with antibodies, washing, and the fluorescein isothiocyanate (FITC)-antiglobulin phase. Nonspecific fluorescence is entirely avoided if labeled $F(ab')_2$ fractions of antiglobulin sera are used. In our hands, the PAIFT is much less laborious than the PSIFT, requires less material, and avoids PFA fixation. It is as sensitive as the PSIFT and, therefore, optimally suited for mass screening. Therefore, we use the PAIFT as the basic assay for all serum investigations. General disadvantages of all immunofluorescent tests pertain to the subjective nature of the endpoint (unless quantitative immunofluorescent microphotometry is employed) and the necessity to read the reactions immediately in the dark to avoid evanescence of fluorescence.

Radioactive Antiglobulin Tests

Platelet radioactive antiglobulin tests have been developed and used for years with excellent results (*see* Table 20-1), but there is general consensus that in the clinical laboratory they should be replaced by ELISAs, which are equally sensitive and quantifiable but employ stable reagents and carry no hazard of radioactivity.

Table 20-1
Synopsis of Recently Published Assays Used for the Detection of Platelet Antibodies

Type of Assay	Refs.
Platelet Immunofluorescent Tests (PIFT)	
Membrane PIFT	v. d. Schans et al, 1977[99]
PSIFT*	v. d. Borne et al, 1978[106]
Modified PSIFT	Andersen et al, 1981[1]
PAIFT*	Schneider and Schnaidt, 1981[83]
Fluorospectrophotometry with lysed platelets	Sugiura et al, 1980[92]
Flowcytometry	Lazarchick and Hall, 1986[50]
Platelet Radioactive Antiglobulin Tests (PRAT)	
Radioactive Coombs test	Soulier et al, 1975[88]
PRAT	Mueller-Eckhardt et al, 1978[71]
Coombs antiglobulin test	Cines and Schreiber, 1979[8]
MSPRIA*	Cheung et al, 1983[6]
SPRIA*	Hotchkiss et al, 1986[33]
Antihuman IgG monoclonal antibody assay	LoBuglio et al, 1983[53]
Fab/anti-Fab–radioimmunoassay using staphylococcal protein A	Pfueller et al, 1981[78]
Enzyme-Linked Immunosorbent Assays (ELISA)	
Immunoperoxidase test	Leporrier et al, 1979[52]
PAP* slide technique	Schmidt et al, 1980[82]
ELISA	Nel and Stevens, 1980[75]
ELISA	Horai et al, 1981[32]
ELISA	Hegde et al, 1981[29]
Competitive solid-phase enzyme immunoassay	Tsubakio et al, 1981[98]
Solid-phase enzyme immunoassay	Follea et al, 1982[19]
Micro-ELISA	Forster and Schmidt, 1983[20]
Microplate ELISA	Taaning, 1985[95]
ELISA	Winiarski and Ekelund, 1986[108]
CELIA*	Kiefel et al, 1987[42]
Radioactive Staphylococcal Protein A (SPA) Assays	
SPA	Kekomäki, 1977[36]
SPA	Berg and Solheim, 1978[4]
Solid-phase SPA	Hymes et al, 1979[34]
SPA-Sepharose	McVeigh and Chesterman, 1981[60]
SPA-sheep red blood cells	Takahashi et al, 1982[96]
SPA-Percoll	Shaw et al, 1984[84]
"sandwich"-SPA	Salama et al, 1985[79]
Various Assays	
Mixed passive hemagglutination	Shibata et al, 1981[85]
Immunobeads rosetting test	Salmassi et al, 1980[80]
Nephelometry of platelet lysates	Morse et al, 1982[62]
Immunoblotting Assays	
Immunoblotting of SDS-lysates	Beardsley et al, 1984[3]
Immunoprecipitation and immunoblotting	Mulder et al, 1984[72]
Immunoblotting	Herman et al, 1986[31]
Immunoblotting	v. d. Schoot et al, 1986[100]
Capture Assays	
Microtiter well assay	Woods et al, 1984[110]
Capture ELISA	Collins and Aster, 1987[9]
	Furihata et al, 1987[21]
Immunobead assay	McMillan et al, 1987[59]
MAIPA*	Kiefel et al, 1987[45]

*Abbreviations: PSIFT, platelet suspension immunofluorescence test; PAIFT, platelet adhesion immunofluorescence test; MSPRIA, microtiter solid-phase radioimmunoassay; SPRIA, solid-phase radioimmunoassay; PAP, peroxidase–antiperoxidase; CELIA, competitive enzyme-linked immunoassay; MAIPA, monoclonal antibody immobilization of platelet antigens

Enzyme-Linked Immunosorbent Assays

A large variety of ELISA modifications have been published in recent years (*see* Table 20-1). Much like the immunofluorescent test, platelets are used in suspension, as a monolayer attached to microtiter wells, or as a detergent lysate. Ligands are primary or secondary antibodies ("sandwich-type") tagged with peroxidase or alkaline phosphatase. Free proteins, as well as platelet-associated proteins bound in vivo can be measured directly (i.e., determination of platelet-fixed antibody activity) or by competitive inhibition of the labeled antiglobulin reagents. In principle, the quantification of platelet-associated immunoproteins can more elegantly be achieved by competitive assays. This is because the consumption of the antiglobulin reagent by platelet-associated immunoproteins can be directly assessed by comparison with appropriate standard curves constructed from inhibition values at a given antiglobulin dilution with known amounts of soluble antigens.

We have recently developed a highly sensitive and specific, competitive ELISA for the quantitation of platelet-associated immunoglobulins (PAIgG, PAIgM, PAIgA) and complement C3 (PAC3c, PAC3d), using both polyclonal and monoclonal reagents.[42]

Staphylococcal Protein A Assays

The staphylococcal protein A (SPA) assays exploit the ability of SPA to specifically adhere to the C_2H-domain of the Fc portion of human IgG1, IgG2, and IgG4, but not IgG3. This limits the usefulness of SPA assays, but that limitation can be overcome if purified IgG rabbit antihuman globulin antibodies are used as secondary antibodies followed by addition of radiolabeled SPA, which also has a strong affinity for rabbit IgG.[79] In general, however, SPA tests are inferior to tests employing other ligands and, therefore, are not as commonly used in clinical laboratories.

Various Assays

Various other assays listed in Table 20-1 have been recommended, but their use has been restricted to a few laboratories. They have no obvious advantages over other tests, and therefore, will not be further discussed.

Immunoblotting Assays

Immunoblotting assays have become an essential tool for the immunochemical analysis of platelet antigens and antibodies and will be described in detail in a separate chapter of this volume.

Capture Assays

The capture assays represent the latest development in the ELISA approach. Their general principle is the application of murine monoclonal antibodies, specific to epitopes on the platelet membrane, for capturing the epitope-carrying molecules from a platelet lysate onto a solid matrix (e.g., microtiter trays or plastic beads). These are then exposed to human antibodies, which are finally detected by a labeled ligand.

The first assay of this type was described by Woods et al.[110,111] in which a platelet lysate was first exposed to microtiter wells coated with monoclonal antibodies specific for GPIb or the GPIIb–IIIa complex, respectively. The respective glycoproteins (GP) were thus specifically bound to the antibody-coated wells and used as antigens in a second-step reaction with human sera containing auto-antibodies and radioactively labeled antihuman IgG antibodies. This assay proved to be specific, but rather insensitive, for the detection of platelet autoantibodies.

An important improvement was the "immunobead assay" reported by McMillan et al.[59] In this assay, specific antibody is first adsorbed onto target platelets. The platelets are then washed and solubilized, and the soluble antigen–antibody complexes are adsorbed onto plastic beads to which the mouse monoclonal antihuman IgG antibody, HB 43 (available from American Type Culture Collection), has been attached. The antigen is then identified by addition of an appropriate radioiodinated murine monoclonal antibody specific for the suspected protein antigen (e.g., AP1 specific for glycoprotein Ib; or AP2 specific for the GPIIb–IIIa complex). The murine monoclonal anti-HLA framework antibody w6.32 was used in this assay to detect anti-HLA antibodies. The main difference between the immunobead assay and the microtiter assay is that, in the former, platelets are first incubated with human antibodies before they are lysed.

Hence, certain protein epitopes are preserved which, by initial platelet solubilization, might have been destroyed and, therefore, would not have been detected by their respective platelet antibodies. The authors applied the immunobead assay successfully for the detection of platelet autoantibodies and HLA antibodies.

A similar approach, but using ELISA, was described by Collins and Aster[9] and by Furihata et al.[21] Murine monoclonal antibodies [e.g., AP1 (anti-GPIb), AP2 (anti-GPIIb–IIIa), AP3 (anti-GPIIIa), or Tab (anti-GPIIb)] are adsorbed onto the wells of microtiter trays and used to capture the corresponding antigen from a detergent lysate of platelets. The bound antigen is, thus, presented in purified form free of nonspecific proteins. The absence of HLA antigen enables detection of glycoprotein-specific antibodies in sera of transfused patients that may be heavily contaminated with HLA-specific antibodies. This assay has proved very useful for screening not only for alloantibodies, but also for autoantibodies and drug-dependent antibodies (discussed later).

Kiefel et al.[45] have developed a similar ELISA, termed monoclonal antibody-specific immobilization of platelet antigens (MAIPA). In contrast to both the aforementioned assays, the MAIPA has one important difference: target platelets are sensitized simultaneously with the human serum to be investigated *and* with the murine monoclonal antibody specific for platelet membrane glycoproteins. The sensitized platelets are then washed and solubilized by detergent. The trimolecular complexes consisting of human platelet-reactive antibodies, murine monoclonal antibodies, and platelet membrane glycoproteins carrying the respective epitopes of either type of antibodies, are then fixed to a solid phase (microtiter wells) by rabbit antimouse antibodies, and the human antibodies attached to membrane molecules held by monoclonal antibodies are then demonstrated by alkaline phosphatase-labeled antihuman antibodies (Fig. 20-1). Because of low background values, specific-binding rates are high. By employing a set of monoclonal antibodies specific for human platelet membrane constituents and a platelet panel with known alloantigens, platelet-reactive antibodies can be characterized, in a single experiment, both by localization of epitopes (e.g., HLA class I molecules, GPIIb–IIIa complex molecules, GPIX–Ib complex molecules) and by serologic specificities. Platelet antibodies of different immunoglobulin classes can also be detected by using class-specific antihuman globulin sera. The MAIPA is a particularly sensitive and practical tool for analysis of sera with ambiguous serologic findings.

USE AND LIMITATIONS OF METHODS FOR THE DEMONSTRATION OF PLATELET ANTIBODIES

The diagnosis of immune thrombocytopenia requires laboratory techniques capable of detecting platelet-reactive antibodies with a high degree of accuracy and reproducibility. To this end, the serologic platelet laboratory should not rely upon any single assay but, instead, should use a number of assays that collectively provide a broad capability for antibody detection. This repertoire of methods should be capable of distinguishing auto- and alloantibodies, platelet-specific, and HLA antibodies, as well as complement-fixing and non–complement-fixing antibodies. Both direct and indirect assays that incorporate elution procedures to differentiate between antibody-mediated and other immunologically mediated thrombocytopenias should be available. This chapter critically reviews the feasibility of various methods for antibody detection as reflected in our own experience.

Platelet Autoantibodies

Platelet autoantibodies play an important pathogenetic role in idiopathic and secondary autoimmune thrombocytopenia (reviewed in Refs. 56 and 107). For the demonstration of autoantibodies, both platelet-associated immunoglobulins (PAIg) and free serum autoantibodies are conventionally determined.

Platelet-Associated Immunoglobulins

The origin and nature of PAIg is discussed in Chapter 16. In this context, we shall merely focus on some diagnostic and methodologic aspects of PAIg determinations.

It has been shown by many workers that PAIgG and, also, more recently, PAIgM, PAIgA, and PAC3 are present on platelets of normal individuals. Normal values differ considerably with the methods used (Table 20-2)

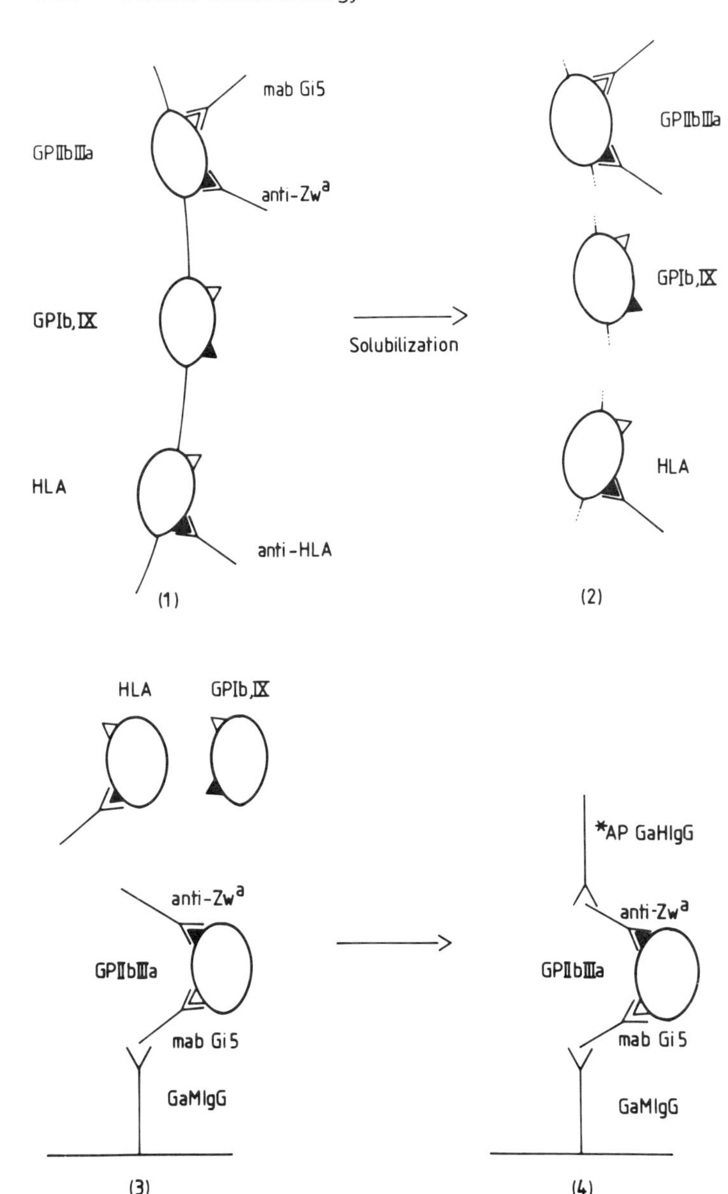

Figure 20-1. Schematic representation of the Monoclonal antibody immobilization of platelet antigens (MAIPA) assay. (*1*) Three different glycoproteins (GP)—the GPIIb-IIIa complex, the GPIX-Ib complex, and HLA antigens (HLA)—in a section of the platelet membrane (line) are illustrated. Platelets are incubated with a monoclonal antibody (MAb) reactive with an epitope on GPIIb-IIIa complex (MAb Gi5) and an antigen on the same GP complex (anti-Zw^a). The HLA antibodies (anti-HLA) also present in the human serum bind to another GP. (*2*) The platelet membrane is disrupted by detergent lysis. (*3*) The GPIIb-IIIa complex carrying the MAb is immobilized into wells of a microtiter plate coated with goat antimouse IgG (GaMIgG). (*4*) The human antibody (anti-Zw^a) fixed to the immobilized GPIIb-IIIa complex is detected by alkaline phosphatase-labeled goat antihuman IgG (*AP GaHIgG).

and, as a rule, are higher if platelet lysates, instead of whole platelets, are measured, probably because of the α-granule immunoglobulins[39,78,107] (*see also* Chap. 16).

Platelet-associated immunoglobulin values are elevated to a variable degree in most cases of autoimmune thrombocytopenia (AITP; for review see Ref. 107) and also in a certain proportion of patients with thrombocytopenias of presumably nonimmunologic origin.[40,68] This has led us[68,70] and others[40,78,85] to question the hypothesis that increased quantities of PAIg represent bound antiplatelet antibodies.

The reason for increased levels of PAIg is not clear. There are two basically different interpretations. One argues that high levels of platelet-associated immune proteins measured in normal and, more so, in pathologic states are real and are partly due to a nonspecific process, possibly by the entrapment of plasma components in the platelet canalicular system or resealed membrane fragments.[33,87] This has been disputed by others.[41] An alternative theory claims that the high amounts of PAIgG, as reported by most authors, are caused by inappropriate technical conditions (prepara-

Table 20-2
Normal Values of Platelet-Associated IgG Determined by Various Assays

Refs.	Assay	Normal Values
Direct Binding Assays		
v. d. Borne et al 1978[106]	PSIFT	Negative
Mueller-Eckhardt et al 1978[77]	PRAT	<2.5% of total radioactivity
Cines and Schreiber 1979[8]	PRAT	1–5 × 10^3 binding sites/platelet
Leporrier et al 1979[52]	ELISA	235 ± 74 binding sites/platelet
LoBuglio et al 1983[53]	PRAT with monoclonal anti-IgG	169 ± 79 binding sites/platelet
Competitive Binding Assays		
McMillan et al 1971[57]	Fab-anti-Fab assay	♂ 0.41–1.74 fg/platelet ♀ 0.49–1.94 fg/platelet
Dixon et al 1975[16]	Hemolysis inhibition assay	200–400 fg/platelet
Nel and Stevens 1980[19]	ELISA	1.3–15.3 fg/platelet
Follea et al 1982[19]	ELISA	2.04 ± 1.1 fg/platelet
Kelton and Denomme 1983[38]	Immunoradiometric assay	0.8 fg/platelet
Assays Measuring PAIgG in Platelet Lysates		
Morse et al 1981[61]	Radial immunodiffusion	1.5–7.0 fg/platelet
Hegde et al 1981[29]	ELISA	5–16 fg/platelet
Kunicki et al 1983[48]	Electroimmunoassay	2.7–7.2 fg/platelet
Winiarski and Holm 1983[109]	ELISA	3.2 ± 1.4 fg/platelet

For abbreviations of assays see legend of Table 20-1; PRAT, platelet radioactive anti-immunoglobulin test.

tion of platelets, application of polyclonal antibodies), and that the normal platelet surface displays only small amounts of IgG (124 ± 86 molecules per platelet) if a specific monoclonal anti-IgG is used[12] (*see also* Chap. 16). It also has been reported that such an assay would allow excellent discrimination between immune and nonimmune thrombocytopenias.[11,53]

We have recently studied these problems in more detail with a quantitative competitive ELISA.[42] Most conspicuous was our finding that PAIgG values, whether assessed by monoclonal or by polyclonal antihuman IgG antibodies, were identical, regardless of whether normal individuals or thrombocytopenic patients were analyzed. Although the binding characteristics of the monoclonal antibody we used were slightly different from the polyclonal (rabbit) anti-IgG, as reflected in the slope of the calibration curve (Fig. 20-2), there was an almost perfect correlation between results obtained with both reagents over a wide range of PAIgG concentrations.[5] (See Fig. 20-3). These data contrast with those published by LoBuglio's group.[11,12,53] We cannot see any theoretical reason why data generated with monoclonal antibodies should be different from those obtained with polyclonal monospecific antibodies, provided both are employed under strictly identical conditions. Furthermore, we believe that the use of monoclonal reagents will not permit better discrimination between immune and nonimmune thrombocytopenias. It is much more likely that the large amount of PAIg measurable on washed normal or diseased human platelets is a biologic fact, rather than a technical artifact. This opinion is consistent with the view of other investigators.[37,87,107] Recent data from George et al.[22] have indicated that a large proportion of PAIgG is localized in α granules (for details *see* Chap. 16). The ultimate question about the role and origin of PAIgG is still unanswered.

An additional source of discrepant results lies in the choice of anticoagulant. It was early reported that EDTA caused increased nonspecific consumption of antihuman globulin by platelets.[46] Blood anticoagulated with EDTA has also been shown to exhibit increased PAIgG levels, either immediately after or within 24 hr of blood collection.[28] Lucas and Holburn[54] have recently demonstrated that blood anticoagulated with solid K_2 EDTA had PAIgG levels fivefold higher than citrated blood, and they presented evidence that this was attributable to low-density particulate material, with an apparent volume of > 33 fl and, therefore, it would seem that these levels are unlikely to be derived from platelets. Conse-

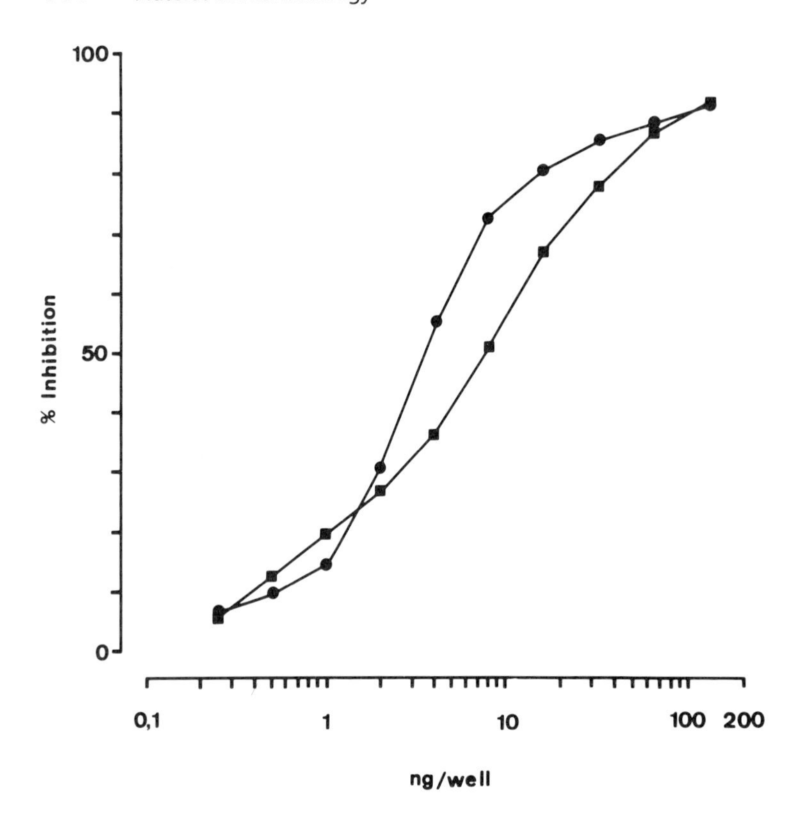

Figure 20-2. Calibration curve of the competitive enzyme-linked immunoassay (CELIA) for quantification of platelet-associated IgG using polyclonal rabbit antihuman IgG γ-chain-specific (dots), and monoclonal mouse antihuman IgG (squares) (Kiefel V, Jäger S, Mueller-Eckhardt C: Vox Sang 53:151, 1987).

quently, the authors recommend that solid K_2 EDTA should not be used to anticoagulate blood destined for PAIgG measurement.

The only reliable method to differentiate between platelet-bound immunoglobulins exhibiting an autoantibody nature and nonspecifically bound immunoglobulins, i.e., immune complexes or aggregated immunoglobulins, is elution and reassociation of antibodies with platelets. Acid and ether elution have been used most extensively.[33,88,107] Von dem Borne and associates[107] found definite positive results in 49 of 118 patients with idiopathic or secondary autoimmune thrombocytopenia (41.5%), but the test failed in approximately 50% to 60% of the patients. This may be related to the insensitivity of the detection systems used or to the nonspecific nature of the major portion of platelet-associated immunoglobulins.[33]

Elutability of PAIgs is particularly mandatory in patients without thrombocytopenia but with platelet functional defects. Niessner et al.[76] have recently described a patient with a thrombasthenialike thrombocytopathy in which the highly elevated PAIgG could be shown to be, at least in part, autoantibodies directed against epitopes on the GPIIb–IIIa complex.

Serum Platelet Autoantibodies

It is now clear that, in uncomplicated cases of autoimmune thrombocytopenia, free serum platelet autoantibodies are, with very few exceptions, of the IgG class and "incomplete" (i.e., noncomplement-fixing). Hence, they literally never agglutinate test platelets (for review *see* Ref. 63). By the same token, all platelet function assays such as aggregometry, serotonin release, and platelet factor 3 release have not stood the test of time and must be considered obsolete.[63] In rare instances, however, sera of patients with secondary AITP may contain antibodylike factors that aggregate platelets directly. Thus, we have described a patient with systemic lupus erythematosus (SLE) and typical immune thrombocytopenia whose serum caused strong agglutination and aggregation of washed platelets and platelet-rich plasma of all panel donors used and induced serotonin release.[64] Among many hundreds of AITP patients now investigated in our laboratory, we have never encountered a similar case.

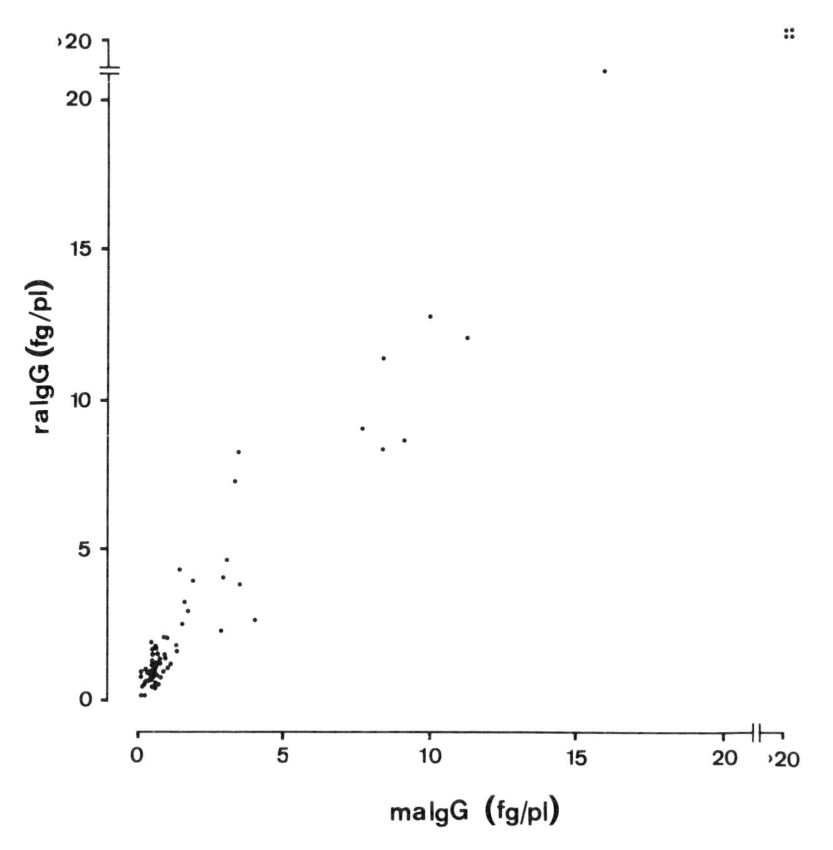

Figure 20-3. PAIgG (fg/platelet) determined simultaneously on normal platelets and on platelets with elevated PAIgG with a polyclonal rabbit antihuman IgG, γ-chain-specific (ra IgG), and a monoclonal mouse antihuman IgG (ma IgG). Each point represents the mean of duplicate determinations at two different platelet concentrations (Kiefel V, Jäger S, Mueller-Eckhardt C: Vox Sang 53:151, 1987).

Complement-fixing platelet autoantibodies are also very unusual, and only a few adequately documented cases have been reported.[35,94] A complement-fixing monoclonal IgM κ-antiplatelet antibody was recently described in a patient with secondary AITP resulting from malignant lymphoreticular disease.[51] Devine et al.[15] studied a patient with severe thrombocytopenia after procainamide therapy who had free complement-fixing platelet autoantibodies in his plasma that were directed against determinants on the GPIb complex. These autoantibodies inhibited ristocetin-induced aggregation, a property of platelets mediated by GPIb. This type of antibody is best demonstrated by direct complement fixation assays, for instance, the microcomplement fixation test[10] that is routinely used in our laboratory, or by the complement-dependent platelet lysis assay used by Aster and associates.[47,94]

For the demonstration of almost all free noncomplement-fixing platelet autoantibodies, one of the antiglobulin-binding assays is recommended. The platelet immunofluorescent test with one of its varied modifications is probably the technique of choice and is used in most laboratories for screening purposes. If monospecific antisera against different immunoglobulin classes or complement components (e.g., C3 or C4) are concomitantly utilized, additional relevant information can be obtained.[109] In our experience, the PAIFT is the easiest test to perform and is very sensitive. The ELISA techniques, although more cumbersome, are similarly useful.[27]

The percentage of positive tests by using serum of AITP patients obtained in the acute thrombocytopenic phase varies greatly. Whereas von dem Borne et al.[102] found 28 of 80 cases (35%) positive, the respective figures reported by Hegde et al.[27] and Dixon et al.[16] were 57% and 100%, respectively. With use of the PAIFT, we found free platelet autoantibodies in only 20% of sera.* All were IgG, and only one serum also contained noncomplement-fixing IgM autoantibodies. Because many patients with chronic AITP are young multiparous women, HLA antibodies are frequently encountered and are usually recognized by microlymphocytotoxicity tests using an appropriate platelet and lymphocyte panel.

Glycoprotein specificity of platelet autoantibodies can be determined by Western blotting,[3] by the microtiter assay,[110,111] by the immunobead assay,[59] by MAIPA,[45] or by the glycoprotein capture assay.[21] Western blotting yields positive results in only a few sera that are positive by other assays, such as the PAIFT. This is probably because of the denaturation of epitopes on glycoprotein molecules by sodium dodecyl sulfate. Most epitopes recognized by platelet autoantibodies have been localized to the GPIIb–IIIa complex. Less frequently, they are found to reside on GPIb. McMillan et al.,[59] using the immunobead assay, recently studied 59 patients with chronic autoimmune thrombocytopenia (AITP) for platelet-associated and plasma autoantibodies against the GPIIb–IIIa complex and GPIb. Platelet-associated autoantibodies were detected in 21 of 28 patients (13 with anti-GPIIb–IIIa and 8 with anti-GPIb), whereas plasma autoantibodies were noted in 34 of 59 patients (21 with anti-GPIIb–IIIa, 11 with anti-GPIb, and 2 with both). In a study conducted in our laboratory, sera from 56 patients with AITP, which had been shown by immunofluorescence to contain platelet-reactive autoantibodies, were investigated by MAIPA. Of these, 14 had autoantibodies reactive with the GPIIb–IIIa complex, 11 with the GPIX–Ib complex, and 3 with both. Twenty-eight sera did not react, indicating that the autoantibodies were directed against epitopes on other glycoproteins. With use of both Western blotting and MAIPA, we have localized platelet autoantigens to GPIb, GPIIb, as well as on GPIIIa.[45,81]

Clinical Conditions Associated with Platelet Alloantibodies

Three well-defined clinical entities require detailed serologic analysis: neonatal alloimmune thrombocytopenic purpura (NATP), post-transfusion purpura (PTP), and refractoriness to platelet transfusion. The major problem in these conditions is the frequent simultaneous occurrence of platelet-specific and HLA antibodies, rendering serologic investigation difficult.

Neonatal Alloimmune Thrombocytopenic Purpura

Neonatal alloimmune thrombocytopenic purpura caused by platelet antibodies is evidently a rare clinical condition (reviewed in Ref. 69, 73, 86, 88). Approximately 80% of established cases with demonstrable platelet-specific alloantibodies are due to Pl^{A1} (Zw^{a}) antibodies. A few cases caused by other antibodies have been reported. Practically all antibodies are of the noncomplement-fixing (blocking) type and belong to the IgG class. Thus, it had already been shown by Shulman et al.[88] in early work that they usually cannot be demonstrated directly by complement fixation but, rather, by their ability to inhibit (block) complement fixation by antibodies of identical specificity. In recent years, platelet-specific alloantibodies in NATP have mostly been assessed by immunofluorescence. In the few larger series published by Shulman's,[86] Aster's,[47] von dem Borne's,[103] Muller's,[73] and our group,[69] the immunofluorescent or the radioactive antiglobulin tests were primarily used.

In our series of more than 120 children with serologically proven NATP, 115 cases were precipitated by anti-Pl^{A1}, 1 each by anti-Pl^{A2} and Bak^{a}, 4 by antibodies of a recently described new specificity, anti-Br^{a}.[43] Most antibodies were initially detected by PAIFT. Weak or doubtful sera were reinvestigated by CELIA.[42] In general, both assays are of comparable sensitivity, but the PAIFT is much less cumbersome and, therefore, is recommended as a first-line test. The MAIPA[45] proved to be of particular value when the maternal sera were contaminated by HLA antibodies, obscuring platelet-specific antibodies, and in patients with a clinical picture suggesting NATP but with negative conventional serology. Thus, we have recently identified four patients with NATP resulting from a new platelet-specific alloantibody, anti-Br^{a}, which did not reliably react in binding assays that used whole platelets.[43] In patients for whom no serologic diagnosis can be made, the alloantibody can sometimes be identified by elution and antibody

*Unpublished data.

concentration.[67] If no antibody can be detected in the maternal serum against selected panel platelets, it is always advisable to use paternal platelets for a crossmatch to avoid missing a new or rare antibody specificity. For crossmatching, the CELIA or MAIPA proved particularly useful in our hands because shipped paternal platelets can be used. Platelet typing of parental and, after recovery, of neonatal platelets is obligatory for establishing the antibody specificity. The method used depends on the availability of appropriate antibodies.

Posttransfusion Purpura

Data describing approximately 150 cases of this rare syndrome have been published (for reviews *see* Refs. 2 and 65). As in NATP, platelet antibodies of Pl^{A1} specificity are responsible for most cases, but HLA antibodies are present more often and at higher titers. In our survey of 25 PTP patients, 22 were due to Pl^{A1} and 1 to Bak^{b} antibodies.[45a] In one patient, only HLA antibodies were detected, despite extensive absorption and elution. More than half of the PTP sera contained HLA antibodies, and complement-fixing Pl^{A1} antibodies were present in 10 of 25 sera. All platelet antibodies were detectable by immunofluorescence, in line with the experience of Pegels et al.[77] and von dem Borne et al.[105] Therefore, we prefer the PAIFT as a primary assay, although ^{51}Cr release, the PRAT, or the ELISA have been successfully used for antibody identification.

Refractoriness to Platelet Transfusion

One of the major problems in platelet immunology lies with detection of alloimmunization against platelets in patients receiving multiple blood transfusions. The incidence of alloimmunization in patients receiving multiple blood transfusions is estimated to be approximately 50% to 70%.[74] The HLA antibodies are thought to be involved in about 70% to 80% of patients, and the frequency of platelet-specific antibodies has been reported as high as 20% to 25%.[74] The specificity of these antibodies, however, has never been elucidated. Hence, many crossmatch procedures have been advocated. The efficacy of such assays is analyzed in Chapter 21. In our experience, none of the available assays, including PAIFT and ELISA, has shown sufficient reliability to predict the platelet increment in refractory patients. However, a new possibility may be opened by the application of the MAIPA or similar techniques (e.g., the immunobead assay[59] or the capture ELISA[21]) for platelet crossmatching. For instance, McMillan et al.[58] have evaluated by the immunobead assay 51 single-donor platelet transfusions given to seven patients refractory to random donors. They reported a correct prediction value of 88%. We have recently analyzed, by MAIPA, a patient's serum that contained two platelet-specific antibodies (anti-Bak^{a} and anti-Pl^{A2}) and polyspecific HLA antibodies.[49] The serologic analysis is outlined in Figure 20-4. The potential for these assays is promising, but their practical usefulness remains to be determined (*see also* Chap. 21).

Drug-Induced Immune Thrombocytopenia

A vast and ever-increasing number of drugs have been implicated in DITP. Most of the proven cases, however, are due to a few compounds, e.g., quinine, quinidine, sulfonamides, gold, and heparin (for review *see* Ref. 66; *see also* Chap. 8). From a serologic point of view, two basic forms of drug-induced platelet antibodies need to be differentiated: drug-dependent platelet antibodies and drug-induced, but drug-independent platelet autoantibodies. Whereas the former react only with platelets if free antigen (drug) is present in the solution, the latter combine with platelets in the absence of drug (or metabolites) and behave serologically as true platelet autoantibodies. Prototypes are quinidine- and gold-induced platelet antibodies.

A plethora of tests have been employed for the serologic determination of drug-induced platelet antibodies. Although strong, particularly complement-fixing drug-dependent antibodies, can be recognized by almost any method, many of the older assays (i.e., clot retraction, platelet agglutination, serotonin release, platelet factor 3 release, platelet migration inhibition) must be regarded as obsolete because of their insensitivity and nonspecificity. Reliable methods include complement fixation, complement-dependent ^{51}Cr release for complement-fixing antibodies, and direct binding assays using labeled antiglobulin reagents (reviewed in Ref. 23, 66, 86). Immunoblotting has been employed successfully for the definition of target antigens of quinidine-dependent antibodies[91] but, in our hands, this assay yields positive results with only a few antibodies. No single assay, therefore, is supe-

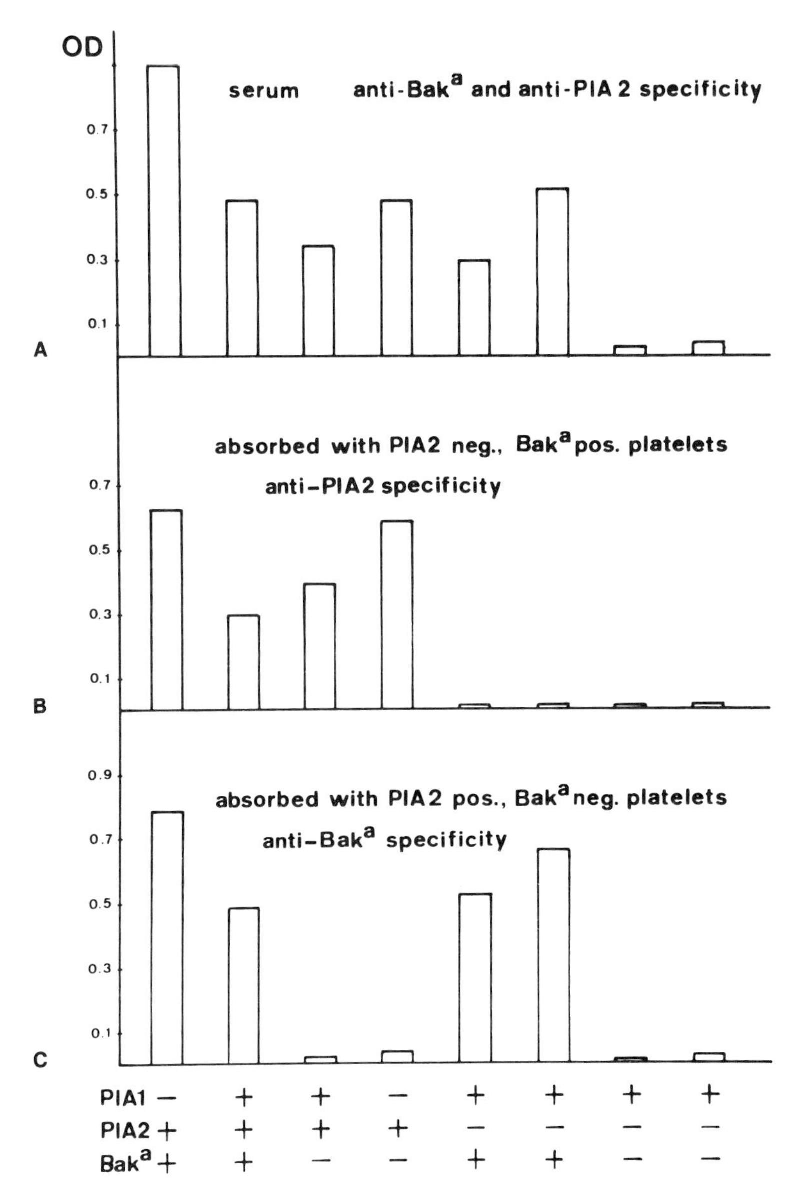

Figure 20-4. Serologic analysis by MAIPA of serum from a patient refractory to random platelet transfusions. The serum contained two rare platelet-specific antibodies (anti-Bak^a and anti-Pl^{A2}) associated with multispecific HLA antibodies. The platelet GPIIb–IIIa complex was immobilized by monoclonal antibody Gi5. Pl^{A1}, Pl^{A2}, and Bak^a antigens of panel donors are shown at the bottom. (*A*) Reaction pattern of unabsorbed serum; (*B*) Serum absorbed with Bak^a-positive platelets showing anti-Pl^{A2} specificity; (*C*) Serum absorbed with Pl^{A2}-positive platelets showing anti-Bak^a specificity. Note the gene-dosage effect of anti-Pl^{A2} with homozygous (donors 1 and 4 from left) and heterozygous Pl^{A2}-positive platelets (donors 2 and 3 from left) (Langenscheidt F, Kiefel V, Mueller-Eckhardt C: Transfusion, in press).

rior for the detection of all antibodies. For instance, Kunicki and Aster[47] reported that 14 of 18 quinine- and quinidine-dependent antibodies gave positive results in both the PSIFT and ^{51}Cr- release assays, but two antibodies were positive in either test alone. In our experience most, but not all, quinine- and quinidine-dependent antibodies are complement-fixing and readily recognizable by platelet complement fixation, whereas weaker, noncomplement-fixing, drug-dependent antibodies (e.g., reactive with *p*-aminosalicylic acid, rifampicin, nomifensine, or sulfamethoxazole) were detected only by immunofluorescence (PAIFT) or CELIA using anti-IgG and anti-IgM.[44] It is also mandatory that "ex vivo antigens" [i.e., plasma or urine samples from individuals obtained before (control) and at appropriate times after ingestion of therapeutic doses of the suspected drug] are employed, because it is now obvious that some drug-dependent antibodies are directed against metabolites of drugs, rather than the original compound.[17,18,44]

Drug-induced, but drug-independent platelet autoantibodies can be best demonstrated by one of the antiglobulin-binding assays. Most authors favor the platelet immunofluorescent test.[47,66,104]

Heparin-induced thrombocytopenia is regarded by some authors as an immune disorder, but definite proof is still lacking (for review *see* Ref. 66; *see also* Chap. 8). The most frequently reported positive laboratory tests are platelet aggregation or [^{14}C]serotonin release using autologous platelet-rich plasma (PRP) or mixtures of the patient's plasma and normal PRP in the presence of heparin. Binding assays and Western blot analysis have also been used, but both the optimal procedure for antibody detection and the ideal method for detection of the platelet antigens involved remain to be determined.

CONCLUDING REMARKS

Platelet serology is still a notoriously difficult task and, to a large extent, has remained the domain of specialized laboratories. Nevertheless, slow but continuous methodologic progress, leading to the development of methods with higher sensitivity, higher specificity, and reduced susceptibility to laboratory errors, have brought platelet laboratory procedures within the realm of clinical immunohematology. Judicious, professional use of these procedures will undoubtedly assist in the diagnosis and treatment of bleeding disorders.

This work was supported by the Deutsche Forschungsgemeinschaft, Mu 277/9-6

REFERENCES

1. Andersen E, Bashir H, Archer GT: Modification of the platelet suspension immunofluorescence test. Vox Sang 40:44, 1981

2. Aster RH: Posttransfusion purpura. In Engelfriet CP (ed): Baillères Clinical Immunology and Allergy. London, Academic Press, 1988

3. Beardsley DS, Spiegel JE, Jacobs MM, Handin RI, Lux SE IV: Platelet membrane glycoprotein IIIa contains target antigens that bind anti-platelet antibodies in immune thrombocytopenias. J Clin Invest 74:1701, 1984

4. Bergh OJ Solheim BG: Detection of thrombocyte antibodies by ^{125}I labeled protein A. Tissue Antigens 12:189, 1978

5. Blumberg N, Masel D, Stoler M: Disparities in estimates of IgG bound to normal platelets. Blood 67:200, 1986

6. Cheung N-KV, McFall P, Schulman I: A microtiter solid-phase radioimmunoassay for platelet-associated immunoglobulin G. J Lab Clin Med 101:392, 1983

7. Cimo PL, Gerber SA: AET-treated platelets: Their usefulness for platelet antibody detection and an examination of their altered sensitivity to immune lysis. Blood 54:1101, 1979

8. Cines DB, Schreiber AD: Immune thrombocytopenia. Use of a Coombs antiglobulin test to detect IgG and C3 on platelets. N Engl J Med 300:106, 1979

9. Collins J, Aster RH: Use of immobilized platelet membrane glycoproteins for the detection of platelet-specific alloantibodies in solid-phase ELISA. Vox Sang 53:157, 1987

10. Colombani J, D'Amaro J, Gabb B, Smith G, Svejgaard A: International agreement on a microtechnique of platelet complement fixation (Pl. C Fix.). Transplant Proc 3:121, 1971

11. Court WS, Bozeman JM, Soong SJ, Saleh MN, Shaw DR, LoBuglio AF: Platelet surface-bound IgG in patients with immune and nonimmune thrombocytopenia. Blood 69:278, 1987

12. Court WS, LoBuglio AF: Measurement of platelet surface-bound IgG by a monoclonal ^{125}I-anti-IgG assay. Vox Sang 50:154, 1986

13. Dacie JV: The Haemolytic Anaemias (Part II), 2nd ed. New York, Grune & Stratton, 1962

14. Dausset J, Malinvaud G: Influence de l'agitation sur l'agglutination thrombocytaire. Sang 25:847, 1954

15. Devine DV, Currie MS, Rosse WF, Greenberg CS: Pseudo-Bernard-Soulier syndrome caused by autoantibody to platelet glycoprotein Ib. Blood 68(Suppl 1):106a, 1986

16. Dixon R, Rosse W, Ebert L: Quantitative determination of antibody in idiopathic thrombocytopenic purpura: Correlation of serum and platelet-bound antibody in clinical response. N Engl J Med 292:230, 1975

17. Eisner EV, Kasper K: Immune thrombocytopenia due to a metabolite of para-amino-salicylic acid (PAS). Am J Med 53:790, 1972

18. Eisner EV, Shaidi NT: Immune thrombocytopenia due to a drug metabolite. N Engl J Med 287:376, 1972

19. Follea G, Mandrand B, Dechavanne M: Simultaneous enzymoimmunologic assay of platelet-

associated IgG, IgM and C3. A useful tool in assessment of immune thrombocytopenias. Thromb Res 26:249, 1982

20. Forster J, Schmidt B: Micro-enzyme-linked immunoassay for the quantitation of platelet-associated IgG (PAIgG). Klin Wochenschr 61:165, 1983

21. Furihata K, Nugent DJ, Bissonette A, Aster RH, Kunicki TJ: On the association of the platelet-specific alloantigen, Pen[a], with glycoprotein IIIa. Evidence for heterogeneity of glycoprotein IIIa. J Clin Invest 80:1624, 1987

22. George JN, Saucerman S, Levine SP, et al: Immunoglobulin G is a platelet alpha granule-secreted protein. J Clin Invest 76:2020, 1985

23. Hackett T, Kelton JG, Powers P: Drug-induced platelet destruction. Semin Thromb Hemost 8:116, 1982

24. Harrington WJ, Minnich V, Hollingsworth JW, Moore CV: Demonstration of a thrombocytopenic factor in the blood of patients with thrombocytopenic purpura. J Lab Clin Med 38:1, 1951

25. Harrington WJ, Sprague CC, Minnich V, Moore CV, Aulvin RC, Dubach R: Immunologic mechanisms in idiopathic and neonatal thrombocytopenic purpura. Ann Intern Med 38:433, 1953

26. Hawker RJ, Hawker LM: A microcytotoxicity assay using ^{111}indium oxine release from platelets. J Immunol Methods 33:45, 1980

27. Hegde UM, Bowes A, Powell DK, Joyner MV: Detection of platelet-bound and serum antibodies in autoimmune thrombocytopenia by enzyme-linked assay. Vox Sang 41:306, 1981

28. Hegde UM, Bowes A, Roter BLT: The effect of storage in different anticoagulants on platelet associated IgG. Clin Lab Haematol 6:51, 1984

29. Hegde UM, Powell DK, Bowes A, Gordon-Smith EC: Enzyme-linked immunoassay for the detection of platelet associated IgG. Br J Haematol 48:39, 1981

30. Helmerhorst FM, Bossers B, de Bruin HG, Engelfriet CP, von dem Borne AEG Kr: Detection of platelet antibodies: A comparison of three techniques. Vox Sang 39:83, 1980

31. Herman JH, Kickler TS, Ness PM: The resolution of platelet serologic problems using Western blotting. Tissue Antigens 28:257, 1986

32. Horai S, Claas FHJ, van Rood JJ: Detection of platelet antibodies by enzyme-linked immunosorbent assay (ELISA). Comparative studies with the indirect immunofluorescence assay. Immunol Lett 3:155, 1981

33. Hotchkiss AJ, Leissinger CA, Smith ME, Jordan JV, Kautz CA, Shulman NR: Evaluation by quantitative acid elution and radioimmunoassay of multiple classes of immunoglobulins and serum albumin associated with platelets in idiopathic thrombocytopenic purpura. Blood 67:1126, 1986

34. Hymes K, Shulman S, Karpatkin S: Solid-phase radioimmunoassay for bound anti-platelet antibody. J Lab Clin Med 94:639, 1979

35. Kayser W, Mueller-Eckhardt C, Budde U, Schmidt RE: Complement-fixing platelet autoantibodies in autoimmune thrombocytopenia. Am J Hematol 11:213, 1981

36. Kekomäki R: Detection of platelet-bound IgG with ^{125}I-labelled staphylococcal protein A. Med Biol 54:112, 1977

37. Kelton JG: Platelet associated IgG. Clin Res 33:383, 1985

38. Kelton JG, Denomme G: An immunoradiometric assay for quantitating platelet-associated IgG. In McMillan R (ed): Immune Cytopenias, pp 197–213. New York, Churchill-Livingstone, 1983

39. Kelton JG, Denomme G, Lucarelli A, Garvey J, Powers P, Carter C: Comparison of the measurement of surface or total platelet-associated IgG in the diagnosis of immune thrombocytopenia. Am J Hematol 18:1, 1985

40. Kelton JG, Powers PJ, Carter CJ: A prospective study of the usefulness of the measurement of platelet-associated IgG for the diagnosis of idiopathic thrombocytopenic purpura. Blood 60:1050, 1982

41. Kelton JG, Sheridan D, Neame PB, Simon GT: Platelet fragments do not contribute to elevated levels of platelet associated IgG. Br J Haematol 61:707, 1985

42. Kiefel V, Jäger S, Mueller-Eckhardt C: Competitive enzyme-linked immunoassay (CELIA) for the quantitation of platelet-associated immunoglobulins (IgG, IgM, IgA) and complement (C3c, C3d) with polyclonal and monoclonal reagents. Vox Sang 53:151, 1987

43. Kiefel V, Santoso S, Katzmann B, Mueller-Eckhardt C: A new platelet-specific alloantigen Br(a). Report of four cases with neonatal alloimmune thrombocytopenia. Vox Sang 54:101, 1988

44. Kiefel V, Santoso S, Schmidt S, Salama A, Mueller-Eckhardt C: Metabolite-specific (IgG) and drug specific antibodies (IgG, IgM) in two cases of trimethoprim-sulfamethoxazole-induced immune thrombocytopenia. Transfusion 27:262, 1987

45. Kiefel V, Santoso S, Weisheit M, Mueller-Eckhardt C: Monoclonal antibody-specific immobilization of platelet antigens (MAIPA): A new tool for the identification of platelet-reactive antibodies. Blood 70:1722, 1987

45a. Kiefel V, Santoso S, Glöckner WM, Katzmann B, Mayr W, Mueller-Eckhardt C: Post-transfusion purpura associated with an antibody against an allele of the Bak[a] antigen. Vox Sanguinis (in press), 1988

46. Kissmeyer-Nielsen F, Jensen KG: Immunology of platelets. Prog Clin Pathol 2:141, 1969

47. Kunicki TJ, Aster RH: Qualitative and quantitative tests for platelet alloantibodies and drug-dependent antibodies. In McMillan R (ed): Immune Cytopenias, pp 49-67. New York, Churchill-Livingstone, 1983

48. Kunicki TJ, Koenig MB, Kristopeit SM, Aster DH: Direct quantitation of platelet-associated IgG by electroimmunoassay. Blood 60:54, 1982

49. Langenscheidt F, Kiefel V, Santoso S, Mueller-Eckhardt C: Platelet transfusion refractoriness due to two rare platelet-specific alloantibodies (anti-Bak[a] and anti-Pl[A2]) associated with multiple HLA antibodies. Transfusion (in press)

50. Lazarchik J, Hall SA: Platelet-associated IgG assay using flow cytometric analysis. J Immunol Methods 87:257, 1986

51. Lehman HA, Lehman LO, Rustagi PK, Rustgi RN, Plunkett, RW, Farolino DL, Conway J, Logue GL: Complement-mediated autoimmune thrombocytopenia. N Engl J Med 316:194, 1987

52. Leporrier M, Dighiero G, Auzemery M, Binet JL: Detection and quantification of platelet-bound antibodies with immunoperoxidase. Br J Haematol 42:605, 1979

53. LoBuglio AF, Court WS, Vinocur L, Maglott G, Shaw GM: Immune thrombocytopenic purpura: Use of a ^{125}I-labeled antihuman IgG monoclonal antibody to quantify platelet-bound IgG. N Engl J Med 309:459, 1983

54. Lucas GF, Holburn AM: The effect of anticoagulant on platelet associated IgG. Br J Haematol 65:111, 1987

55. Magee JM: A study of the effects of treating platelets with paraformaldehyde for use in the platelet suspension immunofluorescence test. Br J Haematol 61:513, 1985

56. McMillan R: Chronic idiopathic thrombocytopenic purpura. N Engl J Med 304:1135, 1981

57. McMillan R, Smith RS, Longmire RL, Yelonosky R, Reid RT, Craddock CG: Immunoglobulin associated with human platelets. Blood 37:316, 1971

58. McMillan R, Tani P, Berchtold P, Millard F: Detection of autoantibodies and alloantibodies against platelet-associated antigens (abstr). Thromb Haemostasis 58:530, 1987

59. McMillan R, Tani P, Renshaw L, Woods VL: Platelet-associated and plasma anti-glycoprotein autoantibodies in chronic ITP. Blood 70:1040, 1987

60. McVeigh DJ, Chesterman CN: The use of a protein A-Sepharose column in the detection of platelet-associated IgG. Thromb Res 23:559, 1981

61. Morse BS, Giuliani D, Nussbaum M: Quantitation of platelet-associated IgG by radial immunodiffusion. Blood 57:809, 1981

62. Morse BS, Giuliani D, Nussbaum M: A rapid quantitation of platelet-associated IgG by nephelometry. Am J Hematol 12:271, 1982

63. Mueller-Eckhardt C: Idiopathic thrombocytopenic purpura (ITP): Clinical and immunologic considerations. Semin Thromb Hemost 3:125, 1977

64. Mueller-Eckhardt C: Clinical significance of immune complex-induced thrombocytopenias. In de Gaetano G, Garattini S (eds): Platelets: A Multidisciplinary Approach, pp 269-282. New York, Raven Press, 1978

65. Mueller-Eckhardt C: Posttransfusion purpura. Br J Haematol 64:419, 1986

66. Mueller-Eckhardt C: Drug-induced immune thrombocytopenia. In Engelfriet CP (ed): Baillière's Clinical Immunology and Allergy, pp 369-389. London, Academic Press, 1987

67. Mueller-Eckhardt C, Kayser W, Förster C, Mueller-Eckhardt G: Improved assay for detection of platelet-specific Pl[A1] antibodies in neonatal alloimmune thrombocytopenia. Vox Sang 43:76, 1981

68. Mueller-Eckhardt C, Kayser W, Mersch-Baumert K, Mueller-Eckhardt G, Breidenbach M, Kugel H-G, Graubner M: The clinical significance of platelet-associated IgG: A study on 298 patients with various disorders. Br J Haematol 46:123, 1980

69. Mueller-Eckhardt C, Küenzlen E: Alloimmune thrombocytopenia of the newborn. In Engelfriet CP, van Loghem JJ, von dem Borne AEG Kr (eds): Immunohematology, pp 165-171. Amsterdam, Elsevier Science Publishers, 1984

70. Mueller-Eckhardt C, Mueller-Eckhardt G, Kayser W, Voss RM, Wegner J, Küenzlen E: Platelet-associated IgG, platelet survival, and platelet sequestration in thrombocytopenic states. Br J Haematol 52:49, 1982

71. Mueller-Eckhardt C, Schulz G, Sauer K-H, Dienst C, Mahn I: Studies on the platelet radioactive anti-immunoglobulin test. J Immunol Methods 19:1, 1978

72. Mulder A, van Leeuwen EF, Veenboer GJM, Tetteroo PAT, von dem Borne AEG Kr: Immunochemical characterization of platelet-specific alloantigens. Scand J Haematol 33:267, 1984

73. Muller JY, Rezinikoff-Etievant MF, Patereau C, Dangu C, Chesnel N: Thrombopénies neo-natales allo-immunes. Etude clinique et biologique de 84 cas. Presse Med 14:83, 1985

74. Murphy MF, Waters AH: Immunological aspects of platelet transfusions. Br J Haematol 60:409, 1985

75. Nel JD, Stevens K: A new method for the simultaneous quantitation of platelet-bound immunoglobulin (IgG) and complement (C3) employing an enzyme-linked immunosorbent assay (ELISA) procedure. Br J Haematol 44:281, 1980

76. Niessner H, Clemetson KJ, Panzer S,

Mueller-Eckhardt C, Santoso S, Bettelheim P: Acquired thrombasthenia due to GPIIb/IIIa-specific platelet autoantibodies. Blood 68:571, 1986

77. Pegels JG, Bruynes ECE, Engelfriet CP, von dem Borne AEG Kr: Post-transfusion purpura: A serological and immunochemical study. Br J Haematol 49:521, 1981

78. Pfueller SL, Cosgrove L, Firkin BG, Tew D: Relationship of raised platelet IgG in thrombocytopenia to total platelet protein content. Br J Haematol 49:293, 1981

79. Salama A, Mueller-Eckhardt C, Bhakdi S: A two-stage immunoradiometric assay with ^{125}I-staphylococcal protein A for the detection of antibodies and complement on human blood cells. Vox Sang 48:239, 1985

80. Salmassi S, Yokoyama MM, Maples JA, Matsui Y: Detection of antiplatelet antibody using rosette technique with anti-IgG antibody-coated polyacrylamide gel. Vox Sang 39:264, 1980

81. Santoso S, Kiefel V, Mueller-Eckhardt C: Redistribution of platelet glycoproteins induced by allo- and autoantibodies. Thromb Haemostasis 58:866, 1987

82. Schmidt GM, Bross KJ, Blume KG, Enders N, Santos S, Novitski M, Chillar RK: Detection of platelet-directed immunoglobulin G in sera using the peroxidase-anti-peroxidase (PAP) slide technique. Blood 55:299, 1980

83. Schneider W, Schnaidt M: The platelet adhesion fluorescence test: A modification of the platelet suspension immunofluorescence test. Blut 43:389, 1981

84. Shaw GM, Axelson J, Maglott JG, LoBuglio AF: Quantification of platelet-bound IgG by ^{125}I-staphylococcal protein A in immune thrombocytopenic purpura and other thrombocytopenic disorders. Blood 63:154, 1984

85. Shibata Y, Juji T, Nishizawa Y, Sakamoto H, Ozawa N: Detection of platelet antibodies by a newly developed mixed agglutination with platelets. Vox Sang 41:25, 1981

86. Shulman NR, Jordan JV: Platelet immunology. In Colman RW, Hirsh J, Marder VJ, Salzman EW (eds): Hemostasis and Thrombosis, 2nd ed, 452-529. Philadelphia, JB Lippincott, 1987

87. Shulman NR, Leissinger CA, Hotchkiss AJ, Kautz CA: The nonspecific nature of platelet-associated IgG. Trans Assoc Am Physicians 95:213, 1982

88. Shulman NR, Marder VJ, Hiller MC, Collier EM: Platelet and leucocyte iso-antigens and their antibodies: Serologic, physiologic and clinical studies. In Moore CV, Brown EB, (eds): Progress in Hematology, pp 222-304. New York, Grune & Stratton, 1964

89. Soulier JP, Patereau C, Drouet J: Platelet indirect radioactive Coombs test. Its utilization for Pl^{A1} grouping. Vox Sang 29:253, 1975

90. Stockman A, Zilko PJ, Major GAC, Tait BD, Property DN, Mathews JD, Hannah MC, McCluskey J, Muirden KD: Genetic markers in rheumatoid arthritis. Relationship to toxicity from D-penicillamine. J Rheumatol 13:269, 1986

91. Stricker RB, Shuman MA: Quinidine purpura: Evidence that glycoprotein V is a target platelet antigen. Blood 67:1377, 1986

92. Sugiura K, Steiner M, Baldini, M: Platelet antibody in idiopathic thrombocytopenic purpura and other thrombocytopenias. J Lab Clin Med 96:640, 1980

93. Svejgaard A: Iso-antigenic systems of human blood platelets—A survey. In Jensen KG, Killmann SA (eds): Series Haematologica, pp 1-88. Copenhagen, Munksgaard, 1969

94. Szatkowski NS, Kunicki TJ, Aster RH: Identification of glycoprotein Ib as a target for autoantibody in idiopathic (autoimmune) thrombocytopenic purpura. Blood 67:310, 1986

95. Taaning E: Microplate enzyme immunoassay for detection of platelet antibodies. Tissue Antigens 25:19, 1985

95. Takahashi A, Ohara S, Imaoka S, Kambayashi J, Kosaki G: A simple and rapid method to detect platelet associated IgG. Thromb Res 28:11, 1982

97. Taylor MA: Cryopreservation of platelets: An in-vitro comparison of four methods. J Clin Pathol 34:71, 1981

98. Tsubakio T, Kurata Y, Yonezawa T, Kitani T: Quantification of platelet-associated IgG with competitive solid-phase enzyme immunoassay. Acta Haematol 66:251, 1981

99. van der Schans GS, Veenhoven WA, Snijder JAM, Nieweg HO: The detection of platelet isoantibodies by membrane immunofluorescence. J Lab Clin Med 90:17, 1977

100. van der Schoot CE, Wester M, von dem Borne AEG Kr, Huisman HG: Characterization of platelet-specific alloantigens by immunoblotting: Localization of Zw and Bak antigens. Br J Haematol 64:715, 1986

101. van der Weerdt DM: Platelet antigens and iso-immunization. In: Thesis, Amsterdam: Drukkerij Aemstelstad, 1965

102. von dem Borne AEG Kr, Helmerhorst FM, van Leeuwen EF, Pegels HG, von Riesz E, Engelfriet CP: Autoimmune thrombocytopenia: Detection of platelet autoantibodies with the suspension immunofluorescence test. Br J Haematol 45:319, 1980

103. von dem Borne AEG Kr, van Leeuwen EF, von Riesz LE, van Boxtel CJ, Engelfriet CP: Neonatal alloimmune thrombocytopenia: Detection and characterization of the responsible antibodies by the platelet immunofluorescence test. Blood 57:649, 1981

104. von dem Borne AEG Kr, Pegels JG, van der Stadt RJ, van der Plas-van Dalen CM, Helmerhorst FM: Thrombocytopenia associated with gold therapy: A drug-induced autoimmune disease. Br J Haematol 63:509, 1986

105. von dem Borne AEG Kr, van der Plas-van Dalen CM: Further observations on post-transfusion purpura (PTP). Br J Haematol 61:374, 1985

106. von dem Borne AEG Kr, Verheugt FWA, Oosterhof F, von Riesz E, Brutel de la Rivière A, Engelfriet CP: A simple immunofluorescence test for the detection of platelet antibodies. Br J Haematol 39:195, 1978

107. von dem Borne AEG Kr: Autoimmune thrombocytopenia. In Engelfriet CP, van Loghem JJ, von dem Borne AEG Kr (eds): Immunohaematology, pp 222–256. Amsterdam Elsevier Science Publishers, 1984

108. Winiarski J, Ekelund E: Antibody binding to platelet antigens in acute and chronic idiopathic thrombocytopenic purpura: A platelet membrane ELISA for the detection of antiplatelet antibodies in serum. Clin Exp Immunol 63:459, 1986

109. Winiarski J, Holm G: Platelet associated immunoglobulins and complement in idiopathic thrombocytopenic purpura. Clin Exp Immunol 53:210, 1983

110. Woods VL, Kurata Y, Montgomery RR, Tani P, Mason D, Oh EH, McMillan R: Autoantibodies against platelet glycoprotein Ib in patients with chronic immune thrombocytopenic purpura. Blood 64:156, 1984

111. Woods VL, Oh EH, Mason D, McMillan R: Autoantibodies against the platelet glycoprotein IIb/IIIa complex in patients with chronic ITP. Blood 63:368, 1984

21

Prevention of Alloimmunization in Platelet Transfusion Recipients

CHARLES A. SCHIFFER

The management of the alloimmunized patient represents the greatest remaining clinical and research challenge in the field of platelet transfusion therapy. Despite increased availability of HLA-typed donors and greater understanding of factors that influence the results of such transfusions, as many as 40% to 60% of allegedly "histocompatible" transfusions administered to alloimmunized patients are unsuccessful.[12,16,52] Although donor selection by platelet antibody crossmatching could theoretically improve upon these results,[22,40,41,55] most available techniques are cumbersome and none have been utilized in multiinstitutional prospective trials.[67] In addition, all approaches to provide histocompatible platelets for alloimmunized patients are costly, the expenses including HLA-typing, computer storage of donor information, the apheresis procedure, hospital costs associated with transfusions, and other costs related to loss of donor time from employment. Lastly, there are no proven approaches to the management of bleeding in alloimmunized patients for whom histocompatible donors cannot be identified. In brief, with the possible exception of massive transfusions of random donor platelets,[56] multiple therapeutic maneuvers, including corticosteroid administration, high-dose intravenous gamma globulin,[48,70] splenectomy,[33] plasma exchange,[3] and single-donor transfusions from "random" donors, have all been shown to be ineffective in such patients.

Thus, any practical means by which the rate of alloimmunization could be minimized would be of enormous clinical importance. Indeed, a recent NIH Consensus Development Conference on Platelet Transfusion Therapy focused, in part, upon this problem and emphasized the need for further investigations in this area.[57] This is particularly true because current approaches to the management of adult acute leukemia are now focused on the administration of intensive, often repetitive courses of postremission chemotherapy administered with curative intent. Similar high-dose approaches are being used with a variety of other tumors as well. In some such patients, alloimmunization and nonavailability of histocompatible donors can potentially preclude the administration of effective chemotherapy. This review will attempt to critically analyze the available preclinical data and clinical trials that have attempted to modify the rate of alloimmunization and will outline the prospects for future research endeavors in this area. To help place the problem in perspective, information about the frequency of alloimmunization, criteria for diagnosis, and factors that can influence the interpretation of clinical studies will be summarized in introductory sections.

INCIDENCE OF ALLOIMMUNIZATION

Estimates of the frequency of the development of alloimmunization vary widely in the literature. Although older reports suggest that alloimmunization is a universal accompaniment of multiple platelet transfusions, most of these studies were either based on projected rather than actual data, or they evaluated small, heterogeneous groups of patients.[27,36,77,85,89] In addition, varying definitions of alloimmunization were utilized. A number of serial studies of the frequency of alloimmunization have been conducted at our institution, primarily in patients with acute nonlymphocytic leukemia.[18,19,73] All patients received prophylactic transfusions of pooled platelet concentrates, along with standard packed red blood cells. Until the early 1980s, serial analyses demonstrated that between 40% and 50% of new patients with acute leukemia became refractory to platelet transfusions on an immune basis.[18,19,73] Of importance is that the development of alloimmunization was independent of the number of transfusions received,[18] an observation since confirmed by other investigators.[26] In addition, it was of interest that patients tended to become alloimmunized relatively early in their treatment course in that if alloimmunization had not occurred within the first 4 to 6 weeks of therapy, it infrequently developed subsequently despite repeated transfusions.[19] It has been impossible to distinguish between these two groups prospectively in terms of a variety of clinical factors, HLA-A or HLA-B type or most importantly, the timing between initial transfusion and cytotoxic and immunosuppressive therapy.[18,73] The latter is of importance because, conceivably, it could be manipulated clinically, if a distinct pattern that induced this apparent tolerance to histocompatibility antigens could be identified. Systematic studies of HLA-DR types in "responders" and non-antibody-producers have not been reported.

More recently, in a group of 88 consecutive patients with acute nonlymphocytic leukemia, treated at the University of Maryland Cancer Center (UMCC) on two successive treatment induction protocols, only 24% of recipients became refractory to random-donor platelet transfusion at any time during their life. It is not clear why or if the incidence of alloimmunization is actually decreasing, although it is possible that more intensive induction therapy administered in the last few years, particularly with higher doses of cytosine arabinoside, may have played a role. A similar lower incidence of immunization has been noted by others in recent years, as well,[1,35,45,53] and these lower incidence figures should be considered when estimating the number of patients necessary in clinical trials of prevention of alloimmunization. Some of these studies, as well as our own experience, also emphasize the need to include homogeneous groups of patients receiving similar treatment in such trials. In particular, it is well accepted that patients with aplastic anemia have higher rates of alloimmunization, probably because of the absence of concomitant cytotoxic/immunosuppressive therapy.[77] In contrast, the immunization rate appears to be lower in patients with acute lymphoblastic leukemia,[35,49] perhaps related to the high doses of corticosteroids administered to these patients as part of their initial therapy. Nonetheless, the incidence of alloimmunization is still appreciable and can limit the ability to safely deliver intensive postremission therapy, therapy which in many patients may result in prolonged disease-free survival and, probably, in a cure.

DEFINITION OF ALLOIMMUNIZATION

Alloimmunization against platelet antigens is characterized clinically by the failure to achieve expected platelet count increments after transfusion. This finding is often accompanied by transfusion reactions and, presumably, leaves the recipient at a continued risk of hemorrhage. A number of other clinical factors, including fever, serious infection, hepatosplenomegaly, disseminated intravascular coagulation, and possibly brisk hemorrhage, can markedly shorten platelet survival as well as decrease platelet recovery. By measuring platelet recovery 1 hr after transfusion, it is usually possible to distinguish between alloimmunization and most of these other factors because, with the exception of splenomegaly and septic shock, all of these factors affect platelet survival more than initial platelet recovery.[13] Alloimmunized patients, thus, have poor increments at both 1 and 24 hr after transfusion, whereas most patients with other complicating clinical factors retain good immediate posttransfusion results, with poor day-to-day increments. Recently, it has been shown that sampling 10 minutes postinfusion produces equivalent results as 1-hr increments.[58] This change in practice represents a considerable savings in time for patients and medical staff and should make posttransfusion counts easier to obtain routinely.

In studies of alloimmunization that rely

heavily on assessment of posttransfusion increments, data should be presented on more than one transfusion, whenever possible, because even apparently stable patients occasionally respond poorly to an individual transfusion but have good increments after subsequent transfusions. There is no uniform explanation for this phenomenon, although it is possible that changes in spleen size occur after chemotherapy for acute leukemia that are not easily detectable by palpation. In addition, it has recently been suggested that circulating immune complexes may bind nonspecifically to platelets and for a period of time decrease responsiveness to platelet transfusion in the absence of antibody directed specifically against platelets.[46,65] In these studies, platelet transfusions produced transient falls in circulating immune complexes (CIC) as well, suggesting a role of platelets in clearing CIC. In contrast, we have studied a total of 40 transfusions administered to both alloimmunized and nonimmunized recipients and noted no apparent effect of different levels of CIC on increments. In addition, CIC were actually slightly higher posttransfusion.[71] It is unclear why these studies produced discrepant results, but these data suggest that any putative negative effect of CIC on platelet transfusions require further documentation.

Because of the variable impact of these poorly understood clinical factors on posttransfusion increments, it is helpful in individual patients, and mandatory in research evaluations, to perform serologic studies as well. Measurement of lymphocytotoxic antibody directed against HLA antigens has been used most frequently to serologically confirm the diagnosis of alloimmunization. *Positive lymphocytotoxicity* is generally (although somewhat arbitrarily) defined as cytotoxicity against greater than 20% of a panel of lymphocytes with broad antigenic representation. When positive, most antibodies tend to react against the majority of cells in the panel. In the largest available study, posttransfusion increments following 210 transfusion sequences in 189 clinically stable patients with acute leukemia treated at our institution were analyzed by Hogge et al. and correlated with lymphocytotoxic antibody levels.[32] In these and other studies,[13,49,58] posttransfusion increments were corrected, according to the following equation, for the number of platelets transfused and recipient size to permit standardized comparisons among different transfusions.

$$\text{CCI} = \frac{\text{Absolute platelet count increment} \times \text{BSA* (m}^2\text{)}}{\text{Number of platelets transfused} \times 10^{11}}$$

Thus, if the platelet count rose from 10,000 to 50,000 after transfusion of 4×10^{11} platelets to a recipient with a BSA of 2 m^2,

$$\text{CCI} = \frac{40{,}000 \times 2}{4} = 20{,}000$$

The mean corrected increments for antibody-negative patients at 1 and 24 hr posttransfusion were 16,100 and 12,000, respectively, whereas the corresponding values for patients with positive lymphocytotoxic antibody were 5600 and 2600 ($p < 0.0005$). We have defined corrected increments of 10,000 at 1-hr posttransfusion and 7500 at 24-hr posttransfusion as "satisfactory" increments.[13] Of patients with highly reactive lymphocytotoxic antibody, 88% had poor platelet count increments at both 1 and 24 hr after transfusion, with only 7% of the antibody-positive patients having good increments at both posttransfusion times. In contrast, only 7% of patients with negative antibody had poor increments at both 1 and 24 hr, whereas 80% of these patients had good increments at 1 and 24 hr. It is noteworthy that a number of patients who had good increments at 1 hr, but poor increments at 24 hr, subsequently developed antibody positivity. This suggests that low levels of antibody might have been present at the time of transfusion, amounts sufficient to affect platelet survival but not to substantially influence platelet recovery. Similarly, a smaller group of patients with less reactive, but nonetheless clearly positive sera, had increments intermediate between these extremes. Some of these patients developed greater "positivity" over time, whereas others probably had developed antibodies directed against a limited number of antigens.[59]

These observations, and other studies,[26,27,35] indicate that measurements of lymphocytotoxic antibody correlate well with responsiveness to random donor platelet transfusion and serve as a good serologic screen for the diagnosis of alloimmunization for both research and clinical purposes. Serial measurements are advisable because antibody activity can fluctuate significantly, over time, in the same patient and, sometimes, disappear.[49] Antibody measurements are particularly helpful in seriously

*BSA = body surface area

ill patients and in patients with splenomegaly, in whom it can be difficult to determine by assessment of count increments alone whether apparent refractoriness is secondary to immune factors, to clinical factors, or to both. In addition, these lymphocytotoxic data support the contention that the bulk of immune refractoriness is a consequence of antibody against HLA antigens.

Although it is likely that many of the large variety of antiplatelet antibody assays could also be used to document alloimmunization, there is less published experience using these techniques for this purpose. In addition to detection of HLA antigens, the use of the platelet as the "target cell" would theoretically also permit assessment of the frequency of antibody against platelet-specific antigens. Antibody against these antigens should be considered in patients refractory to closely HLA-matched transfusions. Although older literature suggests that the failure rate of perfectly HLA-matched platelet transfusions is between 6% and 40%,[6,12,16,25,42,52] there are a number of difficulties in interpreting these data, including: not all of the papers include only stable patients; differentiation is usually not made between family and nonfamily donors; the presence or absence of HLA directed antibody is usually not listed; differing criteria are used to assess the "success" of transfusion; most data are presented as results from donor-recipient pairs so that individual patients, who may, in fact, have had platelet specific antibody, were probably frequently transfused and represented repeatedly in the data points, thereby overcontributing to the apparent incidence because they rejected platelets from most, if not all, of the HLA-matched donors used. Given these comments it would appear that the failure rate of "perfectly" HLA-matched platelet transfusion is less than 20%. Finally, it is also probable that some failures could be due to drugrelated antibody,[76] particularly resulting from antibiotics such as the penicillins or trimethaprim-sulfamethoxazole.

As a means of estimating the percentage of *patients* who fall into this category, we conducted a retrospective analysis of adults with acute nonlymphocytic leukemia treated at our center.[66] Only 7 of 209 patients (3.3%) ever became refractory to random donor and perfectly HLA-A- and HLA-B-matched platelets. This general clinical evaluation could represent an underestimate because perfectly matched donors could not be located for all of the alloimmunized patients studied. Three of the seven patients did not have lymphocytotoxic or detectable antiplatelet antibodies, whereas four of the seven had high-titer lymphocytotoxic antibody. Recently, using more sensitive Western blot techniques that can detect antiplatelet antibody in the presence of HLA antibody, Herman et al. arrived at a similar conclusion.[30] None of seven patients unresponsive to HLA-matched platelets had antibodies demonstrable against Pl^{A1} or Bak^{a} by this technique. This low estimate of refractoriness resulting from antibody against platelet-specific antigens is in keeping with the known very high gene frequencies of most of the platelet-specific antigens in that, presumably, only recipients who lack these antigens would be capable of mounting such an alloantibody response. Similarly, Brand et al., in a recent large study, found that only 5 of 335 multiply transfused patients developed detectable antiplatelet antibody that appeared to be a cause of clinical transfusion failures. Four of these five patients also had HLA antibodies.[5]

These data would suggest that attempts to modify the occurrence of refractoriness to platelet transfusion should focus primarily on prevention of HLA antibody formation. This is not an academic distinction. The well-characterized platelet-specific antigens have been shown to be transmembrane glycoproteins, often functioning as specific receptors and intrinsic to platelet structure and function.[10,44] In contrast, HLA antigens are also found in plasma and need not be intrinsic to the platelet in that it has been shown that these class I histocompatibility antigens can be passively adsorbed onto the platelet surface from suspending plasma.[39,47] Although some HLA antigens can be chemically removed from the platelet in vitro,[4] the antigen elution is incomplete and damaging to the platelets. Because of these differences, it is quite possible that processing of HLA- and platelet-specific antigens by the recipient immune system may differ considerably.

GUIDELINES FOR CLINICAL STUDIES

A variety of approaches to prevent, or modify, the rate of alloimmunization have been tested in clinical trials in humans. These will be discussed in detail in the following sections. These are cumbersome trials to perform, particularly because of the serious intercurrent problems such patients frequently develop. Nonetheless, because of the critical impact of the results of such trials could have on the type and cost of transfusion practice, it is important to reiterate a number of criteria to which an "ideal" trial should conform. These include

- Prospective randomization with a control group receiving standard (pooled platelet concentrates) transfusion support.
- Inclusion of a patient population with the same underlying disease, receiving identical chemotherapy. In general, patients with acute nonlymphocytic leukemia (ANLL) probably represent the best group of patients to study. In addition, patients with ANLL represent the largest group of patients receiving repetitive platelet transfusions in most centers.
- Stratification for known "risk factors" for the development of alloimmunization (prior pregnancies or transfusions).
- Restriction of eligibility for randomization to patient receiving initial treatment for their leukemia. This is important because of the demonstration that the development of HLA antibody occurs early in the patient's transfusion history and infrequently thereafter.[19]
- Objective criteria for alloimmunization: because such patients frequently develop confounding clinical factors that affect platelet count increments, it is mandatory that serologic endpoints, which are monitored at fixed (generally weekly) intervals be employed. Standard lymphocytotoxicity assays, possibly supplemented by screens using antiplatelet antibody tests, should be done.
- Exclusion of alloimmunized patients from randomization.
- A standard approach to red blood cell transfusion policy. It is probably preferable to utilize leukocyte-free red blood cell transfusions to limit the comparison of "immunogenicity" to the different platelet preparations being studied.
- Careful prestudy statistical assessment to guarantee registration of a sufficient number of patients to demonstrate either significant differences or equivalence. In general, one should utilize the most conservative estimate of the rate of alloimmunization to determine if a sufficient number of patients would be available in a given center to answer the question being posed. In addition, so-called protocol violations, usually a consequence of an inability to provide the specific platelet or red blood cell preparations under emergency conditions, are an inevitable feature of studies of this type. Patients must survive at least 3 to 4 weeks to guarantee a sufficient time for antibody production. In most leukemia treatment trials, some patients die before this because of complications of pancytopenia. Decisions about statistical disposition of such events should be made before beginning the study.
- Appropriate quality control of the platelet product to determine that the "maneuver" being tested remains consistent over the duration of the study.
- Lastly, the modalities selected for study should be as simple as possible to allow their wide-spread utilization in blood banks of differing size and sophistication. It would be silly to study methodologies that are either prohibitively time-consuming or cumbersome, or that cannot be utilized consistently to produce a homogeneous product from transfusion to transfusion.

MANEUVERS TO PREVENT ALLOIMMUNIZATION

Single-Donor Platelet Transfusion

Background

A number of different cytopheresis technologies now permit the rapid, safe, and efficient procurement of functionally normal platelets from single donors.[31,34] Transfusions of platelets collected from single donors are a well-accepted feature of the management of alloimmunized patients. In parallel with the proliferation of these blood cell separators, there has been increasing interest in the use of single-donor platelets to be given in preference to the more readily available pooled, random-donor products. In particular, there has been considerable interest in the use of single-donor platelets as a means of preventing or delaying alloimmunization. Theoretically, exposure to fewer donors and, hence, fewer donor antigens might be associated with either a reduced or more restricted pattern of alloimmunization, because antibodies might be formed against a smaller number of antigens. Thus, it may be possible, should alloimmunization develop, to switch to platelets from donors of different HLA types.

Slichter et al. have recently reported the results of a study in which groups of dogs received weekly, serial platelet transfusions, using a variety of different donor selection strategies.[81] Twenty of 21 dogs, receiving transfusions from the same single donor, became alloimmunized, three-quarters becoming immunized after three or fewer transfusions. Immunization in these "clinically stable" animals was defined as profound shortening of survival of chromium-labeled platelets. When a single DLA (analogous to HLA)-identical littermate was used as the donor, 31% of 13 dogs developed alloimmunization. Although platelet antibody-testing results were not reported, this suggests that these closely matched transfusions may have selected for the development of antibodies against platelet-specific antigens. In a situation perhaps more analogous to what could represent transfusion practice in humans, groups of recipient dogs were transfused with platelets from six random donors, which were administered either in a pooled fashion or sequentially. When the single donors were used sequentially, animals received platelets from a single donor until refractoriness to that donor developed. This was then followed by platelets from a second single donor, to be followed by a third single donor should refractoriness develop, and so on. Although the overall immunization rates were similar using the two techniques (77% with pooled transfusions, 60% for sequential single-donor transfusions; $p =$ NS), there was a significant delay in onset of refractoriness with the sequential approach. Animals receiving the sequential program required an average of 14 transfusions before becoming refractory to all six donors, whereas 5.5 transfusions of pooled platelets from the same six donors sufficed to induce refractoriness. Of note, however, is that the animals refractory to pooled random-donor platelets could then be supported with DLA-matched platelets from littermates. The authors concluded that platelet support in their study was equivalent with use of either pooled, unrelated random transfusions followed by DLA-identical platelets in refractory recipients, sequential single unrelated donors, or transfusions from a DLA-identical or nonidentical littermate also followed by DLA-identical platelets, should refractoriness develop.

Caution must be utilized in extrapolating the results from this carefully performed experiment to transfusion practice in patients with cancer for the following reasons:

- A weekly transfusion schedule is generally not sufficient for leukemia patients, particularly if other complicating clinical conditions are present.
- The effect of concurrently administered immunosuppressive therapy was not assessed in this model—this obviously is of importance because the overall rate of immunization in leukemia patients is lower than reported in this canine model.
- Although DLA antigens are felt to be class I antigens, similar to HLA antigens, the genetics, polymorphism, and cross-reactivity among these antigens has not been studied as clearly as it has for the HLA antigens. Because of the marked antigenic cross-reactivity in the HLA system, it may not be possible to easily switch from unselected single donors used in sequence, because it is possible that recipients exposed to even a few HLA antigens will also develop antibody directly against the many HLA antigens that share so-called public epitopes.[59]

Thus, even the most comprehensive animal studies can only serve to provide "leads," which must then be pursued in carefully designed clinical trials.

Clinical Trials

Only two clinical trials comparing single-donor versus pooled random-donor platelet transfusions have been published. The first such study by Sintincolaas et al., randomized 34 patients to receive either multiple- or single-donor platelets, primarily utilizing platelet recovery as the endpoint of alloimmunization.[78] Only two transfusions per patient were reported and, based on a deterioration in increments following the second compared with the first multiple-donor transfusion, the authors concluded that single-donor platelets may delay the onset of alloimmunization. This study included patients who were previously transfused, it did not specify if the patients were clinically stable (a critical feature if increments are to be analyzed), and it contained patients with a variety of diseases, presumably, receiving different treatment. The major statistical difference between the results of the single- and multiple-donor transfusions was a consequence of extremely poor and unexplained low increments after the first transfusion in the single-donor group, which then improved after the second transfusion. Because of these considerations, the data from this small study are not interpretable and do not provide guidance for the proper use of single-donor platelets.

A more compelling study was performed in Zurich by Gmur et al.[26] Fifty-four previously untransfused leukemia patients were randomized to receive either multiple-donor or single-donor platelet concentrates, beginning with their initial induction therapy. Refractoriness was documented by lymphocytotoxicity assays, as well as by posttransfusion increments. Statistical analysis using Kaplan-Meier calculations suggested that alloimmunization was delayed, particularly in a subgroup of recipients of single-donor platelets. Approximately 50% of the patients receiving pooled, random-donor transfusions became refractory at a median of 21 days after initiation of transfusion. There was no relationship between the number of transfusions received and the development of refractoriness. In a subsequent study, the same group compared single-donor platelets with a lower leukocyte content resulting from preparation with a different apheresis apparatus. The results in both arms of this latter study were similar and were essentially identical with the incidence of refractoriness (approximately 15% to 20%) noted in the original study.[23,24]

These studies were carefully performed and analyzed and are quite provocative. There are a number of questions about the data that should be addressed. In particular, only 54 patients were studied, and a statistically significant benefit was most prominent in women who had had prior exposure to histocompatibility antigens through pregnancy, a somewhat surprising finding in that, in general, it is extremely difficult to block secondary or anamnestic antibody responses. In addition, entry to the study was limited to patients with no past or recent transfusions; this is not representative of the leukemia patient population in most referral centers, because many, if not most, patients have been previously transfused at least with red blood cell products. In addition, it is possible that the donor pool in Switzerland might be more genetically homogeneous than the wide racial and ethnic distribution found in other countries and in the United States, in particular. If this were the case, one might theorize that randomly selected donors are more likely to be fortuitously HLA compatible with the recipient than might be so elsewhere. Nonetheless, this is an important study that fulfills essentially all of the foregoing study guideline criteria. Another study, reported only in an abstract form, could not demonstrate a similar benefit for single-donor platelets.[38] Only 16 patients were studied, and the information provided is insufficient to definitively evaluate the results, although it is of interest that the recipients of single-donor platelets actually had twice the alloimmunization rate (as assessed by development of lymphocytotoxic antibody) as the patients receiving pooled random-donor platelets.

Conclusions

Although the results reported by Gmur et al. are intriguing, they are insufficient in my estimation, to justify the use of single-donor platelets as a routine approach to the transfusion management of patients with leukemia. On a "scientific" basis, it is generally accepted that small studies of this type should be duplicated in other settings before being generalized. There are also a number of critical, practical considerations. Because of the relatively small numbers of apheresis or HLA-matched donors available,[17,72] even in large centers, the exclusive use of single-donor platelets would be difficult to implement and could reduce the number of donors available for patients who are already alloimmunized. Furthermore, if only donors closely matched for HLA antigens are used, it is possible that one could select for the development of antibody against platelet-specific antigens (analogous to the canine setting described earlier) that are now extremely difficult to detect. It is also difficult for most blood centers to adhere to the rigorous requirements for supplying only single-donor platelets on weekends and during emergencies. The Swiss study was conducted in a center in which the patients' oncologists also were directors of the blood transfusion service. I am aware of at least two studies in other large regional blood centers in which the investigators found it impossible to provide either the single-donor platelets or the leukocyte-poor red blood cells at all times for the patients randomized to these products. Protocol violations occurred in up to 50% of the patients on study. It would obviously be inappropriate to use a complex and expensive modality such as single-donor platelets only part of the time. Widespread implementation of this approach would require much greater coordination between blood transfusion services and clinicians than now exists in most centers. Although it is possible to store platelets obtained from some apheresis machines for up to 5 days, thereby potentially easing the logistics of continually supplying such platelets, there is no published experience documenting the clinical effectiveness and increments following storage. Finally, in most centers, the cost of single-donor platelets is considerably higher than the charges for pooled random-platelets and does not include the "hidden cost" to society of donors missing work for at least half a day because of travel and donation time. Such costs are not incurred in the preparation of platelets prepared as a byproduct of routine whole-blood donations. As will be discussed later, exclusive use of this expensive modality will also benefit only a fraction of leukemia patients because only a few such patients ever become immunized using standard approaches.

Thus, it is likely that the exclusive use of single-donor platelets would strain the apheresis capabilities of most blood centers, so that it would be more difficult to supply histocompatible platelets and granulocytes for patients who clearly need these products. Because the number of apheresis donors and, in particular, HLA-typed donors, is usually limited, one has to question whether or not this is an appropriate use of this valuable resource. Although the scientific question about the prevention of alloimmunization by the use of single-donor platelets remains open, it would appear that practical considerations would dictate that other, less-expensive and simpler maneuvers would represent more desirable approaches.[75]

Leukocyte-Depleted Platelet Transfusion

Background

It has been known since the 1960s that administration of purified platelet preparations is insufficient to stimulate a primary antibody response against histocompatibility antigens. Dausset and Rappaport demonstrated that highly purified platelet preparations injected intradermally failed to induce sensitization to skin grafts from the same human donors, whereas lymphocytes from the same donors reliably induced sensitization with rejection of subsequent skin grafts.[14] Similar results were reported in murine models by Welsh et al., who also noted that after sensitization by lymphocytes, injection of platelets is capable of producing a brisk secondary antibody response.[88] In addition, repetitive administration of purified platelet preparations only, without prior lymphocytic injection, produced a state of tolerance. Essentially identical observations were made more recently in murine models by Claas and colleagues.[8,9]

Platelets lack class II (Ia) antigens, and it was initially felt that the absence of Ia precluded appropriate recognition and processing of the class I major histocompatibility (MHC; HLA) platelet antigens. Further experiments suggested, however, that copresentation of Ia and HLA antigens alone was insufficient, as immunization with lymphocyte membrane preparations did not result in antibody production.[2] Rather, it appeared that the antigen had to be presented by intact, probably viable leukocytes, although it appeared that these cells did not have to be capable of further division, as sensitization could also be produced after prior irradiation of the immunizing cells. Lastly, experiments in canines have demonstrated that, although rejection of bone marrow occurs almost uniformly after prior exposure to donor whole blood or skin epithelial cells, buffy coat-free red blood cell transfusions or "buffy coat-depleted" platelet transfusions produced graft rejection in less than 50% of recipients of DLA-identical marrow.[84]

All of these studies indicate that in many species, platelets alone are very poor immunogens, although they are capable of inducing a secondary antibody response in previously exposed animals. More importantly, repetitive administration of leukocyte-depleted platelets seemed capable of inducing a state of tolerance in terms of antibody production against MHC antigens.

Clinical Studies

Investigators from Leiden, the Netherlands, were probably the first to extend these observations to clinical studies of platelet transfusion in humans. Eernisse and Brand administered leukocyte-depleted platelets and red blood cells to 68 patients with "bone marrow depression" (primarily acute leukemia and aplastic anemia) and compared the rate of alloimmunization with that in a group of patients treated a few years earlier with standard blood products.[20] The rate of alloimmunization, as documented by the presence of lymphocytotoxic antibody and refractoriness to platelet transfusion, was 24% compared with 93% in the historical control group. Although the immunization rate was unusually high in this "control" group, possibly because of a higher rate of prior sensitization by previous pregnancies or by transfusions in these patients, these results were, nonetheless, quite provocative. Of note is that only approximately 5×10^6 leukocytes were administered per transfusion using a somewhat unorthodox platelet preparation technique. In some centers in the Netherlands, platelets are prepared from buffy coats that have been separated from whole blood and stored in small volumes at 4°C. When platelets are needed, multiple buffy coats are pooled and slowly centrifuged after addition of a saline solution. The platelet-rich supernatant is then recentrifuged and administered. This procedure is markedly different and incompatible with blood banking practice in the United States. Because of the high metabolic activity of the leukocytes in the buffy coat preparation, platelets prepared in this fashion must be stored at 4°C, with the well-described decline in post-transfusion platelet survival associated with storage at this temperature.[54]

As a consequence, we elected to initiate a prospectively randomized study of the effect of leukocyte-depleted platelet transfusions in a group of patients with newly diagnosed acute nonlymphocytic leukemia who were receiving identical, initial induction chemotherapy.[69] All patients received frozen red blood cells and pooled platelet concentrates prepared from random donors. Leukocyte depletion was performed by slow centrifugation of the pooled platelet concentrates, which resulted in removal of approximately 80% of the contaminating leukocytes and a final white cell blood count of 0.12×10^8/unit or somewhat less than 10^8 leukocytes per platelet transfusion. A total of 98 patients were randomized. These are difficult studies to perform, and it is instructive that a number of patients had to be excluded from analysis because of early death (7 patients), granulocyte transfusions (15 patients), positive lymphocytotoxic antibody on admission (14 patients), or protocol violations (5 patients—generally consisting of administration of nonleukocyte-depleted products because of emergency conditions). Although the randomization was stratified for prior exposure through pregnancy or transfusions, the exclusions resulted in an imbalance between the two groups with respect to prior sensitization.

The rate of alloimmunization was identical in the two randomized groups in the "cleanest" cohort of patients, i.e., those who had never been exposed to histocompatibility antigens. The overall rate of alloimmunization, as documented by the formation of lymphocytotoxic antibody, was approximately 30%. In patients whose only transfusion history consisted of red blood cells administered before referral to our center, the results were the same. Because of these observations, the study was closed to further accrual. It was noteworthy that there was a trend toward a reduced rate of alloimmunization in patients receiving leukocyte-depleted products who had received prior transfusions or had been pregnant. Overall, only 18% of patients required HLA-matched platelet transfusions during initial induction therapy, with no difference between the two groups. This relatively low requirement for single-donor platelets was related to the fact that antibody usually developed during the third or fourth week after initiation of therapy at a time when most patients were either in remission or had rising blood counts and no longer required platelet transfusion. Because of the marked heterogeneity in degree and type of prior antigenic exposure in the "presensitized" group, we did not feel that it would be interpretable to continue observations in this subset of patients. In addition, because of failure to demonstrate an overall benefit, the similar requirements for HLA-matched platelet transfusions in the two groups, and the cumbersome, time-consuming, and expensive technology required for leukocyte depletion at that time, it was felt that leukocyte-depleted platelet transfusions could not be recommended for patients with leukemia.

A third comparative study was recently reported by Murphy et al. from London.[53] In this study, patients with newly diagnosed acute leukemia who did not have HLA antibodies at presentation received either single-donor platelets prepared from the Haemonetics Model 30 or IBM 2997 Blood Cell Separators, single-donor platelets subjected to an additional centrifugation, or HLA-matched single donor platelets. The number of leukocytes administered with the platelets varied rather widely with mean WBC yields between 0.09 and 0.22×10^9, depending on the collection apparatus used. This was not a randomized study, and patients were placed in one of the three groups depending on "availability" of specific blood components or donors. A total of 61 evaluable patients were studied, half in the control group. Somewhat surprisingly, the alloimmunization rate seemed to be independent of prior antigenic exposure, a finding that is discrepant from most other studies. The alloimmunization rate was significantly lower in the leukocyte-depleted patients (3 of 19, 16%) and the recipients of HLA-matched transfusions (0 of 11), compared with the controls (15 of 31 patients, 48%) as assessed by the development of lymphocytotoxic antibody. Not all such patients, apparently, became refractory (23% of control versus 5% of leukocyte-depleted recipients). The authors felt that it is extremely difficult, if not impossible, to provide HLA-matched products for most patients and recommended that further studies of leukocyte-depleted platelets be pursued, making use of newer and more effective means of leukocyte depletion.

Although many details of the study are not provided in the abstract, Sniecinski and O'Donnell also noted a decline in immunization rate in a randomized study conducted in an apparently heterogeneous group of patients with "hematologic malignancy or marrow aplasia."[83] Both clinical refractoriness and the formation of lymphocytotoxic antibodies were reduced in recipients of "filtered blood products" (3/23, 13%) compared with recipients of standard products (10/20, 50%). No patient developed platelet specific antibodies.

Lastly, the group from Leiden have recently updated and expanded their previous observations.[5] Of 335 patients receiving multiple leukocyte-depleted platelet transfusions, only 31 patients developed broadly reactive alloantibodies and eventually required HLA-matched platelet transfusions. Approximately twice that number of patients developed lymphocytotoxic antibodies, but some of these antibodies were either transient or did not seem to impair the response to platelet transfusions. The development of refractoriness to platelet transfusion was significantly higher in female patients who had prior pregnancies. These results are particularly intriguing because the same low rate of immunization was also noted in patients with aplastic anemia, although it should be kept in mind that many of these patients received immunosuppressive therapy in the form of antithymocyte globulin and corticosteroids.

Conclusions

The very large experience from the Netherlands, albeit nonrandomized, as well as two of the randomized trials, strongly suggest that effective leukocyte depletion can decrease the rate of alloimmunization after platelet transfusion, particularly in patients who have not been previously sensitized. Certainly, the bulk of preclinical data support this conclusion. Although these results were not confirmed in the randomized trial conducted in our institution, leukocyte contamination was approximately 1 to 2 logs higher with the centrifugation technique that was used in our study. It is somewhat surprising that Murphy et al. were able to demonstrate an apparent major benefit of leukocyte depletion because the level of white cell contamination was even higher in their study[53] than in ours. There was a major difference between the two studies, however, in that pooled random-donor platelets were used in ours, whereas Murphy et al. used only single-donor platelet transfusions.

It would seem to be an inescapable conclusion that if a simple, reproducible, and inexpensive means of leukocyte depletion were available, a randomized trial with that approach would be of great importance and might very well be successful. Centrifugation of either single-donor platelets or pooled random-donor platelets is a tedious technique that is associated with considerable platelet loss (generally greater than 20%) and is probably insufficient to reproducibly result in adequate levels of leukocyte depletion.[11,69] The technique is highly "operator"-dependent, and quality control is extremely difficult. Recently, a modified centrifugation technique has been developed that uses a specially designed bag with a small pocket at the bottom in which leukocytes are concentrated after centrifugation.[74] More than 90% of leukocytes are removed using this technique. This requires an extra step, however, and although easier to standardize, is time-consuming and potentially expensive. There are also a number of new filters, either commercially available or in the process of being tested, that deplete more than 90% of leukocytes in the platelet product.[50,79] Any study using these techniques must include administration of leukocyte-depleted red cells, an additional considerable expense that is technically difficult for many blood banks to routinely accomplish.

Nonetheless, there are both adequate experimental and provocative clinical data suggesting that leukocyte-depleted platelets can decrease the rate of alloimmunization. The practical importance of this finding remains to be determined, but it would appear that it is time for the "technology" of leukocyte depletion to "catch up" with the available science to permit further clinical experimentation.

Miscellaneous Approaches

Immunosuppressive Regimens

A variety of immunosuppressive treatments are now available for use in recipients of organ transplants. Some of these approaches are now being tested as a means of preventing or modifying alloimmunization to platelet transfusion. Slichter et al. administered daily oral cyclosporine to dogs receiving weekly transfusions of platelets from a single-donor dog.[80] As judged by decrements in platelet recovery and survival, 86% of control dogs became sensitized to their donor, most after only two to three transfusions. In contrast, none of nine recipients receiving concurrent cyclosporine became refractory. Although these results are intriguing, there is considerable concern about cyclosporine administration to patients with malignancy who are receiving additional immunosuppressive and cytotoxic therapy. Such patients often also receive nephrotoxic antibiotics, and there is concern that cyclosporine may add to this side effect. Recognizing these problems, the authors also tested platelets that had been preincubated with small amounts of cyclosporine before transfusion. There was no detectable cyclosporine after transfusion and the "cyclosporine-loaded platelets" circulated normally. There may have been some benefit using this approach, as only four of nine recipients became refractory. Both sets of the experiments are intriguing, although, as yet, there are no prospective studies in humans.

Antithymocyte globulin (ATG) has also been studied in a very limited fashion. A few patients with aplastic anemia have been described in whom preexisting alloimmunization disappeared after the administration of variable amounts of ATG prepared from different sources.[64] Antibodies against other antigens were not apparently affected and it was unclear whether this was a selective immunosuppressive effect of the ATG or whether the disappearance of the antibodies was even related to the ATG administration. Slichter et al. have prospectively administered ATG to both baboons and dogs, sometimes in combination with prednisone, in an attempt to prevent alloimmunization.[82] Alloimmunization seemed to be delayed in the baboons, but there was no apparent benefit in the dogs. Because of this gross difference between species, it is unclear whether or not these observations have any relevance to human transfusion practice. Prospective studies in patients have not been done. Antithymocyte globulin is a somewhat heterogeneous product that has a number of associated side effects, including thrombocytopenia. A number of patients have now been treated with ATG as their initial therapy for aplastic anemia,[7] and it would be of considerable interest to review the transfusion histories of these patients to determine whether or not there was any obvious effect on the rate of refractoriness to platelet transfusion. Such observations might be important before considering prospective studies in patients with malignant diseases.

Patients with leukemia and other malignancies are treated with a variety of cytotoxic and immunosuppressive regimens, given in a variety of doses and schedules. It has been difficult to systematically dissect out whether or not any of these approaches have been associated with differing rates of alloimmunization. In particular, we attempted to determine if there was an association between the timing of initial chemotherapy with respect to the first platelet transfusion and subsequent antibody formation.[19] If, in fact, tolerance was being induced by chemotherapeutic modulation or suppression of clones that had been activated by the initial platelet transfusion, then this could conceivably be capitalized upon clinically as a means of preventing alloimmunization. Unfortunately, it was impossible to demonstrate such a relationship. It should be kept in mind, however, that it is usually quite difficult to determine when the first "antigenic" exposure occurs in many patients, and it is possible that the sequence of antigenic exposure and subsequent chemotherapy is of some importance in preventing refractoriness.

Ultraviolet Irradiation

Background. The formation and secretion of antibody against neoantigens is one of the final steps of a complex process involving serial interactions among macrophages and other Ia-bearing, antigen-processing cells, subclasses of helper and suppressor T-lymphocytes and, eventually, B-lymphocytes (reviewed in Ref. 87). Recently, it has been demonstrated that ultraviolet (UV) irradiation can modify some of these processes both in vitro and in vivo. Ultraviolet irradiation of lymphocytes abrogates their ability to serve as either stimulatory or responding cells in a mixed lymphocyte culture reaction (MLR) and also alters the function of antigen-presenting cells, reducing their immunogenicity.[28,43,51,86] Ultraviolet-irradiated mice have an increased rate of skin cancer and have reduced immunologic reactivity against injected allogeneic cells.[21] This suppressed reactivity seems specific for antigens on the cells to which they have been exposed. Finally, it has been demonstrated that UV irradiation of pancreatic tissue permits successful transplantation of these tissues in a murine model.[37] Similar results were obtained with UV irradiation of the recipient, suggesting that this modality can have an immunomodulatory effect both by immunosuppression of the recipient and by alteration of the antigen-presenting cell, a situation analogous to its effect in the MLR.

In vitro experiments have demonstrated that doses of UV irradiation sufficient to abolish lymphocyte reactivity, as assessed by MLR, do not affect either platelet function in vitro[37] or the posttransfusion survival of such UV-exposed platelets as assessed in a canine model.[80] Only 1 of 12 canine recipients of UV-irradiated platelets became refractory to such platelets, compared with 86% of control dogs.[80] In addition, dogs who had failed to become sensitized to UV-irradiated platelets from their original donor, also did not become sensitized to platelet transfusions from approximately half of other subsequent donors. Lastly, UV irradiation of donor blood administered before bone marrow transplant, permitted successful engraftment with rescue from aplasia induced by total body irradiation.[15] In contrast, in previous studies, the same group had demonstrated that pretransfusion with donor blood uniformly results in rejection of bone marrow grafts from such donors.[15,84] The mechanisms resulting in suppression of sensitization are unknown, but they are unlikely to be simply a reduction or alteration in the class II antigens themselves.

Clinical Studies/Conclusions. There are no clinical studies now available that have used UV-irradiated platelets. There are many practical problems involved in UV irradiation of platelets, and the canine and in vitro studies were performed with small aliquots of blood or platelets that had been irradiated in open dishes. Obviously, this is not compatible with transfusion practice. There is intense ongoing research to develop methodologies and appropriate plastics that will permit sufficient penetration by UV waves to inactivate lymphocytes placed in plastic bags that are also biocompatible with platelets. It is hoped that such materials will be available in the near future and permit clinical testing.

There are many potential advantages to this approach, perhaps the most compelling of which is the ease with which UV irradiation could be applied to all blood products, should appropriate technical advances occur. One could imagine a "box" analogous to that used for gamma irradiation of blood products in many centers, which could be routinely utilized with a minimum of technologist time, advance preparation and, hopefully, cost. The simplicity of this approach makes it much more attractive than single-donor platelets or leukocyte-depleted platelets, even if relatively reliable means of leukocyte depletion became available. It is hoped that clinical trials using this approach can be initiated in the next year or two to test these extremely exciting preliminary findings in humans.

Soluble HLA Antigens

As described earlier, a situation analogous to the development of specific humoral tolerance against histocompatibility antigens develops in most platelet transfusion recipients. In addition to depletion or alteration of antigen-presenting cells, other methods have been studied that could also theoretically affect the frequency of antibody production. Osborne and Grumet have demonstrated, in a murine model, that repetitive intraperitoneal injection of allogeneic liver membrane preparations induced tolerance to platelet transfusions administered subsequently to these mice.[61] These liver membrane preparations lack class II (Ia) antigens, perhaps accounting for the nonreactivity to the class I HLA antigens. More recently, Grumet has theorized that administration of soluble HLA antigens could similarly induce tolerance to subsequent platelet transfusions.[29] Certain of the HLA-A and HLA-B locus genes have been cloned, potentially allowing manufacture of purified, homogeneous HLA molecules that can be produced in a soluble form for experimental use. Theoretically, one could conceive that injection of a variety of such cloned products could produce tolerance against a wide range of HLA antigens.

Obviously, this approach must first be verified in murine models before its consideration for clinical studies. In addition, it has been shown that the administration of carefully prepared leukocyte-free plasma can boost antibody reactivity in presensitized individuals and, perhaps more importantly, stimulate apparent de novo antibody production in previously nonsensitized recipients.[62] These studies were performed in patients with renal insufficiency who were deliberately exposed to plasma from histoincompatible donors. In fact, although only a few of the recipients developed antibody, it is very likely that the antibody was produced as a consequence of exposure to soluble HLA antigens in the plasma. Because some of the recipients also developed antibody against Ia antigens, however, it may be that the plasma contained these antigens, as well, and that it was this combination that resulted in the development of antibodies against HLA antigens. Nonetheless, this small experience may have some relevance to the consideration of using soluble HLA antigens to induce tolerance.

CONCLUSION

Thus, it would appear that a variety of lines of evidence suggest that modification of the manner by which platelet transfusions are administered holds promise for decreasing the rate of alloimmunization. Efforts have been focused on either reducing the number of antigen-presenting cells (leukocyte depletion or single-donor transfusion) or modifying the fashion in which these antigens are presented to the recipient immune system. As noted earlier, further clinical studies are required in both areas. Additional research is also necessary to determine why given individuals become tolerant to particular antigens. There is considerable controversy about the roles of suppressor T cells and the idiotypic antibody network in this process, and complicated leukemia patients receiving multiple transfusions and other therapeutic modalities are probably not the ideal population in whom to perform evaluations of this type. A recent observation in renal transplant patients may be of some interest, however. Reed et al. studied a group of transplant recipients who had previously formed antibodies to HLA antigens.[63] The circulating level of these antibodies had subsequently declined before transplant, and the kidney graft was accepted and functioned well. Of note was that nine of the ten patients studied had anti-idiotype antibodies at the time of transplantation, suggesting that it was the development of these "anti anti-HLA antibodies" that contributed to the success of the graft. Fluctuations and disappearance of lymphocytotoxic antibody frequently occur in patients with chronic renal insufficiency[60] and have also been documented in leukemia patients. In a recent evaluation of 224 patients in our institution, approximately one-quarter of patients had either transient or permanent reductions in HLA antibody levels.[49] It is intriguing to speculate that the development of a series of anti-idiotypic antibodies may play a role either in the development of tolerance or in the subgroup of patients in whom antibodies develop and subsequently disappear permanently. Studies of this type in alloimmunized patients would be of considerable interest. Such studies should, however, take into account that tolerance has apparently developed for whole classes of antigens (i.e., MHC antigens) in addition to specific antigenic epitopes.

Finally, it is important to consider exactly what fraction of patients with leukemia or other cancers might benefit from any approach that has been proved to reduce the rate of alloimmunization. For example, of 100 patients with newly diagnosed disease, approximately 10% will be alloimmunized on admission or after their first transfusion because of an anamnestic antibody response. This would leave a total of approximately 90 patients who might benefit from any approach to modify alloimmunization. If one assumes a final alloimmunization rate of approximately 40%, the number of patients is reduced to 36. Not all patients who achieve complete remission are candidates for aggressive subsequent therapy. If one assumes a complete response rate of 75% with approximately 75% of complete responders warranting intensive consolidation therapy, the number of patients is further reduced to approximately 21. At our institution, approximately 10% of patients receive granulocyte transfusions, which are not routinely HLA matched, during induction reducing the number of "beneficiaries" to approximately 19 patients. Finally, it is unlikely that any approach to modify alloimmunization would be 100% effective. If one, perhaps generously, assumes a halving of the alloimmunization rate, one is left with approximately ten patients who might benefit from any approach to modify alloimmunization. Because it is impossible to distinguish prospectively between those patients who are more or who are less likely to become alloimmunized, it would be necessary to "treat" 100 patients to benefit only ten of these patients. Furthermore, most of these alloimmunized patients can be managed successfully with HLA-matched platelets or in some centers with autologous frozen platelet transfusions.[68]

Although it is possible to quibble with some of the estimates used in this analysis, these factors must be taken into consideration when considering the costs and potential effectiveness of any approach used to decrease alloimmunization. This simply reiterates the point that such methodology must be as simple as possible to be routinely applicable. Perhaps the method that, at least in theory, approaches this ideal is UV irradiation. Clinical trials in this area, therefore, would be particularly exciting.

This investigation was supported in part by National Heart, Lung, and Blood Institute DHHS grant RO1-HL35322-02.

REFERENCES

1. Baldwin M, Scott D, Ness PM, Kickler T, Braine H: Alloimmunization $\mathbf{Rh_0}$(D) and HLA in oncology patients. Transfusion 25:446, 1985

2. Batchelor JR, Welsh KI, Burgos H: Transplantation antigens per se are poor immunogens within a species. Nature 273:54, 1978

3. Bensinger WI: Plasma exchange in the treatment of patients with cancer. In Schiffer CA, (ed): Clinics in Oncology, pp 739–754. Philadelphia, WB Saunders, 1983

4. Blumberg N, Masel D, Mayer T, Horan P, Heal J: Removal of HLA-A,B antigens from platelets. Blood 63:448, 1984

5. Brand A, Claas FHJ, Voogt PJ, Wasser MNJM, Eernisse JG: Alloimmunization after leucocyte depleted multiple random donor platelet transfusions. Vox Sang 54:160, 1988

6. Brand A, van Leeuwen A, Eernisse JG, van Rood JJ: Platelet transfusion therapy. Optimal donor selection with a combination of lymphocytotoxicity and platelet fluorescence tests. Blood 51:781, 1978

7. Champlin R, Winston H, Gale RP: Antithymocyte globulin treatment in patients with aplastic anemia: A prospective randomized trial. N Engl J Med 308:113, 1983

8. Claas FHJ, Blankert JJ, Ruigrok R, Moerel L: Platelet transfusions can induce transplantation tolerance. Immunol Lett 5:35, 1982

9. Claas FHJ, Smenk RJT, Schmidt R, van Steenbrugge GJ, Eernisse JG: Alloimmunization against the MHC antigens after platelet transfusions is due to contaminating leukocytes in the platelet suspension. Exp Hematol 9:84, 1981

10. Clemetson KJ, McGregor, James E, Dechavanne M, Luscher EJ: Characterization of the platelet membrane glycoprotein abnormalities in Bernard-Soulier syndrome and comparison with normal by surface-labeling techniques and high-resolution two-dimensional gel electrophoresis. J Clin Invest 70:304, 1982

11. Cott ME, Oh JH, Vroon DH: Isolation of leukocyte-free platelets from standard platelet concentrates by centrifugation. Transfusion 26:272, 1986

12. Dahlke MB, Weiss KL: Platelet transfusion from donors mismatched for crossreactive HLA antigens. Transfusion 24:299, 1984.

13. Daly PA, Schiffer CA, Aisner J, Wiernik PA: Platelet transfusion therapy—one hour post-transfusion increments are valuable in predicting the need for HLA-matched preparations. J Am Med Assoc 243:435, 1980

14. Dausset J, Rapaport FT: Transplantation antigen activity of human blood platelets. Transplantation 4:182, 1966

15. Deeg HJ, Aprile J, Graham TC, Appelbaum FR, Storb R: Ultraviolet irradiation of blood prevents transfusion-induced sensitization and marrow graft rejection in dogs. Blood 67:537, 1986

16. Duquesnoy RJ, Filip DJ, Rodey GE, Rimm AA, Aster RH: Successful transfusion of platelet "mismatched" for HLA antigens to alloimmunized thrombocytopenic patients. Am J Hematol 2:219, 1977

17. Duquesnoy RJ, Vieira J, Aster RH: Donor availability for platelet transfusion support of alloimmunized thrombocytopenic patients. Transplant Proc 9:519, 1977

18. Dutcher J, Schiffer CA, Aisner J, Wiernik PH: Alloimmunization following platelet transfusion: The absence of a dose response relationship. Blood 57:395, 1980

19. Dutcher JP, Schiffer CA, Aisner J, Wiernik PH: Long-term follow-up of patients with leukemia receiving platelet transfusions: Identification of a large group of patients who do not become alloimmunized. Blood 58:1007, 1981

20. Eernisse JG, Brand A: Prevention of platelet refractoriness due to HLA antibodies after administration of leukocyte-poor blood components. Exp Hematol 9:77, 1981

21. Fisher MS, Kripke ML: Suppressor T lymphocytes control the development of primary skin cancers in ultraviolet-irradiated mice. Science 216:1133, 1982

22. Freedman J, Hooi C, Garvey MB: Prospective platelet crossmatching for selection of compatible random donors. Br J Haematol 56:9, 1984

23. Gmur J: Random single-donor platelet transfusions: Pros and cons. Plasma Ther Transfusion Technol 7:463, 1986

24. Gmur JP: Random single-donor platelets compared to random multiple-donor platelet concentrates. In Proceeding NIH Consensus Development Conference on Platelet Transfusion Therapy, 1986

25. Gmur J, von Felten A, Frick P: Platelet support in polysensitized patients: Role of HLA specificities and crossmatch testing for donor selection. Blood 51:903, 1978

26. Gmur J, von Felten A, Osterwalder B, Honegger H, Hormann A, Sauter C, Deubelbeiss K, Berchtold W, Metaxas M, Scali G, Frick PG: Delayed alloimmunization using random single donor platelet transfusions: A prospective study in thrombocytopenic patients with acute leukemia. Blood 62:473, 1983

27. Green D, Tiro A, Basiliere J, Mittal KK: Cytotoxic antibody complicating platelet support in acute leukemia. J Am Med Assoc 236:1044, 1976

28. Greene Mi, Sy MS, Kripke ML, Benacerraf B: Impairment of antigen-presenting cell function by ultraviolet radiation. Proc Natl Acad Sci USA 76:6591, 1979

29. Grumet FC: Prevention and management of the refractory state: Induction of tolerance to allogenic platelet transfusions. In Proceeding NIH Consensus Development Conference on Platelet Transfusion Therapy, 1986.

30. Herman JH, Kickler TS, Ness PM: Western blot analysis of HLA compatible platelet transfusion failures. Blood 66 (Suppl 1):279a, 1985

31. Hester JP, Kellogg RM, Mulzet AP, Kruger VR, McCredie KB, Freireich EJ: Principles of blood separation and component extraction in a disposable continuous-flow single-stage channel. Blood 54:254, 1979

32. Hogge DE, Dutcher JP, Aisner J, Schiffer CA: Lymphocytotoxic antibody is a predictor of response to random donor platelet transfusion. Am J Hematol 14:363, 1983

33. Hogge DE, Dutcher JP, Aisner J, Schiffer CA: The ineffectiveness of random donor platelet transfusion in splenectomized, alloimmunized recipients. Blood 62:253, 1984

34. Hogge DE, Schiffer CA: Collection of platelets depleted of red and white cells with the "surge pump" adaptation of a blood cell separator. Transfusion 23:177, 1983

35. Holohan TV, Terasaki PI, Deisseroth AB: Suppression of transfusion-related alloimmunization in intensively treated cancer patient. Blood 58:122, 1981

36. Howard JE, Perkins HA: The natural history of alloimmunization to platelets. Transfusion 18:496, 1978

37. Kahn RA, Duffy BF, Rodey GG: Ultraviolet irradiation of platelet concentrate abrogates lymphocyte activation without affecting platelet function in vitro. Transfusion 25:547, 1985.

38. Kakaiya RM, Hezzey AJ, Bove JR, Katz AJ, Genco PV, Buchholz DH, Blumberg N: Alloimmunization following apheresis platelets vs. pooled platelet concentrates transfusion—A prospective randomized study. Transfusion 21:600, 1981

39. Kao KJ: Plasma and platelet HLA in normal individuals: Quantitation by competitive enzyme-linked immunoassay. Blood 70:282, 1987

40. Kelton JG: The measurement of platelet-bound immunoglobulins: An overview of the methods and the biological relevance of platelet-associated IgG. Prog Hematol 13:163, 1983

41. Kickler TS, Braine HG, Ness PM: Selection of platelet donors for alloimmunized patients by crossmatching. Transfusion 24:422, 1984

42. Kickler TS, Briane H, Ness PM: The predictive value of crossmatching platelet transfusion for alloimmunized patients. Transfusion 25:385, 1985

43. Kripke ML: Immunologic unresponsiveness induced by ultraviolet radiation. Immunol Rev 80:87, 1984

44. Kunicki TJ, Aster RH: Deletion of the platelet-specific alloantigen Pl^{A1} from platelets in Glanzmann's thrombasthenia. J Clin Invest 61:1225, 1978

45. Kutti J, Zaroulis CG, Dinsmore RE, Reich L, Clarkson BD, Good RA: A prospective study of platelet-transfusion therapy administered to patients with acute leukemia. Transfusion 22:44, 1982

46. Kutti J, Zaroulis CG, Safai-Kutti S, Dins-

more RE, Day NK, Good RA: Evidence that circulating immune complexes remove transfused platelets from the circulation. Am J Hematol 11:255, 1981

47. Lalezari P, Driscoll AM: Ability of thrombocytes to acquire HLA specificity from plasma. Blood 59:167, 1982

48. Lee EJ, Papenberg D, Schiffer CA: Intravenous gammaglobulin for patients alloimmunized to random donor platelet transfusion. Transfusion 27:245, 1987

49. Lee EJ, Schiffer CA: Serial measurement of lymphocytotoxic antibody and response to nonmatched platelet transfusions in alloimmunized patients. Blood 70:879, 1987

50. Lichtiger B, del Valle L, Armintor M, Trujillo JM: Use of Imugard IG500 filters for preparation of leukocyte-poor blood for cancer patients. Vox Sang 46:136, 1984

51. Lindahl-Kiessling K, Safwenberg J: Inability of UV-irradiated lymphocytes to stimulate allogeneic cells in mixed lymphocyte culture. Int Arch Allergy 41:670, 1971

52. Lohrmann HP, Bull MI, Decter JA et al: Platelet transfusions from HLA compatible unrelated donors to alloimmunized patients. Ann Intern Med 80:9, 1974

53. Murphy MF, Metcalfe P, Thomas H, Eve J, Ord J, Lister TA, Waters AH: Use of leukocyte-poor blood components and HLA-matched-platelet donors to prevent HLA alloimmunization. Br J Haematol 62:529, 1986

54. Murphy S: Platelet storage for transfusion. Semin Hematol 22:165, 1985

55. Myers TJ, Kim BK, Steiner M et al: Selection of donor platelets for alloimmunized patients using a platelet-associated IgG assay. Blood 58:444, 1981

56. Nagasawa T, Kim BK, Baldini MG: Temporary suppression of circulating platelet antiplatelet alloantibodies by the massive infusion of fresh, stored or lyophilized platelets. Transfusion 18:429, 1978

57. NIH Consensus Development Conference Statement: Platelet transfusion therapy. 6:1, 1986

58. O'Connell B, Lee EJ, Schiffer CA: The value of 10-minute posttransfusion platelet counts. Transfusion 28:66, 1988

59. Oldfather JW, Phelan DL, Rodey GE. Preselection of platelet donors based on the identification of HLA antibodies in multiply transfused hematology patients. Blood 64:(Suppl):229a, 1984

60. Opelz G, Graver B, Mickey MR, Terasaki PI: Lymphocytotoxic antibody responses to transfusions in potential kidney transplant recipients. Transplantation 32:177, 1981

61. Osborne RM, Grumet FC: Platelet transfusion tolerization by liver membrane treatment. Transplantation 28:96, 1979

62. Pellegrino MA, Indiveri F, Fagiolo U, Antonello A, Ferrone S: Immunogenicity of serum HLA antigens in allogeneic combinations. Transplantation 33:530, 1982

63. Reed E, Hardy M, Benvenisty A, Lattes C, Brensilver J, McCabe R, Reemstma K, King DW, Suciu-Foca N: Effect of antidiotypic antibodies to HLA on graft survival in renal allograft recipients. N Engl J Med 316:1450, 1987

64. Sabbe LJM, Claas FHJ, Haak HL, van Gemert GW, Jansen J, Zwaan FE, Tricot G, Niterink A, Langerak J, van Rood JJ: Anti-thymocyte globulin (ATG) can eliminate platelet refractoriness. Blut 42:331, 1981

65. Safai-Kutti S, Zaroulis CG, Day NK, Good RA, Kutti J: Platelet transfusion therapy and circulating immune complexes. Von Sang 39:22, 1980

66. Schiffer CA: Clinical importance of antiplatelet antibody testing for the blood bank. In Bell C (ed): Seminar on Antigens on Blood Cells and Body Fluids, pp 189–208. American Association of Blood Banks, 1980

67. Schiffer CA: Donor selection for patients refractory to platelet transfusion. In Brown EB (ed): Progress in Hematology, pp 91–114. New York, Grune & Stratton, 1987

68. Schiffer CA, Aisner J, Wiernik PH: Frozen autologous platelet transfusion for patients with leukemia. N Engl J Med 229:7, 1978

69. Schiffer CA, Dutcher JP, Aisner J, Hogge D, Wiernik PH, Reilly JP: A randomized trial of leukocyte depleted platelet transfusion to modify alloimmunization in patients with leukemia. Blood 62:815, 1983

70. Schiffer CA, Hogge DE, Aisner J, Dutcher JP, Lee EJ, Papenberg D: High dose intravenous gammaglobulin in alloimmunized platelet transfusion recipients. Blood 64:937, 1984

71. Schiffer CA, Johnson J, Lee EJ, Reich L, O'Connell B: Complement activation following platelet transfusion (abstr). Blood 70(suppl):334, 1987

72. Schiffer CA, Keller C, Dutcher JP, Aisner J, Hogge DE, Wiernik PH: Potential HLA matched platelet donor availability for alloimmunized patients. Transfusion 23:286, 1983

73. Schiffer CA, Lichtenfeld JL, Wiernik PH, Mardiney MR, Joseph JM: Antibody response in patients with acute non-lymphocytic leukemia. Cancer 37:2177, 1976

74. Schiffer CA, Patten E, Reilly J, Patel S: Effective Leukocyte removal from platelet preparations by centrifugation in a new pooling bag. Transfusion 27:162, 1987

75. Schiffer CA, Slichter SJ: Platelet transfusion from single donors. N Engl J Med 307:245, 1982

76. Schiffer CA, Weinstein HJ, Wiernik PH: Methicillin-associated thrombocytopenia. Ann Intern Med 85:3, 1976

77. Shulman NR: Immunological considerations attending platelet transfusion. Transfusion 6:39, 1966

78. Sintnicolaas K, Sizoo W, Haije WG, Abels J, Vriesendorp HM, Kroese WFS, Hop WCJ, Lowenberg B: Delayed alloimmunisation by random single donor platelet transfusions: A randomised study to compare single donor and multiple donor platelet transfusions in cancer patients with severe thrombocytopenia. Lancet 1:750, 1981

79. Sirchia G, Parravicini A, Rebulla P, Bertolini F, Morelati F, Marconi M: Preparations of leukocyte-free platelets for transfusion by filtration through cotton wool. Vox Sang 44:115, 1983

80. Slichter SJ, Deeg HJ, Kennedy MS: Prevention of platelet alloimmunization in dogs with systemic cyclosporine and by UV-irradiation or cyclosporine-loading of donor platelets. Blood 69:41, 1987

81. Slichter SJ, O'Donnell MR, Weiden PL, Storb R, Schroeder ML: Canine platelet alloimmunization: The role of donor selection. Br J Haematol 63:713, 1986

82. Slichter SJ, Weiden P, Kane P, Storb R: Approaches to preventing or reversing platelet alloimmunization using animal models. Transfusion 28:103, 1988

83. Sniecinski I, O'Donnell M: Preventing refractoriness to random donor platelet transfusion. Transfusion 26:582, 1986

84. Storb R, Deeg HJ, Weiden PL, Graham TC, Atkinson KA, Slichter SJ, Thomas ED: Marrow graft rejection in DLA-identical canine littermates: Antigens involved are expressed on leukocytes and skin epithelial cells but probably not on platelets and red blood cells. Transplantation Proc 11:504, 1979

85. Tejada F, Bias WB, Santos GW, Zieve PD: Immunologic response of patients with acute leukemia to platelet transfusions. Blood 42:405, 1973

86. Ullrich SE: Suppression of the immune response to allogeneic histocompatibility antigens by a single exposure to ultraviolet radiation. Transplantation 42:287, 1986

87. Unanue ER, Allen PM: The basis for the immunoregulatory role of macrophages and other accessory cells. Science 551, 1987

88. Welsh KI, Burgos H, Batchelor JR: The immune response to allogeneic rat platelets: Ag-B antigens in matrix form lacking Ia. Eur J Immunol 7:267, 1977

89. Wu KK, Thompson JS, Koepke JA, Hoak JC, Flink R: Heterogeneity of antibody response to human platelet transfusion. J Clin Invest 58:432, 1976

22

Platelet-Specific Antibodies as in vivo Therapeutic Reagents: A Baboon Model

STEPHEN R. HANSON

Numerous reports have described monoclonal antibodies that interact specifically with platelet membrane constituents, inhibit the binding of fibrinogen and other adhesive glycoproteins, and produce significant inhibition of platelet function in vitro.[1,5,15-17,21,26,28,33] However, there have been relatively few experimental studies of the effects of platelet-specific antibodies on thrombosis and hemostasis in vivo.

Coller et al. have described an IgG1 murine monoclonal antibody (7E3) against the platelet glycoprotein (GP) IIb–IIIa receptor that blocks fibrinogen binding to platelets and inhibits ADP-induced platelet aggregation.[2,4,6] Infusion of the $F(ab')_2$ fragment of this antibody into dogs (0.17–0.81 mg/kg) caused a dose-dependent inhibition of ADP-induced platelet aggregation ex vivo and a decreased ability of the platelets to subsequently bind radiolabeled 7E3, presumably reflecting occupancy of the GPIIb–IIIa sites by the unlabeled $F(ab')_2$ fragments.[6] The capacity of platelets to aggregate and bind antibody reverted toward normal within 1 day.[6]

Further studies by these investigators have employed a well-established animal model of platelet thrombus formation in partially stenosed arteries.[3,4] Mechanical stenosis of the circumflex coronary artery in dogs, or of the carotid artery in monkeys, resulted in cyclic variations in arterial blood flow because of the repetitive accumulation and embolization of platelet thrombi.[4] Infusion of 0.7 to 0.8 mg/kg of the $F(ab')_2$ fragment of 7E3 completely blocked new thrombus formation, which could not be restored by epinephrine infusions, repeated mechanical trauma to the vessel intima, electrical current, or a combination of these stimuli. 7E3 was the most potent antithrombotic agent tested in this model, and its use was not associated with significant changes in heart rate or blood pressure. In a preliminary report, 7E3 has also been found to be effective for preventing coronary reocclusion in dogs after thrombolysis with tissue plasminogen activator.[34]

Although these studies document the potential usefulness of platelet-specific antibodies for antithrombotic therapy, the hemostatic consequences of antibody infusion have not been fully defined. Although 7E3 has been administered without clear evidence of spontaneous bleeding, excessive hemorrhage, or significant acute thrombocytopenia,[4,6] no objective data on blood loss or bleeding tendency have been reported. Other possible consequences of antibody infusion, including increased platelet destruction or the development of late thrombocytopenia, have not been systematically studied.

We, therefore, have used a baboon animal model to quantitatively assess the effects of injected antibodies against platelet membrane glycoproteins considering the following variables: platelet count, bleeding time, platelet aggregation ex vivo, content of platelet storage granules, antibody pharmacokinetics, and platelet deposition onto arterial vascular grafts. A baboon animal model was used in this study because this species is hemostatically similar to humans with respect to coagulation factors, platelets and their granular contents, and immunologic characteristics of platelet and plasma proteins.[9,11,12,19,30] The antithrombotic efficacy of injected antibody was assessed using a gamma scintillation camera to measure ^{111}In-labeled platelet deposition onto vascular grafts surgically placed in the femoral artery, or incorporated into an externalized femoral arteriovenous shunt.[12,31]

ANTIBODY PREPARATION AND CHARACTERIZATION

The murine monoclonal antibodies used in these studies are described in Table 22-1 and were all prepared and characterized as described previously.[13,22,25] AP1 recognizes GPIb[8,23] and, when added at saturating concentrations, totally abolishes the ristocetin-induced aggregation of baboon platelets in stirred suspensions of platelet-rich plasma (PRP). AP2 and LJ-CP8 recognize the GPIIb–IIIa complex,[22,25] and both AP2 and LJ-CP8 inhibited the binding of baboon fibrinogen, purified as described previously,[32] to thrombin-stimulated baboon platelets. AP2 inhibited the binding by 55%, whereas LJ-CP8 inhibited the binding completely. Similar results were obtained with human fibrinogen and human platelets. The methods used to measure the binding of antibody and fibrinogen to platelets have been previously reported in detail.[13,27] Both LJ-CP8 and AP2 IgG, when added at saturating concentrations, completely inhibited aggregation of human or baboon PRP induced by ADP, collagen, or γ-thrombin.[13]

For each antibody, bivalent $F(ab')_2$ fragments were prepared from IgG by papain digestion, as described.[18] Contaminating Fc fragments were removed using protein A-Sepharose, and the material was homogeneous as determined by sodium dodecyl sulfate–polyacrylamide gel electrophoresis (SDS–PAGE). The number of antibody molecules bound per platelet was calculated on the basis of the specific activity after separating the platelets from PRP by means of centrifugation through 20% sucrose, as described.[27] The binding was always saturable. Binding isotherms were analyzed by Scatchard-type analysis to determine the dissociation constant and number of binding sites.

Each antibody recognized approximately 50,000 binding sites on resting baboon platelets (*see* Table 22-1) and exhibited a dissociation constant ranging from approximately 3×10^{-7} M to 2×10^{-9} M. The doses of antibodies injected ranged from 0.2 to 10 mg/kg. At the highest doses injected, saturating amounts of antibody were attained, as determined from the in vitro aggregation studies and estimates of baboon plasma volume.

ANIMALS STUDIED

Normal male baboons (*Papio anubis*) were used in these studies. The animals weighed 8 to 12 kg and had been observed to be disease-free for at least 6 weeks before use. All animals had a chronic arteriovenous (AV) shunt surgically implanted between the femoral artery and vein.[11,12,29]

As described in detail previously, the permanent Teflon-Silastic shunt does not detectably shorten platelet survival or produce measurable platelet activation.[12,29] Dacron vascular grafts were interposed between the segments of

Table 22-1
Antibodies Studied in Baboons

Antibody	K_d(M)	Number of Binding Sites	Dose (mg/kg)
AP1 IgG			10
AP1 $F(ab')_2$	2×10^{-8}	47,000	1
AP2 IgG	2×10^{-9}	50,000	0.2–1.0
AP2 $F(ab')_2$	3×10^{-9}	53,000	1
LJ-CP8 IgG	3×10^{-7}	45,000	10
LJ-CP8 $F(ab')_2$	1×10^{-7}	48,000	10

the permanent AV shunt. This method was chosen because measurements of platelet incorporation into forming arterial thrombi are quantitative and reproducible and the graft materials used have clinical applications in man.[12]

In a separate group of animals, expanded Teflon vascular grafts were inserted into the right superficial femoral artery.[31] All grafts were 30-μm fibril length, 4.0-mm ID (Gore-Tex, W.L. Gore and Associates, Inc., Flagstaff, Az). Under general anesthesia and using standard surgical techniques, the artery was dissected and the animals were given 100 units/Kg of heparin. In the treated group, antibody was also injected at this time. The artery was then clamped, divided, and replaced with a 4.0-cm length of graft. End-to-end anastomoses were performed using continuous 6-0 polypropylene suture. Surgical hemostasis was achieved after approximately 5 to 10 min in the antibody-treated group. The surgical site was then closed in two layers, and the animals were allowed to recover for 3 hr before graft imaging. All procedures were performed in accordance with the *Principles of Laboratory Care* and the *Guide for the Care and Use of Laboratory Animals* (NIH Publication No. 80-23, revised 1978).

EXPERIMENTAL METHODS

Platelet count and hematocrit determinations were performed on whole blood collected in 2 mg/ml disodium EDTA. Before the antibody studies began, whole-blood platelet counts averaged 370,000 ± 86,000/μl (± 1 SD), and hematocrits averaged 34 ± 5%. Bleeding time measurements were performed on the shaved volar surface of the forearm using the standard template method as previously described for studies in baboons.[19] Bleeding time measurements were performed in duplicate and were averaged.

Platelet aggregation was measured, using a Chrono-Log aggregometer, by recording the increase in light transmission through a stirred suspension of PRP maintained at 37°. Platelet-rich and platelet-poor plasmas were prepared as previously described.[19] All platelet concentrations in PRP were adjusted to 200,000/μl. At each dose of injected antibody, platelet aggregation was assessed in at least three different animals within 2 hr and at daily intervals, thereafter.

The platelet content of PF-4 and β-TG were measured by radioimmunoassay of Triton X-100 platelet lysates as previously described.[12,19] Plasma levels of PF-4 and β-TG were also determined by radioimmunoassay on blood samples collected and processed as described previously.[12,19]

For the imaging studies, autologous baboon platelets were labeled with ^{111}In-labeled oxine as described.[12,13] In several studies, platelets harvested according to the same method were simultaneously labeled with ^{111}In-labeled oxine and [^{14}C]serotonin, as reported elsewhere.[20] These studies were included to examine the possibility that, after exposure to antibody, platelet granular serotonin might be lost preferentially, compared with cytoplasmic ^{111}In.

All imaging was performed with a gamma scintillation camera and a computer-assisted image-processing system, as previously described.[12,13,31] Dacron grafts were placed in the baboon AV shunt for 1 hr with images acquired at 5-min intervals. Deposited ^{111}In platelet activity, calculated by subtracting the blood pool activity from all dynamic study images, increased monotonically over the exposure period. The total number of platelets deposited after 1 hr (labeled plus unlabeled cells) was calculated by dividing the deposited platelet activity (cpm) by the blood-specific activity (cpm/ml) and multiplying by the circulating platelet count (platelets/ml).[12,13] In animals with expanded Teflon vascular grafts surgically placed in the femoral artery, 5-min static images of the grafted artery, contralateral limb, and freshly drawn whole-blood standards were acquired at 3, 24, and 48 hr postoperatively.[14,31]

CLEARANCE OF INJECTED ANTIBODIES

To assess levels of platelet-associated antibody and its clearance from plasma, ^{125}I-labeled LJ-CP8 IgG was injected into normal baboons at a dose of 10 mg/kg. Typical results are shown in Figure 22-1. Immediately after antibody injection, 50,000 IgG molecules were bound per platelet, representing approximately 4% of the total injected antibody. Platelet-associated antibody disappeared in a linear fashion over 4 days, with an apparent half-life that

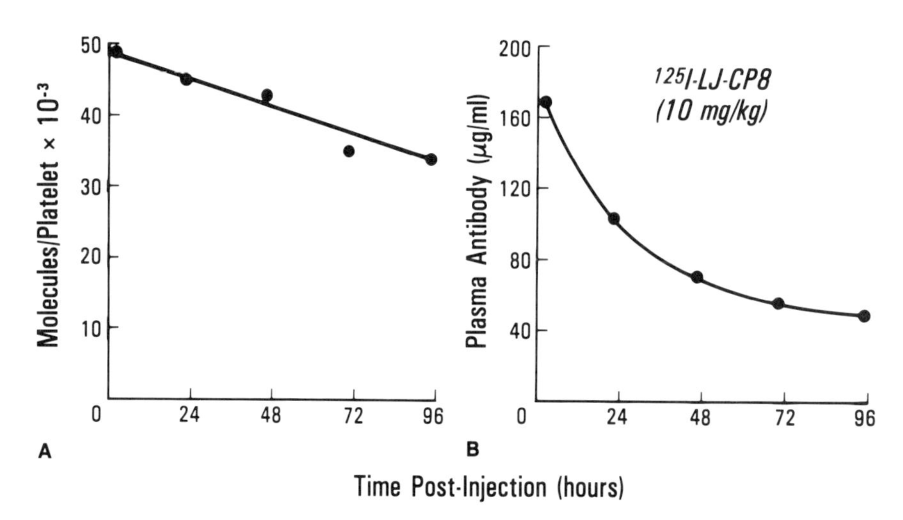

Figure 22-1. Disappearance pattern of ^{125}I-labeled LJ-CP8 (10 mg/kg) injected into a normal baboon. Initially, an average of 50,000 LJ-CP8 molecules were bound per platelet (*A*). The level of platelet-associated antibody decreased in a linear fashion over 4 days. Levels of plasma antibody decreased more quickly in a nonlinear fashion (*B*), exhibiting a half-life in plasma of approximately 2 days.

exceeded 4 days. Because the half-life of baboon platelets in the circulation is only 2.5 to 3.0 days,[12,29] this result suggests that continued binding of plasma antibody to newly formed platelets was occurring. Plasma antibody was cleared in an exponential fashion with a half-life of approximately 2 days (*see* Fig. 22-1)

After the injection of ^{131}I-labeled AP2 IgG at the highest dose used, 1.0 mg/kg, approximately 33,000 molecules per platelet were initially bound, representing approximately 25% of the total amount of antibody injected.[13] With 0.2 mg/kg and 0.4 mg/kg IgG, 10,000 to 15,000 sites per platelet were initially occupied (59% and 34% of total injected dose). Platelet-associated IgG invariably decreased progressively to less than 2000 molecules per platelet after 4 days. Analysis of the platelets by SDS–PAGE at various times after antibody infusion revealed that the platelet-bound radioactivity was indeed associated with intact IgG molecules.[13] Plasma AP2 levels ranged from approximately 0.5 μg/ml to 10 μg/ml after the injection of 0.2 mg/kg and 1.0 mg/kg, respectively. Most of the plasma IgG was cleared within the first 24 hr, with a more gradual reduction to less than 0.5 μg/ml by 96 hr.

The ^{125}I-labeled F(ab′)$_2$ fragments of AP2 and LJ-CP8 were injected at doses of 1.0 mg/kg and 10.0 mg/kg, respectively, and were cleared more quickly than the intact IgG. Both F(ab′)$_2$ fragments exhibited a plasma half-life of 3 to 5 hr. It should be noted that the interpretation of the pharmacokinetic data obtained with AP2 was complicated by the fact that both intact IgG and F(ab′)$_2$ fragments produced moderate thrombocytopenia, as discussed later.

ANTIBODY-INDUCED THROMBOCYTOPENIA

The effects of injected antibodies on circulating platelet counts are shown in Table 22-2, in which values have been normalized for measurements of platelet count made before antibody administration (pre-Ab). Initial platelet counts for each study group averaged approximately 400,000/μl. Infusion of AP2 IgG (0.2–1.0 mg/kg) caused dose-dependent reductions of platelet counts that were apparent by 2 hr, and that appeared largely irreversible, persisting for at least 48 hr. At the highest dose (1.0 mg/kg), the reduction in platelet numbers averaged 40% to 50%. Comparable results were also observed with the F(ab′)$_2$ fragment of AP2, suggesting that the effect was independent of the Fc portion of the antibody molecule. No thrombocytopenia was observed over 48 hr in animals given 10 mg/kg LJ-CP8, i.e., an amount ten times greater than the dose of AP2 administered. Since we subsequently excluded the possibility that AP2 caused a direct

Table 22-2
Effect of Injected Antibodies on Circulating Platelet Count

Dose (mg/kg)	Pre-Ab	% Platelets Remaining 2 hr	24 hr	48 hr
0	100	92 ± 2 (4)	102 ± 4 (4)	102 ± 3 (4)
AP2 IgG				
0.2	100	67 ± 7 (5)	80 ± 5 (4)	81 ± 5 (4)
0.4	100	78 ± 2 (5)	83 ± 3 (5)	76 ± 15 (4)
1.0	100	54 ± 8 (8)	56 ± 6 (8)	53 ± 6 (8)
AP2 F(ab')$_2$				
1.0	100	55 ± 3 (3)	59 ± 4 (3)	
LJ-CP8 IgG				
10.0	100	98 ± 4 (5)	94 ± 3 (5)	107 ± 9 (5)

The number of observations is shown in parenthesis. Values are mean ± 1 SEM

activation of platelets in vivo (*see* later discussion), the explanation for the differential effects of AP2 versus LJ-CP8 on circulating platelet levels remains enigmatic.

When the anti-GPIb antibody AP1 was injected, either as whole IgG (10 mg/kg) or as F(ab')$_2$ fragments (1.0 mg/kg), immediate and profound thrombocytopenia was observed within 10 min, with platelet counts in the two animals studied averaging less than 30,000/μl. Because this effect was not investigated further, we cannot exclude the possibility that AP1 caused a direct activation of platelets in vivo. Alternatively, these data suggest that intact or accessible GPIb may be important for maintaining platelet viability in the general circulation.

Determination of platelet survival was not appropriate in animals given AP2 IgG or F(ab')$_2$ because these antibodies caused marked fluctuations in the circulating platelet count. Although platelet counts were largely unchanged after administration of LJ-CP8, this result did not preclude the possibility of some increase in platelet turnover. Therefore, in three animals, platelet survival was measured over 4 days in animals given 10 mg/kg LJ-CP8. Results are shown in Figure 22-2. The labeled platelets exhibited a disappearance pattern typical of the normal pattern for baboons, as previously described.[12] Thus, over the experimental interval, LJ-CP8 caused no increase in platelet turnover.

Serial platelet counts over 10 days in baboons given LJ-CP8 are shown in Figure 22-3. Severe thrombocytopenia occurred 4 to 6 days after infusion of LJ-CP8 IgG (10 mg/kg) into four animals, and a similar time course was

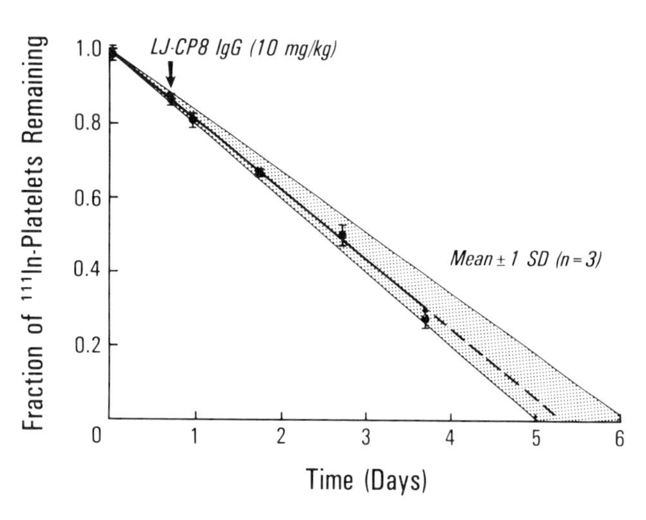

Figure 22-2. Disappearance pattern of ^{111}In-labeled platelets in three baboons given LJ-CP8 IgG (10 mg/kg). The fraction of labeled platelets remaining in the circulation over time (closed symbols) was within normal limits for untreated animals (shaded area), indicating no increase in the rate of platelet destruction resulting from antibody infusion. All values are ± 1 SEM.

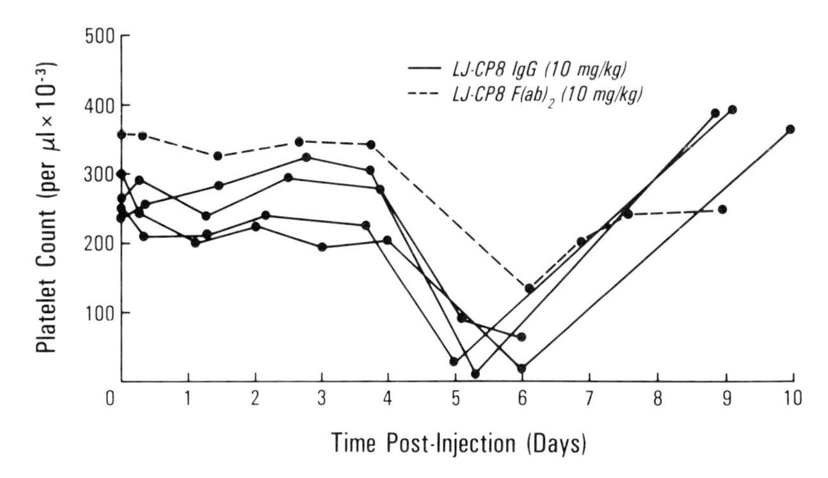

Figure 22-3. Delayed thrombocytopenia after antibody infusion. Whereas normal platelet counts were maintained over 4 days in four animals given LJ-CP8 IgG (10 mg/kg), severe thrombocytopenia was observed between 4 and 6 days, with platelet counts rebounding to higher than normal values by 8 to 10 days. A similar time course was also observed in one animal given the $F(ab')_2$ fragment of LJ-CP8 (10 mg/kg).

observed in one animal given LJ-CP8 $F(ab')_2$. The effect was transient, with counts returning to normal, or higher than normal, values by 8 days. These results document the importance of serial platelet counts for identifying episodes of transient thrombocytopenia, and perhaps rebound thrombocytosis, which may be associated with the use of platelet-specific antibodies or their Fab fragments.

EFFECTS ON PLATELET GRANULAR RELEASE

To determine whether AP2 or LJ-CP8 caused a depletion of platelet α-granule or dense-granule contents, platelet PF-4, β-TG, and [^{14}C]serotonin were measured before and after antibody administration. No reductions in platelet PF-4 or β-TG were observed over the 24-hr period following the injection of either antibody (Table 22-3). Similarly, platelet [^{14}C]serotonin radioactivity, expressed as a percentage of the pre-IgG values, was not preferentially reduced relative to platelet cytoplasmic ^{111}In radioactivity. Also, 2 hr after the injection of 1.0 mg/kg AP2 IgG into three animals, plasma levels of PF-4 and β-TG were normal and equivalent to control values obtained in untreated animals, as reported previously.[12,29] These results suggest that circulating platelets have not undergone either α-granule or dense-granule release, and they are also in accord with the observed inability for AP2 IgG to induce platelet release in vitro.[13]

EFFECTS OF INJECTED ANTIBODIES ON THE BLEEDING TIME

Measurements of the standard template bleeding time are shown in Figure 22-4. In normal animals, the bleeding times averaged 4.6 ± 0.1 min and were not prolonged significantly by the infusion of 0.2 mg/kg AP2 IgG (5.2 ± 0.4 min). AP2 IgG at 0.4 mg/kg caused a transient prolongation of the bleeding time (9.8 ± 1.5 min; $p = 0.05$), which returned to normal by 24 hr (4.6 ± 0.3 min). The highest dose of AP2 IgG, 1.0 mg/kg, initially prolonged the bleeding time to 19.2 ± 3.4 min ($p = 0.01$), and values were still abnormal at 24 hr (15.8 ± 3.9 min, $p < 0.05$) but not at 48 hr (12.0 ± 4.0 min; $p = 0.14$). AP2 $F(ab')_2$ (1.0 mg/kg) also increased the bleeding time initially (16.5 ± 1.8 min, $p < 0.05$), but values at later time points were statistically normal.

Infusion of LJ-CP8 (10.0 mg/kg) initially prolonged the bleeding time to longer than 30 min in five animals (*see* Fig. 22-4B). Values were significantly prolonged at 24 hr (12.6 ± 0.9 min; $p < 0.001$), and modestly prolonged at 48 hr (8.8 ± 1.8; $p = 0.07$). Despite the marked increase in bleeding tendency, none of

Table 22-3
Effect of Injected Antibodies on Platelet Granular Release

Measurement	Pre-IgG	2 hr	24 hr
AP2 IgG (1.0 mg/kg):			
Platelet count (per μl × 10^{-3})	454 ± 18	214 ± 82	277 ± 52
Platelet PF-4 (μg per 10^9 plats)	10.6 ± 1.5	8.2 ± 1.5	
Platelet β-TG (μg per 10^9 plats)	11.2 ± 0.8	17.1 ± 3.4	
^{111}In-labeled platelets (% baseline)	100	35.5 ± 20.3	36.6 ± 10.6
[^{14}C]serotonin (% baseline)	100	41.0 ± 18.7	47.3 ± 10.7
LJ-CP8 IgG (10.0 mg/kg):			
Platelet count (per μl × 10^{-3})	305 ± 46	297 ± 34	290 ± 39
Platelet PF-4 (μg per 10^9 plats)	7.6 ± 0.6	7.2 ± 0.7	7.2 ± 0.8*
Platelet β-TG (μg per 10^9 plats)	8.8 ± 0.3	9.2 ± 0.3	10.4 ± 0.6*
^{111}In-labeled platelets (% baseline)	100	0.96 ± 0.07	0.68 ± 0.04
[^{14}C]serotonin (% baseline)	100	0.95 ± 0.05	0.72 ± 0.04

The platelet contents of PF-4, β-TG, ^{111}In-labeled platelet activity and [^{14}C]serotonin–platelet activity were measured before (Pre-IgG) and at 2 hr and 24 hr following antibody injection in three animals (AP2 IgG) or four animals (LJ-CP8 IgG) unless otherwise indicated. All values are mean ± 1 SEM. *Measurements in three animals.
(Hanson SR, Pareti FI, Ruggeri ZM, Marzec UM, Kunicki TJ, Montgomery RR, Zimmerman TS, Harker LA: J Clin Invest 81:149, 1988, by copyright permission of The American Society for Clinical Investigation.)

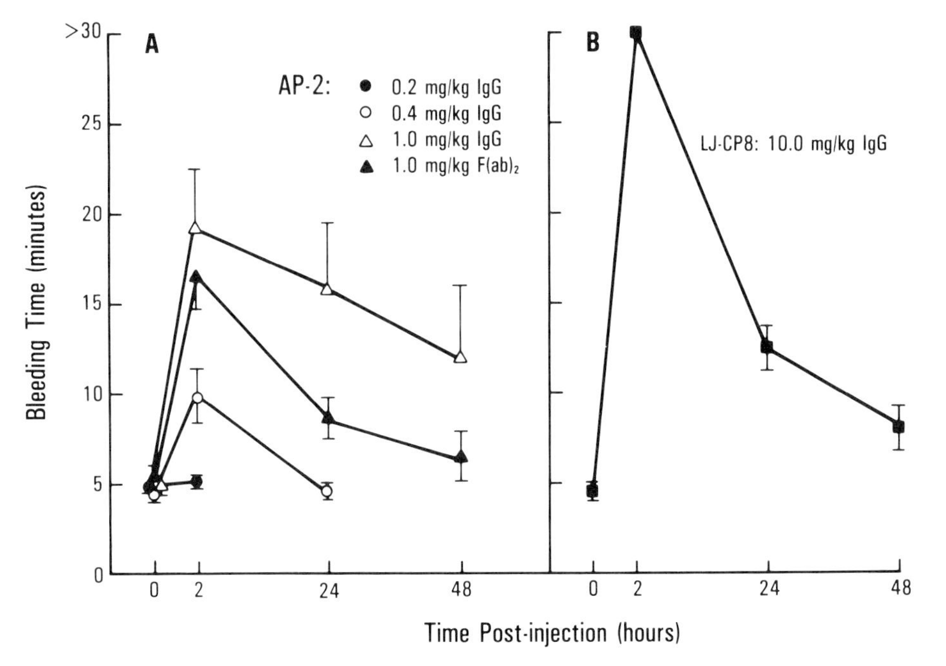

Figure 22-4. Measurements of standard template bleeding times in animals given anti-GPIIb–IIIa antibodies. (*A*) Bleeding times were prolonged in a dose-response fashion over 48 hr in animals given AP2 IgG (0.2–1.0 mg/kg). A significant acute prolongation of bleeding was also observed in animals given the F(ab′)$_2$ fragment of AP2 (1.0 mg/kg). (*B*) LJ-CP8 IgG (10 mg/kg) caused bleeding times to be initially prolonged to more than 30 min, with values returning toward normal by 48 hr. All values are mean ± 1 SEM of measurements in three to five animals (Hanson SR, Pareti FI, Ruggeri ZM, Marzec UM, Kunicki TJ, Montgomery RR, Zimmerman TS, Harker LA: J Clin Invest 81:149, 1988. With permission).

the treated animals exhibited spontaneous bleeding or hemorrhage from surgical sites.

EFFECTS ON PLATELET AGGREGATION EX VIVO

Serial measurements of platelet aggregation in response to ADP, collagen, and γ-thrombin were performed after the antibody infusions. Typical aggregation tracings are shown in Figure 22-5. The data were expressed quantitatively in terms of the maximum extent of light transmission through stirred PRP suspensions relative to control values taken before antibody infusion.[13]

AP2 IgG (0.2 – 1.0 mg/kg) caused a dose-dependent inhibition of aggregation with all agonists tested. Measurements in response to 10 μM ADP are given in Figure 22-6. Whereas 0.2 mg/kg AP2 caused only a transient impairment of platelet function which reverted toward normal by 24 hr, aggregation was still reduced at 48 hr in animals given 1.0 mg/kg of

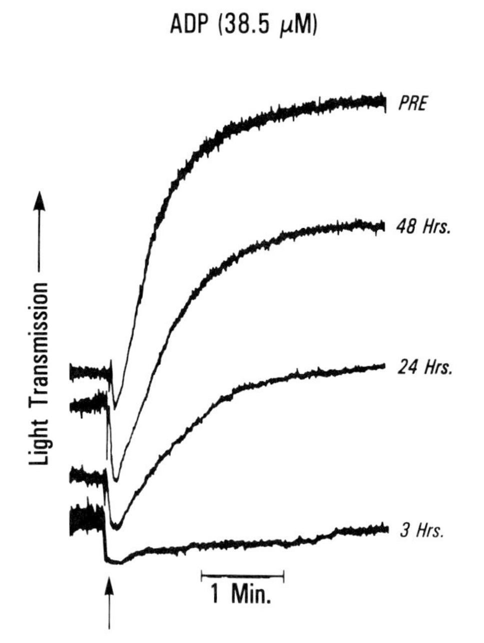

Figure 22-5. Platelet aggregation *ex vivo* following infusion of LJ-CP8 (10 mg/kg) into a normal baboon. In response to a fixed amount of ADP (38.5 μM) platelet aggregation in PRP (increase in light transmittance) was totally abolished at 3 hr but returned over 48 hr toward normal values, taken before antibody infusion (PRE).

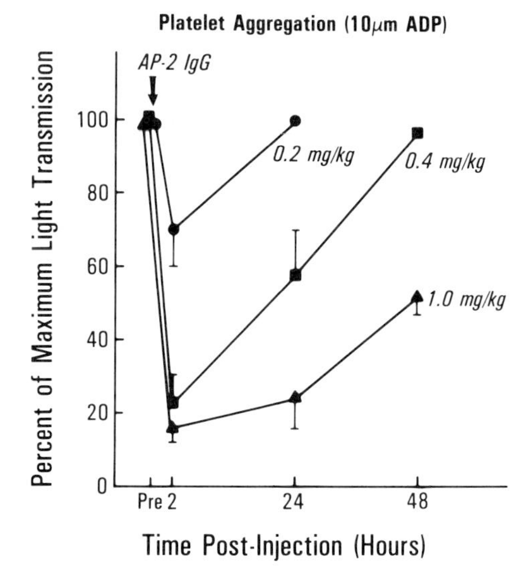

Figure 22-6. Inhibition of platelet aggregation after administration of AP2 IgG. Platelet aggregation in response to 10 μM ADP was measured quantitatively in terms of the percentage of maximum light transmission through stirred suspensions of PRP. Aggregation was markedly inhibited at 2 hr after AP2 infusion but returned to normal by 24 hr (0.2 mg/kg), 48 hr (0.4 mg/kg), or remained impaired over 48 hr (1.0 mg/kg). A clear dose-response effect was evident. Error bars represent 1 SEM of observations in three animals.

this antibody. Interestingly, the lowest dose of AP2 IgG (0.2 mg/kg) caused a transient impairment of platelet aggregation but had no detectable effect on bleeding time (*see* Fig. 22-4). Similarly, in animals given 0.4 mg/kg AP2 IgG, bleeding times at 24 hr were normal, but aggregation in response to all three agonists was still reduced. These results suggest that, at least under some conditions, measurements of abnormal platelet aggregation ex vivo do not necessarily predict changes in platelet hemostatic function in vivo.

LJ-CP8 IgG (10 mg/kg) was an even more potent inhibitor of platelet aggregation ex vivo (Fig. 22-7). Aggregation in response to ADP and collagen was abolished sharply, with only partial recovery of function over 48 hr.

In general, with all monoclonal antibodies studied, platelet aggregation in response to collagen was suppressed to the greatest extent, and aggregation in response to γ-thrombin was suppressed the least.[13] In several additional studies, platelet aggregation and bleeding times were assessed as early as 10 min after the injec-

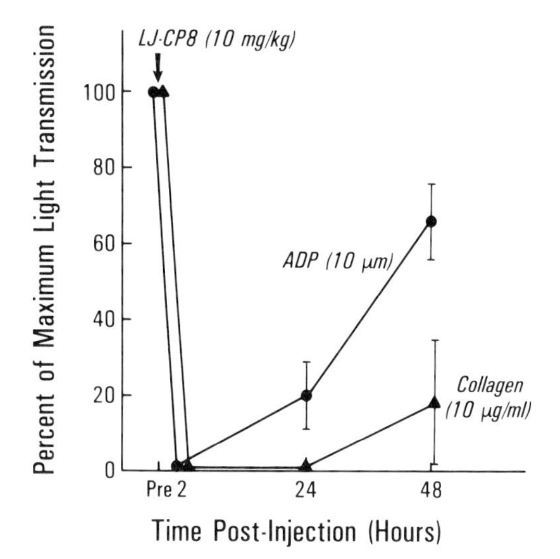

Figure 22-7. Inhibition of platelet aggregation after administration of LJ-CP8. The anti-GPIIb–IIIa antibody (10 mg/kg) initially abolished platelet aggregation in response to ADP (10 μM) and collagen (10 μg/ml). Aggregation in response to collagen was markedly impaired over 48 hr. Aggregation in response to ADP showed a moderate recovery of function over this interval. All values are mean ± 1 SEM of observations in five animals.

tion of antibody. The results of these studies were equivalent to those obtained at 2 hr postinfusion, implying that the maximal effects of the injected antibodies were virtually immediate.

STUDIES WITH DACRON VASCULAR GRAFTS

Measurements of platelet deposition onto Dacron grafts inserted 10 min after antibody infusion, and exposed for 1 hr, are given in Figure 22-8. Because we have previously shown that graft platelet deposition depends, in an approximately linear fashion, on the circulating platelet count,[10] the experimental groups were chosen to have comparable mean platelet counts in the range of 307,000 to 389,000/μl. After 60 min of blood exposure, AP2 IgG reduced graft platelet deposition in a dose-dependent fashion. Thus, the accumulation of platelets was reduced by an average of 41% by 0.2 mg/kg AP2, 51% by 0.4 mg/kg AP2, and 73% by 1.0 mg/kg AP2 ($p < 0.001$). Platelet accumulation over 60 min was also reduced 55% by AP2 $F(ab')_2$ (1.0 mg/kg). In five animals given 10.0

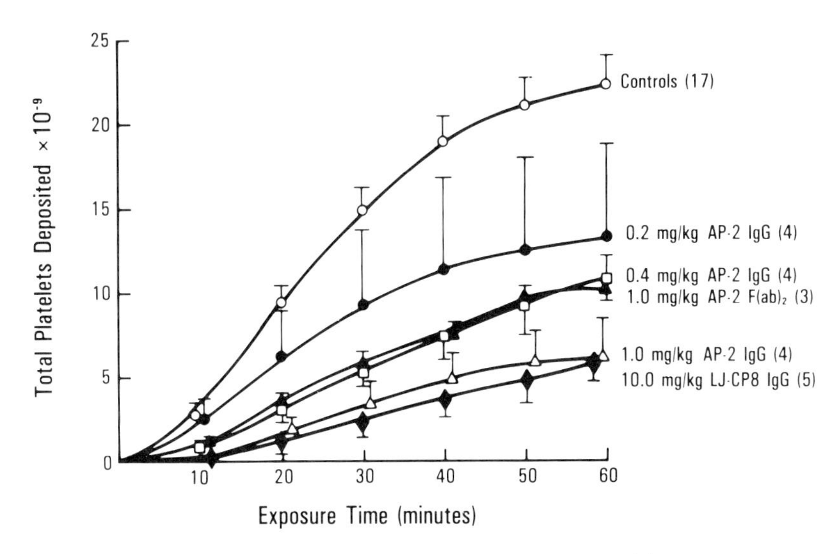

Figure 22-8. Effects of AP2 and LJ-CP8 on platelet deposition onto acutely placed Dacron vascular grafts. Antibodies were administered 10 min before graft placement in femoral AV shunts. The time course (0–60 min) of platelet accumulation was reduced in a dose-dependent fashion by AP2 IgG. Significant antithrombotic effects were also observed in animals given AP2 $F(ab')_2$ and LJ-CP8 IgG. The number of observations with each antibody is given in parenthesis. All values are mean ± SEM (Hanson SR, Pareti FI, Ruggeri ZM, Marzec UM, Kunicki TJ, Montgomery RR, Zimmerman TS, Harker LA: Clin Invest 81:149, 1988, by copyright permission of The American Society for Clinical Investigation).

mg/kg LJ-CP8, graft platelet deposition was reduced 73% versus the control studies ($p < 0.001$), a value equivalent to the result observed in animals treated with the highest dose of AP2 IgG.

Although the results obtained with Dacron grafts evaluated on subsequent days after AP2 infusion were ambiguous, because of the observed reductions in circulating platelet count (*see* Table 22-2), platelet counts were relatively stable over 48 hr following LJ-CP8 administration. Thus 24 hr after LJ-CP8 injection, platelet accumulation onto freshly inserted grafts in four animals averaged $7.5 \pm 2.2 \times 10^9$ platelets per graft at 1 hr, which represented a 66% reduction in platelet numbers versus the control results ($p < 0.01$). In two animals studied at 48 hr, graft platelet deposition over 1 hr was still reduced by an average of 46%.

Three additional groups of animals were also studied after administration of heparin (100 U/kg), oral aspirin (32.5 mg/kg *b.i.d.*) or the combination of heparin and aspirin at these doses (Fig. 22-9). These study groups had comparable mean circulating platelet counts, ranging from 365,000 to 450,000/μl. Neither heparin, aspirin, nor the combination was effective in reducing platelet deposition over the 60-min period after graft placement.[13]

In another group of five animals not given antibody, we observed that all of five Dacron vascular grafts irreversibly occluded, because of platelet thrombus accumulation, at an average time of 1.2 hr. In five animals given 10 mg/kg LJ-CP8, all five grafts remained patient after 2 hr. Four of these grafts left in place for 24 hr were also patent, demonstrating that the antibody protected not only against acute platelet deposition but also prevented acute occlusion resulting from platelet thrombus formation.

Thus, in this arteriovenous shunt model of acute thrombosis and occlusion associated with Dacron vascular grafts, the monoclonal antibodies studied were found to be highly potent antithrombotic agents, compared with more conventional therapeutic strategies.[10,13]

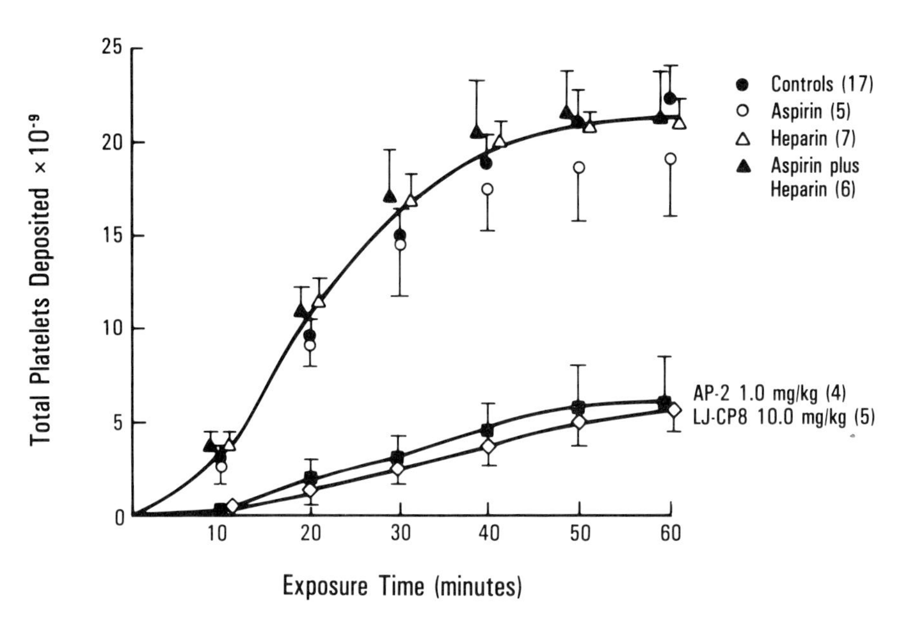

Figure 22-9. Effect of heparin and aspirin therapies on graft platelet deposition in baboons. Neither heparin (100 U/kg), aspirin (32.5 mg/kg *b.i.d.*), nor the combination at these dosages was effective relative to control values in reducing platelet deposition onto Dacron vascular grafts incorporated into AV shunts for 1 hr. For comparison, the results obtained with AP2 IgG and LJ-CP8 IgG are also shown (*see* Fig. 22-8). The number of observations is in parenthesis. All values are mean ± 1 SEM.

EFFECTS OF LJ-CP8 ON THROMBOSIS ASSOCIATED WITH SURGICAL GRAFT PLACEMENT

These studies employed ten normal baboons. Five served as controls, and five animals were given 10 mg/kg LJ-CP8 intraoperatively, after exposing the superficial femoral artery but before restoration of flow through the grafted segment.[31] After the graft procedures, variable hematoma formation was noted at the surgical sites in the animals given intravenous antibody. Therefore, before imaging at 3 hr postoperatively, the surgical sites in the treated animals were reopened and approximately 2 to 4 ml of blood evacuated. Thereafter, no further hematoma formation was noted, and the sites were closed and imaged. The surgical sites in control animals were also opened with no evidence of blood leakage. All grafts were patent at this time, as demonstrated by direct Doppler scanning of the distal artery using a pencil probe. All sites subsequently remained closed until the grafts were removed 8 days later.

Serial measurements, by scintillation camera imaging, of the ratio of graft ^{111}In-labeled platelet radioactivity to circulating platelet radioactivity are shown in Figure 22-10. For determinations made at 3, 24, and 48 hr postoperatively, no differences were seen between the treated and untreated groups ($p > 0.5$ at all times). Total platelet accumulation (labeled plus unlabeled cells) was also calculated from images taken 3 hr postoperatively.[31] Platelet deposition onto grafts placed in the treated animals ($5.1 \pm 1.0 \times 10^9$ platelets per graft) was equivalent to values obtained in the control group ($4.8 \pm 0.8 \times 10^9$ platelets per graft, $p > 0.5$). All grafts were removed after 8 days. None of the grafts placed in untreated animals was patent, and only one graft from a treated animal was found to be patent. No technical problems were noted with any of the graft anastomoses.

Thus, we unexpectedly observed no significant benefit of the injected monoclonal antibody with respect to immediate graft thrombus formation or graft patency, despite the profound inhibition of platelet function shown by measurements of bleeding time and platelet aggregation ex vivo[31] and despite the efficacy of this same antibody regimen for blocking platelet deposition onto Dacron vascular grafts exposed in the AV shunt system.[13] These results, in part, may be reconciled by observations that platelets exposed to strong agonists, such as thrombin, exhibit markedly increased numbers of surface-oriented binding sites associated with platelet GPIIb–IIIa.[22] With unstimulated platelets, these sties would be inaccessible to extracellular antibodies. Upon activation, platelets also release intracellular fibrinogen and von Willebrand factor, which may be bound to the GPIIb–IIIa receptor and subsequently support platelet aggregation.[7,24] Thus, under the conditions of this study involving vessel trauma and altered flow conditions at the graft–vessel anatomoses, platelet aggregation may have been favored by the close proximity of activated cells and local high concentrations of adhesive glycoproteins and physiologic agonists. Conversely, bleeding times

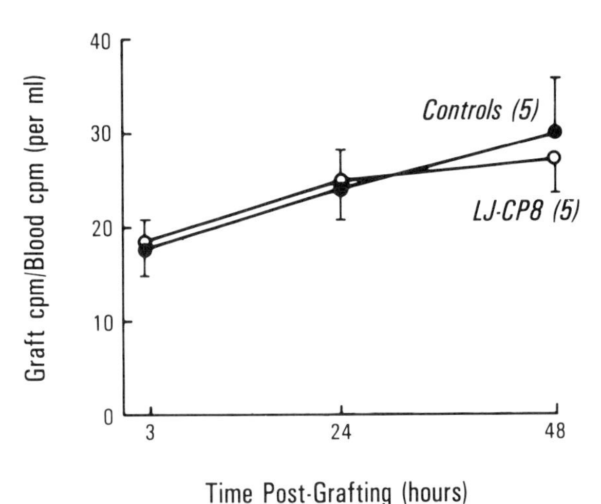

Figure 22-10. Ratio of graft-deposited platelet ^{111}In activity/circulating ^{111}In-labeled platelet activity (per ml whole blood) in animals having expanded Teflon vascular grafts surgically placed in the baboon superficial femoral artery. LJ-CP8 anti-GPIIb–IIIa antibody (10 mg/kg) was injected intraoperatively before restoration of blood flow through the grafted segment. No differences in graft platelet accumulation were seen over 48 hr in treated vs. untreated animals as measured by noninvasive scintillation camera imaging. All values are mean ± 1 SEM of observations in five animals (Torem S, Schneider PA, Hanson SR: J Vasc Surg 7:172, 1988. With permission).

may have been prolonged by the antibody as a consequence of particular modulating effects of vessel injury at the capillary level and microenvironmental factors influencing the intensity of platelet stimulation and local concentrations of relevant blood elements.

CONCLUSIONS

We conclude that antibodies against platelet GPIIb-IIIa have potentially significant antithrombotic and antihemostatic effects in vivo. However, on the basis of these preliminary studies, it seems likely that the antithrombotic efficacy of antiplatelet antibodies may depend strongly on those factors regulating thrombus formation in a particular clinical or experimental setting. Such factors could include the nature and extent of vessel injury, differences in mechanisms of thrombus formation on natural versus artificial surfaces, rheologic effects, and perhaps levels of plasma versus platelet-associated antibody.

The use of platelet-specific antibodies, in general, either as whole IgG or Fab fragments, may be complicated by moderate or severe thrombocytopenia occurring either acutely or at later times by mechanisms that remain to be defined. Such antibodies may also cause a quantitative and dose-dependent increase in bleeding tendency, which could limit their use in association with surgical procedures. The antithrombotic effectiveness of antibodies against platelet GPIIb-IIIa may not always be predicted by tests of platelet hemostatic competence, such as measurements of platelet aggregation *ex vivo* or bleeding time. Although we observed no benefit by using an anti-GPIIb-IIIa monoclonal antibody in a surgical model of vascular graft thrombosis, these results do not preclude the usefulness of this strategy in other settings. Indeed, it is anticipated that this approach might be most appropriate in situations requiring potent, transient, yet immediate inhibition of platelet function, such as percutaneous arterial angioplasty or postreperfusion arterial occlusion. Therefore, further studies are warranted.

The antibodies used in these studies were generously provided by Drs. Thomas Kunicki and Robert Montgomery (AP1, AP2), and by Dr. Zaverio Ruggeri (LJ-CP8). This work was supported by National Institutes of Health research grants HL-31469 and HL-31950.

This is publication number 5137-BCR from the Research Institute of Scripps Clinic, La Jolla, California.

REFERENCES

1. Bennett JS, Hoxie JA, Leitman SF, Vilaire G, Cines DB: Inhibition of fibrinogen binding to stimulated human platelets by a monoclonal antibody. Proc Natl Acad Sci USA 80:2417, 1983

2. Coller BS: A new murine monoclonal antibody reports an activation-dependent change in the conformation and/or microenvironment of the platelet glycoprotein IIb/IIIa complex. J Clin Invest 76:101, 1985

3. Coller BS, Folts JD, Scudder LE: A potent new antithrombotic agent: The $F(ab')_2$ fragment of a monoclonal antibody to the platelet GPIIb/IIIa receptor (abstr) Blood 66:288a, 1985

4. Coller BS, Folts JD, Scudder LE, Smith SR: Antithrombotic effect of a monoclonal antibody to the platelet glycoprotein IIb/IIIa receptor in an experimental animal model. Blood 68:783, 1986

5. Coller BS, Peerschke EI, Scudder LE, Sullivan CA: A murine monoclonal antibody that completely blocks the binding of fibrinogen to platelets produces a thrombasthenic-like state in normal platelets and binds to glycoprotein IIb and /or IIIa. J Clin Invest 72:325, 1983

6. Coller BS, Scudder LE: Inhibition of dog platelet function by in vivo infusion of $F(ab')_2$ fragments of a monoclonal antibody to the platelet glycoprotein IIb/IIIa receptor. Blood 66:1456, 1985

7. Courtois G, Ryckewaert J-J, Woods VL, Ginsberg MH, Plow EF, Marguerie GA: Expression of intracellular fibrinogen on the surface of stimulated platelets. Eur J Biochem 159:61, 1986

8. George JN, Pickett EB, Saucerman S, McEver RP, Kunicki TJ, Kieffer N, Newman P: Platelet surface glycoproteins. Studies on resting and activated platelets and platelet membrane microparticles in normal subjects, and observations in patients during adult respiratory distress syndrome and cardiac surgery. J Clin Invest 78:340, 1986

9. Hampton JW, Matthews C: Similarities between baboon and human blood clotting. J Appl Physiol 21:1713, 1966

10. Hanson SR, Harker LA: Studies of suloctidil in experimental thrombosis in baboons. Thrombo Haemostasis 53:423, 1985

11. Hanson SR, Harker LA, Bjornsson TD: Effects of platelet-modifying drugs on arterial thromboembolism in baboons: Aspirin potentiates the antithrombotic actions of dipyridamole and sulfinpyrazone by mechanism(s) independent of platelet cyclooxygenase inhibition. J Clin Invest 75:1591, 1985

12. Hanson SR, Kotze HF, Savage B, Harker LA: Platelet interactions with Dacron vascular grafts: A model of acute thrombosis in baboons. Arteriosclerosis 5:595, 1985

13. Hanson SR, Pareti FI, Ruggeri ZM, Marzec UM, Kunicki TJ, Montgomery RR, Zimmerman TS, Harker LA: Effects of monoclonal antibodies against the platelet glycoprotein IIb/IIIa complex on thrombosis and hemostasis in the baboon. J Clin Invest 81:149, 1988

14. Hanson SR, Paxton LD, Harker LA: Iliac artery mural thrombus formation: Effect of antiplatelet therapy on ^{111}In-platelet deposition in baboons. Arteriosclerosis 6:511, 1986

15. Henrich D, Scharf T, Santoso S, Clemetson KJ, Mueller-Eckhardt C: Monoclonal antibodies against human platelet membrane glycoproteins IIb/IIIa. II. Different effects on platelet function. Thromb Res 38:547, 1985

16. Jennings LK, Phillips DR, Walker WS: Monoclonal antibodies to human platelet glycoprotein IIbα that initiate distinct platelet responses. Blood 65:1112, 1985

17. Kornecki E, Tuszynski GP, Niewiarowski S: Inhibition of fibrinogen receptor-mediated platelet aggregation by heterologous antihuman platelet membrane antibody. J Biol Chem 258:9349, 1983

18. Lombardo VT, Hodson E, Roberts JR, Kunicki TJ, Zimmerman TS, Ruggeri ZM: Independent modulation of von Willebrand factor and fibrinogen binding to the platelet membrane glycoprotein IIb/IIIa complex as demonstrated by monoclonal antibody. J Clin Invest 76:1950, 1985

19. Malpass TW, Hanson SR, Savage B, Hessel EA II, Harker LA: Prevention of acquired transient defect in platelet plug formation by infused prostacyclin. Blood 57:736, 1981

20. Malpass TW, Savage B, Hanson SR, Slichter SJ, Harker LA: Correlation between prolonged bleeding time and depletion of platelet dense granule ADP in patients with myelodysplastic and myeloproliferative disorders. J Lab Clin Med 103:894, 1984

21. McPherson J, Brownlea S, Zucker MB: Effect of monoclonal antibodies against von Willebrand factor and platelet glycoproteins IIb/IIIa on the platelet retention test. Blood 70:546, 1987

22. Niiya K, Hodson E, Bader R, Byers-Ward V, Koziol JA, Plow EF, Ruggeri ZM: Increased surface expression of the membrane glycoprotein IIb/IIIa complex induced by platelet aggregation. Blood 70:475, 1987

23. Okita JR, Pidard D, Newman PJ, Montgomery RR, Kunicki TJ: On the association of glycoprotein Ib and actin-binding protein in human platelets. J Cell Biol 100:317, 1985

24. Parker RI, Gralnick HR: Identification of platelet glycoprotein IIb/IIIa as the major binding site for released platelet–von Willebrand factor. Blood 68:732, 1986

25. Pidard P, Montgomery RR, Bennett JS, Kunicki TJ: Interaction of AP-2, a monoclonal antibody specific for the human platelet glycoprotein IIb/IIIa complex with intact platelets. J Biol Chem 258:12582, 1983

26. Ruan C, Tobelem G, McMichael AJ, Drouet L, Legrand Y, Degos L, Keifer N, Lee, H, Caen JP: Monoclonal antibody to human platelet glycoprotein I. II. Effects on human platelet function. Br J Haematol 49:511, 1981

27. Ruggeri ZM, DeMarco L, Gatti L, Bader R, Montgomery RR: Platelets have more than one binding site for von Willebrand factor. J Clin Invest 72:1, 1983

28. Sakariassen KS, Nievelstein PFEM, Coller BS, Sixma JJ: The role of platelet membrane glycoproteins Ib and IIb–IIIa in platelet adherence to human artery subendothelium. Br J Haematol 63:681, 1986

29. Savage B, McFadden PR, Hanson SR, Harker LA: The relation of platelet density to platelet age: Survival of low and high density ^{111}indium-labeled platelets in baboons. Blood 68:386, 1986

30. Todd ME, McDevitt E, Goldsmith EI: Blood-clotting mechanisms of nonhuman primates: Choice of the baboon model to simulate man. J Med Primatol 1:132, 1972

31. Torem S, Schneider PA, Hanson SR: Monoclonal antibody-induced inhibition of platelet function: Effects on hemostasis and vascular graft thrombosis in baboons. J Vasc Surg 7:172, 1988

32. Weathersby PK, Horbett TA, Hoffman AS: Solution stability of bovine fibrinogen. Thromb Res 10:245, 1977

33. Weiss HJ, Turitto VT, Baumgartner HR: Platelet adhesion and thrombus formation on subendothelium in platelets deficient in glycoproteins IIb–IIIa, Ib, and storage granules. Blood 67:322, 1986

34. Yasuda T, Gold HK, Leinbach PC, Kanke M, Fallon J, Scudder LE, Coller BS: A monoclonal anti-platelet antibody prevents acute coronary reocclusion (RO) following thrombolysis in dogs despite residual high-grade stenosis (abstr) Clin Res 34:634A, 1986

Index

Page numbers followed by *f* indicate figures; page numbers followed by *t* indicate tabular material.

ISBN 0-397-50872-7